Pharmacology
and Therapeutics
of Airway Disease

LUNG BIOLOGY IN HEALTH AND DISEASE

Executive Editor

Claude Lenfant

Former Director, National Heart, Lung, and Blood Institute
National Institutes of Health
Bethesda, Maryland

For information on volumes 25–182 in the *Lung Biology in Health and Disease* series, please visit www.informahealthcare.com

The opinions expressed in these volumes do not necessarily represent the views of the National Institutes of Health.

Pharmacology and Therapeutics of Airway Disease

Second Edition

edited by

Kian Fan Chung
National Heart and Lung Institute
Imperial College
London, UK

Peter J. Barnes
National Heart and Lung Institute
Imperial College
London, UK

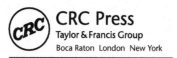

CRC Press
Taylor & Francis Group
Boca Raton London New York

CRC Press is an imprint of the
Taylor & Francis Group, an **informa** business

CRC Press
Taylor & Francis Group
6000 Broken Sound Parkway NW, Suite 300
Boca Raton, FL 33487-2742

First issued in paperback 2019

© 2010 by Taylor & Francis Group, LLC
CRC Press is an imprint of Taylor & Francis Group, an Informa business

No claim to original U.S. Government works

ISBN-13: 978-1-4200-7000-2 (hbk)
ISBN-13: 978-0-367-38499-9 (pbk)

Library of Congress Cataloging-in-Publication Data

Pharmacology and therapeutics of airway disease / edited by Kian Fan Chung, Peter J. Barnes. – 2nd ed.
    p. ; cm. – (Lung biology in health and disease ; v. 234)
    Rev. ed. of: Pharmacology of the respiratory tract / edited by K. Fan Chung, Peter J. Barnes. c1993.
    Includes bibliographical references and index.
    ISBN-13: 978-1-4200-7000-2 (hardcover : alk. paper)
    ISBN-10: 1-4200-7000-2 (hardcover : alk. paper)   1. Respiratory organs—Pathophysiology. 2. Respiratory organs—Effect of drugs on. 3. Respiratory organs—Diseases—Molecular aspects. I. Chung, K. Fan, 1951- II. Barnes, Peter J., 1946- III. Pharmacology of the respiratory tract. IV. Series: Lung biology in health and disease ; v. 234.
    [DNLM: 1.   Lung Diseases, Obstructive—drug therapy. 2.   Anti-Asthmatic Agents—therapeutic use. W1 LU62 v.234 2009 / WF 600 P5357 2009]
    RC711.P49 2009
    616.2'00471—dc22
                                                                                   2009031208

Visit the Taylor & Francis Web site at
http://www.taylorandfrancis.com

and the CRC Press Web site at
http://www.crcpress.com

Introduction

In 1993, volume 67, *Pharmacology of the Respiratory Tract*, appeared as part of this series of monographs Lung Biology in Health and Disease. In the preface, the editors, K. Fan Chung and Peter J. Barnes, indicated that the volume combined two concepts and stated "one deals with basic mechanisms of cell activation and pathophysiology, and the other with several functional aspects of specific cell types found in the normal and abnormal respiratory tract."

There is no doubt that volume 67 opened the window to a new world of research on the treatment of airway dysfunctions and pathological alterations. This expose of new knowledge significantly departed from what had been investigated for decades before, relative to the treatment of asthma, chronic bronchitis, and emphysema.

New hypotheses presented in volume 67 stimulated many investigations adding knowledge at a pace never seen before in research of the respiratory tract with regard to asthma and chronic obstructive pulmonary disease, or COPD—the term that is now widely used; this series of monographs became an important vehicle for the transfer of new advances. In fact, 31 monographs about asthma, 12 about COPD, and 13 that cover both conditions have appeared since 1993—and more are in preparation!

This new volume, also edited by K. Fan Chung and Peter J. Barnes, has a different title from that of their first monograph, *Pharmacology and Therapeutics of Airway Disease*. This is because a new array of therapeutic approaches often derived from very basic research advances can be described and are utilized clinically. Many alter the natural history of asthma and COPD, and more importantly, have considerably improved the quality of life for patients who are diagnosed with these airways diseases.

In the preface of this new volume, the editors state, "This volume is addressed to respiratory physicians, respiratory investigators, and respiratory allied professionals," the readers who have the most opportunity to provide help to the patients. Thus, it is a privilege to introduce this new volume. As the executive editor of this series of monographs, I thank the editors and the authors for the opportunity to present it to our readership.

Claude Lenfant, MD
Vancouver, Washington, U.S.A.

Preface

Since the publication of the first edition, there have been many significant advances in the pharmacology and therapeutics of the respiratory tract. This has been evident by the introduction of a number of new entities in the treatment of many respiratory tract diseases. In parallel, there have been advances in the assessment and evaluation of new drugs, and in understanding of the pathophysiology of respiratory tract diseases and of the methods of measuring airway and clinical responses such that potential targets for therapy have been identified and are being investigated, together with new therapeutic uses of already-available drugs.

Airway diseases comprise asthma and chronic obstructive pulmonary disease (COPD), which cause much chronic respiratory disability and death in the world. They are characterized by intermittent and/or chronic airflow obstruction, which in severe asthma and COPD can be poorly responsive to available treatments. The morbidity and mortality caused by these diseases are increasing, in particular COPD, which is now the sixth most common cause of death worldwide but predicted to become the third commonest cause within the next 10 years. There is therefore a pressing need to obtain even more effective treatments than that we currently have.

This volume is addressed to the respiratory physician, respiratory investigators, and respiratory allied professions. It not only provides the concepts upon which many treatments are used for these conditions, but also emphasizes the way in which these treatments work, and how new treatments can be discovered and tested in different patient groups. The book focuses on the state-of-the-art pharmacologic and therapeutic approaches in controlling pathophysiological processes in the airways, and reviews normal and abnormal physiologic, biochemical, and molecular aspects of the respiratory tract. It explores the basic mechanisms of inflammatory cell activation and pathophysiology in disease, and therapeutic ways of controlling inflammation, ways of reversing or preventing airflow obstruction, and symptomatic treatments for advanced disease.

We hope that this volume will be useful to those who deal with the many patients who suffer from airway disease. We would like to thank all the contributors to this volume and the editors at Informa Healthcare for their encouragement and help during the inception of this book.

Kian Fan Chung
Peter J. Barnes

Contributors

Ian M. Adcock National Heart and Lung Institute, Imperial College, and Royal Brompton Hospital, London, U.K.

Neil Barnes The London Chest Hospital, Barts and The London NHS Trust and School of Medicine and Dentistry, London, U.K.

Peter J. Barnes National Heart and Lung Institute, Imperial College, London, U.K.

John D. Brannan Firestone Institute for Respiratory Health, St. Joseph's Hospital and McMaster University, Hamilton, Ontario, Canada

Gaetano Caramori Research Centre for Asthma and COPD, University of Ferrara, Ferrara, Italy

Kian Fan Chung National Heart and Lung Institute, Imperial College, and Royal Brompton Hospital, London, U.K.

William Cookson National Heart and Lung Institute, Imperial College, London, U.K.

Chris J. Corrigan MRC and Asthma UK Centre for Allergic Mechanisms of Asthma, King's College London School of Medicine, London, U.K.

James F. Donohue University of North Carolina at Chapel Hill, Chapel Hill, North Carolina, U.S.A.

Sophe G. Fuika Hospital de Santiago, Vitoria-Gasteiz, Basque Country, Spain

Trevor T. Hansel Imperial Clinical Respiratory Research Unit (ICRRU), St. Mary's Hospital, Imperial College, London, U.K.

J. R. Hurst Academic Unit of Respiratory Medicine, UCL Medical School, University College, London, U.K.

David P. Johns Menzies Research Institute, University of Tasmania, Tasmania, Australia

Onn Min Kon St. Mary's Hospital, Imperial College, London, U.K.

Miriam Moffatt National Heart and Lung Institute, Imperial College, London, U.K.

Alyn H. Morice University of Hull and Castle Hill Hospital, Cottingham, East Yorkshire, U.K.

Paul M. O'Byrne Firestone Institute for Respiratory Health, St. Joseph's Hospital and McMaster University, Hamilton, Ontario, Canada

Jill Ohar Wake Forest University School of Medicine, Winston-Salem, North Carolina, U.S.A.

William Pease University of Nebraska Medical Center, Omaha, Nebraska, U.S.A.

Stephen I. Rennard University of Nebraska Medical Center, Omaha, Nebraska, U.S.A.

Andrew J. Tan Imperial Clinical Respiratory Research Unit (ICRRU), St. Mary's Hospital, Imperial College, London, U.K.

Neil C. Thomson University of Glasgow, Glasgow, U.K.

Omar S. Usmani National Heart and Lung Institute, Imperial College, and Royal Brompton Hospital, London, U.K.

E. Haydn Walters Menzies Research Institute, University of Tasmania, Tasmania, Australia

Chris Ward Institute of Cellular Medicine, Freeman Road Hospital, Newcastle University, Newcastle-upon-Tyne, U.K.

J. A. Wedzicha Academic Unit of Respiratory Medicine, UCL Medical School, University College, London, U.K.

Youming Zhang National Heart and Lung Institute, Imperial College, London, U.K.

Contents

1

Principles of Airway Pharmacology and Therapeutics

PETER J. BARNES
National Heart and Lung Institute, Imperial College, London, U.K.

I. Introduction

Airway pharmacology is concerned with the action of drugs on target cells of the airways and improving our understanding of the mechanism of action of drugs used to treat airway diseases. This should lead to advances in drug development, so that treatment may be more specific and maximizes the beneficial effects. Drugs may also be used as specific probes to analyze pathophysiological processes in airway disease. This chapter concerns the general pharmacological principles of drug action in the airways, with particular emphasis on the application of pharmacology to understanding obstructive airway diseases and their therapy.

II. Receptors

Most hormones, neurotransmitters, mediators, cytokines, and growth factors produce their effects by interacting with specific protein recognition sites or receptors on target cells. Because receptors are specific, they allow a cell to recognize only selected signals from the myriad of molecules that come into contact with the cell. They play an important role in disease, since their function may be altered, resulting in abnormal cellular responsiveness. Many drugs used in the treatment of airway diseases stimulate (agonists) or block (antagonists) specific receptors.

There have been major advances in elucidating the function, regulation, and structure of receptors, made possible by the development of radioligand binding, in which highly potent radiolabeled agonists or antagonists are used to characterize and directly quantify and map receptors. Many receptors have now been cloned, making it possible to deduce their amino acid sequence and structure and to determine the critical parts of the receptor protein that are involved in ligand binding and interaction with intracellular second messengers. Receptor cloning and production of pure receptor proteins have also made it possible to produce specific antibodies for use in immunocytochemical studies. Furthermore, advances in molecular biology have made it possible to study the regulation of receptor genes. Some receptors termed orphan receptors have been cloned, but their endogenous ligands have not been identified. This has led to the discovery of new endogenous ligands and identification of novel drug targets. The cloning of the human genome has revealed many orphan receptors.

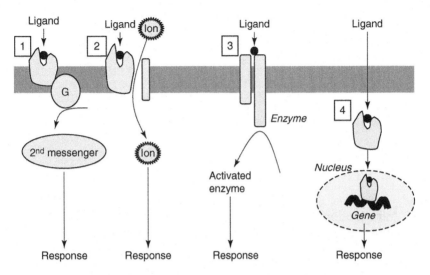

Figure 1 Several classes of receptor are recognized. (1) G protein–coupled receptors, which activate second messengers to induce a response; (2) receptor-operated ion channels; (3) enzyme-linked receptors; and (4) intracellular receptors, which translocate to the nucleus to regulate gene expression.

A. Receptor Classification

Most receptors are proteins located within the cell membrane, which interact with specific ligands outside the cell, leading to a conformational change, which results in activation of a second messenger system within the cell and subsequently to the typical cellular response. Cell surface receptors include (Fig. 1)

- guanine nucleotide–binding protein (G protein)–coupled receptors (GPCRs, e.g., β-adrenergic receptors, chemokine receptors),
- ion channel–linked receptors (e.g., nicotinic receptors),
- enzyme-linked receptors [e.g., platelet-derived growth factor (PDGF) receptors],
- cytokine and growth factor receptors, which usually have at least two subunits (e.g., interleukin-5 receptors), and
- intracellular receptors, such as steroid and thyroid receptors, where the ligand diffuses into the cell and usually binds to cytosolic receptors, which translocate to the nucleus and interact with recognition binding sites on DNA to regulate the transcription of target genes.

Molecular cloning techniques have made it possible to recognize several families of receptor that share a common structure and to trace the evolutionary lineage of receptors within receptor families.

B. G Protein–Coupled Receptors

Many different receptors interact with G proteins, which act as a coupling mechanism linking receptor activation to intracellular signal transduction pathways. All of these receptors have structural similarities and constitute a large supergene family. Over 1000 GPCRs, making up >1% of the human genome, have now been cloned and sequenced (1,2). Each receptor is a single polypeptide chain, ranging in size from ∼400 to >1000 amino acids, with seven hydrophobic sequences that cross the cell membrane. Many drugs used in the treatment of airway diseases interact with GPCRs. In addition, many unknown (orphan) GPCRs have been discovered, which are now targets for the development of novel drugs (3). For example, polymorphisms of the orphan G protein–coupled receptor for asthma susceptibility (GPRA) was discovered when polymorphisms of its gene were linked to increased asthma susceptibility and airway hyper-responsiveness (4). The endogenous agonist of this receptor has now been identified as neuropeptide S, which has been linked to anxiety and arousal, but the function of neuropeptide S in asthma has not yet been defined (5).

Rhodopsin as a Model Receptor

The first and most carefully characterized GPCR was rhodopsin in light-sensitive rods of the retina, which is coupled to a unique G protein called transducin, and this has served as a useful structural model for other receptors in this superfamily. Analysis of the amino acid sequence of rhodopsin revealed seven hydrophobic (lipophilic) stretches of 20 to 25 amino acids, which are linked by hydrophilic regions of variable length. The most likely spatial arrangement of the receptor in the cell surface membrane is for the seven hydrophobic sections (each of which is in the form of an α-helix) to span the cell membrane. The intervening hydrophilic sections are exposed alternately, intracellularly and extracellularly, with the amino (N)-terminal exposed to the outside and the carboxy (C)-terminal within the cytoplasm. The extracellular regions of rhodopsin recognize the specific ligand (retinal), and the intracellular regions interact with transducin. More recently, the three-dimensional (3D) structures of other GPCRs, including the β_2-adrenergic receptor, have been characterized, and these generally conform to the rhodopsin model (6).

Structure

All GPCRs share the common feature of seven similar hydrophobic transmembrane segments (7TM). There is also some sequence homology of the intracellular loops (which interact with various species of G protein) but less similarity in the extracellular domains. For example, there is a 50% homology between rat β_2-adrenergic and muscarinic M_2 receptors. There is also close homology between the same receptor in different species. Thus, there is 95% homology between rat and pig heart M_2 receptors. These similarities demonstrate that G receptor–linked receptors form part of a supergene family that may have a common evolutionary origin.

　　　Members of the G protein receptor supergene family are generally 400 to 500 amino acids in length, and the receptor cDNA sequence consists of 2000 to 4000 nucleotide bases (2–4 kb) (Fig. 2) (2). The molecular weight of the cloned receptors predicted from the cDNA sequence is 40 to 60 kDa, which is usually less than the molecular mass of the native receptor, when assessed by sodium dodecyl sulfate poly-acrylamide gel electrophoresis. This discrepancy is explained as due to *glycosylation* of the native receptor. For example, β_2 receptors contain two sites for glycosylation on asparagine (Asn/N) residues near the N-terminus, and it is estimated that N-glyco-sylation accounts for 25% to 30% of the molecular mass of the native receptor. Receptor

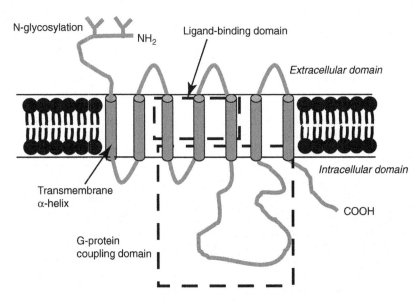

Figure 2 Structure of a G protein–coupled receptor. The peptide chain is folded seven times across the cell membrane. The hydrophobic segments that cross the cell membrane are in the form of an α-helix. Small ligands interact deep within the cell membrane between the α-helices, whereas peptide ligands interact with the extracellular parts of the receptor. Intracellular loops (especially the third intracellular loop) are important in interaction with the G protein. Most of these receptors are glycosylated at extracellular loops.

glycosylation does not affect receptor affinity for ligand or coupling to G proteins, but may be important for the trafficking of the receptor through the cell during down-regulation, or for keeping the receptor correctly orientated in the lipid bilayer.

Another feature of these receptors is palmitoylation, when cysteine residues covalently bind palmitic acid via a thioester bond, thus anchoring the receptor chain to the cell membrane. This confers 3D stability to the receptor, and disruption of this bond in β receptors (by mutation of Cys341) alters both binding characteristics and coupling to G proteins and may affect desensitization of the receptor (7).

Deletion mutagenesis (deleting sections of the peptide sequence) and site-directed mutagenesis (substitution of single amino acids in the polypeptide chain) have established that the ligand-binding domain is well conserved between members of the same family. In the case of β-adrenoceptors, there is good evidence for a ligand-binding cleft between the transmembrane-spanning domains within the cell membrane (7). Critical amino acids for the interaction of endogenous adrenergic agonists (norepinephrine and epinephrine) are asparagine (Asp) in the third transmembrane loop (TM3, Asp113) and serines in TM5 (Ser204, Ser207), which interact with the hydroxy groups on the catechol ring (Fig. 3).

The binding site for antagonists differs from those of naturally occurring ligands, and for antagonist binding to β receptors, 7TM appears to be critical. Binding of substance P

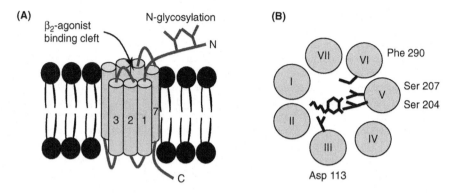

Figure 3 Ligand binding domain of the β_2-adrenergic receptor, showing the clustering of the seven transmembrane domains to form a binding cleft (**A**) and the interaction between the catecholamine and critical amino acids in the transmembrane domains (**B**).

to the NK_1 receptor occurs to extracellular domains of the receptor, whereas antagonist binding of the nonpeptide NK_1 antagonist CP96,345 binds to a transmembrane domain (His197) (8).

One special type of GPCR is the proteinase-activated receptor (PAR), exemplified by receptors for thrombin and tryptase (9). There are currently four PARs recognized; thrombin activates PAR1, 3, and 4, whereas trypsin, mast cell tryptase, and other serine proteases activate PAR2. Activators of these receptors are enzymes that cleave a site on the extracellular domain of the receptor, thus revealing an active site that then binds to and activates the remaining receptor protein (Fig. 4). PAR may play an important role in lung diseases, leading to a search for specific antagonists (9).

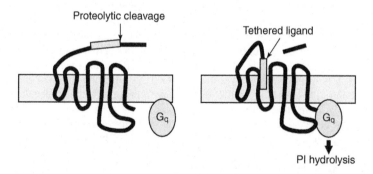

Figure 4 PARs are G protein–coupled receptors that are activated by proteinases, such as thrombin (PAR1, 2, 4) and tryptase (PAR2). Cleavage occurs at the N-terminal end of the receptor to reveal a tethered ligand sequence that then inserts into the binding cleft of the receptor, resulting in coupling of a G protein (usually G_q) to effector mechanisms such as PI hydrolysis. *Abbreviations*: PARS, proteinase-activated receptors; PI, phosphoinositide.

C. Receptor Dimerization

Most GPCR undergo physical association not only with themselves (homodimerization) but also with other GPCR (heterodimerization), and this may influence receptor function and interaction with signaling pathways, providing a novel mechanism of receptor interactions that may be relevant to airway diseases (10–12). Recognition of GPCR heterodimers might also lead to the development of novel drugs that only recognize the heterodimers and therefore have a greater selectivity. For example, heterodimerization between prostaglandin E (EP$_1$) receptors and β_2 receptors in airway smooth muscle cells results in uncoupling of β_2 receptors and a diminished bronchodilator response to β_2-agonists (13). β_2 Receptors are also known to dimerize with β_1, β_3, opioid, and angiotensin AT$_1$ receptors. Heterodimerization of chemokine receptors may be important in determining cell recruitment and may account for why selective antagonist of one receptor may inhibit responses to other chemokines that signal through different receptors (14). For example, CXCR1/CXCR2 and CCR2/CCR4 heterodimers have been identified and appear to be induced when the chemokine ligands for both receptors are present together.

D. G Proteins

G proteins link activation of 7TM receptors to enzymes or ion channels that then mediate the characteristic response (15). All G proteins have GTPase intrinsic activity and catalyze the conversion of guanosine triphosphate (GTP) to guanosine diphosphate (GDP). G proteins are made up of three separate units and are termed heterotrimeric G proteins; the α-subunit interacts with the receptor, binds GTP, and interacts with the effector enzyme, such as adenylyl cyclase and phospholipase C (PLC). The β- and γ-subunits are hydrophobic and are associated as a $\beta\gamma$ complex within the cytoplasmic surface of the cell membrane. G proteins are freely diffusible within the cell membrane, and the pool of G proteins may interact with several receptors. In the resting state, the G protein exists as a $\alpha\beta\gamma$ heterotrimer with GDP occupying the binding site on the α-subunit. When a receptor is occupied by an agonist, a conformational change occurs and the intracellular loops of the receptor protein acquire a high affinity for $\alpha\beta\gamma$, resulting in the dissociation of GDP and its replacement with GTP, which in turn causes α-GTP to dissociate from the $\beta\gamma$-subunits (Fig. 5). α-GTP is the active form of the G protein and diffuses to associate with effector molecules, such as enzymes and ion channels. This process is terminated by hydrolysis of GTP to GDP via the GTPase activity of the α-subunit. The resulting α-GDP dissociates from the effector molecule and reassociates with $\beta\gamma$, in readiness for activation again (16).

In addition to the classical heterotrimeric G proteins with $\alpha\beta\gamma$-subunits, there are several other small G proteins with GTPase activity, such as the Rho, Rab, and Rac subfamilies, which are not activated directly by GPCR but play a key role in regulating actin and cytoskeletal organization (17). Rho activates specific Rho kinases, leading to a cascade of interacting signals within the cell. For example, Rho GTPases are involved in contractile responses in airway smooth muscle and in fibrosis so that Rho kinase inhibitors might have therapeutic potential in asthma (18). Rab GTPases are involved in secretion and may therefore play a role in mucus secretion and in mast cell degranulation (19).

Several receptors, such as β receptors and vasoactive intestinal polypeptide (VIP)-receptors, stimulate adenylyl cyclase via a stimulatory G protein, G$_s$, whereas other

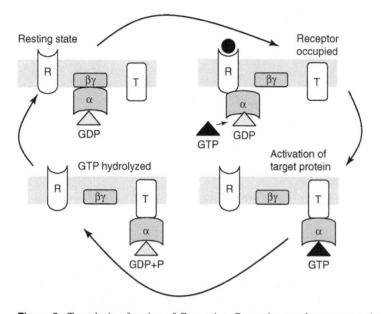

Figure 5 Transducing function of G proteins. G proteins couple receptor activation to a target membrane protein, such as an enzyme (e.g., adenylyl cyclase) or an ion channel (T). Each G protein is made up of three subunits (α, β, and γ). In the inactive state, GDP binds to the α-subunit, but when a receptor (R) is activated it interacts with the α-subunit, displacing GDP for GTP, and resulting in the association of the α-subunit with the effector system. GTP is then hydrolyzed by the intrinsic GTPase activity of the α-subunit, resulting in activation of T. This then allows the α-subunit to associate with the $\beta\gamma$-subunits that remain fixed in the hydrophobic cell membrane. The α-subunit is therefore believed to act as a "shuttle" coupling receptor activation to stimulation of the target protein. *Abbreviations*: GDP, guanine diphosphate; GTP, guanine triphosphate

receptors, such as muscarinic M_2 receptors, inhibit adenylyl cyclase via G_i (Fig. 6) (15). G_s may be stimulated directly by cholera toxin, whereas Gi is inhibited by *pertussis* toxin, and these toxins have proved to be useful in elucidating the involvement of a particular G protein in a specific receptor-mediated response. Other G proteins are now recognized that couple receptors that activate phosphoinositide hydrolysis (G_0, G_q) and particular ion channels in the cell membrane (e.g., G_k, which is coupled to potassium channels). G proteins may play a very important role in the regulation of cell responsiveness, and there is evidence that receptors may become uncoupled from G proteins under certain conditions. For example, in fatal asthma there is evidence for a reduced responsiveness of airway smooth muscle to β-agonists, yet the number and affinity of β receptors on airway smooth muscle is not reduced and the response to other smooth muscle relaxants is not impaired, suggesting that the receptors have become *uncoupled* from G_s in severe asthma (20).

While receptors affect the function of G proteins, G proteins also influence the interaction of ligands with their receptors. Thus, when coupled to an inactive G protein, the receptor exists in a state of high affinity for the agonist. Agonist binding releases G_α

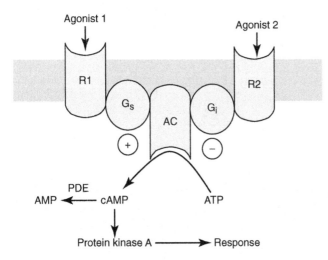

Figure 6   G proteins and adenylyl cyclase. Receptors (R_1 and R_2) are coupled to G proteins that stimulate (G_s) or inhibit (G_i) adenylyl cyclase (AC), resulting in increased or decreased formation of the second messenger, cAMP from ATP. cAMP is degraded to AMP via PDE. cAMP activates protein kinase A, which phosphorylates target proteins leading to a response. *Abbreviations*: cAMP, cyclic adenosine $3',5'$-monophosphate; ATP, adenosine triphosphate; AMP, adenosine monophosphate; PDE, phosphodiesterases.

from contact with the receptor, resulting in a reduction in agonist affinity, referred to as the "guanine nucleotide shift."

E.   Second Messengers
The ligand that activates a receptor is described as the first messenger and leads, via activation of a G protein, to the typical cellular response via a second messenger, such as a change in intracellular calcium ion (Ca^{2+}) concentration or cyclic $3',5'$ adenosine monophosphate (cAMP) concentration. While the number of surface receptors that may respond on any particular cell is very large, only a very limited number of signal transduction and second messenger systems have been described. Thus, the surface receptors determine cellular responsiveness and sensitivity, rather than the intracellular mechanisms that are activated by the receptor-ligand interaction. Great progress has been made in understanding the intracellular mechanisms involved in receptor-mediated effects, through the development of techniques, such as intracellular dye indicators, which reflect intracellular concentrations of ions (e.g., fura-2 that detects intracellular Ca^{2+} concentrations), by more sensitive biochemical assays, and by the development of patch-clamping techniques.

Adenylyl Cyclase
Many receptors produce their effects by interaction with the membrane-bound enzyme adenylyl cyclase to either increase or decrease production of cyclic $3',5'$ adenosine monophosphate (cAMP) (Fig. 6). At least nine closely related forms of adenylyl cyclase

have now been differentiated, and there is increasing evidence that these isoforms may be differentially regulated (21). Thus, protein kinase C (PKC) phosphorylates and activates certain isoforms (types 1, 2, and 3), which may be a mechanism for the interaction of different receptors, whereas it has no effect on other isoforms (4–6). The formation of cAMP leads to the characteristic cellular response via the activation of a specific protein kinase, protein kinase A (PKA), by dissociating a regulatory (inhibitory) subunit. PKA then phosphorylates serine and threonine residues on specific proteins such as regulatory proteins, ion channels, and enzymes within the cell, which lead to the characteristic response. For example, in airway smooth muscle cells PKA phosphorylates large-conductance calcium-activated potassium (K^+) channels, which open leading to K^+ efflux from the cell, hyperpolarization and relaxation (22). PKA also phosphorylates and therefore inactivates myosin light-chain kinase, resulting in a direct relaxant effect on the contractile machinery.

It is now increasingly recognized that cAMP also actives signaling mechanisms other than PKA, such as ion channels and the ubiquitous guanine nucleotide exchange factors Epac 1 and 2 (23). For example, cAMP-induced inhibition of IL-5 in human T lymphocytes is independent of PKA (24). On the other hand, β_2-agonists inhibit the release of certain cytokines from airway smooth muscle cells via an effect on PKA, since these responses are completely inhibited by transfection with the selective endogenous PKA inhibitor called PKA inhibitor-α.(25)

Phosphodiesterases

cAMP is hydrolyzed within cells by a family of enzymes termed phosphodiesterases (PDEs). At least 12 PDE families have now been distinguished on the basis of substrate specificity, inhibition by selective inhibitors, and molecular cloning (26). In airway smooth muscle, PDE3 and PDE4 isoenzymes are involved in cAMP-mediated relaxation, whereas in inflammatory cells (mast cells, eosinophils, neutrophils, macrophages, T lymphocytes) and airway epithelium, PDE4 predominates. This has led to the development of several selective PDE4 inhibitors to treat asthma and chronic obstructive pulmonary disease (COPD), although side effects after oral administration are a major problem that has limited development (27). Each PDE has several subtypes encoded by different genes, and each subtype of PDE has several splice variants, so multiple forms of PDE exist in the cell. This may allow precise control of intracellular cyclic nucleotide concentrations. For example, there are four distinct PDE4s, PDE4A, PDE4B, PDE4C, and PDE4D, each of which has several splice variants that are differentially expressed and regulated (28). This may be relevant in drug design as inhibition of one subtype may mediate the desired effect and another may be responsible for side effects. For example, PDE4B appears to mediate the anti-inflammatory effect of PDE4 inhibitors, whereas PDE4D mediates the nausea and vomiting that are often dose-limiting (29,30).

Phosphatidylinositol Hydrolysis

Another signaling system involves breakdown of a membrane phospholipid, phosphatidylinositol (PI), which results in increased intracellular Ca^{2+} concentration. Over 100 receptors are coupled via G_q or G_i to the membrane-associated enzyme phosphoinositidase or PLC, which converts phosphoinositide(4,5)bisphosphate (PIP_2) to inositol

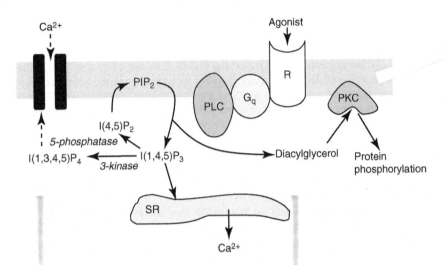

Figure 7 Phosphoinositide hydrolysis. Occupation of a surface receptor leads to activation of the enzyme PLC via a G protein (G_q). PLC converts phosphoinositide 4,5,-bisphosphate (PIP_2) to inositol (1,4,5) trisphosphate and diacylglycerol. $I(1,4,5)P_3$ binds to receptors on sarcoplasmic/ endoplasmic reticulum (SR) to release Ca^{2+}, resulting in a rise in intracellular Ca^{2+} concentration and cell activation. $I(1,4,5)P_3$ is dephosphorylated to $I(4,5)P_2$, inositol phosphate, and inositol, which is then reincorporated into membrane phophoinositides. In some cells it is further phosphorylated to $I(1,3,4,5)P_4$, which may be involved with calcium entry and refilling of intracellular stores. Diacylglycerol activates PKC, which phosphorylates various regulatory proteins in the cell. *Abbreviations*: PLC, phospholipase C; PKC, protein kinase C.

(1,4,5)trisphosphate (IP_3) and 1,2-sn-diacylglycerol (DAG) (Fig. 7). Four main groups of PLC have now been identified (PLC-β, PLC-γ, PLC-δ, PLC-ε), each of which has subclasses (PLC-β1, PLC-β2, PLC-β3, etc.) based on amino acid structure of different cloned genes (31). These isoenzymes are differentially coupled to different receptors and are subject to differential regulation.

IP_3 binds to a specific receptor on endoplasmic/sarcoplasmic reticulum, which leads to the release of Ca^{2+} from intracellular stores. Thus, PI hydrolysis links occupation of a surface receptor to intracellular Ca^{2+} release. Most of the mediators that contract airway smooth muscle act on receptors that activate PI hydrolysis in airway smooth muscle (32). IP_3 is broken down into the inactive IP_2 by IP_3 kinase and subsequently to inositol, which is reincorporated into phophoinositides in the cell membrane. IP_3 may also be phosphorylated by IP_3 kinase to IP_4, which may be involved in opening receptor-operated calcium channels and the refilling of intracellular stores. Calcium release in response to agonists or IP_3 occurs in a series of oscillations, which is probably mediated via calcium-induced calcium release and the opening of calcium channels on the cell membrane, and the frequency of oscillation may be important in the type of cell activation that ensues (33).

The formation of DAG activates PKC by causing it to translocate to the cell membrane and by dramatically increasing its sensitivity to Ca^{2+}. Activated PKC is then capable of phosphorylating various cell membrane–associated proteins, including receptors, G proteins, and regulatory proteins. Several isoenzymes of PKC are now recognized and play a critical role in the regulation of inflammatory and structural cells of the airways, although the role of individual isoenzymes in regulating cell function is not yet clear as selective inhibitors have been difficult to find (34). PKC may be activated directly by tumor-promoting phorbol esters, such as phorbol myristate acetate (PMA). In some species, PMA and other phorbol esters cause prolonged contractile responses in airway smooth muscle, but in other species, bronchodilatation is observed. It has been suggested that PKC may be important for the prolonged contractile responses seen in asthmatic airways. Several PKC isoenzymes have been identified in human airway smooth muscle (35). PKC inhibitors, such as staurosporine (which is not very selective) and Ro 31-8220, may be useful in elucidating the role of PKC but have no selectivity for different isoforms.

Guanylyl Cyclase

It was previously believed that, while relaxation of smooth muscle is brought about by receptors that activate cAMP, contraction is due to the production of another cyclic nucleotide, cyclic $3',5'$ guanosine monophosphate (cGMP), formed by the activation of guanylyl cyclase (36). This is now known to be incorrect and the increase in cGMP is secondary to a rise in intracellular Ca^{2+} concentration. Indeed cGMP causes relaxation of smooth muscle and is the major mechanism of vasodilatation after nitrovasodilators (such as sodium nitroprusside) and dilators (such as acetylcholine), which release nitric oxide (NO) from endothelial cells. cGMP is also involved in the relaxant response of airway smooth muscle to nitrovasodilators and to atrial natriuretic peptide (ANP), which is a potent bronchodilator in vitro (37). Guanylyl cyclase exists in particulate form, binds natriuretic peptides, and also exists as a soluble form that binds NO (38). cGMP is broken down by PDEs, and in particular the PDE5 isoenzyme (39). PDE5 inhibitors, such as sildenafil, have potent vasodilator effects on pulmonary vessels and weak bronchodilator effects.

Ion Channel–Coupled Signaling

G proteins may also couple receptors to ion channels, including K^+, Na^+, and Ca^{2+} channels. Thus, certain muscarinic receptors are coupled via G proteins (G_0) to K^+ channels and Ca^{2+} channels. In airway smooth muscle, β_2 receptors are directly coupled via G_s to the opening of large-conductance K^+ (maxi-K) channels, and the same channels are inhibited by M_2 receptors via G_i (22). These G proteins allow rapid cell activation by GPCR, in contrast to the slower responses mediated by changes in cyclic nucleotides.

F. Cytokine Receptors

The effects of cytokines are mediated via specific surface receptors, many of which have now been cloned. There is a very complex network of cytokines and chemokines (small chemotactic cytokines) that orchestrate the inflammation in asthma, COPD, and interstitial lung disease, and all of their complex effects are mediated by surface receptors (40).

Chemokine Receptors

Chemokines, such as CXCL8 (IL-8), CCL5 (RANTES), and CCL11 (eotaxin), bind to receptors that are coupled to G proteins, and their receptors have the typical 7TM GPCR structure (41,42). Many chemokines have overlapping activities and interact with common receptors on target leukocytes. Over 20 chemokine receptors have now been characterized and they appear to be differentially expressed on different inflammatory cells, thus explaining the differential chemotactic effects of these cytokines. For example eosinophils express CCR3 that is activated by CCL5, CCL13 (MCP-4), CCL11, CCL24 (eotaxin-2), and CCL26 (eotaxin-3), thus accounting for the selective chemotactic effects of these chemokines on eosinophil migration. Because of the 7TM structure of chemokine receptor, small molecule inhibitors are feasible. This has led to the development of several chemokine antagonists for the treatment of asthma and COPD (43,44).

Cytokine Receptor Superfamilies

Most cytokine receptors have a primary structure that is quite different from the 7TM spanning segments associated with GPCR. Many cytokine receptors have at least two subunits that interact to activate signal transduction pathways within the cell (45). For example IL-5, IL-4, and IL-13 receptors have an α- and β-chain. The tumor necrosis factor α (TNF-α) receptor is a 55-kDa peptide (p55) that has a single transmembrane-spanning helical segment, an extracellular domain that binds TNF-α, and an intracellular domain (46). The intracellular domain leads to activation of several kinases and ceramide, which subsequently lead to the activation of transcription factors, such as nuclear factor–kappaB (NF-κB) and activator protein 1 (AP-1). A second TNF receptor (p75) has also been cloned, but differs markedly in sequence and may be linked to different intracellular pathways (46). There are now almost 30 receptors and 20 cytokines in the TNF superfamily, which have complex and interacting signal transduction pathways (47).

Molecular cloning has now revealed that although cytokines may be structurally diverse, their receptors may be grouped into various families that share structural homology (48). The immunoglobulin superfamily of receptors includes the receptors for IL-1 and PDGF, T-cell antigen receptors, and certain cell-surface adhesion molecules. The hematopoietin receptor superfamily includes receptors for IL-2, IL-3, IL-4, IL-5, IL-6, IL-7, interferons, granulocyte-macrophage colony-stimulating factor (GM-CSF), growth factor, and erythropoietin receptors. The receptor proteins are orientated with an extracellular N-terminal domain and a single hydrophobic transmembrane-spanning segment. There is striking homology in the extracellular ligand–binding domain with four conserved cysteine residues. There is very close homology between the receptors for IL-3, IL-5, and GM-CSF, all of which stimulate growth of eosinophils. Molecular cloning has demonstrated that each of these receptors consists of α- and β-chains and share a common β-chain, which may explain why they have overlapping biological activities.

The second messenger system used by cytokines are highly complex, involving many interacting pathways that allow for the possibility of signal splitting, so that the same activating signal may result in the activation of several parallel pathways. Which signal pathways predominate is determined by other signals impinging on the cell. Most cytokines activate a group of transcription factors and result in prolonged cellular activation and gene transcription, in contrast to the relatively rapid and transient signaling of most GPCR.

G. Enzyme-Linked Receptors

Some receptors contain an enzyme domain within their structure so that when the enzyme is activated by a ligand the enzyme becomes activated, leading to signal transduction through the formation of a specific substrate within the cell. The best characterized of these enzyme-linked receptors is receptor tyrosine kinases (RTKs) that have intrinsic protein tyrosine kinase activity.

Receptor Tyrosine Kinases

Activation of RTKs results in phosphorylation of tyrosine residues on certain target proteins that are usually associated with cell growth and chronic activation of cells. More than 50 different RTKs belonging to at least 14 distinct families have now been identified (49). These receptors include epithelial growth factor (EGF), PDGF, vascular endothelial growth factor (VEGF), and insulin receptors (Fig. 8). Small molecule inhibitors, such as gefitinib and erlotinib, which block EGF receptors, have been developed for treating lung cancer (50).

RTKs share a similar general structure, consisting of a large extracellular N-terminal portion that contains the ligand recognition domain, a single short membrane-spanning region (α-helix), and a cytoplasmic C-terminal portion (~250 amino acids) that contains the tyrosine kinase activity and autophosphorylation sites. The extracellular

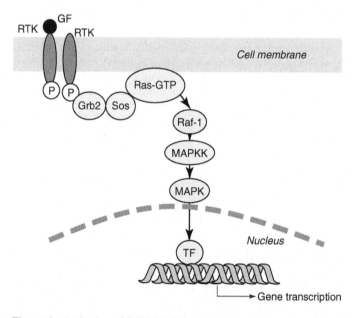

Figure 8 Activation of RTK by GF results in a cascade of enzyme activation, involving the adaptor proteins Grb2, Sos, and Ras-GTP, leading to the activation of MAPK, which then activate TFs to regulate expression of genes involved in cell proliferation. *Abbreviations*: RTK, receptor tyrosine kinase; GF, growth factors; MAPK, mitogen-activated protein kinases; TFs, transcription factors; MAPKK, MAPK kinase.

domain usually contains cysteine-rich regions and/or immunoglobulin-like motifs, with a large number of disulfide bonds forming a highly specific tertiary structure that is needed to establish ligand-binding specificity. All RTK (with the exception of the insulin receptor family) undergo a transition from a monomeric to a dimeric state (either homodimers or heterodimers) following binding of their specific ligands. Another characteristic of RTK is that they undergo internalization into two types of intracellular vesicles: pitted vesicles coated with the protein clathrin and smooth vesicles lacking clathrin. There is a spontaneous internalization, but this is rapidly accelerated when the receptor is occupied by a ligand. A proportion of the receptors is degraded, whereas others are recycled to the cell surface.

Signal Transduction

RTKs phosphorylate intracellular molecules containing Src homology 2 and 3 (SH2 and SH3) domains. These SH2 and SH3 domains are short sequences of about 100 and 50 to 60 amino acids, respectively, which function to specify the interaction with a target protein (51). The SH2 motifs recognize phosphotyrosine residues and are responsible for interactions with autophosphorylated RTK, the specificity of which depends on the amino acid sequences surrounding both the tyrosine autophosphorylation site on the RTK and the substrate's SH2 domain. RTK substrate proteins containing SH2 and SH3 motifs may contain enzymatic activity.

Most RTK stimulate the mitogen-activated protein kinase (MAPK) pathways through a complex multistep signaling cascade initiated by translocation of the adaptor protein Grb2 to the cytoplasmic membrane. This results in the activation of Ras proteins, small molecular weight GTPases, in turn activate Raf, which is a serine/threonine kinase that activates the MAPK pathway (52). There is increasing evidence that RTK may interact with several cell signaling pathways to elicit their effects, and it now seems likely that specific pathways are selected under certain conditions. For example, PDGF, which may exist in the dimeric forms AA, BB, or AB, may interact with different receptor dimers ($\alpha\alpha$, $\alpha\beta$, $\beta\beta$), resulting in activation of different signal transduction pathways.

MAP Kinase Pathways

RTK and other extracellular signals activate several MAP kinase cascades, resulting in a cascade of kinase activation that result in activation of transcription through the transcription factors Jun, Elk-1, and ATF2 (53,54).

Receptor Serine/Threonine Kinases

Similar to RTK, there are some receptors that are linked to serine/threonine kinase activity. The best-known example is transforming growth factor β (TGF-β), which exists in three mammalian isoforms encoded by separate genes, all of which may have complex and divergent effects on cell activity (55). TGF-β receptors signal through regulatory Smad pathways within the cell, including Smad2 and Smad3, together with coactivator Smads, whereas inhibitory Smads, such as Smad6 and Smad7, act as a feedback inhibitory mechanism. Some of the effects of TGF-β are mediated via inhibition of cyclins that regulate the cell cycle, and this may account for the diverse effects of TGF-β depending on the stage of the cell cycle (56).

Receptor Protein Tyrosine Phosphatases

Little is known about the third type of enzyme-linked receptors, which have a high level of intrinsic enzyme activity (57). Occupation by a ligand may turn this enzyme activity off, thus resulting in cell suppression. These receptors appear to be important in cell differentiation and include CD45 (also known as leukocyte common antigen) that is involved in T-lymphocyte signaling (58).

H. Ion Channel Receptors

Although several receptors are linked via G proteins to ion channels, such as Ca^{2+} and K^+ channels as discussed above, other receptors are ion channels themselves. Ion channel receptors are oligomeric proteins containing about 20 transmembrane segments arranged around a central aqueous channel. Binding of the ligand and channel opening occur very rapidly (within milliseconds). This is in contrast to the *slow* receptors, such as GPCR, which involve a series of catalytic steps. The best-characterized example is the nicotinic acetylcholine receptor (nAChR), which is made up of four subunits that form a cation channel. When activated by Ach, the channel opens to allow the passage of Na^+ ions (59). This type of receptor, which can respond rapidly as no intracellular mechanisms are involved, is known as a fast receptor and is usually involved in synaptic transmission (Fig. 9). nAChR are involved in ganglionic transmission in parasympathetic ganglia within the airways and are blocked by hexamethonium, which therefore blocks ganglionic transmission and cholinergic reflex bronchoconstriction. nAChR are widely distributed and $\alpha 4 \beta 2$ nAChR in the brain are responsible for nicotine addiction. Varenicline is a partial antagonist of $\alpha 4 \beta 2$ nAChR, acting to block the addictive effects of nicotine and its withdrawal symptoms (60). Other examples include glutamate and γ-aminobutyric acid ($GABA_A$) receptors.

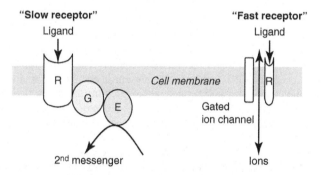

Figure 9 Fast and slow receptors. Some receptors are ion channels and consist of several subunits grouped round an aqueous channel through which ions (e.g., Na^+, K^+, Ca^{2+}, Cl^-) enter or leave the cell when agonists bind to one or more of the subunits. Such receptors function very rapidly (in milliseconds) and are involved in neurotransmission (e.g., nicotinic receptors in airway ganglia). Other receptors, which are coupled via G proteins (G), produce their effects more slowly, since a sequence of enzymatic events is necessary before a response occurs. *Abbreviations*: E, enzyme; R, receptor.

I. Intracellular Receptors

Several ligands cross the cell membrane to interact with intracellular (cytosolic) receptors rather than surface receptors. There is a family of steroid receptors that recognize different endogenous steroids such as glucocorticoids, mineralocorticoids, androgens, and estrogens. Indeed, steroid receptors belong to a supergene family that also includes thyroid hormone, retinoic acid (vitamin A), and vitamin D receptors (61). The exploration of cDNA libraries for related sequences has led to the discovery of over 40 "orphan" nuclear receptors whose ligands are now being identified (62). One new class of nuclear receptor so identified is the peroxisome proliferator-activated receptor (PPAR), with α, γ, and β/δ subtypes, for which selective ligands have now been identified. PPAR may be involved in metabolism and inflammation and may be endogenously activated by lipid mediators (63). For example, PPARγ agonists, such as rosiglitazone, appear to have anti-inflammatory effects on lung inflammation and are also potentially anti-fibrotic, so they have the potential for treating small airway fibrosis in COPD as well as interstitial lung diseases. Several other orphan receptors, including liver X receptors (LXR), farnesoid X receptors (FXR), pregnane X receptors (PXR) and retinoic acid X receptors (RXR) appear to play a role in the inflammatory process and may lead to the discovery of novel anti-inflammatory treatments (64).

Intracellular receptors share a common general structure with a central DNA-binding domain, characterized by the presence of two "zinc fingers," which are loops stabilized by four cysteine/histidine residues around a zinc ion. These zinc fingers anchor the receptor to the double helix at specific hormone response elements in the promoter region of target genes. Ligands bind in the C-terminal domain, which also contains sequences important for binding of associated chaperone proteins (e.g., heat shock proteins) and a nuclear localization signal involved in transporting the receptor from the cytoplasm into the nucleus. The N-terminal domain is involved in transcriptional regulation (*trans*-activation) and in the interaction with other transcription factors.

Steroid Receptors

Several steroid receptors have now been cloned, and their structures have been shown to differ. However, there is some homology between these receptors since they all interact with nuclear DNA, where they act as modulators of the transcription of specific genes. For example, glucocorticoid receptors (GRs) are normally present in the cytosol in an inactive form bound to two molecules of a 90-kDa heat shock protein (hsp90), which cover the DNA binding domain. Binding of a corticosteroid to its receptor results in the dissociation of hsp90, and the occupied receptor then undergoes a conformational change that allows it to bind to DNA (65,66).

The DNA-binding domain of steroid receptors is rich in Cys residues. Formation of a complex with zinc is able to fold the peptide chain into a finger-shaped conformation and the zinc is coordinated by four Cys residues. GRs have two zinc fingers that are loops of approximately 15 residues, each of which is held in shape by four cysteine residues surrounding an atom of zinc. Zinc fingers are essential for the interaction with the DNA double helix. Steroid receptors recognize specific DNA sequences—in the case of GR, glucocorticoid response elements (GREs), which have the consensus sequence GGTAnnnTGTTCT. Dimers of GR occupied by steroid bind to the GRE on the DNA double helix and either *increase* (+GRE) or much less commonly *decrease* (−GRE) the rate of transcription by influencing the promoter sequence in the target gene. Indeed repression of target genes may be the most important aspect of corticosteroid action in inflammatory diseases, such as asthma, since corticosteroids may inhibit the transcription of many cytokines that are involved in chronic inflammation. The major mechanism of gene repression is mediated via an interaction between the activated GR and transcription factors, such as NF-κB and AP-1 that are activated via inflammatory signals such as cytokines. NF-κB activates inflammatory genes by recruiting coactivator molecules that have histone acetyltransferase activity, leading to acetylation of core histones associated with inflammatory genes, which results in increased gene transcription. Activated GRs inhibit coactivator molecules and also recruit histone deacetylase-2 (HDAC2), which deacetylate the hyperacetylated histones, resulting in switching off of the activated inflammatory genes (66) (Fig. 10).

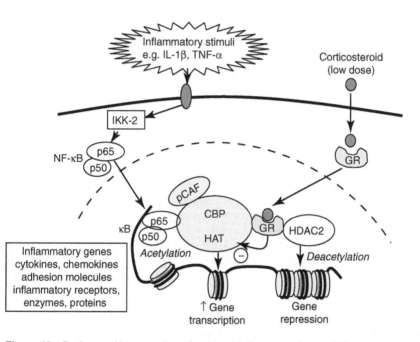

Figure 10 Corticosteroid suppression of activated inflammatory genes. Inflammatory genes are activated by inflammatory stimuli, such as IL-1β or TNF-α, resulting in activation of IKK2 (inhibitor of I-κB kinase-2), which activates the transcription factor NF-κB. A dimer of p50 and p65 NF-κB proteins translocates to the nucleus and binds to specific κB recognition sites and also to coactivators, such as CBP, which have intrinsic HAT activity. This results in acetylation of core histone H4, resulting in increased expression of genes encoding multiple inflammatory proteins. GRs after activation by glucocorticoids translocate to the nucleus and bind to coactivators to inhibit HAT activity directly and recruit HDAC2, which reverses histone acetylation leading to suppression of these activated inflammatory genes. *Abbreviations*: IL-1β, interleukin 1β; TNF-α, tumor necrosis factor α; NF-κB, nuclear factor kappa B; CBP, CREB-binding protein; HAT, histone acetyltransferase; GRs, glucocorticoid receptors; HDAC2, histone deacetylase-2.

J. Receptor Subtypes

The existence of receptor subtypes is often first indicated by differences in the potency of a series of agonists in different tissues. This could be due to differing proportions of coexistent receptor subtypes, or may indicate the existence of a novel receptor subtype. Molecular biology can resolve these possibilities since molecular techniques can clearly discriminate between different subtypes of receptor and show that they are encoded by different genes. Thus, the human β_1 receptor is clearly different from the β_2 receptor in its amino acid sequence, with a 54% homology, and the NK_1 receptor, which is selectively activated by substance P, has a 48% homology with the NK_2 receptor that is activated by the related tachykinin neurokinin A. A third tachykinin receptor, NK_3 receptor, which is selectively activated by neurokinin B, has also been cloned.

Using cross-hybridization in which a known receptor cDNA sequence is hybridized with a genomic library, it has also been possible to detect previously unknown subtypes of a receptor. For example, an atypical β receptor, which does not clearly fit into the β_1 or β_2 receptor subtypes, has been suspected in adipose tissue and some smooth muscle preparations. A distinct β_3 receptor was subsequently identified, cloned, sequenced, and expressed (67). The β_3 receptor is clearly different from either β_1 or β_2 receptors (about 50% amino acid sequence homology) and appear to be important in the regulation of metabolic rate, but has not been detected in lung homogenates (68).

Molecular biology has been particularly useful in advancing our understanding of muscarinic receptors. Five distinct muscarinic receptors have been cloned from rat and human tissues (69). The m1, m2, and m3 receptor genes correspond to the M_1, M_2, and M_3 receptors identified pharmacologically, whereas m4 and m5 receptors are previously unrecognized pharmacological subtypes that occur predominantly in the brain and for which no selective drugs have yet been developed. Interestingly m4 receptors have been demonstrated in rabbit lung using antibodies against the cloned m4 receptor, and their presence confirmed by cDNA probes for the m4 receptor. These m4 receptors are localized to vascular smooth muscle and alveolar walls, but have not been observed in lungs of other species, including humans (70). The reason for so many different subtypes of a receptor that recognize a single agonist is still not certain, but it seems likely that they are linked to different intracellular pathways and that the regulation of the intracellular portion of the amino acid sequence may be unique to each subtype. The m1, m2, and m5 receptors stimulate PI hydrolysis through a *pertussis*-insensitive G protein, whereas m2 and m4 receptors inhibit adenylyl cyclase via G_i. It is possible that the difference in protein structure may reflect regulation at a transcriptional level from DNA through different promoters, leading to variations in tissue or developmental expression, or to differences at a posttranslational level, allowing regulation by intracellular mechanisms, such as phosphorylation at critical sites on intracellular loops.

K. Receptor Interactions

Activation of one receptor may influence the function of a separate receptor via a number of interacting mechanisms. The opposing effects of receptors, which increase and decrease adenylyl cyclase activity via G_s and G_i, respectively, are well described. In airway smooth muscle, M_2 receptors inhibit adenylyl cyclase, whereas β_2 receptors stimulate this enzyme, so that there are opposing effects. This may explain why it is more difficult for β agonists to reverse contraction of airway smooth muscle induced by cholinergic agonists compared with histamine. Conversely, β-agonists may also

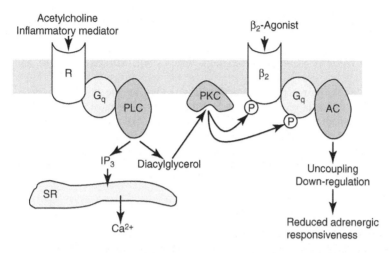

Figure 11 Receptor interactions ("cross talk"). The activation of one surface receptor may affect the function of a different receptor type via interaction of intracellular mechanisms. For example, activation of an inflammatory mediator or muscarinic receptor (R) on airway smooth muscle cells may stimulate phosphoinositide hydrolysis, with activation of PKC via diacylglycerol formation. This may result in phosphorylation (P) of other receptors, such as β_2 receptors (β_2) or a stimulatory G protein (G_s), resulting in downregulation and uncoupling of β_2 receptors, with reduced responsiveness to β_2-agonists. *Abbreviations*: PKC, protein kinase C; G_q, receptor-coupled G protein that activates phosphoinositide hydrolysis; PLC, phospholipase C; AC, adenylyl cyclase; IP_3, inositol (1,4,5) trisphosphate; SR, sarcoplasmic/endoplasmic reticulum; Ca^{2+}, calcium ions.

influence the expression of M_2 receptors (71). Several other interactions between receptors are recognized. Receptors that increase cAMP will oppose the effects of receptors that elevate intracellular Ca^{2+} via several mechanisms, including stimulation of Ca^{2+} sequestration and exchange (72).

PI hydrolysis leads to activation of PKC, which then phosphorylates receptors and G proteins, resulting in uncoupling and impaired receptor function (73) (Fig. 11). In airway smooth muscle, this may be an important interaction in inflammation since inflammatory mediators will stimulate PI hydrolysis in airway smooth muscle cells and via activation of PKC will phosphorylate G proteins, leading to uncoupling of β_2 receptors. This may explain the reduced bronchodilator response to β agonists in vitro observed in airways taken from patients with fatal asthma attacks. G protein receptor kinases (GRK) may be activated by GPCR occupation and then phosphorylate other receptors, leading to altered signaling in heterologous GPCR (74). Receptor interactions may also occur through receptor heterodimerization as discussed above.

An additional type of interaction may operate at the level of gene transcription. Cytokines may activate transcription factors that have an effect on a target gene, and steroid receptors may interact with the same gene with an opposing effect. There may also be a direct interaction between transcription factors within the cytoplasm. For example, activated GRs bind directly to the AP-1 complex and thereby prevent its interaction with the target gene. In human lung, for example, cytokines such as TNF-α

and phorbol esters, which activate PKC, lead to activation of AP-1 and NF-κB binding to DNA; this effect may be blocked by corticosteroids. cAMP may exert a profound modulatory effect on MAPK signaling pathways and may activate the transcription factor CREB (cAMP response element binding), which itself interacts with GRs and with AP-1 (75).

A good example of receptor interaction is provided by the interaction of β_2 receptors and GRs, which is relevant to the treatment of asthma and COPD, as combination inhalers containing a long-acting β_2-agonist and a corticosteroid are now commonly used as first-line therapy. Corticosteroids increase the expression of β_2 receptors in lungs and so enhance the effects of β_2-agonists and prevent receptor downregulation (76,77). In turn, β_2-agonists increase the action of GRs by facilitating nuclear translocation for the cytoplasm and increasing the binding of GRs to GRE, thus increasing the effects of corticosteroids.

III. Drug-Receptor Interactions

The binding of a drug to its receptor is a dynamic process and follows the laws of mass action. At equilibrium, there is a balance between the rate of association and the rate of dissociation of a drug. The concentration of drug giving half maximal activation is the EC_{50}, which describes the potency of the drug. The *affinity* of the drug describes the balance between association and dissociation and can be quantified as the dissociation constant, K_d, which is the logarithm of the concentration of drug needed to occupy 50% of the receptors. Drugs with a low K_d therefore have a high affinity for their receptor.

A. Radioligand Binding

Binding between a hormone or drug and its receptor may be studied directly by radioligand binding. A radiolabeled ligand (usually a high-affinity antagonist, such as $[^{125}I]$ iodocyanopindolol for β receptors) is incubated with a receptor preparation (either a membrane preparation from the tissue of interest or, in the case of some ligands, with intact cells). The binding interaction between ligand and receptor obeys the law of mass action. As the concentration of ligand is increased, the proportion of ligand binding to receptors increases until saturation occurs when all the receptors are occupied. Nonspecific binding to nonreceptor sites is determined by parallel incubations with radioligand in the presence of an excess of unlabeled agonist or antagonist (e.g., 200 μM isoproterenol or 1 μM propranolol for β receptors). Specific binding (i.e., total − nonspecific binding) may be analyzed by a Scatchard plot, which will give a straight line if a single class of binding site is involved, the slope of which is related to binding affinity ($1/K_d$), and the intercept on the x-axis gives the maximum number of binding sites (B_{max})—a measure of receptor density. Radioligand binding studies can also be used to investigate selectivity of drugs for the receptor using competition between the competitor drug and a fixed concentration of radioligand. Receptors may be characterized in this way, using the rank order of potency of agonists or antagonists.

Binding studies can also be used to determine the distribution of receptors in tissues, using autoradiography. The radioligand is incubated with frozen sections of the tissue of interest using optimal conditions and using an excess of nonradiolabeled competitor to define nonspecific binding, as in membrane-binding studies. The distribution of specific binding is then used to map tissue localization of receptors.

B. Agonists and Antagonists

After binding to the receptor, the response is activated via second messenger systems described above. Different agonists may elicit variable degrees of response, which is described as *efficacy*. A drug that produces less than a maximal response (E_{max}) is known as a *partial agonist*. In airway smooth muscle, isoproterenol (isoprenaline) is a full agonist and produces a maximal response, whereas albuterol (salbutamol) and salmeterol act as partial agonists, giving less than 50% of the maximal relaxation seen with isoproterenol.

Antagonists have zero efficacy. They block the effects of an agonist by interfering with its binding to the receptor. When antagonists interact with agonists at a common receptor, the antagonism is competitive. This can be demonstrated by a rightward shift in the log concentration-response curve (Fig. 12). For true competitive antagonism (e.g., between a β_2-antagonist and β-agonist in airway smooth muscle), the shift is parallel. The amount of shift observed with each concentration of agonist can be used to calculate the affinity of the antagonist for the particular receptor.

Sometimes a drug interferes with an agonist effect in a noncompetitive manner by inhibiting any of the steps that lead to the typical agonist effect. This results in a nonparallel shift in the agonist dose-response curve and a reduced maximal response (Fig. 12). Studies with overexpressed GPCR or mutated receptors have demonstrated that there may be constitutive activation of the receptor in the absence of any agonist. Drugs that reduce this constitutive activation by binding to the receptor are known as *inverse agonists* (78). It is now clear that many drugs that were assumed to be antagonists of GPCR act as inverse agonists, and this may be explained by stabilization of the inactive state of the receptor (79). There may be constitutive overactivity of GPCR in disease, and this could account for phenomena such as bronchoconstriction after

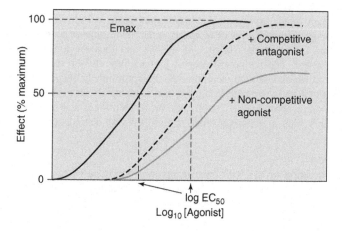

Figure 12 Dose-response curve to an agonist is affected by the presence of antagonists. A competitive antagonist causes a parallel rightward shift in the dose-response curve, with an increase in the concentration of drug that yields half-maximal activation (EC_{50}) but no change in the maximal response (E_{max}), whereas a noncompetitive antagonist shifts the dose response to the right in a nonparallel fashion and also decreases E_{max}.

β-adrenergic blockers in asthma but not in normal individuals as a result of the inverse agonism of certain β-blockers (78).

Another type of antagonism, which is relevant to lung diseases is *functional antagonism*, which describes an interaction between two agents that have opposite functional effects on the same cellular response. Thus, β-agonists act as functional antagonists in airway smooth muscle since they counteract the contractile effects of any spasmogen, including histamine, leukotriene D_4, thromboxane, bradykinin, and acetylcholine.

Two drugs may interact to produce effects that are more than additive. If two drugs given together produce an effect that is greater than the additive effect of the drugs given separately, this is known as *synergy*. *Potentiation* is when one drug given alone has no effect, but increases the response to a second drug. *Tolerance* refers to a diminishing response to a drug that is administered repeatedly, whereas *tachyphylaxis* usually describes tolerance of rapid onset, so that it may be seen after only one administration of the drug. *Desensitization* is a term that includes rapid and long-term loss of response.

The interaction between a ligand and its receptor has several characteristics. Binding is rapid reversible and is temperature dependent. There is stereoselectivity with the *levo*-isomer (*R*-isomer) usually binding more effectively than the *dextro*-isomer (*S*-isomer). Many ligands are a mixture of the active *R*-isomer with the inactive *S*-isomer, so that the racemic mixture has half of the activity. It is claimed that for some racemates the inactive isomer is actually detrimental. For example, *S*-albuterol (levalbuterol) has been reported to increase airway hyperactivity in animal models so that the *R*-albuterol is more effective than *RS*-albuterol (80). However, no clear advantage of *R*-albuterol over *RS*-albuterol has been demonstrated in clinical studies (81).

IV. Receptor Regulation

Receptors are subject to many regulatory factors that may operate at several sites (Fig. 13). Some factors influence the gene transcription of receptors, either increasing or decreasing transcription. Other factors influence the stability of mRNA and thus the amount of receptor protein that is formed. Translation of receptor protein may also be regulated. Once the receptor protein is inserted into the membrane, the receptor may be regulated by phosphorylation as a result of various receptor kinases, and receptor phosphorylation is one of the major means of receptor regulation (82). Some receptors are also tyrosine nitrated or ubiquitinated, resulting in abnormal function and increased degradation.

A. Desensitization

Tachyphylaxis or desensitization occurs with most receptors when exposed to an agonist. This phenomenon has been studied in some detail with β_2 receptors and involves several distinct processes that may operate simultaneously or sequentially (83).

G Protein Receptor Kinases

In the short term, desensitization involves *phosphorylation*, which uncouples the GPCR from G_s, via the action of enzymes called GRK, of which seven are now identified (84). This has been studied in most detail for β receptors that are phosphorylated by GRK2, also known as β-adrenergic receptor-specific kinase (βARK). The site of this

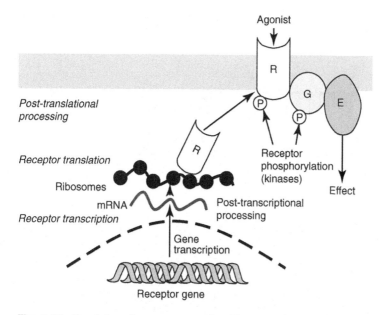

Figure 13 Regulation of receptor expression. The expression and function of surface receptors may be regulated in several ways, including effects on receptor synthesis (gene transcription, posttranscriptional processing/mRNA stability, protein translation and posttranslational processing). Once the receptor is inserted in the membrane it may be inactivated and uncoupled by phosphorylation via various kinases. *Abbreviations*: R, receptor; G, G protein; E, effect; P, phosphorylation.

phosphorylation appears to be on the Ser/Thr-rich region of the third intracellular loop and the C-terminal tail, since their replacement reduces the rate of desensitization. GRK2 is also involved in the phosphorylation of several other receptors, including muscarinic and tachykinin receptors. The expression of GRK2 varies between cells. There is low expression of GRK2 in airway smooth muscle cells that show resistance to desensitization, whereas expression of this enzyme is high in mast cells that are much more easily desensitized (85). GRK2 expression is increased in lungs after exposure to β_2-agonists, thus contributing to uncoupling of β_2 receptors (86) and is increased by corticosteroids, which therefore reverse uncoupling and restore responsiveness to β_2-agonists (87). GPCR are also regulated by other kinases, including PKA and PKC (82). For β_2 receptors, this appears to be via phosphorylation of GRK2, enhancing its ability to uncouple receptors rather than direct phosphorylation of β_2 receptors.

Arrestins
Another protein, β-arrestin, is also involved in uncoupling the phosphorylated β receptor from the G protein and in resensitization of receptors (Fig. 14). There are two β-arrestins and they appear to be universally expressed and involved in the coupling of many GPCRs. β-Arrestins determine whether β_2 receptors are degraded within the cell by

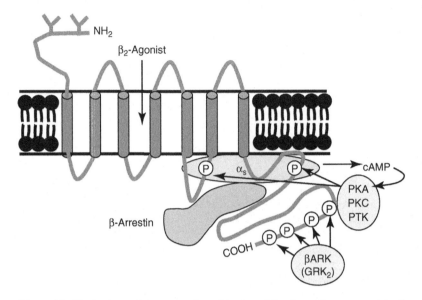

Figure 14 Mechanisms of short-term desensitization of β_2-adrenergic receptors. The β receptor is phosphorylated by βARK and other GRK on its C tail (COOH), resulting in increases in binding of β-arrestin, which leads to uncoupling of the receptor from the α-subunit of the stimulatory G protein (α_s) and internalization of the receptor. PKA, activated by an increase in cAMP phosphorylates the receptor at other sites on the third intracellular loop or may phosphorylate GRK. PKC and PTK may also phosphorylate the receptor, resulting in uncoupling. *Abbreviations*: βARK, beta-adrenergic receptor kinase; GRK, G protein receptor kinases; PKA, protein kinase A; cAMP, cyclic $3',5'$ adenosine monophosphate; PKC, protein kinase C; PTK, protein tyrosine kinases.

endocytosis or are recycled to the cell membrane (88) (Fig. 15). β-Arrestins terminate receptor function and also allow receptors to interact with signal transduction pathways [such as MAPK and PI3K (phosphoinositide-3-kinase)] independently and therefore allow the receptor to regulate different responses in the cell. Ligands that preferentially stimulate the interaction between receptor and β-arrestins have now been identified, and these drugs may have a different spectrum of activity to the classical drugs that activate receptor–G protein coupling. Ligands that are biased toward receptor–G protein interaction with less effect on β-arrestins do not desensitize the receptor and thus have greater and more prolonged effects.

Downregulation
Longer-term mechanisms of desensitization include downregulation of surface receptor number, a process that involves internalization (*sequestration*) of the receptor and its subsequent degradation. Downregulation of β_2 receptors results in a rapid decline in the steady-state level of β_2-receptor mRNA. This suggests that downregulation is achieved in part, either by inhibiting the gene transcription of receptors or by increased posttranscriptional processing of the mRNA in the cell. Using actinomycin D to inhibit

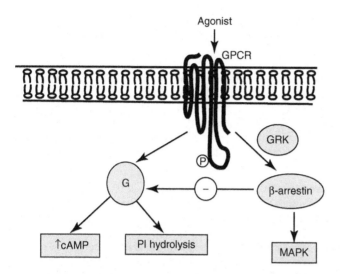

Figure 15 G protein–coupled receptors signal through G proteins and also via β-arrestins. When the receptor is occupied by its agonist, signal transduction pathways are activated, such as changes in cAMP or increased PI hydrolysis. Agonists also O-phosphorylate the receptor via GRK, which recruit β-arrestin that then stimulates other signaling pathways, such as MAPK, and also inhibits G protein–mediated signal transduction. *Abbreviations*: cAMP, cyclic $3',5'$ adenosine monophosphate; PI, phosphoinositide; GRK, G protein receptor kinases; MAPK, mitogen-activated protein kinases.

transcription, it has been found that β_2-receptor mRNA stability is markedly reduced in these cells after exposure to β-agonists (89). Furthermore, by isolating nuclei and performing a nuclear run-on transcription assay, it is apparent that β-agonist exposure does not directly alter receptor gene transcription. Longer-term exposure to β agonists may also result in inhibition of β-receptor gene transcription, mediated via the effects of a cAMP-specific transcription factor (CREB). Long-term exposure to β-agonists results in reduced transcription of β_2 receptors in the airways (90,91).

B. Corticosteroid Modulation

Certain G protein–linked receptors are also influenced by corticosteroids. Thus, pulmonary β receptors are increased in density by pretreatment with corticosteroids (92). Corticosteroids increase the steady-state level of β_2-receptor mRNA in cultured smooth muscle cells, thus indicating that steroids may increase β-receptor density by increasing the rate of gene transcription. The increase in mRNA occurs rapidly (within 1 hour), preceding the increase in β receptors, and then declines to a steady-state level about twice the normal. The cloned β-receptor gene contains three potential GRE, and incubation of human lung with corticosteroids results in a doubling of the rate of transcription (92). By contrast, corticosteroids decrease transcription of tachykinin NK_2 receptors (93).

C. Receptor Ontogeny

Another area in which molecular biology of receptors may be relevant is in studying the development of receptors and the factors that determine expression of particular receptor genes during development. In fetal lung, there is a marked increase in the expression of β_2 receptors in the perinatal period and this is critically dependent on glucocorticoids (94). There may be differential expression of receptor subtypes during development. For example, muscarinic receptor subtypes in the lung show differential changes around the perinatal period (95). Receptors also play an important role in lung development. For example, receptors for hepatocyte growth factor are expressed in airway epithelium during lung development and appear to mediate branching of the airways (96).

D. Pulmonary Disease

There are several pulmonary diseases in which altered expression of receptors may be relevant to understanding their pathophysiology. Molecular biology offers a new perspective in investigating these abnormalities of receptor expression by providing insights into whether the abnormality arises through altered transcription of the receptor gene or due to abnormalities in posttranscriptional or posttranslational processing. There is some evidence that β-adrenoceptor function may be impaired in airway smooth muscle of patients with fatal asthma (97). However, binding and autoradiographic studies have not demonstrated any reduction in β receptors in airway smooth muscle, suggesting that the reduced bronchodilator responses to β-agonists may be due to uncoupling of the receptor (98). Similarly no differences in muscarinic receptors have been detected in asthmatic lungs using binding approaches (98).

Relatively few studies have explored whether there are any differences in the expression of mediator receptors in asthmatic airways. There is some evidence for increased expression of platelet-activating factor (PAF) receptor mRNA in lungs of asthmatic patients, although whether this has functional significance is not known (99). Bradykinin B_1 and B_2 receptors are upregulated by inflammatory stimuli such as TNF-α, and this effect appears to be due to prolongation of mRNA half-life (100). There is also evidence for increased NK_1 receptor expression in the lungs of patients with asthma and COPD (101,102).

E. Transcriptional Control

Receptor genes, like any other genes, may be regulated by transcription factors, which may be activated within the cell under certain conditions, leading to increased or decreased receptor gene transcription, which may in turn alter the expression of receptors at the cell surface. Little is known about the transcription factors that regulate receptors, but these may be relevant to diseases, such as chronic inflammation. The transcription factor AP-1, a Fos-Jun heterodimer, may be activated via PKC. AP-1 increased transcription of several genes, including some receptor genes. For example, the gene coding for the NK_1 receptor has an AP-1 site, which leads to increased gene transcription and a GRE that conversely results in decreased transcription (103). Chronic cell stimulation, via activation of PKC, may therefore lead to an increase in NK_1 receptor gene expression, which could lead to increased neurogenic inflammation. An increased NK_1 receptor gene expression is present in asthmatic airways (101). By contrast, corticosteroids reduce NK_1-specific mRNA in human lung, probably via an inhibitory effect of GR on AP-1.

V. Ion Channels

Movement of ions across the cell membrane is important in determining the state of cell activation. Ions cross the cell membrane through protein-lined pores called channels, several of which have now been cloned and characterized electrophysiologically. Most channels are made up of distinct subunits that are grouped together in the cell membrane (for example, nAChR as discussed above). Whether the channel is open or closed depends on different factors for each channel, but may be determined by receptor activation, the polarization of the cell membrane, or the presence of particular ligands that interact directly with the channel.

A. Calcium Channels

Voltage-Gated Channels

Several types of Ca^{2+} channel have now been identified and characterized electrophysiologically by molecular cloning and by the use of antagonists and toxins. Voltage-gated channels mediate Ca^{2+} entry into cells in response to membrane depolarization. Electrophysiological studies reveal different Ca^{2+} currents designated L-, N-, P-, Q-, R-, and T-type. High-voltage-activated Ca^{2+} channels that have been characterized biochemically are complexes of a pore-forming $\alpha1$-subunit of approximately 190 to 250 kDa, a transmembrane, disulfide-linked complex of $\alpha2$-and δ-subunits, an intracellular β-subunit and in some cases a transmembrane γ-subunit. Ten $\alpha1$-subunits, four $\alpha2\delta$ complexes, four β-subunits, and two γ-subunits are now identified (104). The Cav1 family of $\alpha1$-subunits conduct L-type Ca^{2+} currents, which initiate muscle contraction, endocrine secretion, and gene transcription, and are regulated by protein phosphorylation. The Cav2 family of $\alpha1$-subunits conducts N-type, P/Q-type, and R-type Ca^{2+} currents, which initiate rapid synaptic transmission and are regulated primarily by direct interaction with G proteins and SNARE proteins and secondarily by protein phosphorylation. The Cav3 family of $\alpha1$-subunits conducts T-type Ca^{2+} currents, which are activated and inactivated more rapidly and at more negative membrane potentials than other Ca^{2+} current types.

L-type channels (for long lasting) open in response to depolarization of the cell, resulting in influx of Ca^{2+} to increase intracellular Ca^{2+} concentration (Fig. 16); these channels are blocked by dihydropyridines, such as nifedipine, and by verapamil. Voltage-sensitive calcium channels are important in contractile responses of pulmonary vascular smooth muscle, but are less important in the contractile response of airway smooth muscle or in the activation of inflammatory cells. T-type calcium channels are also opened by depolarization but are insensitive to dihydropyridines. Electrophysiological studies have revealed the presence of both L- and T-channels in airway smooth muscle, although the L-channels are less sensitive to dihydropyridines than the L-channels in the myocardium (105). N-type channels, which are largely restricted to neurons, are also sensitive to depolarization and insensitive to dihydropyridines, but are blocked by ω-conotoxin.

Receptor-Operated Channels

Receptor-operated channels (ROCs) are channels that open in response to activation of certain receptors; these receptors are not well defined, but recently blockers have been developed. Contraction of airway smooth muscle in response to agonists such as acetylcholine and histamine is independent of external Ca^{2+} and is not associated with ^{45}Ca uptake, suggesting that calcium entry is not important for initiation of contractile

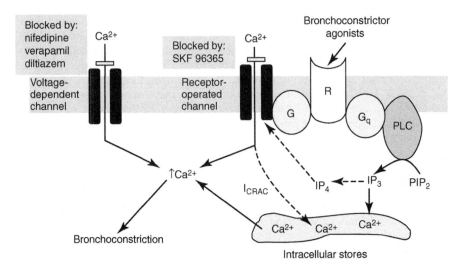

Figure 16   Calcium ion (Ca^{2+}) channels. There are at least two classes of calcium channel in the cell membrane. One is activated by depolarization (voltage-dependent channels) and the other via receptors (ROC). Ca^{2+} are also released from intracellular stores via phosphoinositide hydrolysis and the action of IP_3. Intracellular stores are refilled by calcium release-activated calcium current (I_{CRAC}). IP_4 generated from IP_3 may activate calcium entry via receptor-operated channels. *Abbreviations*: IP_3, inositol (1,4,5) trisphosphate; IP_4, inositol (1,3,4,5) tetrakis phosphate; G, G protein; PLC, phospholipase C; PIP_2, phosphoinositide 4,5,-bisphosphate.

responses. Entry of Ca^{2+} via ROCs may be important in refilling intracellular stores. ROCs are members of an increasing group of calcium channels called transient receptor potential (TRP) cation channels, which is a superfamily of at least over 30 channel proteins divided into six main groups. TRP channels are involved in regulation of inflammatory cells, structural cells, and sensory nerves and may be important novel targets for drug discovery (106). For example, transient receptor potential vanilloid (TRPV) channels on sensory nerves mediate to response to capsaicin and acids. TRPC3 and TRPC6 are expressed in human airway smooth muscle and may correspond to ROCs involved in Ca^{2+} entry (107).

A rise in intracellular Ca^{2+} concentration is associated with cell activation, but recovery depends on removal of Ca^{2+} by sequestration or by pumping out of the cell in exchange for Na^+. In airway smooth muscle, there is a pump that exchanges $3Na^+$ for each Ca^{2+} that is linked to the activity of $Na^+–K^+$ ATPase, which maintains the inwardly directed Na^+ gradient by exchanging intracellular Na^+ for extracellular K^+. In airway smooth muscle, there is also an active uptake of Ca^{2+} into intracellular stores, which may be stimulated by cAMP (32).

I_{CRAC}

When Ca^{2+} are released from intracellular stores via the action of IP_3, these stores are refilled by calcium entry via specific channels called CRAC, measured as a current called I_{CRAC} (Ca^{2+} release-activated Ca^{2+} current) that is activated by depletion of intercellular stores (store-operated calcium entry) (108). This is an important mechanism in inflammatory cells, such as mast cells and T lymphocytes. Inhibitors of I_{CRAC} are therefore potential immunomodulators or anti-allergy drugs. TRPC1 is thought to function as a component of store-operated calcium channels (109).

In airway smooth muscle, several types of calcium channel have been identified and these may lead to contraction via different spasmogens. L-channels respond to depolarization and ROCs are activated by various spasmogens, but contraction initially is independent of Ca^{2+} entry and due to release of Ca^{2+} from internal stores in response to IP_3. These internal stores are then refilled via store-operated calcium channels. In addition, cyclic ADP-ribose also mobilizes calcium from the sarcoplasmic reticulum by acting on ryanodine receptors (32).

B. Potassium Channels

Recovery of cells after depolarization depends on the movement of potassium ions (K^+) out of the cell via K^+ channels in the cell membrane. This results in hyperpolarization of the cell with relaxation of smooth muscle and inhibition of cell activity. Conversely, blockade of K^+ channels with drugs such as tetraethylammonium and 4-aminopyridine results in increased excitability or hyperresponsiveness of cells. Over 50 different K^+ channel genes have been identified in humans, using selective toxins, patch-clamping techniques, and cloning (110). K^+ channels may be subdivided into four main classes:

1. *Voltage-gated channels* that open on depolarization of the membrane, which are rectifying channels that return the cell membrane to its previous polarized state. This is a diverse group of channels, some of which are blocked by α-dendrotoxin.
2. Ca^{2+}*-activated channels* open in response to elevation of intracellular Ca^{2+} concentration. Large-conductance (maxi-K or big) K^+ channels are found in smooth muscle and neurons and are blocked by the scorpion venoms charybdotoxin and iberiotoxin, as well as several small molecules (111). Small conductance channels, some of which are blocked by apamin are found in neurons.
3. *Receptor-coupled channels* are opened by certain receptors via a G protein, but no specific blockers have been found.
4. *ATP-sensitive channels* are opened by a fall in intracellular ATP concentration. These channels are found in smooth muscle and in the islet cells of the pancreas. They are blocked by sulfonylureas, such as glibenclamide, and are opened by drugs such as cromakalim (BRL 34915), its active enantiomer lemakalim (BRL 38227), RP 53891, and HOE 245.

K^+ channels play an important role in relaxation of airway smooth muscle (112,113). β-Agonist-induced bronchodilatation is markedly inhibited by charybdotoxin (114), indicating that opening a maxi-K channel is involved in the relaxant response. K^+ channel openers, such as cromakalim and levcromakalim, act on ATP-sensitive K^+ channels and are dilators of animal and human airways (115). K^+ channel openers therefore have potential as bronchodilators and vasodilators, although when given orally they may cause cardiovascular side effects due to systemic vasodilatation, which limit their usefulness in asthma therapy. K^+ channels are also involved in neurotransmitter release (112). Cromakalim inhibits cholinergic neurotransmission and the release of neuropeptides from sensory nerves in airways (116). Modulation of neurotransmission is also mediated by opening of maxi-K channels, since charybdotoxin reverses the modulatory effect of many agonists on sensory and cholinergic nerves (117). K^+ channels are also involved in mucus secretion (118). K^+ channel openers therefore have several potential applications in the therapy of airway disease (119).

C. Sodium Channels

Na^+ channels are involved in depolarization and release of neurotransmitters. Drugs that block Na^+ channels, such as tetrodotoxin and local anesthetics, act as nerve blockers. However, tetrodotoxin has no direct effect on smooth muscle. Na+ channels in airway epithelium (ENaC) play an important role in regulating mucus hydration and mucociliary clearance and play a key role in alveolar fluid absorption. ENaC dysfunction is important in acute respiratory disease syndrome and in cystic fibrosis (120,121). Each channel is comprised of three subunits designated α, β, and γ and several new drugs that target these channels are in development of the treatment of lung disease.

D. Chloride Channels

Although less well characterized than other ion channels, it is increasingly recognized that chloride (Cl^-) channels play an important role in pulmonary physiology and pathology. The cystic fibrosis transmembrane regular (CFTR) that is functionally abnormal in cystic fibrosis plays a critical role in airway hydration and has been extensively investigated. Calcium-activated Cl^- channels (CLCA) play an important role in mucus secretion and are now targeted to treat mucus hypersecretion (122). Volume and voltage-dependent Cl^- channels appear to play a role in airway responses to indirect bronchoconstrictors and are blocked by furosemide and cromolyn (cromoglycate) sodium (123).

VI. Enzymes

Many drugs produce their therapeutic effect by inhibition of particular enzymes. Most commonly the drug molecule is a substrate analog that acts as a *competitive inhibitor*. The interaction between drug and enzyme obeys the law of mass action and may be analyzed in the same way as drug-receptor interactions. An example is L-N^G-nitro arginine, which acts as a competitive inhibitor of NO synthase by substituting for the natural substrate L-arginine. The enzyme blockade may be overcome by increasing the concentration of L-arginine, whereas D-arginine, which is not a substrate for this enzyme, has no effect. Many drugs act noncompetitively. An example is aspirin, which noncompetitively blocks cyclooxygenase by acetylating the active catalytic site of the enzyme. Another type of interaction involves a false substrate, where the drug undergoes chemical transformation by the enzyme to form a product that subverts the normal metabolic pathway. The best example of this is α-methyldopa, which mimics DOPA, causing norepinephrine to be replaced by methylnorepinephrine, which is inactive.

Enzymes are increasingly recognized as playing an important part in the pathophysiology of various diseases and are increasingly a target for drug therapy. Drugs that inhibit 5'-lipoxygenase, which generates leukotrienes, such as zileuton, are now used in the treatment of asthma. Drugs that inhibit neutrophil elastase may be useful in the future management of cystic fibrosis and COPD, whereas drugs that inhibit tryptase and chymase from mast cells may be potential treatments in asthma.

A. Protein Kinases

Signal transduction within cells is regulated by *kinases*, which phosphorylate substrate molecules that are often themselves kinases, so that there is a cascade of phosphorylation. Over 700 kinases are now recognized in the human genome. Kinase cascades link the activation of surface receptors to functional responses, including secretion, differentiation, and gene expression. For example, multiple kinases are activated when cells are exposed to the proinflammatory cytokines IL-1β and TNF-α (124,125). MAPK and PI3K cascades are of particular importance in inflammatory responses, as well as cell proliferation and survival, as discussed above. Many novel kinase inhibitors are now in development and are predicted to be the major development in drug therapy in the future (126).

MAP Kinases

Over 10 MAPK have been identified and these kinase cascades include a MAPK kinase (MAPKK or MEK) and a MAPKK/MEK kinase (MAPKKK/MEKK) (Fig. 17). These signaling pathways serve as a means of connecting cell-surface receptors to specific transcription factors and other regulatory proteins, thus allowing extracellular signals to

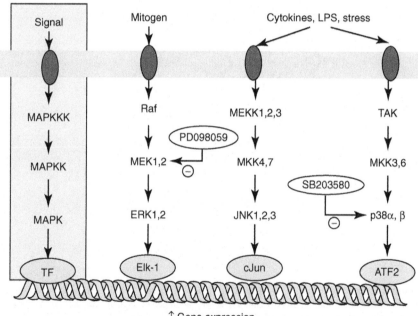

↑ Gene expression

Figure 17 MAPK pathways. Extracellular signals activate MAP kinase kinase kinase (MAPKKK), MAP kinase kinase (MAPKK), MAP kinase (MAPK), and then TF. Three major cascades are now recognized. *Abbreviations*: MAPK, mitogen-activated protein kinase; MAP, mitogen-activated protein; TF, transcription factors; LPS, lipopolysaccharide, MEK, MAP/ERK kinase; ERK, extracellular signal-regulated kinase; JNK, Jun N-terminal kinase; TAK, transforming growth factor-β-activating kinase; ATF, activating transcription factor.

regulate the expression of specific genes. There is now increasing recognition that there are interactions between the MAPK pathways resulting in different cellular responses to the same activating stimuli. MAPK may be activated by several types of stress and other extracellular stimuli. Selective inhibitors, such as SB203580, which block the p38α pathway, and PD098059, which blocks the extracellular signal–regulated kinase (ERK) pathway, have now been developed; this has resulted in a better understanding of these complex signaling pathways. p38α MAPK inhibitors are now in clinical development for the treatment of inflammatory diseases, such as COPD and asthma, but may have to be delivered by inhalation as there is a high risk of systemic side effects (53,125).

Phosphoinositide 3-Kinases

PIP_2 is converted to PI(1,4,5)trisphosphate (PIP_3) by the enzyme PI3K, which results in phosphorylation of the downstream kinases Akt (protein kinase B) and mammalian target of rapamycin (mTOR) (Fig. 18). This signal transduction pathway is of critical importance in the regulation of cell proliferation and inhibition of apoptosis, as well as many other cellular functions such as metabolism, chemotaxis, and cytokine secretion.

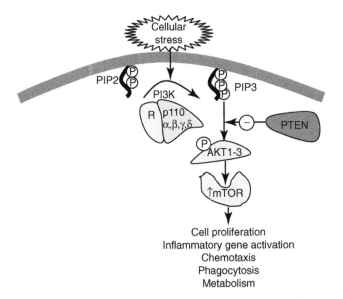

Figure 18 PI3K converts PIP_2 to PIP_3 in response to various cellular stresses, including oxidative stress and inflammatory mediators, acting on receptor tyrosine kinases or G protein–coupled receptors. PI3K consists of a regulatory subunit (R, p85 or p101) and a catalytic domain (p110) of the α, β, γ, or δ subtype. Activated PI3K then phosphorylates Akt1-3 (protein kinase B), which then phosphorylates mTOR. Further, kinase cascades lead to a variety of cellular responses, including proliferation, activation of inflammatory genes, chemotaxis, phagocytosis, and metabolic functions. The activation of PI3K is inhibited by PTEN (phosphatase and tensin homolog deleted on chromosome 10). *Abbreviations*: PI3K, phosphoinositide-3-kinase; PIP_2, phosphoinositide (4,5) diphosphate; PIP_3, phosphoinositide (3,4,5) triphosphate; mTOR, mammalian target of rapamycin.

Several isoforms of PI3-kinase are now recognized, which are differentially regulated and expressed. For example, PI3K-γ is expressed in monocytes and granulocytes and play as key role in chemotactic responses and inflammatory cytokine release, whereas PI3K-δ is involved in mediating corticosteroid resistance induced by oxidative stress (127). An endogenous inhibitor of the PI3K pathway PTEN (phosphatase and tensin homolog deleted on chromosome 10) is an important feedback mechanism, and this enzyme is often defective and mutated in cancers, including lung cancer (128). PI3K inhibitors, such as wortmannin and LY294002, have proved to be useful in elucidating the role of PI3K-Akt signaling pathways, but isoenzyme-selective inhibitors are now in development for the treatment of inflammatory diseases, such as asthma and COPD.

B. Protein Phosphatases

The effects of kinases are counteracted by phosphatases that dephosphorylate the protein targets of kinase activity. While there are approximately 700 protein kinases, only approximately 200 protein phosphatases have been identified, and these tend to have a broader specificity than kinases. Their regulation is less well understood than that of kinase pathways, and there are few useful inhibitors. Approximately 100 protein tyrosine phosphatases have been identified and several of these inhibit inositol phosphates. Several MAPK phosphatases have now been identified; the best characterized is MAPK phosphate-1 (MKP-1), which is also known as dual-specificity kinase-1 as it dephosphorylates both threonine and tyrosine residues (54). MKP-1 inhibits p38, JNK, and ERK-MAPK pathways and its gene is rapidly induced by corticosteroids, contributing to their anti-inflammatory effects (129). As discussed above, PTEN appears to be the major phosphatase regulating the PI3K pathways, whereas *Src* homology 2 domain–containing tyrosine phosphatases-1 and -2 (SHP-1, SHP-2) regulate multiple inflammatory growth factor and metabolic pathways, including PI3K signaling.

VII. Pharmacokinetics

To achieve the intended pharmacological response, it is necessary to achieve an effective concentration of a drug at its site of action in the lung. Several steps are involved in determining the concentration of a drug at its site of action; these include *absorption, distribution* to various tissues, *metabolism,* and finally *excretion.* The crucial properties of drugs are often summarized as an ADMET (absorption, distribution, metabolism, excretion, and toxicity) profile.

A. Absorption

Absorption of drugs involves their passage across a cell membrane. For some drugs this may involve specially mediated transport systems or movement through specific channels, but for most drugs this involves simple diffusion down a concentration gradient. The rate of transport depends on the lipid solubility of the drug. Most drugs exist in solution as weak acids or weak bases, and there is, therefore, an equilibrium between the ionized form, which does not readily penetrate lipid membranes, and the nonionized fraction, which is lipophilic and may cross the cell membrane. The equilibrium between ionized and nonionized forms is determined by the *pKa* of the drug, which is defined as the pH at which 50% of the drug is in the ionized state. As an example, cromolyn sodium is a weak acid with a pKa of 2. At physiological pH, it exists almost entirely in an ionized state and is therefore not absorbed from the gastrointestinal tract, which is why it must be delivered directly to the lungs.

Lipid solubility is also important in determining whether absorbed drugs may cross the blood-brain barrier and exert central effects. Highly lipophilic compounds such as ethanol and nicotine readily cross the blood-brain barrier. Atropine also crosses the blood-brain barrier that results in central nervous system side effects such as hallucinations, but its quaternary derivatives ipratropium bromide and tiotropium bromide are ionized and have low lipid solubility so that they are not able to cross the blood-brain barrier and so central side effects, such as hallucinations, which limit the use of atropine, are not seen. Similarly, the nonsedative antihistamine cetirizine differs from its parent drug hydroxazine by the presence of a C group that makes the drug less lipophilic so that central side effects such as sedation are avoided.

B. Distribution

The concentration of a drug that is obtained at the site of action is determined by the volume of distribution of the drug, its clearance, and the half-life of the drug. The volume of distribution (V_d) describes the body space available to contain the drug. Thus, for parenteral drugs, which are extensively bound to plasma proteins, the volume of distribution will be largely confined to the vascular space, whereas for drugs that are lipid soluble, the volume of distribution (V_d) will be much greater as the drug is taken up into adipose tissues throughout the body. The concentration of a drug in the blood (C) is determined by the equation:

$$C = \frac{\text{Drug dose}}{V_d}$$

For example, the V_d for theophylline is approximately 35 L in a 70-kg person. An approximate loading dose required to give a plasma concentration of 15 mg/L would therefore be $C \times V_d$ or 15 mg/L $\times$ 35 L = 525 mg. If V_d is reduced by disease such as cardiac or renal failure, then a correspondingly lower dose is necessary to give the same plasma concentration and to avoid toxic doses.

C. Clearance

The clearance of a drug describes its elimination from biological fluids; the half-life ($t_{1/2}$) is the time required to eliminate 50% of a drug from the body, after absorption and distribution are complete. Although clearance and half-life may readily be established for systemically administered drugs, little is known about the clearance of inhaled drugs since the local concentrations in the lungs are not known.

Systemically administered drugs are biotransformed to an inactive state that usually involves oxidation, reduction, or hydrolysis, converting the drug to more polar forms that may be more readily excreted by the kidney. Biotransformation usually takes place in the liver, but for inhaled drugs, biotransformation may also take place in the lungs. Hepatic metabolism of drugs may be increased if metabolizing enzymes are induced by drugs such as phenobarbitone and rifampicin, which increase the activity of cytochrome P450 (CYP)-related oxidative enzymes. This results in more rapid elimination of theophylline and will require an increased dose of theophylline to maintain therapeutic levels. Decreased clearance of theophylline is seen with certain drugs, including erythromycin, certain quinolone antibiotics (ciprofloxacin but not ofloxacin), allopurinol, cimetidine (but not ranitidine), serotonin uptake inhibitors (fluvoxamine), and the 5-lipoxygenase inhibitor zileuton, which interfere with P450 (especially CYP 1A2) function (130).

VIII. Routes of Drug Delivery

Drugs may be delivered to the lungs not only by oral or parenteral routes, but also by inhalation. The choice depends on the drug and on the respiratory disease.

A. Inhaled Route

Inhalation is the preferred mode of delivery of many drugs with a direct effect on airways, particularly for asthma and COPD (131). It is the only way to deliver some drugs such as cromolyn sodium and anticholinergics and is the preferred route of delivery for β_2-agonists and corticosteroids. Antibiotics may also be delivered by inhalation in patients with chronic respiratory sepsis (e.g., in cystic fibrosis). The major advantage of inhalation is the delivery of drug to the airways in doses that are effective with a much lower risk of side effects. This is particularly important with the use of inhaled corticosteroids that largely avoid systemic side effects. In addition, drugs such as bronchodilators have a more rapid onset of action than when taken orally so that more rapid control of symptoms is achieved.

Particle Size

The size of particles for inhalation is of critical importance in determining the site of deposition in the respiratory tract. The optimum size for particles to settle in the airways is 2 to 5 μm mass median aerodynamic diameter (MMAD). Larger particles settle out in the upper airways, whereas smaller particles (<1 μm) remain suspended and are therefore exhaled. There is increasing interest in delivering drugs to small airways, particularly in COPD and severe asthma (132). This involves delivering drug particles of approximately 1- to 2-μm MMAD, which is now possible using drugs formulated in hydroxyfluoroalkane (HFA) propellant (133).

Pharmacokinetics

Of the total drug delivered, only 5% to 20% enters the lower airways with a pressurized metered-dose inhaler (pMDI). The fate of the inhaled drug is poorly understood. Drugs are absorbed from the airway lumen and have direct effects on target cells of the airway. Drugs may also be absorbed into the bronchial circulation and distributed to more peripheral airways. Whether drugs are metabolized in the airways is often uncertain and there is little understanding of the factors that may influence local absorption and metabolism of inhaled drugs. Drugs with higher molecular weights tend to be retained more in the airways. Nevertheless, it is known that several drugs have great therapeutic efficacy when given by the inhaled route. The novel inhaled corticosteroid ciclesonide is an inactive prodrug that is activated by esterases in the respiratory tract to the active principle des-ciclesonide (134). More peripheral distribution of a drug with smaller MMAD also increases alveolar deposition and is thus likely to increase absorption from the lungs into the general circulation resulting in more systemic side effects. Thus, although HFA pMDIs deliver more inhaled corticosteroid to smaller airways, there is also increased systemic absorption.

Delivery Devices

Several ways of delivering inhaled drugs are possible (135). These are described in the following sections.

Metered Dose Inhalers

Drugs are propelled from a canister previously with a chlorofluorocarbon (freon) propellant but now replaced by HFA, which is an "ozone friendly" propellant (136). These devices are convenient, portable, and deliver 100 to 400 doses of drug. They are usually easy to use, although it is necessary to coordinate inhalation with action of the device, so it is important that patients are taught to use these devices correctly (137).

Spacer Chambers

Large-volume spacer devices between the metered dose inhaler (MDI) and the patient reduce the velocity of particles entering the upper airways and the size of the particles by allowing evaporation of liquid propellant. This reduces the amount of drug that impinges on the oropharynx and increases the proportion of drug entering the lower airways. The need for careful coordination between activation and inhalation is also avoided since the pMDI can be activated into the chamber and the aerosol subsequently inhaled from the one-way valve. Perhaps the most useful application of spacer chambers is in the reduction of the oropharyngeal deposition of inhaled corticosteroids and thus the local side effects of these drugs. Large volume spacers also reduce the systemic side effects of drugs as less drug is deposited in the oropharynx and therefore swallowed, since it is the swallowed fraction of the drug that is absorbed from the gastrointestinal tract that makes the greatest contribution to the systemic fraction. This is of particular importance in the use of certain inhaled steroids, such as beclomethasone dipropionate, which can be absorbed from the gastrointestinal tract. Spacer devices are also useful in delivering inhaled drugs to small children who are not able to use a pMDI. Children as young as three years are able to use a spacer device fitted with a face mask.

Dry Powder Inhalers

Drugs may also be delivered as a dry powder using devices that scatter a fine powder dispersed by air turbulence on inhalation. These devices may be preferred by some patients, since careful coordination is not as necessary as with the MDI, but some patients find the dry powder to be irritant. Several multiple dose dry powder inhalers (DPIs) are now available, which are more convenient (138). Some devices deliver doses of pure drug and therefore avoid the problems of additives, such as surfactants, which are necessary in pMDIs and which may provoke throat irritation, coughing, and even a fall in lung function in sensitive asthmatic patients. DPIs are also easier to use in children. DPIs have been developed to deliver peptides and proteins, such as insulin, systemically.

Nebulizers

Two types of nebulizer are available. Jet nebulizers are driven by a stream of gas (air or oxygen), whereas ultrasonic nebulizers utilize a rapidly vibrating piezoelectric crystal and thus do not require a source of compressed gas. The nebulized drug may be inspired during tidal breathing and it is possible to deliver much higher doses of drug. Nebulizers are therefore useful in treating acute exacerbations of asthma and COPD, for delivering drugs when airway obstruction is extreme (e.g., in severe COPD), for delivering inhaled drugs to infants and small children who cannot use the other inhalation devices, and for delivering drugs such as antibiotics when relatively high doses must be delivered. Small hand-held nebulizers are now in development.

B. Oral Route

Drugs for treatment of pulmonary diseases may also be given orally. The oral dose is much higher than the inhaled dose required to achieve the same effect (by a ratio of more than 20:1), so that systemic side effects are far more common. When there is a choice of inhaled or oral route for a drug (e.g., β-agonist or corticosteroid), the inhaled route is always preferable and the oral route should be reserved for the few patients unable to use inhalers (e.g., small children, patients with physical problems such as severe arthritis of the hand). Theophylline is ineffective by the inhaled route and therefore must be given orally. Corticosteroids may have to be given orally for parenchymal lung diseases (e.g., in interstitial lung diseases and emphysema), although it may be possible in the future to deliver such drugs into alveoli using specially designed inhalation devices with a small particle size.

C. Parenteral Route

The intravenous route should be reserved for delivery of drugs in the severely ill patient who is unable to absorb drugs from the gastrointestinal tract. Side effects are generally frequent due to the high plasma concentrations.

IX. Summary

The pharmacology of the lung concerns the action of drugs on target cells in the lung, the use of drugs to better understand the pathophysiology of lung diseases, and understanding the mechanism of action of current and future drugs used to treat pulmonary diseases. Pulmonary pharmacology is complex as there are many different cell types in the lung and these interact in a complex manner so that drugs may have direct and indirect effects on lung function. Many drugs act by interacting with specific receptors, which may be GPCR, cytokine receptors, enzyme-linked receptors, ion channel receptors, or intracellular receptors. Much more is now understood about how these receptors are regulated and how they produce differential effects. There are also many signal transduction pathways activated by receptors that usually involve activation of a cascade of specific interacting kinases. These kinases may activate transcription factors that then regulate the expression of genes within the nucleus and the molecular basis for gene regulation is now being elucidated, giving insights into how drugs such as corticosteroids and cyclosporin work. The pharmacokinetics of drugs involves absorption, distribution, metabolism, and excretion. Many drugs used to treat airway diseases are given by inhalation, so the pharmacokinetics and distribution of inhaled drugs is important. Many drugs used to treat airway disease interact with the autonomic nervous system, which regulates many aspects of lung function, through cholinergic, adrenergic, and sensory nerves, and the release of neurotransmitter and neuropeptides. Many inflammatory mediators are involved in pulmonary diseases and there are now many selective receptor antagonists and synthesis inhibitors that provide insights into the pathophysiological role of these mediators in disease. These mediators include amines, lipid, peptides, chemokines, cytokines, and growth factors.

References

1. Hermans E. Biochemical and pharmacological control of the multiplicity of coupling at G-protein-coupled receptors. Pharmacol Ther 2003; 99:25–44.
2. Lagerstrom MC, Schioth HB. Structural diversity of G protein-coupled receptors and significance for drug discovery. Nat Rev Drug Discov 2008; 7:339–357.
3. Howard AD, McAllister G, Feighner SD, et al. Orphan G-protein-coupled receptors and natural ligand discovery. Trends Pharmacol Sci 2001; 22:132–140.
4. Laitinen T, Polvi A, Rydman P, et al. Characterization of a common susceptibility locus for asthma-related traits. Science 2004; 304:300–304.
5. Bernier V, Stocco R, Bogusky MJ, et al. Structure-function relationships in the neuropeptide S receptor: molecular consequences of the asthma-associated mutation N107I. J Biol Chem 2006; 281:24704–24712.
6. Huber T, Menon S, Sakmar TP. Structural basis for ligand binding and specificity in adrenergic receptors: implications for GPCR-targeted drug discovery. Biochemistry 2008; 47:11013–11023.
7. Lefkowitz RJ. Seven transmembrane receptors: something old, something new. Acta Physiol (Oxf) 2007; 190:9–19.
8. Fong TM, Cascieri MA, Yu H, et al. Amino-aromatic interaction between histidine 197 of the neurokinin-1 receptor. Nature 1993; 362:350–353.
9. Kawabata A, Kawao N. Physiology and pathophysiology of proteinase-activated receptors (PARs): PARs in the respiratory system: cellular signaling and physiological/pathological roles. J Pharmacol Sci 2005; 97:20–24.
10. Prinster SC, Hague C, Hall RA. Heterodimerization of g protein-coupled receptors: specificity and functional significance. Pharmacol Rev 2005; 57:289–298.
11. Barnes PJ. Receptor heterodimerization: a new level of cross-talk. J Clin Invest 2006; 116:1210–1212.
12. Dalrymple MB, Pfleger KD, Eidne KA. G protein-coupled receptor dimers: functional consequences, disease states and drug targets. Pharmacol Ther 2008; 118:359–371.
13. McGraw DW, Mihlbachler KA, Schwarb MR, et al. Airway smooth muscle prostaglandin-EP1 receptors directly modulate β2-adrenergic receptors within a unique heterodimeric complex. J Clin Invest 2006; 116:1400–1409.
14. Wang J, Norcross M. Dimerization of chemokine receptors in living cells: key to receptor function and novel targets for therapy. Drug Discov Today 2008; 13:625–632.
15. Oldham WM, Hamm HE. Heterotrimeric G protein activation by G-protein-coupled receptors. Nat Rev Mol Cell Biol 2008; 9:60–71.
16. Perez DM, Karnik SS. Multiple signaling states of G-protein-coupled receptors. Pharmacol Rev 2005; 57:147–161.
17. Sah VP, Seasholtz TM, Sagi SA, et al. The role of Rho in G protein-coupled receptor signal transduction. Annu Rev Pharmacol Toxicol 2000; 40:459–489.
18. Schaafsma D, Gosens R, Zaagsma J, et al. Rho kinase inhibitors: a novel therapeutical intervention in asthma? Eur J Pharmacol 2008; 585:398–406.

19. Collins RN. Rab and ARF GTPase regulation of exocytosis. Mol Membr Biol 2003; 20:105–115.
20. Bai TR, Mak JCW, Barnes PJ. A comparison of beta-adrenergic receptors and in vitro relaxant responses to isoproterenol in asthmatic airway smooth muscle. Am J Respir Cell Mol Biol 1992; 6:647–651.
21. Hanoune J, Defer N. Regulation and role of adenylyl cyclase isoforms. Annu Rev Pharmacol Toxicol 2001; 41:145–174.
22. Kume H, Hall IP, Washabau RJ, et al. Adrenergic agonists regulate K_{Ca} channels in airway smooth muscle by cAMP-dependent and -independent mechanisms. J Clin Invest 1994; 93:371–379.
23. Bos JL. Epac proteins: multi-purpose cAMP targets. Trends Biochem Sci 2006; 31:680–686.
24. Staples KJ, Bergmann M, Barnes PJ, et al. Stimulus-specific inhibition of IL-5 by cAMP-elevating agents and IL-10 reveals differential mechanisms of action. Biochem Biophys Res Commun 2000; 273:811–815.
25. Kaur M, Holden NS, Wilson SM, et al. Effect of β2-adrenoceptor agonists and other cAMP-elevating agents on inflammatory gene expression in human airways smooth muscle cells: a role for protein kinase A. Am J Physiol Lung Cell Mol Physiol 2008; 295:L505–L514.
26. Soderling SH, Beavo JA. Regulation of cAMP and cGMP signaling: new phosphodiesterases and new functions. Curr Opin Cell Biol 2000; 12:174–179.
27. Currie GP, Butler CA, Anderson WJ, et al. Phosphodiesterase 4 inhibitors in chronic obstructive pulmonary disease: a new approach to oral treatment. Br J Clin Pharmacol 2008; 65:803–810.
28. Houslay MD. PDE4 cAMP-specific phosphodiesterases. Prog Nucleic Acid Res Mol Biol 2001; 69:249–315.
29. Jin SL, Conti M. Induction of the cyclic nucleotide phosphodiesterase PDE4B is essential for LPS-activated TNF-alpha responses. Proc Natl Acad Sci U S A 2002; 99:7628–7633.
30. Robichaud A, Stamatiou PB, Jin SL, et al. Deletion of phosphodiesterase 4D in mice shortens alpha(2)-adrenoceptor-mediated anesthesia, a behavioral correlate of emesis. J Clin Invest 2002; 110:1045–1052.
31. Rhee SG. Regulation of phosphoinositide-specific phospholipase C. Annu Rev Biochem 2001; 70:281–312.
32. Jude JA, Wylam ME, Walseth TF, et al. Calcium signaling in airway smooth muscle. Proc Am Thorac Soc 2008; 5:15–22.
33. Tsien RW, Tsien RY. Calcium channels, stores, and oscillations. Ann Rev Cell Biol 1990; 6:715–760.
34. Dempsey EC, Cool CD, Littler CM. Lung disease and PKCs. Pharmacol Res 2007; 55:545–559.
35. Webb BJL, Lindsay MA, Barnes PJ, et al. Protein kinase C isoenzymes in airway smooth muscle. Biochem J 1997; 324:167–175.
36. Lucas KA, Pitari GM, Kazerounian S, et al. Guanylyl cyclases and signaling by cyclic GMP. Pharmacol Rev 2000; 52:375–414.
37. Hamad AM, Clayton A, Islam B, et al. Guanylyl cyclases, nitric oxide, natriuretic peptides, and airway smooth muscle function. Am J Physiol Lung Cell Mol Physiol 2003; 285:L973–L983.
38. Kuhn M. Structure, regulation, and function of mammalian membrane guanylyl cyclase receptors, with a focus on guanylyl cyclase-A. Circ Res 2003; 93:700–709.
39. Rybalkin SD, Yan C, Bornfeldt KE, et al. Cyclic GMP phosphodiesterases and regulation of smooth muscle function. Circ Res 2003; 93:280–291.
40. Barnes PJ. Cytokine networks in asthma and chronic obstructive pulmonary disease. J Clin Invest 2008; 118:3546–3556.
41. Jin T, Xu X, Hereld D. Chemotaxis, chemokine receptors and human disease. Cytokine 2008; 44:1–8.
42. Allen SJ, Crown SE, Handel TM. Chemokine: receptor structure, interactions, and antagonism. Annu Rev Immunol 2007; 25:787–820.

43. Palmqvist C, Wardlaw AJ, Bradding P. Chemokines and their receptors as potential targets for the treatment of asthma. Br J Pharmacol 2007; 151:725–736.
44. Donnelly LE, Barnes PJ. Chemokine receptors as therapeutic targets in chronic obstructive pulmonary disease. Trends Pharmacol Sci 2006; 27:546–553.
45. Grotzinger J. Molecular mechanisms of cytokine receptor activation. Biochim Biophys Acta 2002; 1592:215–223.
46. Sprang SR. The divergent receptors for TNF. Trends Biochem Sci 1990; 15:366–368.
47. Aggarwal BB. Signalling pathways of the TNF superfamily: a double-edged sword. Nat Rev Immunol 2003; 3:745–756.
48. Kishimoto T, Taga T, Akira S. Cytokine signal transduction. Cell 1994; 76:253–262.
49. van der Geek P, Hunter T, Lindberg RA. Receptor protein-tyrosine kinases and their signal transduction pathways. Annu Rev Biol 1994; 10:251–337.
50. Ciardiello F, Tortora G. EGFR antagonists in cancer treatment. N Engl J Med 2008; 358:1160–1174.
51. Pawson T. Regulation and targets of receptor tyrosine kinases. Eur J Cancer 2002; 38(suppl 5): S3–S10.
52. Burgering BMT, Bos JL. Regulation of Ras-mediated signalling: more than one way to skin a cat. Trends Biochem Sci 1995; 20:18–22.
53. Cuenda A, Rousseau S. p38 MAP-kinases pathway regulation, function and role in human diseases. Biochim Biophys Acta 2007; 1773:1358–1375.
54. Boutros T, Chevet E, Metrakos P. Mitogen-activated protein (MAP) kinase/MAP kinase phosphatase regulation: roles in cell growth, death, and cancer. Pharmacol Rev 2008; 60: 261–310.
55. Shi Y, Massague J. Mechanisms of TGF-beta signaling from cell membrane to the nucleus. Cell 2003; 113:685–700.
56. Clarke DC, Liu X. Decoding the quantitative nature of TGF-beta/Smad signaling. Trends Cell Biol 2008; 18:430–442.
57. Walton KM, Dixon JE. Protein tyrosine phosphatases. Annu Rev Biochem 1993; 12:101–120.
58. Mustelin T, Rahmouni S, Bottini N, et al. Role of protein tyrosine phosphatases in T cell activation. Immunol Rev 2003; 191:139–147.
59. Steinlein OK, Bertrand D. Neuronal nicotinic acetylcholine receptors: from the genetic analysis to neurological diseases. Biochem Pharmacol 2008; 76:1175–1183.
60. Cahill K, Stead LF, Lancaster T. Nicotine receptor partial agonists for smoking cessation. Cochrane Database Syst Rev 2007; CD006103.
61. Evans RM. The steroid and thyroid hormone receptor superfamily. Science 1988; 247:889–895.
62. Shi Y. Orphan nuclear receptors in drug discovery. Drug Discov Today 2007; 12:440–445.
63. Straus DS, Glass CK. Anti-inflammatory actions of PPAR ligands: new insights on cellular and molecular mechanisms. Trends Immunol 2007; 28:551–558.
64. Wang K, Wan YJ. Nuclear receptors and inflammatory diseases. Exp Biol Med (Maywood) 2008; 233:496–506.
65. Rhen T, Cidlowski JA. Antiinflammatory action of glucocorticoids—new mechanisms for old drugs. New Engl J Med 2005; 353:1711–1723.
66. Barnes PJ. How corticosteroids control inflammation. Br J Pharmacol 2006; 148:245–254.
67. Emorine LJ, Marullo S, Briend-Sutren M-M, et al. Molecular characterization of the human b_3-adrenergic receptor. Science 1989; 245:1118–1121.
68. Kriff S, Lonnqvist F, Raimbault S, et al. Tissue distribution of b_3-adrenergic receptor mRNA in man. J Clin Invest 1993; 91:344–349.
69. Eglen RM, Choppin A, Dillon MP, et al. Muscarinic receptor ligands and their therapeutic potential. Curr Opin Chem Biol 1999; 3:426–432.
70. Mak JCW, Haddad E-B, Buckley NJ, et al. Visualization of muscarinic m_4 mRNA and M_4-receptor subtypes in rabbit lung. Life Sci 1993; 53:1501–1508.

71. Rousell J, Haddad E-B, Webb BLJ, et al. β-Adrenoceptor-mediated down-regulation of M_2-muscarinic receptors: role of cAMP-dependent protein kinases and protein kinase C. Mol Pharmacol 1996; 49:629–635.
72. Werry TD, Wilkinson GF, Willars GB. Mechanisms of cross-talk between G-protein-coupled receptors resulting in enhanced release of intracellular Ca2+. Biochem J 2003; 374:281–296.
73. Grandordy BM, Mak JCW, Barnes PJ. Modulation of airway smooth muscle b-receptor function by a muscarinic agonist. Life Sci 1994; 54:185–191.
74. Vazquez-Prado J, Casas-Gonzalez P, Garcia-Sainz JA. G protein-coupled receptor cross-talk: pivotal roles of protein phosphorylation and protein-protein interactions. Cell Signal 2003; 15:549–557.
75. Adcock IM, Stevens DA, Barnes PJ. Interactions between steroids and b₂-agonists. Eur Respir J 1996; 9:160–168.
76. Barnes PJ. Scientific rationale for combination inhalers with a long-acting b2-agonists and corticosteroids. Eur Respir J 2002; 19:182–191.
77. Giembycz MA, Kaur M, Leigh R, et al. A Holy Grail of asthma management: toward understanding how long-acting beta₂-adrenoceptor agonists enhance the clinical efficacy of inhaled corticosteroids. Br J Pharmacol 2008; 153:1090–1104.
78. Parra S, Bond RA. Inverse agonism: from curiosity to accepted dogma, but is it clinically relevant? Curr Opin Pharmacol 2007; 7:146–150.
79. Strange PG. Mechanisms of inverse agonism at G-protein-coupled receptors. Trends Pharmacol Sci 2002; 23:89–95.
80. Ameredes BT, Calhoun WJ. (R)-albuterol for asthma: pro [a.k.a. (S)-albuterol for asthma: con]. Am J Respir Crit Care Med 2006; 174:965–969.
81. Barnes PJ. Treatment with (*R*)-albuterol has no advantage over racemic albuterol. Am J Respir Crit Care Med 2006; 174:969–972.
82. Tobin AB. G-protein-coupled receptor phosphorylation: where, when and by whom. Br J Pharmacol 2008; 153(suppl 1):S167–S176.
83. Kohout TA, Lefkowitz RJ. Regulation of G protein-coupled receptor kinases and arrestins during receptor desensitization. Mol Pharmacol 2003; 63:9–18.
84. Ribas C, Penela P, Murga C, et al. The G protein-coupled receptor kinase (GRK) interactome: role of GRKs in GPCR regulation and signaling. Biochim Biophys Acta 2007; 1768:913–922.
85. McGraw DW, Liggett SB. Heterogeneity in beta-adrenergic receptor kinase expression in the lung accounts for cell-specific desensitization of the beta2-adrenergic receptor. J Biol Chem 1997; 272:7338–7344.
86. Finney PA, Donnelly LE, Belvisi MG, et al. Chronic systemic administration of salmeterol to rats promotes pulmonary b2-adrenoceptor desensitization and down-regulation of Gsa. Br J Pharmacol 2001; 132:1261–1270.
87. Mak JC, Hisada T, Salmon M, et al. Glucocorticoids reverse IL-1β-induced impairment of β-adrenoceptor-mediated relaxation and up-regulation of G-protein-coupled receptor kinases. Br J Pharmacol 2002; 135:987–996.
88. Violin JD, Lefkowitz RJ. Beta-arrestin-biased ligands at seven-transmembrane receptors. Trends Pharmacol Sci 2007; 28:416–422.
89. Hadcock JR, Wang HY, Malbon CC. Agonist-induced destabilization of b-adrenergic receptor mRNA: attenuation of glucocorticoid-induced up-regulation of β-adrenergic receptors. J Biol Chem 1989; 264:19928–19933.
90. Nishikawa M, Mak JCW, Shirasaki H, et al. Long term exposure to norepinephrine results in down-regulation and reduced mRNA expression of pulmonary β-adrenergic receptors in guinea pigs. Am J Respir Cell Mol Biol 1994; 10:91–99.
91. Mak JCW, Nishikawa M, Shirasaki H, et al. Protective effects of a glucocorticoid on down-regulation of pulmonary β₂-adrenergic receptors in vivo. J Clin Invest 1995; 96:99–106.

92. Mak JCW, Nishikawa M, Barnes PJ. Glucocorticosteroids increase β_2-adrenergic receptor transcription in human lung. Am J Physiol 1995; 12:L41–L46.
93. Katsunuma T, Mak JCW, Barnes PJ. Glucocorticoids reduce tachykinin NK_2-receptor expression in bovine tracheal smooth muscle. Eur J Pharmacol 1998; 344:99–107.
94. Hislop AA, Mak JC, Kelly D, et al. Postnatal changes in b-adrenoceptors in the lung and the effect of hypoxia induced pulmonary hypertension of the newborn. Br J Pharmacol 2002; 135:1415–1424.
95. Hislop AA, Mak JCW, Reader JA, et al. Muscarinic receptor subtypes in porcine lung during postnatal development. Eur J Pharmacol 1998; 359:211–221.
96. Ohmichi H, Koshimizu U, Matsumoto K, et al. Hepatocyte growth factor (HGF) acts as a mesenchyme-derived morphogenic factor during fetal lung development. Development 1998; 125:1315–1324.
97. Bai TR. Abnormalities in airway smooth muscle in fatal asthma: a comparison between trachea and bronchus. Am Rev Respir Dis 1991; 143:441–443.
98. Haddad E-B, Mak JCW, Barnes PJ. Expression of β-adrenergic and muscarinic receptors in human lung. Am J Physiol 1996; 270:L947–L953.
99. Shirasaki H, Nishikawa M, Adcock IM, et al. Expression of platelet activating factor receptor mRNA in human and guinea-pig lung. Am J Resp Cell Mol Biol 1994; 10:533–537.
100. Haddad EB, Fox AJ, Rousell J, et al. Post-transcriptional regulation of bradykinin B_1 and B_2 receptor gene expression in human lung fibroblasts by tumor necrosis factor-a: modulation by dexamethasone. Mol Pharmacol 2000; 57:1123–1131.
101. Adcock IM, Peters M, Gelder C, et al. Increased tachykinin receptor gene expression in asthmatic lung and its modulation by steroids. J Mol Endocrinol 1993; 11:1–7.
102. Bai TR, Zhou D, Weir T, et al. Substance P (NK_1)- and neurokinin A (NK_2)-receptor gene expression in inflammatory airway diseases. Am J Physiol 1995; 269:L309–L317.
103. Ihara H, Nakanishi S. Selective inhibition of expression of the substance P receptor mRNA in pancreatic acinar AR42J cells by glucocorticoids. J Biol Chem 1990; 36:22,441–22,445.
104. Catterall WA. Structure and regulation of voltage-gated Ca2+ channels. Annu Rev Cell Dev Biol 2000; 16:521–555.
105. Kotlikoff MI. Calcium currents in isolated canine airway smooth muscle cells. Am J Physiol 1988; 254:C793–901.
106. Li S, Westwick J, Poll C. Transient receptor potential (TRP) channels as potential drug targets in respiratory disease. Cell Calcium 2003; 33:551–558.
107. Corteling RL, Li S, Giddings J, et al. Expression of TRPC6 and related TRP family members in human airway smooth muscle and lung tissue. Am J Respir Cell Mol Biol 2004; 32(2):145–154.
108. Parekh AB. Store-operated Ca^{2+} entry: dynamic interplay between endoplasmic reticulum, mitochondria and plasma membrane. J Physiol 2003; 547:333–348.
109. Ambudkar IS, Ong HL, Liu X, et al. TRPC1: the link between functionally distinct store-operated calcium channels. Cell Calcium 2007; 42:213–223.
110. Shieh CC, Coghlan M, Sullivan JP, et al. Potassium channels: molecular defects, diseases, and therapeutic opportunities. Pharmacol Rev 2000; 52:557–594.
111. Nardi A, Olesen SP. BK channel modulators: a comprehensive overview. Curr Med Chem 2008; 15:1126–1146.
112. Black JL, Barnes PJ. Potassium channels and airway function: new therapeutic approaches. Thorax 1990; 45:213–218.
113. Kotlikoff MI. Potassium currents in canine airway smooth muscle cells. Am J Physiol 1990; 259:L384–L395.
114. Miura M, Belvisi MG, Stretton CD, et al. Role of potassium channels in bronchodilator responses in human airways. Am Rev Respir Dis 1992; 146:132–136.

115. Black JL, Armour CL, Johnson PRA, et al. The action of a potassium channel activator BRL 38227 (lemakalim) on human airway smooth muscle. Am Rev Respir Dis 1990; 142:1384–1389.
116. Ichinose M, Barnes PJ. A potassium channel activator modulates both noncholinergic and cholinergic neurotransmission in guinea pig airways. J Pharmacol Exp Ther 1990; 252:1207–1212.
117. Stretton CD, Miura M, Belvisi MG, et al. Calcium-activated potassium channels mediate prejunctional inhibition of peripheral sensory nerves. Proc Natl Acad Sci U S A 1992; 89:1325–1329.
118. Rogers DF, Lei Y, Kuo H-P, et al. A K+ channel activator, lemakalin, inhibits cigarette smoke-induced plasma exudation and goblet cell secretion in guinea pig trachea. Am Rev Respir Dis 1991; 143:A754.
119. Pelaia G, Gallelli L, Vatrella A, et al. Potential role of potassium channel openers in the treatment of asthma and chronic obstructive pulmonary disease. Life Sci 2002; 70:977–990.
120. Eaton DC, Helms MN, Koval M, et al. The contribution of epithelial sodium channels to alveolar function in health and disease. Annu Rev Physiol 2009; 71:403–423.
121. Donaldson SH, Boucher RC. Sodium channels and cystic fibrosis. Chest 2007; 132:1631–1636.
122. Patel AC, Brett TJ, Holtzman MJ. The role of CLCA proteins in inflammatory airway disease. Annu Rev Physiol 2009; 71:425–449.
123. Norris AA, Alton EW. Chloride transport and the action of sodium cromoglycate and nedocromil sodium in asthma. Clin Exp Allergy 1996; 26:250–253.
124. Saklatvala J, Dean J, Finch A. Protein kinase cascades in intracellular signalling by interleukin-I and tumour necrosis factor. Biochem Soc Symp 1999; 64:63–77:63–77.
125. Adcock IM, Chung KF, Caramori G, et al. Kinase inhibitors and airway inflammation. Eur J Pharmacol 2006; 533:118–132.
126. Cohen P. Protein kinases—the major drug targets of the twenty-first century? Nat Rev Drug Discov 2002; 1:309–315.
127. Ito K, Caramori G, Adcock IM. Therapeutic potential of phosphatidylinositol 3-kinase inhibitors in inflammatory respiratory disease. J Pharmacol Exp Ther 2007; 321:1–8.
128. Carracedo A, Pandolfi PP. The PTEN-PI3K pathway: of feedbacks and cross-talks. Oncogene 2008; 27:5527–5541.
129. Clark AR, Martins JR, Tchen CR. Role of dual specificity phosphatases in biological responses to glucocorticoids. J Biol Chem 2008; 283:25765–25769.
130. Pelkonen O, Turpeinen M, Hakkola J, et al. Inhibition and induction of human cytochrome P450 enzymes: current status. Arch Toxicol 2008; 82:667–715.
131. Newhouse MT, Dolovich MB. Control of asthma by aerosols. New Engl J Med 1986; 315: 870–874.
132. Sturton G, Persson C, Barnes PJ. Small airways: an important but neglected target in the treatment of obstructive airway diseases. Trends Phamacol Sci 2008; 29:340–345.
133. Usmani OS, Biddiscombe MF, Barnes PJ. Regional lung deposition and bronchodilator response as a function of b2-agonist particle size. Am J Respir Crit Care Med 2005; 172:1497–1504.
134. Derendorf H. Pharmacokinetic and pharmacodynamic properties of inhaled ciclesonide. J Clin.Pharmacol 2007; 47:782–789.
135. Virchow JC, Crompton GK, Dal Negro R, et al. Importance of inhaler devices in the management of airway disease. Respir Med 2008; 102:10–19.
136. McDonald KJ, Martin GP. Transition to CFC-free metered dose inhalers—into the new millennium. Int J Pharm 2000; 201:89–107.
137. Smaldone GC. Advances in aerosols: adult respiratory disease. J Aerosol Med 2006; 19:36–46.
138. Chan HK. Dry powder aerosol delivery systems: current and future research directions. J Aerosol Med 2006; 19:21–27.

2

Clinical Trials in Asthma and COPD: Trial Designs, Clinical Endpoints, and Biomarkers

TREVOR T. HANSEL and ANDREW J. TAN
Imperial Clinical Respiratory Research Unit (ICRRU), St. Mary's Hospital, Imperial College, London, U.K.

PETER J. BARNES
National Heart and Lung Institute, Imperial College, London, U.K.

ONN MIN KON
St. Mary's Hospital, Imperial College, London, U.K.

I. Introduction: summary

The incidence of asthma and chronic obstructive pulmonary disease (COPD) is increasing throughout the world and acts as a major incentive for the development of new and improved drug therapy. However, the cytokine storm caused in human volunteers after administration of TGN1412 (TeGenero, Würzburg, Germany) has emphasized the need for caution in dose selection in phase I with biologics and the need for predictive assays based on human cells. For first-in-man studies, ex vivo whole blood stimulation can be employed with systemic therapies to establish specific target pharmacology, pharmacokinetic/pharmacodynamic modeling, and an optimal dosage regimen. For the large range of bronchodilator and anti-inflammatory agents entering studies in human, reliable decision making is imperative in phase II before entering large scale phase III clinical studies. In phase II studies, it is important to establish the clinical efficacy and tissue anti-inflammatory properties of the new therapy. Many studies have been performed utilizing the inhaled allergen challenge (IAC) in asthmatics as a proof of concept study, although the latest methods of nasal allergen challenge (NAC) in subjects with allergic rhinitis offer advantages in terms of repeated direct sampling of the nasal lining fluid. Airway hyperreactivity (AHR) is commonly measured as provocative concentration to cause a 20% fall in forced expiratory volume in one second (FEV_1) (PC_{20}) in relation to methacholine, adenosine monophosphate (AMP), or mannitol. It is also possible to directly study clinical effects of new therapies on limited numbers of symptomatic asthma patients through morning and evening electronic monitoring of lung function and symptoms. Alternative clinical trial designs in asthma include studies to assess bronchodilation and bronchoprotection, exercise tolerance, add-on and titration studies with inhaled and oral corticosteroids, and a considerable recent focus in phase III on prevention and treatment of exacerbations. In contrast, there is a major challenge for the development of new anti-inflammatory drugs for COPD, as phase II studies have been poorly predictive of efficacy in phase III trials, resulting in difficulties for oral phosphodiesterase (PDE)4 inhibitors to achieve registration after large clinical development. In COPD, clinical trial designs range from studies on lung function, symptoms and exercise performance, inflammatory biomarkers, natural history of chronic stable disease, prevention and treatment of exacerbations, and effects on the BODE score and cachexia and muscle function. Compared with asthma, inclusion criteria, monitoring parameters, comparator therapies, and trial design are less well established for COPD. The large variety of potential clinical endpoints includes lung function, symptoms, walking tests, hyperinflation, health-related quality of life (HRQOL), frequency and severity of exacerbations, natural history, and mortality. In addition, for both asthma and COPD, surrogate biomarkers may be assessed in blood, exhaled breath, induced sputum, bronchial mucosal biopsy, bronchoalveolar lavage (BAL), and through advanced radiographic imaging. There have been considerable recent advances in the development of noninvasive biomarkers and novel clinical trial designs, as well as clarification of regulatory requirements, that will facilitate the clinical development of new therapies for patients with asthma and COPD.

II. Background

The health burden of asthma and COPD is increasing globally at an alarming rate, providing a strong impetus for the development of new therapeutics (1–3). Despite the availability of effective inhaled therapy for asthma, many patients are inadequately treated, while the severe asthmatics who do not respond to inhaled and oral corticosteroids have a major need for supplementary or alternative therapy. The licensing of anti-IgE for use in severe allergic asthma illustrates the successful introduction of a specific biologic for asthma (4,5). An interesting feature of the clinical trials with anti-IgE is that exacerbations have been the major endpoint. In both asthma and COPD there is the need to prevent exacerbations and provide more effective treatment for acute severe exacerbations.

The need for new drugs is more urgent in COPD since bronchodilators have relatively small effects and anti-inflammatory therapy has only limited action in certain patients (6). There has been considerable clinical trial activity in the use of oral PDE4 inhibitors to treat COPD (7,8). In a six-week study, the highest dose of cilomilast (Ariflo, GlaxoSmithKline Pharmaceuticals, Research Triangle Park, North Carolina, U.S.) resulted in a maximum mean difference in trough clinic FEV_1 compared with placebo of 160 mL (9). However, despite showing anti-inflammatory effects in COPD (10), a six-month placebo-controlled study in 431 COPD patients receiving cilomilast has been disappointing (11). Indeed it has been noted that in four separate 26-week studies in COPD, the improvement in trough FEV_1 was only 40 mL versus placebo (12). Hence, encouraging phase II data did not translate into phase III, and cilomilast may never become licensed, and this has major implications for studies of novel anti-inflammatory agents in COPD.

The PDE4 inhibitor, roflumilast (Daxas®, Nycomed, Zurich, Switzerland), has been demonstrated to be efficacious in causing inhibition of the late asthmatic response (LAR) following IAC (13,14), has achieved comparable efficacy to beclomethasone in asthma (15–17), and has effects in exercise-induced asthma (18). Roflumilast has modest effects on FEV_1 in COPD (19) and has been studied in 24-week (20) and 1-year studies (21). The results of studies looking at effects of roflumilast on exacerbations of COPD in phase III studies with suitably severe patients are awaited with interest (22).

A long-term goal for asthma is to develop disease-modifying therapy to alter the natural history and airway remodeling (23); this is analogous to the aim to prevent or inhibit the progressive fall in lung function that contributes to morbidity and mortality in COPD. However, it is proving difficult to develop new drugs for human disease, and in 2007, only 17 new molecular entities (NMEs) and 2 biologics were approved by the FDA (24). There have been considerable efforts to provide new drugs for the treatment of asthma and COPD, and we recommend recent reviews on the various approaches (23,25–31). Many new targets have been identified through scientific studies of the molecular basis of asthma and COPD (32,33).

III. Trial Designs

Textbooks of pharmaceutical medicine contain useful background information on the design and conduct of clinical trials and the development of medicines (34,35). Clinical studies within a drug development program should be carried out according to Good Clinical Practice (GCP) (36). GCP specifically relates to the conduct of clinical research trials with potential new therapies for human use. A clinical development program may take over 10 years, involve thousands of patients, and cost a billion U.S. dollars (including preclinical research spending).

The European Medicines Evaluation Agency (EMEA) has issued general considerations for clinical trials in asthma and COPD (37,38), with recent Federal Drug Agency (FDA) guidelines for studies with new drugs for COPD (39). Indeed there is an expanding literature of regulatory and task force guidelines on various aspects of respiratory clinical trials (Table 1). We summarized a range of clinical endpoints in respiratory studies in patients with asthma and COPD (Table 2) and have provided a selection of representative clinical trials with licensed drugs for asthma and COPD (Table 3).

There are particular ethical issues in carrying out clinical studies in patients with asthma, since challenge tests may be proposed, and treatment may need to be withdrawn or not given when strictly indicated. Patients with asthma may sometimes be required to be off inhaled corticosteroids (ICS) and symptomatic in a run-in phase before being offered either a potential treatment or placebo in a double-blind manner (121).

Inclusion criteria for patients with asthma and COPD in clinical trials can generally be based on definitions provided by international guidelines. Recently, the Global Initiative on Asthma (GINA) (40) and the Global Initiative on Chronic Obstructive Lung Disease (GOLD) (41) have released evidence-based guidelines that cover the definition and management of patients with asthma and COPD (Table 1).

A. Trial and Error with Herbal Remedies

In ancient times, assessment of effects of herbal extracts was based on trial and error, and many subjects were harmed before useful agents could be identified. *Ma huang* extract is an ephedrine-containing adrenaline-like substance with bronchodilator properties, while extracts of *Datura stramonium* (thorn apple or jimson weed) and *Atropa belladonna* (deadly nightshade) have anticholinergic bronchodilator activity (122).

B. Safety Issues in Respiratory Studies

On March 13, 2006, a fully humanized monoclonal antibody (MoAB) directed against CD28, produced by the German biotechnology company TeGenero (TGN1412), was first administered to human subjects. Following infusion of MoAB to six subjects and

Table 1 Background to Respiratory Studies: Clinical, Regulatory, Safety, Endpoint, and Biomarker Considerations

	Asthma	COPD	Rhinitis
Global clinical management guidelines	Global Initiative on Asthma (GINA, 2007) (40)	Global Initiative on Chronic Obstructive Lung Disease (GOLD, 2007) (41)	Allergic Rhinitis and its Impact on Asthma (ARIA, 2001) (42) 2006 update (43)
Regulatory aspects of Good Clinical Practice (GCP)	Clinical Trials Directive (2001/20/EC) (36)		
Regulatory documents for development of new drugs	EMEA, 2002 (37)	EMEA, 1999 (38) FDA, 2007 (39)	Allergic rhinitis (WHO, 2001) (44)
Bioequivalence	ICS, Canada, 2007 (45) ICS, EMEA, 2007 (46)		
Drug safety: adverse events and regulation	Death of a healthy volunteer from bronchoscopy, 1998 (47) Death of a healthy volunteer from inhaling hexamethonium, 2001 (48) TGN1412 (monoclonal antibody vs. CD28), cytokine storm, 2003 (49–51) Salmeterol Multicenter Asthma Research Trial (SMART) (52)		
Clinical endpoints — Symptoms Health status	Asthma QOL Questionnaire (53)	St. George's Respiratory Questionnaire (54) Short-Form 36 (55)	Rhinosinusitis: developing guidance for clinical trials (56)
Biomarkers general	NIH Biomarkers Definitions Working Group, 2001 (57) ATS/ERS Taskforce COPD Biomarkers, 2008 (58)		
Specific biomarkers and endpoints	Spirometry. ATS/ERS Task Force, 2005 (59) Guidelines for methacholine and exercise challenge testing ATS 1999 Indirect airway challenges. ERS Task Force, 2003 (60) 6-Minute walk test. ATS Statement 2002 (61) Exercise testing in clinical practice. ERS Task Force, 2007 (62) Exhaled NO. ATS/ERS, 2005 (63) Exhaled breath condensate. ATS/ERS Task Force, 2005 (64) Sputum induction and processing. ATS/ERS Task Force, 2002 (65) Diagnosis and management of chronic cough. ERS Task Force, 2004 Bronchoprovocation and bronchoscopy. NHLBI/NIAID Workshop, 2005 (66) Endobronchiobiopsy (67) Exacerbations of COPD (68–70) Rhinosinusitis (56)		

Table 2 Endpoints for Clinical Studies in Asthma and COPD

Asthma	COPD

Lung function
- PEF and FEV_1
- Reversibility and variability
- Airways hyperresponsiveness (AHR) to methacholine, histamine, AMP

- FEV_1 % predicted (pre/post bronchodilator)
- FEV_1/forced vital capacity, FVC ratio
- FIV_1
- TLCO, transfer factor for carbon monoxide

Symptom diary
Asthma Control Questionnaire
To include rescue short-acting
  β_2-agonist usage

Symptoms and smoking rate diary
For patient-reported outcomes are reviewed by the ATS/ERS Task force (71)
- MRC scale
- Baseline dyspnea index (BDI)
- Transitional dyspnea index

Health status
Health-Related Quality of Life
Asthma Quality of Life Questionnaire

St. George's Respiratory Questionnaire
Chronic Respiratory Disease Questionnaire

Challenge model and airway hyper-reactivity (AHR)
Inhaled allergen challenge, leukotrienes
Inhaled methacholine, AMP, mannitol

Lipopolysaccharide (LPS, endotoxin), cigarette, ozone, diesel exhaust particle inhalation

Exercise responses
Exercise-induced asthma

Dynamic hyperinflation
Six-minute walk test
Incremental shuttle walk test
Endurance shuttle walk test

Systemic effects

Weight, fat-free mass
Respiratory and skeletal muscle function
BODE score
Endocrine function
Cardiovascular disease

Laboratory tests
- Skin prick tests
- Blood
- Sputum
- Exhaled breath
- BAL and bronchial biopsy

- Arterial blood gases
- Blood (cells and serum)
- Sputum
- Exhaled breath
- BAL and bronchial biopsy
- Urine elastin/collagen degradation products

(Continued)

Table 2 Endpoints for Clinical Studies in Asthma and COPD (*Continued*)

Asthma	COPD
Imaging	HRCT scans for emphysema
Natural History	
Rate of FEV_1 decline	Rate of FEV_1 decline
Airway remodeling	Development of emphysema on HRCT
Pharmacoeconomics and pharmacogenetics	
Exacerbations	
Mortality	

Abbreviations: PEF, peak expiratory flow; FEV_1, forced expiratory volume in one second; FIV_1, forced inspiratory volume in one second; AMP, adenosine monophosphate; HRCT, high-resolution computerized tomography.

placebo to two, six previously healthy young males developed a systemic inflammatory response with induction of proinflammatory cytokines, at the Parexel Clinical Pharmacology Research Unit in Harrow, North West London (49). All subjects survived, but one individual has permanent ischemic damage to his toes and finger tips, while all six subjects may be vulnerable to develop malignancies and autoimmune disease. In retrospect, TGN1412 probably caused widespread activation of T cells, leading to a cytokine storm and then to a capillary leak syndrome and organ system failure. It remains an urgent issue to develop human blood and tissue predictive in vitro tests for the capacity of biologics to cause a cytokine storm (123).

We highlight three other serious clinical incidents with relevance to the conduct of respiratory studies:

- The death in 1999 of the 18-year-old Jesse Gelsinger in a gene transfer trial at the University of Pennsylvania (48).
- The death in 2001 of 24-year-old Ellen Roche in a Johns Hopkins study involving inhalation of hexamethonium (124).
- The observation of an increased number of malignancies in patients with COPD receiving an anti-TNF MoAB (Remicade, Johnson & Johnson, New Jersey, U.S.) (125).

C. Phase I Tolerability Studies

Rising dose tolerability studies generally take place in healthy volunteers and then patients with asthma or COPD. For some inhaled agents, it may be preferable to proceed directly to patients, and tolerability studies in younger patients with asthma are generally more sensitive and have greater safety reserve than initial studies in patients with COPD. Incremental ascending dose studies in asthma are performed with serial FEV_1, generally the preferred endpoint, without the need for plethysmography. Many inhaled agents are well tolerated in nonasthmatic volunteers, but may be poorly tolerated in asthmatics. Novel inhaled therapies for COPD are often best studied in volunteers with mild asthma, since these subjects have responsive airways, and may be more sensitive to potential bronchoconstrictor effects.

Table 3 A Selection of Major Recent Clinical Trials with Licensed Drugs in Asthma, COPD, and Allergic Rhinitis

Asthma and allergic rhinitis	COPD
Symbicort Symbicort Maintenance and Rescue Therapy (SMART), 8 studies:	*Tiotropium natural history studies* One year analysis of tiotropium changes on spirometry (83) Investigating New Standards for Prophylaxis in Reduction of Exacerbations (INSPIRE) (84, 85) Understanding the Potential Long-Term Impacts on Function with Tiotropium in COPD (UPLIFT): a 4-year study (86, 87)

Asthma and allergic rhinitis:

Symbicort
Symbicort Maintenance and Rescue Therapy (SMART), 8 studies:

- STEP (72)
- STAY (73)
- STEAM (74)
- COSMOS (75)
- SMILE (76)
- COMPASS (77)
- AHEAD (78)
- PAEDIATRICS (79)

Sublingual immunotherapy (SLIT)
Grazax (80–82)

Seretide
Gaining Optimal Asthma ControL Study (GOLD) (88–92)

Anti-IgE (Xolair, Novartis) (112–118)

COPD:

Tiotropium natural history studies
One year analysis of tiotropium changes on spirometry (83)
Investigating New Standards for Prophylaxis in Reduction of Exacerbations (INSPIRE) (84, 85)
Understanding the Potential Long-Term Impacts on Function with Tiotropium in COPD (UPLIFT): a 4-year study (86, 87)

Tiotropium combination studies
Tiotropium and formoterol in COPD (91–93)
Triple therapy with tiotropium, LABA and ICS (94, 95)

ICS as monotherapy in COPD

- ERS Study on COPD (EuroSCOP) (96)
- Inhaled steroids in obstructive lung disease in Europe (ISOLDE) (97)
- Lung Health Study (LHS) (98)
- Copenhagen (99)
- Prevention of exacerbations over 6 mo (100)
- Withdrawal of fluticasone: COSMIC (101) primary care (102)

ICS/LABA in COPD

- TRial of Inhaled STeroids ANd LABAs (TRISTAN) (103–107)
- Toward a Revolution in COPD Health (TORCH): mortality (108, 109) natural history (110)
- Bronchial biopsies and sputum, 12 wk, $n = 140$ (111)

Mucolytics in COPD

- Bronchitis Randomized on *N*-acetyl cysteine Cost-Utility Study (BRONCUS) (119)
- PEACE study (120)

D. Bronchodilators in Asthma

Asthma can be rapidly and numerically assessed on the basis of peak expiratory flow (PEF) or FEV_1. Acute bronchodilation can be studied in patients with mild asthma who have sufficient bronchoconstriction at baseline, so that there is "room to improve" FEV_1 following single-dose administration.

E. Bronchodilators in COPD

The prolonged effects of the inhaled anticholinergic agent, tiotropium bromide, have been demonstrated in terms of bronchoprotection against methacholine-induced bronchoconstriction in asthma (126), and the dose-response relationship established in COPD (127). Acute bronchodilator trials in COPD have special clinical trial requirements (128,129), there is the need for additional measurements of exercise dynamic hyperinflation, exercise endurance, assessment of dyspnea, and HRQOL (130).

F. Inhaled Allergen Challenge

IAC responses have been extensively studied in relation to drugs, and effects on the early and late asthmatic reactions (EAR and LAR) as well as AHR provide important mechanistic insights. The IAC offers the opportunity to study effects on the EAR and LAR, blood and sputum eosinophils, exhaled breath nitric oxide (NO), and methacholine airway responsiveness (PC20). The reproducibility of the IAC is excellent, and outcome of 12 patients is adequate to reliably demonstrate 50% attenuation of the EAR or LAR with >90% power (131). Recently, the method of bolus as opposed to incremental allergen challenge has been validated (132,133). IAC should ideally not be repeated at less than three-week intervals, because of residual AHR (134). The use of bolus dose allergen challenge for repeated tests in the same patient is a safe and validated method to administer inhaled allergen in clinical trials with valid responses when compared with incremental dose allergen challenge (132,133).

Of the anti-inflammatory drugs effective in controlling asthma, all inhibit the LAR to allergen: this includes steroids, theophyllines, leukotriene antagonists, cromones, cyclosporin A, anti-IgE (see Table 4 with references attached) (184,185). Indeed when considering a range of representative clinical trials with novel unlicensed drugs (Table 5), the IAC design is the classical model for initial assessment of anti-inflammatory therapies in human.

However, a number of other agents that are not effective therapy in asthma also cause some inhibition of the LAR: including furosemide, heparin, and PGE2 (false positives). Hence, when studying the effects of a new therapeutic on the IAC LAR, it is useful for positioning a drug relative to established asthma therapy, but offers a relatively low hurdle due to the false positives. However, there are no anti-inflammatory therapeutics for asthma that are "false negatives," in which there is no effect on the LAR but clinical efficacy.

Of special interest in relation to IAC responses has been a MoAB directed against interleukin-5 (IL-5), since IL-5 has an established role as the major terminal differentiation factor during eosinopoiesis in the bone marrow (261,262). An initial study in human involved a single intravenous infusion of a humanized MoAb directed against IL-5 (SB240563) given to mild allergic asthmatics in a parallel group double-blind clinical trial (169), the design of which has been criticized (263,264). There was pronounced

Table 4   Effects of Selected Therapeutics on Inhaled Allergen Challenge Responses

Therapeutic agent	Comment	Reference
Inhaled corticosteroids	Fluticasone 250 µg has equivalent effects to 250 µg b.i.d. for 2 wk on LAR	135
	Fluticasone (1000 µg daily for 2 wk) causes an 80% decrease in LAR by maximum fall in FEV_1	136
	Budesonide (400 µg daily for 8 days) causes 94% decrease in LAR AUC	137
Prednisone		138
Theophyllines		139,140
Leukotriene antagonists	Montelukast: 3 oral doses, 75% inhibition of EAR and 57% inhibition of LAR	141
		142–145
Cromones	Nedocromil 4 mg by pressurized aerosol inhibits causes a 64% decrease in EAR and a 58.8% decrease in LAR by maximum fall in FEV_1	146–149
Salbutamol		149–151
Terbutaline		152
Salmeterol		153–161
Ipratropium bromide		151
Formoterol		162,163
Cyclosporin A	50% decrease in LAR by AUC	164,165
Anti-IgE	Intravenous anti-IgE inhibits the EAR by 37% and LAR by 62%	166,167
	Inhaled anti-IgE fails to inhibit LAR	
IL-12	No significant effect on LAR	168
Anti-IL-5	No significant effect on LAR	169
Anti-histamine		170
Aspirin like agents	Sodium salicylate: 23% inhibition in LAR	171
	Indomethacin: 39% inhibition of LAR	
	Lysine acetylsalicylate: 44% inhibition of LAR	
Prostaglandin E2		172–174
Heparin	36% inhibition of LAR	175
Furosemide	Inhaled furosemide: inhibition of EAR and LAR	176
Phosphodiesterase 4 inhibitor	CDP840: 30% inhibition of LAR	177,178
	Roflumilast: 43% inhibition of LAR	13,14
Mast cell tryptase inhibitor		179
Platelet-activating factor antagonist	UK-74,505: no significant effect on EAR or LAR	180
	WEB 2086: no significant effect on EAR or LAR	181
	SR27417A: 26% inhibition of LAR	182
IL-4 variant		183

Abbreviations: LAR, late asthmatic response; EAR, early asthmatic response; FEV_1, forced expiratory volume in one second; IL, interleukin.

Table 5 Clinical Trials with Novel Unlicensed Drugs in Asthma, Allergy, and COPD

	Asthma and allergy	COPD and other indications
General reviews including cytokine-directed therapy	186,187,188,189 • Immunomodulators (23) • Peptide immunotherapy (190) • CpG (191) (acts on TLR9) • CRTH2 (DP2) antagonism (192) • Allergen avoidance: (193)	Review of large drug treatment trials in COPD (6)
Novel bronchodilators and allergen avoidance	Ultra-LABAs and LAMAs (25, 194–196)	
PDE4 inhibitors	General review (197) Roflumilast: • Inhaled allergen challenge (198) • Exercise-induced asthma (18) • Comparison with beclomethasone over 12 wk (15) • Dose ranging over 12 wk (16) • Roflumilast in allergic rhinitis (199)	Roflumilast • RECORD 24-wk study in COPD (20) • 1-yr study in severe COPD, $n = 1513$ (21) Cilomilast • 6-wk study in COPD (9) • 24-wk study in COPD (11)
MoAB anti-IL-5	• Inhaled allergen challenge (169) • Asthma bronchoscopy studies (200–203) • Larger asthma clinical studies (204, 205)	• Cutaneous allergen challenge (206) • Atopic dermatitis (207) • Angio-lymphoid hyperplasia (208) • Eosinophilic esophagitis (209) • Hypereosinophilic syndrome (210–212)
IL-4 and IL-13	Soluble IL-4 receptor (213, 214) IL-4 variant (183)	
TNF-α-directed therapy	Severe asthma (215–217) Moderate asthma (218)	Pilot COPD study, $n = 22$ (219) Larger COPD study, $n = 234$ over 6 mo (125) Sarcoidosis (220)
Other cytokine-directed therapy and targets	IFN-α in • Atopic dermatitis (10576) (221) • Childhood asthma (222)	

(Continued)

Table 5 Clinical Trials with Novel Unlicensed Drugs in Asthma, Allergy, and COPD (*Continued*)

	Asthma and allergy	COPD and other indications
	IFN-γ in	
	• AR (223)	
	• Atopic dermatitis (224)	
	• Asthma (225)	
	• Lung fibrosis (226)	
	IL-12 (168, 227)	
Cell surface receptor/kinase targets	CSF/KIT (228): imatinib	MoAB vs. CD4 (234, 235) MoAB vs. CD23 (236, 237)
	• Hypereosinophilic syndrome (229, 230)	
	• Systemic mastocytosis (231)	
	R112 (232, 233)	
Chemokine receptor and adhesion molecule antagonists	VLA-4 antagonist in asthma (238) Selectin inhibitor (239–242)	MoAB vs. IL-8 (243) CXCR2 CCR2 CXCR3
Signal transduction and transcription factors	STAT6 is the common transcription factor for IL-4 and IL-13: inhibitory peptide (244)	
Statins Lung regeneration for emphysema		245–249 Retinoids (250, 251) Clinical studies in emphysema (252, 253) Stem cell therapy (254, 255)
Antibiotics and mucolytics	Antibiotics for exacerbations: Clarithromycin (256) Telithromycin (257)	Mucus secretion review (258)
		• rhDNAse 1 (Pulmozyme) for treatment of severe exacerbations (259)
		• *N*-acetyl cysteine
		Bronchitis Randomized on NAC Cost-Utility Study (BRONCUS) (119) PEACE study (120)
Anti-sense DNA and siRNA (small interference RNA)	Anti-sense CCR3 and β-chain receptor for IL-3, IL-5, and GM-CSF (260)	

Abbreviations: COPD, chronic obstructive pulmonary disease; PDE4, phosphodiesterase type 4; IL, interleukin; LABA, long-acting-β-agonists; LAMA, long-acting muscurinic antagonists; PGE2, prostaglandin E2; ANP, atrial natriuretic peptide; KCO, carbon monoxide transfer coefficient; IFN, interferon; MoAB, monoclonal antibody; GM-CSF, granulocyte-macrophage colony-stimulating factor.

suppression of peripheral blood eosinophil levels for 16 weeks and considerably reduced numbers of sputum eosinophils after allergen challenge. However, despite these clear effects, anti-IL-5 did not protect against the allergen-induced LAR and did not inhibit baseline or postallergen AHR.

Interpretation of the anti-IL-5 effects on IAC must be made with caution, because although eosinophil numbers in blood and sputum were dramatically reduced by anti-IL-5, there are still residual eosinophils in mucosal bronchial biopsies, with a halving of numbers (201). In addition, anti-IL-5 reduces deposition of extracellular matrix proteins in bronchial subepithelial basement membrane (200) and tenascin in skin (206).

However, there are large scale clinical studies that have found that anti-IL-5 is not clinically effective in treating severe asthma (265), moderate asthma (205), and atopic dermatitis (207). However, further clinical studies are ongoing to see effects of anti-IL-5 in selected severe asthmatics with eosinophilia (Ian Pavord, personal communication) and to study the effects on the prevention and treatment of eosinophilic asthma exacerbations (Paul O'Byrne, personal communication). In contrast to asthma, anti-IL-5 is proving to be useful in a variety of eosinophilic conditions: hypereosinophilic syndrome (HES) (210,212,266), eosinophilic esophagitis (209), angiolymphoid hyperplasia with eosinophilia (ALHE) (208).

G. Nasal Allergen Challenge

There is a functional and immunological relationship between the nose and bronchi, both have a ciliated respiratory epithelium and both can be used to study mechanisms of eosinophil influx (267–270). The nose and bronchi can be challenged with allergens, chemokines, and a variety of stimuli.

There are a large number of targets and novel drugs that are of interest as therapy for asthma but require evaluation in reliable disease models in human (Table 6). For a number of reasons, NAC is replacing or supplementing the IAC model. It is much easier to recruit subjects with grass pollen allergic rhinitis (quarter of young adults) for nasal allergen studies than it is to find mild asthmatic subjects for an IAC study. In addition, nasal challenge is less clinically stressful than inhaled challenge, and the nose can be more readily sampled than the bronchi. Nasal papers can be used to absorb nasal lining fluid and an hourly series of samples taken to 10-hour post NAC. In this way, the profile of mast cell mediators, as well as Th2 cytokines (IL-4, IL-5, and IL-13) can be established following NAC, giving considerable statistical power when assessing the effects of a new therapy.

A variety of noninvasive techniques can be used to study changes in the nose following challenge (317). Nasal lavages permit studies on the cellular influx and release of cytokines and chemokines (318). Following NAC, the kinetics of eotaxin release has been studies in nasal fluid (319,320). Following topical nasal budesonide, NAC caused decreased levels of granulocyte-macrophage colony-stimulating factor (GM-CSF) and IL-5 in nasal fluids collected on filter paper strips (321). Nasal challenges have also been performed with eotaxin (322) and IL-8 (323). Nasal rhinomanometry and nasal symptoms and health status can also be determined (324,325). Nasal corticosteroids have effects on nasal late reactions (326–328), but it is difficult to characterize a well-defined late response as obtained in the bronchi (329).

Nasal abnormalities are found in patients with COPD, and especially during exacerbations (330–334). To test new drugs directed against the neutrophil, models of lipopolysaccharide (LPS) nasal challenge are under development (335–338).

Table 6 Novel Drugs and Targets for Asthma and COPD

	Asthma	Severe asthma and COPD
General reviews including cytokine-directed therapy	186,187 (10519) 188,189	25–27 188,271 Treatment of systemic COPD (272)
Novel bronchodilators and ICS	Ultra-LABAs and LAMAs (25, 194–196) VIP, PGE2, ANP, KCO	Soft and dissociated steroids
Mediator antagonists	Antihistamines Leukotriene modifiers iNOS inhibitors Adenosine antagonists Tryptase inhibitors	
Immunotherapy Costimulator blockade Allergen avoidance Anti-IgE/CD23	Allergy and asthma immunomodulators (23) Peptide immunotherapy (190) CpG (191) CRTH2 (DP2) antagonism (192) MoAB vs. CD28	Allergen avoidance: (193)
IL-4, IL-5, IL-9, IL-13 inhibitors	Soluble IL-4 receptor (213, 214) IL-4 variant (183) IL-9 (273–275) IL-13 (276–278)	
TNF-α-directed therapy	Severe asthma (215, 216) Moderate asthma (218)	Pilot COPD study, $n = 22$ (219) Larger COPD study, $n = 234$ over 6 mo (125) Sarcoidosis (220)
Other cytokine-directed therapy and targets	New cytokine targets in asthma and allergy (23): • IL-10 (279–281) • IL-12 (168, 227) • IL-15 (282) • IL-17/23 (283–287) • IL-18 (288–290) • IL-21 (291, 292) • IL-31 (293) • IL-33 (294)	Therapy directed against fibrosis (295): • PAR1 antagonists (296) • TGF-β (297, 298) • CTGF • PDGF (including imatinib) • IL-13 (278, 299)
Cell surface receptor/kinase targets	CSF or KIT (228): imatinib (229, 300) and R112 (232, 233)	Anti-CD23 (236, 237)

(Continued)

Table 6 Novel Drugs and Targets for Asthma and COPD (*Continued*)

	Asthma	Severe asthma and COPD
Chemokine receptor antagonists	Review (301) CCR3, CCR4, CCR8 CXCR4	CXCR2 CCR2 CXCR3
Adhesion molecule blockers		
PDE4 inhibitors		
Signal transduction and transcription factors	Review (302–304) GATA3 P38MAPK (activates GATA3) IKK2 (NFKB kinase 2) (305–308)	STAT6 is the common transcription factor for IL-4 and IL-13: Inhibitory peptide (244)
Statins		245–249
Lung regeneration for emphysema		Stem cell therapy (254, 255)
New targets	Epithelium (309) TSLP (310–313) Fibrosis (295)	Oxidative stress (314) Resveratrol (315) Matrix metalloproteases (21)
Mucolytics		Mucus secretion review (258)
Anti-sense DNA and siRNA (small interference RNA)	Anti-sense CCR3 and β-chain receptor for IL-3, IL-5, and GM-CSF (260)	RNAi (316)

Abbreviations: COPD, chronic obstructive pulmonary disease; PDE4, phosphodiesterase type 4; IL, interleukin; IFN, interferon; MoAB, monoclonal antibody; GM-CSF, granulocyte-macrophage colony-stimulating factor.

H. Exercise-Induced Asthma

For patients with asthma, the American Thoracic Society (ATS) has issued guidelines for exercise challenge (339). After a two-minute warm-up, patients generally exercise for a six-minute period on a treadmill while inhaling compressed dry air at room temperature through a facemask, with a noseclip in place. Exercise is performed at a level that increases the heart rate to 80% to 90% of the age predicted maximum. Spirometry is then performed at intervals up to 90 minutes after exercise, with the area under the curve (AUC) estimated for the first 60 minutes after challenge. Leukotriene antagonists have been demonstrated to be effective in exercise-induced bronchoconstriction (340–342). However, H_1-receptor antagonism with loratidine does not protect against exercise-induced bronchoconstriction (343,344).

I. Symptomatic Asthma

A range of recent studies have documented effects of anti-leukotrienes on patients with symptomatic mild-to-moderate asthma that are on inhaled β_2-agonists only (339). These study designs provide a more clinically relevant "wild-type" population for studying potential efficacy than utilizing an allergen challenge. An important study was to demonstrate that regular use of an ICS (budesonide) is superior to regular use of inhaled β_2-agonist (terbutaline) (345), but that discontinuation of therapy is often accompanied by exacerbation of asthma (346). Convincing efficacy of ICS can be demonstrated in groups of less than 12 symptomatic patients within four weeks of therapy (347,348).

J. Studies with Inhaled Corticosteroids

A whole range of important clinical studies are still being performed on ICS themselves; these address questions such as dose-response finding (348–351), the possibility of once-a-day steroids, establishing a therapeutic index (350,351) and effects on bones and growth (352). Acute anti-inflammatory effects of inhaled budesonide can be demonstrated by a single dose of 2500 µg (353).

K. Corticosteroid Add-on Studies

Since many patients with asthma are treated with ICS, it is important to consider a range of trial designs in these subjects. Theophylline and montelukast have been studied as add-on agents in asthmatics already receiving inhaled and oral corticosteroids (354,359). A major clinical development in the past decade is the recognition of "add-on" therapy with long-acting β_2-agonists and moderate doses of ICS (355) and the availability of combination products with these agents in a single inhaler (356,357). The leukotriene antagonists have been demonstrated to be of lesser efficacy than long-acting β_2-agonists as add-on therapy (358,359).

L. Corticosteroid Titration Studies

Corticosteroid titration is a system for stepwise reduction in the dose of ICS (360,361). Patients with asthma may need to be screened for this type of study, since only some asthmatics become immediately symptomatic on decreasing their dose of inhaled steroids. Many asthmatics will remain nonsymptomatic even on complete withdrawal of ICS, but can suddenly have an exacerbation due to infection, allergen, or other triggers. In patients with COPD, ICS withdrawal studies have also been carried out (101,102).

M. Corticosteroid Abrupt Discontinuation Studies

Soluble IL-4 receptor (Nuvance, Immunex Corp., Seattle, Washington, U.S.) binds IL-4 before it can bind to the cell receptor, suppressing IgE production by B cells and eosinophil migration into the airways. Inhaled Nuvance proved very promising in preliminary studies involving abrupt withdrawal of ICS in patients with asthma (213,214), but larger-scale clinical studies in both mild and moderate asthma were discontinued in 2001 because of lack of efficacy. Discontinuation of inhaled fluticasone in COPD has been shown to cause higher risk of exacerbations (362).

N. Severe Asthma

Patients with severe asthma have disease involving more fixed airways obstruction, airways remodeling, and a tendency for neutrophilic as well as eosinophilic and IgE-mediated disease. A chimeric MoAB against CD4 has recently been shown to be effective in chronic severe asthma (235).

Clinical studies have been carried out in patients with severe asthma to assess cyclosporin A (363) and recently with anti-IgE (112–114,364). Novel therapies in the future will need to be tested on patients receiving both ICS and long-acting β2-agonists. This is because combined use of inhaled steroids and inhaled long-acting β2-agonists is now established as therapy for moderate persistent asthma (40).

O. Natural History and Disease Modification

It is a major challenge to study long-term effects of drugs on the airways in the context of structural changes in the airways that comprise airways remodeling (365–367). Current asthma therapy is palliative and neither curative nor disease modifying, and only a minority of asthmatics achieve a long-lasting remission (368). There are considerable ethical and clinical trial issues in studying the influence of immunomodulatory agents in the context of allergen and peptide immunotherapy. Agents such as IL-12, CpG oligodeoxynucleotides, and *Mycobacterium vaccae* (SRL 172) have potential as adjuvants, but therapy may be required in childhood for genetically susceptible individuals in the context of allergen therapy (369–371). As with disease-modifying anti-rheumatoid drugs (DMARDs), it is important to demonstrate disease modification in terms of prolonged efficacy following cessation of treatment.

So far no therapeutic intervention except for smoking cessation has been shown to reduce the rate of loss of lung function in COPD (372). Studies on the natural history of COPD involve monitoring postbronchodilator FEV_1 in considerable numbers of patients over a number of years. Four major studies have recently been performed on effects of ICS on the longitudinal decline in postbronchodilator FEV_1 in patients with mild (96,99) or moderate-to-severe COPD for over three years (97,98,373). Although effects on FEV_1 are modest, ICS are effective in preventing exacerbations in the moderate-to-severe group and cause improvement in health status. The European points to consider on COPD studies suggest that studies on symptomatic relief should be for at least six months, while to claim that a therapy prevents disease progression will require prolonged studies (38). They also suggest that one design to assess effects on disease progression is to randomize patients to continue or stop treatment after a long period of treatment and then examine the rapidity and extent at which benefit is lost. Design strategies for longitudinal spirometry have recently been elegantly reviewed (374).

P. Weight Loss and Muscle Wasting in COPD

There is increasing evidence for a role for tumor necrosis factor (TNF)-α in asthma (375), and a soluble TNF receptor construct (Nuvance, Immunex) and a MoAB (Remicade, Centocor, Pennsylvania, U.S.) are licensed for use in severe rheumatoid arthritis and Crohn's disease (376). These agents are attractive candidates as add-ons for severe asthma as well as the treatment of cachexia associated with COPD. Should efficacy be demonstrated in proof of concept studies, synthetic low molecular weight chemicals could be used to target TNF-α. Wouters and colleagues have performed extensive studies on subjects with weight loss and nutritional depletion in patients with COPD (377–380). Indeed it would be possible to study relatively small numbers of well-defined patients with extrapulmonary systemic nutritional depletion in clinical trials.

Q. Exacerbations in Asthma: Prevention and Treatment

At present we do not have a universally accepted definition of an exacerbation of asthma (381,382). The FACET study with inhaled formoterol is an important example of a large-scale 12-month study that prospectively studied exacerbations of asthma (383,384). A humanized anti-IgE MoAB (Xolair, Novartis-Genentech) is the first biotechnology product to be licensed for treatment of severe asthma (385). Subcutaneous injections of recombinant human anti-IgE (rhuMAb-E25) have now completed a range of studies in moderate-to-severe asthma that have noted efficacy in terms of prevention of exacerbations and a decreased need for oral and inhaled steroids (112–114,364). Anti-IgE causes a reduction in the early and late phases following allergen challenge and decreased eosinophil counts in the sputum (167).

Treatment of emergency asthma is a distinct clinical need with a requirement for more rapidly acting therapy, since hospitalization generally occurs for a period of at least four days (386). Children with acute severe asthma should be treated with oral prednisone and not ICS (387). Therapies that target TNF have the potential to cause rapid onset of anti-inflammatory effects in emergency asthma. It is important to stress that asthmatics may be vulnerable to exacerbations even when asthma is brought under control (388).

An interesting design to assess the effects of therapy in *preventing* exacerbations in COPD was to employ inhaled fluticasone propionate for six months over the winter in COPD patients with a history of at least one winter exacerbation per year for the past three years (100). In addition, ICS have been demonstrated to prevent exacerbations in a three-year study on patients with moderate-to-severe COPD (97).

With regard to *treatment* of exacerbations, there has been documented moderate improvement in clinical outcome when using oral prednisolone or nebulized budesonide (389,390). However, a major disappointment was that a clinical study on treatment of exacerbations of COPD with recombinant human DNase (dornase alfa, Genentech Inc., San Francisco, California, U.S.) had to be stopped, since a trend for increased mortality was noted on interim analysis (259).

IV. Clinical Endpoints
A. Lung Function

PEF and FEV_1 are fundamental to the monitoring of patients with asthma (391–393). With the advent of hand-held portable electronic lung function meters combined with clinical diaries, it is now possible to perform more reliable home monitoring of PEF, FEV_1, and forced vital capacity (FVC).

FEV_1 has long been established as a major outcome measure in the monitoring of patients with COPD (394–397). There are, however, limitations in the use of this measurement, since changes in FEV_1 over time are small in relation to repeatability of the measurement. Thus, it can take serial measurements over several years to demonstrate a declining trend in FEV_1 in one individual. In addition, the earliest changes in smokers' lungs occur in the peripheral airways (398), and may already be present while the FEV_1 remains normal. At present, post bronchodilator FEV_1 is commonly measured in studies of the effects of drugs on the natural history of COPD, but new endpoints such as systemic features and exacerbation parameters are commonly employed.

Several investigators have attempted to identify sensitive tests of small airways function (maximum mid-expiratory flow, MMEF) that may be used to monitor progression of smoking-related lung disease. Unfortunately, it has been found that the reproducibility of the majority of these tests is low, and, in the main, abnormalities of these tests do not appear to predict the subsequent development of clinically significant airflow obstruction (399–401). Indices of the presence of emphysema include measurements reflecting air trapping (increased total lung capacity, functional residual capacity, and residual volume) and loss of alveolar-capillary membrane [transfer factor, TLCO (Europe) or DLCO (United States)] (393). These tests may be useful in individual patient assessments, but have been shown to correlate weakly with prognosis.

Measurement of exercise dynamic hyperinflation and exercise endurance, together with health-related quality of life and subjective measurement of dyspnea are important additional measures of bronchodilator efficacy in COPD (300,402,403). In addition, reduction in dyspnea following inhalation of β_2-agonists is closely correlated with the forced inspiratory volume in one second (FIV$_1$) (404).

B. Symptom Diary Scores and Asthma Control Questionnaires

Daytime and nocturnal asthma symptom diaries have been found to be appropriate for use as outcome measures in clinical trials of asthma therapy (405). These symptom diaries can now be recorded on portable electronic devices that also include lung function. The Asthma Control Questionnaire (ACQ) consists of seven questions and has strong evaluative properties (406). Daily symptom diaries have been used to a lesser extent in studies on patients with COPD.

C. Health Status

Health status has become a major feature of studies in COPD (407). The St. George's Respiratory Questionnaire (SGRQ) is a standardized self-completed questionnaire for measuring HRQOL in airways disease (54,408). The final version has 76 items divided into three sections: "symptoms," "activity," and "impacts" and provides a total score. Scores range from 0 (perfect health) to 100 (worst possible state), with a four-point change in score considered a worthwhile treatment effect. The SGRQ and the Chronic Respiratory Disease Questionnaire (CRDQ) have been found equivalent in a comparative study (409). Generic questionnaires have a place in COPD studies, but are relatively insensitive, and include the Sickness Impact Profile (SIP) and SF-36 (410).

The Asthma Quality of Life Questionnaire (AQLQ) has 32 questions and takes 5 to 10 minutes to complete (411). In mild asthma, symptom diary scores have been found less sensitive than the AQLQ and SGRQ (412,413). More recently a standardized version, the AQLQ(S), comprising five generic activities instead of five patient-specific activities, has been validated in asthma (414).

D. Airway Hyperresponsiveness

The classical methods of assessment of AHR are to establish the provocative concentration required to cause a 20% fall (PC$_{20}$) in FEV$_1$ to inhaled histamine or methacholine. Both agents cause direct constriction of airway smooth muscle and are said to reflect nonspecific AHR. Guidelines have been published by the ATS for methacholine bronchoprovocation (339), and commercial sources of methacholine produced by Good Manufacturing Practice (GMP) are available.

AMP is a purine nucleoside that causes bronchoconstriction by indirect mediator release from human mast cells (415,416), since it is unlikely that AMP acts on smooth muscle cells in vivo (417). AMP reactivity has been usefully employed in clinical trials with ICS (418,419) and effects of even a single inhaled dose can be demonstrated (349,353,420). AMP is not currently available as GMP material, but mannitol has recently become available as a useful kit to measure airway reactivity (421,422), and reactivity to mannitol and AMP are closely related (423,424).

E.   Exercise Testing in COPD: 6MWT, ISWT, ESWT

For the design of studies on exercise-induced asthma, see earlier in this chapter. The ATS has published recent guidelines for the six-minute walk test (6MWT), since this is an important component in the functional assessment of patients with COPD (61,425). The 6MWT is performed indoors on a long, flat, straight corridor of at least 30 m in length, and the use of a treadmill is not recommended. It has been found that the 6MWT is easier to administer and more reflective of activities of daily living than other walk tests (426). The 12-level incremental shuttle walking test (ISWT) provokes a symptom limited maximal performance exercise, but it uses an audio signal from a tape cassette to guide the speed of walking of the patient back and forth between two traffic cones on a 10-m course (427,428). The shuttle walking test has an incremental and progressive structure to assess functional capacity, and maximum heart rates are significantly higher than that for the 6MWT. The endurance shuttle walk test (ESWT) also uses a 10-m course, but has an externally controlled constant walking speed (429).

F.   Dynamic Hyperinflation

Dynamic lung hyperinflation has been shown to improve after bronchodilator therapy in COPD (430,431). Dyspnea ratings and measurements of inspiratory capacity and endurance time are highly reproducible and responsive to change in disease status (432).

G.   High-Resolution Computerized Tomography

High-resolution computerized tomography (HRCT) is defined as thin section CT (1–2 mm collimation scans), whereas spiral (helical) CT provides continuous scanning while the patient is moved through the CT gantry. HRCT is useful in studies on patients with COPD to assess the extent of airway, interstitial, and vascular diseases (433); as well as detecting bronchiectasis (434) and early cancerous lesions. HRCT is sufficiently sensitive to monitor longitudinal changes in the extent of emphysema (435–437), and it has been shown that annual changes in lung density and percentage of low attenuation area are detectable with inspiratory HRCT (438). Inflammatory infiltration of the lung parenchyma is associated with ground glass attenuation, bronchiolitis can be visualized as parenchymal micronodules, bronchial wall thickening may occur, and emphysema is indicated by areas of decreased attenuation. Progression from parenchymal micronodules (bronchiolitis) to emphysema has been demonstrated in a proportion of smokers over five years (439,440). It appears that subtle changes in progression of lung disease related to α_1-antitrypsin deficiency may be more readily detected with CT imaging than with pulmonary function testing (441,442), and with α_1-antitrypsin augmentation therapy annual CT has proved useful in disease assessment (443,444). In addition, quantitative CT has also been used as an outcome measure in a study of all-*trans*-retinoic acid (ATRA) therapy (445). Finally, HRCT can be used to visualize the small airways and interstitium (446,447), and has been used in studies on patients with asthma (448,449). Nevertheless, there are considerable challenges in the standardization of CT and in the development of methodology for image processing and analysis.

H.   Muscle Testing

An ATS/ERS statement has recently been made on respiratory muscle testing (450). Cellular adaptations in the diaphragm have been reported in COPD (451,452), and skeletal muscle apoptosis can occur in conjunction with cachexia in COPD (453,454), with weakness and dysfunction of voluntary skeletal muscle (455–457). Mid-thigh muscle cross-sectional area is found to be a predictor of mortality in COPD (458).

I. BODE Score

The body mass index (BMI), airflow obstruction, dyspnea, and exercise capacity index (BODE) has been found to be better than FEV_1 at predicting the risk of death from any cause and from respiratory causes in patients with COPD (459). Furthermore, longitudinal changes in the index predict mortality in severe COPD (460). A modified BODE index replaces the 6MWT with peak oxygen uptake (VO_2) and this simpler index has recently been introduced (461).

J. Mortality

In severe COPD, mortality is an important endpoint, and the recent TORCH study with combined fluticasone and salmeterol in a single inhaler has utilized mortality as a primary endpoint (108,109). FEV_1 was originally considered to correlate with mortality in COPD (462). However, weight loss and particularly loss of fat-free mass are independently unfavorable for survival of COPD patients (378), as reflected in the BODE score, a useful predictor of mortality from respiratory causes in patients with COPD (459). Furthermore, the regular use of low-dose ICS is associated with a decreased risk of death from asthma (463).

V. Biomarkers

A biomarker is a characteristic that is objectively measured and evaluated as an indicator of a disease process, and a more complete definition has been provided by the U.S. National Institute of Health (NIH) in 2001 (57). There has recently been a major focus by academics, the pharmaceutical industry, and formation of consortia (464–467). There is an especial need for biomarkers for COPD, and this has been addressed by an ATS/ERS Task Force (71) and by the Evaluation of COPD Longitudinally to Identify Predictive Surrogate Endpoints (ECLIPSE) (468). Characterization of the severe asthma phenotype is within an National Heart Lung and Blood Institute (NHLBI) research program (469), while the Global Allergy and Asthma European Network (470) has a range of biomarker and phenotype issues to study (471).

A. Blood Analysis

Pharmacokinetics

Peripheral blood tests are generally performed in phases I and II of drug development for pharmacokinetics evaluation of the amount of drug substance and its metabolites in the blood. Before the end of phase III it is usual to have established absorption, distribution, metabolism, and excretion (ADME) profiles for oral drugs, although for inhaled drugs distribution in the lung is often more relevant than systemic exposure.

Pharmacodynamics

The utility of pharmacokinetic/pharmacodynamic modeling can be illustrated by taking the example of a hypothetical chemokine antagonist, since a large range of oral compounds have been developed against the numerous chemokine receptors. In relation to allergy and asthma, the chemokine C-C receptor 3 (CCR3) is an interesting target expressed on a range of cells including eosinophils and activated Th2 cells, and a range of synthetic low molecular weight chemicals have been developed that antagonize this receptor (472). Clinical testing of CCR3 antagonists can be performed in terms of whole blood flow cytometric assays to establish the pharmacodynamic duration of chemotactic inhibitory activity on eosinophils. The GAFS (gated autofluorescence forward scatter) assay makes use of the changes seen in the forward scatter of light due to eosinophil shape change in response to chemokines (473,474). It can be used in laboratory screening in the preclinical workup, when dose-response curves can be determined on volunteer or macaque monkey blood to which the novel CCR3 antagonist is added ex vivo, and then the response to a specific stimulus determined (475). The assay can then be used in clinical studies for assisting dose range finding, since serial whole blood samples taken following CCR3 antagonist ingestion can be stimulated ex vivo to give sequential pharmacodynamic capacity. Since the pharmacodynamics can last longer than the pharmacokinetics (hysteresis), this assay will be useful in monitoring the lasting effects of chemokine antagonists on leukocytes in the blood even if the drug is no longer detectable in the plasma.

In the case of PDE4 inhibitors, whole blood stimulation assays (e.g., LPS-induced neutrophil upregulation (476), or LPS-induced TNF-α production) would permit the positioning of levels of systemic efficacy in peripheral blood relative to drug doses that may cause a side effect such as nausea.

Blood Biomarkers in Asthma

It is very frustrating that a whole range of studies have demonstrated peripheral blood immunological abnormalities in asthma, yet these parameters have been little used in the assessment of new therapies. In asthma it is possible to assess inflammation in blood by measuring parameters reflecting eosinophilic inflammation (477): eosinophil numbers, hypodense eosinophils, eosinophil cationic protein (ECP), and plasma cytokines associated with eosinophils (IL-5 and RANTES) (478).

A range of studies have shown peripheral blood T-cell inflammation in asthma and allergy (479).

- Surface marker studies demonstrated T-cell activation in peripheral blood through increased expression of CD25 and HLA-DR (480,481). Recently, blood from allergic subjects has been shown to have a Th2-like signature (IL-4, -5, -9, and -13) on microarray (482), and BAL T cells in atopic asthma have a Th2 phenotype (483). IL-13 stimulation of blood cells in conjunction with microarray has been used to define potential biomarkers (484).
- Peripheral blood Tregs and regulatory NK cells have been studied in relation to allergy and immunotherapy (485–487). A recent longitudinal study has studied T-cell activation in blood and sputum in asthma, showing decreased numbers and activity of Tregs during exacerbations (488).
- Th17 cells have been studied in human blood (489), sputum (490), and BAL (491). IL-17 may be a critical mediator in severe neutrophilic asthma (492), and in mice it is a negative regulator of established allergic asthma (493).

Blood Biomarkers in COPD
A range of peripheral blood abnormalities are found in COPD.

- Neutrophil chemotaxis (494), oxidative burst (495) adhesion molecules are increased (496).
- C-reactive protein (CRP) is slightly elevated in stable COPD populations (497), and this can be lowered by inhaled and oral corticosteroids (498). CRP becomes more elevated during COPD exacerbations (332,499).
- IL-6 and IL-8 are not reliably elevated in plasma during COPD exacerbations (500).
- Protein microarray platform (PMP) technology has been used to profile 143 serum biomarkers in patients with COPD, and associations made with a selected panel of 24 biomarkers and FEV_1 and BODE score (501). Prominent markers of COPD were Th1 cytokines (IL-12, TNF-α, IFN-γ), chemokines (ITAC, eotaxin-2, IL-8), markers of repair (MMP-9, TIMP-1, VEGF), and novel markers (PA1-11 and prolactin).
- After in vitro stimulation of peripheral blood neutrophils from COPD patients, there is increased gene array signal for a range of cytokines [including IL-1β and IL-8 (502)].
- Smokers with preserved lung function have increased BAL (not blood) Tregs than COPD patients (503). COPD patients have BAL T cells with a Tc-2 profile (IL-4/10/13) (504).

B. Exhaled Breath

Exhaled NO has been extensively studied since levels of this gas were found to be increased in asthma (505,506). Standardized measurements of fractional exhaled NO (FE_{NO}), through differential flow analysis, provides a noninvasive means of monitoring of airway inflammation and anti-inflammatory treatment in asthma (507,508). Differential flow analysis of FE_{NO} in adults with asthma has been used to measure alveolar NO and in this way distal inflammation has been demonstrated in refractory asthma (509–511). Exhaled NO has been the subject of an ATS/ERS Task Force (63) and has potential application in asthma, although this remains controversial (512,513).

Changes in serial FE_{NO} have higher predictive values for diagnosing deterioration of asthma (514) than single measurements (515,516). Reproducibility of FE_{NO} measurements within a single day in both adults (ICC 0.94) and children (ICC 0.94) is superior to any conventional methods of airway inflammation monitoring in asthma. This adds significantly to other advantages of FE_{NO} measurements, such as their strong association with airway inflammation (517), elevation even in nonsymptomatic asthma patients (518), high sensitivity to steroid treatment (519), and insensitivity to β_2-agonists (517).

Dose range finding is an important issue in the development of new therapies, and there is high sensitivity and reproducibility of FE_{NO} measurements in relation to inhaled corticosteroids. Recently, a dose-dependent onset of anti-inflammatory action of inhaled corticosteroids has been demonstrated on FE_{NO} and asthma symptoms in a small number of mild asthma patients (520,521). Long-term prospective clinical studies have shown that FE_{NO} can be used to guide inhaled steroid therapy ion chronic asthma (512).

The technical issues involved in exhaled breath condensate (EBC) analysis have been the subject of a recent review by an ATS/ERS Task Force (64). Within this document there is a list of the many factors that affect the collection of EBC. The Task Force also considers the source of EBC. Much of EBC consists of water vapor that may arise from the respiratory tract and ambient air, and mixing droplets of proteinaceous fluid with large volumes of water may cause proteins to precipitate. Volatiles are largely present as gaseous vapors, while proteins are present in droplets that may be derived from the large airways and oropharynx.

It is important to establish intra-assay and inter-assay reproducibility (coefficients of variation and Bland-Altman test), sensitivity (lower limit of detection) and specificity, dilution factors and contamination influences of EBC measures (63). A detailed validation of assays for inflammatory mediators in EBC found that levels of EBC mediators are generally below the level of assay detection (outside the straight line part of the sigmoid standard curve (522).

When measuring EBC, there are variability and other issues due to influences from the following factors:

- Ambient inspired air (523)
- Condensed water vapor causing dilution (524,525)
- Saliva (526–528)
- Dietary factors (529)
- Oropharyngeal flora (529)
- Breath condenser coatings (530)

EBC may be particularly helpful in the situation of lung cancer where proteins specific to the malignancy may be detectable in breath (531,532), could be analyzed from a bronchoscope, or form an intubated patient. In a detailed cross-sectional analysis of EBC in patients with COPD and control healthy smokers, no statistical differences were found between levels of EBC mediators (ERS Munich 2007, poster from I Kilty and colleagues).

C. Sputum Analysis

The analysis of induced sputum is employed as a relatively noninvasive method to measure inflammation in a range of respiratory diseases. Induction of sputum by the inhalation of nebulized hypertonic saline has been shown to be a safe and effective method in asthma (533), COPD (534), and sarcoidosis (535). Despite being derived from different compartments, inflammatory cell counts in asthma are related in sputum, BAL, and biopsies (536,537). Reflecting the increasing importance of sputum analysis, an European Respiratory Society (ERS) Task Force has published a detailed review of the literature and standardized methodology for sputum induction and processing (65,538).

In terms of assessment of cells, measuring the sputum eosinophil percentage and count on induced sputum leukocyte differential has been extensively performed in asthma (539,540). In clinical practice, a treatment strategy aimed at normalization of the induced sputum eosinophil count has been shown to reduce asthma exacerbations without the need for additional anti-inflammatory therapy (541). In addition, analysis of induced sputum has been employed in older children with asthma (542–545).

However, although the sputum eosinophil count is established as a biomarker in asthma, the analysis of sputum inflammatory mediators—including cytokines and chemokines—has been problematic. Problems with sampling induced sputum include it being derived from a particular compartment of the airways and the variable expectoration of this material mixed with saliva. Within the inspissated sputum sample material there is commonly microbial contamination, with variable amounts of mucous and proteases. The presence of dead and dying cells can potentially result in intracellular proteins being released into the extracellular phase.

There have been four recent important studies in COPD:

- In a large study on patients with stable COPD ($n = 140$), Seretide was shown to decrease the sputum neutrophil percentage (111).
- In a longitudinal study of 56 patients with chronic bronchitis studied over four years, sputum myeloperoxidase (MPO) correlated with decline in FEV_1 while sputum IL-8 correlated with progression of lung densitometry CT changes.
- In the context of a repeatability study using spontaneously expectorated sputum, it has been estimated that for a putative therapy that causes a 50% fall in neutrophil count, 23 patients would be required with three data points in a two-way cross-over design (546).
- In exacerbations of COPD, there is elevation of sputum neutrophilia and IL-8 (332,547)

A number of groups have reported elevated levels of IL-8 in induced sputum from asthmatics (548–550); while TNF-α, GRO-α, MCP-1, and IL-8 are elevated in COPD (548,551,552). MMP-9 and TIMP-1 molar ratios have been studied in the sputum of patients with mild asthma in response to inhaled fluticasone (553).

Dithiothreitol (DTT) is effective for liquefaction of sputum, releasing cells and permitting cytospin preparations to determine the cell differential. However, the reducing and denaturant effects of DTT, especially in breaking disulfide bonds, diminish the detectable levels of mediators in immunoassay (554,555). A comprehensive table summarizing the effects of DTT on inflammatory proteins has been published (556). Effects of DTT have been shown to be variable depending on the soluble mediator being studied (554), and DTT has also been shown to affect cell surface marker levels (557,558). In addition, elegant work on the validity of fluid phase detection of IL-5 has demonstrated that in induced sputum there is a problem with proteases as opposed to DTT in causing decreased detectable levels (559) and that IL-5 levels can be significantly increased by adding protease inhibitors (560).

Removal of DTT by dialysis of sputum supernatants has been employed to measure IL-13 in induced sputum supernatants from subjects with mild and severe asthma (561,562), but IL-13 was not detected in COPD (563). In addition, optimized dialysis and protease inhibition of sputum DTT supernatants has been used to increase detectable levels of a range of chemokines and cytokines in sputum (564). Dialysis removes low molecular weight DTT, and this facilitates the reforming of disulfide bonds in sputum proteins, increasing detectable levels of some mediators. However, dialysis is a cumbersome, time-consuming, and variable process.

Various physical methods of sputum processing would escape the effects of DTT, and have included homogenization (565), ultracentrifugation (548,566,567), and ultrasonication (546,565,568,569) prior to analysis of levels of soluble mediators including cytokines and chemokines. If sputum is solubilized with either phosphate buffered saline (PBS) or DTT or DNAse-alpha, there are differences in detectable levels of mediators (570). Sputum proteomics (mass spectroscopy) have been employed successfully in inflammatory and suppurative respiratory diseases: COPD, CF, and bronchiectasis, all have elevated calgranulins A to C (571).

D. Bronchoscopy

Conventional flexible bronchoscopy is normally performed on patients with respiratory disease to perform BAL, mucosal biopsy, and bronchial brushings. This gives important mechanistic insight into the evaluation of inflammation in asthma (66,67,572). An European Society Task Force has issued guidelines for measurements of acellular components and standardization of BAL (573). However, BAL sampling has the major problem of unknown dilution and variable yield that makes accurate detection and quantification of soluble mediators difficult. In our study proposal, we shall perform bronchoscopy within British Thoracic Society (BTS) guidelines (574), using American College of Chest Physicians (ACCP) guidance to prevent infection (575). Bronchoscopy has been shown to be safe when performed by trainees on pulmonary fellowship programs (576), and bronchoscopy with bronchial thermoplasty has been recently safely performed in symptomatic severe asthma (577). Dilution and failure to retrieve is a major problem with BAL (578) and fever is an acknowledged complication (579).

Studies with BAL and mucosal bronchial biopsy are important mechanistic studies for the evaluation of anti-inflammatory therapies for asthma and COPD (572,580). An European Society Task Force has issued guidelines for measurements of acellular components and standardization of BAL (573), while the reproducibility of endobronchial biopsy has been established (581). Fluticasone has been shown to lack effects on neutrophils and CD8+ T cells in biopsies from patients with COPD, but have subtle effects on mast cells (582). Fluticasone has had more convincing effects on biopsies from patients with asthma, reducing eosinophils, macrophages, and T cells (583,584). There is high reproducibility of repeat measures of airway inflammation in stable atopic asthma (581), and the area of BAL-based biomarkers in asthma has been reviewed by Zhang and Wenzel (580).

Bronchoscopic microsampling (BMS) is a new procedure for bronchoscopic diagnosis, capable of collecting local bronchial epithelial lining fluid (ELF) that utilizes a polyester fiber probe in a polyethylene hollow sheath (585–587). The polyester fiber rod of diameter 1.1 mm is placed on the bronchial wall for 15 seconds, and becomes moist, obtaining an average of 18 μL of ELF. BMS is performed while observing the bronchial lumen using a fiberoptic bronchoscope; when the target site is reached, the probe is pushed out of the sheath tip and absorbs bronchial epithelial fluid present in the bronchial lumen.

Applications of BMS:

- Acute respiratory distress syndrome (ARDS): increased levels of endothelin-1, IL-6, neutrophil elastase, KL-6 (585,586,588).
- Bacterial respiratory infection diagnosis (589)
- Small peripheral lung carcinoma (590)
- Measurement of local drug levels (pharmacokinetic) (591–593)
- In COPD there is a single report on BMS of increased levels of xanthine oxidase (XO), TNF-α, IL-1β, and IFN-γ (587)
- In asthma the probe causes bleeding due to epithelial fragility and increased vascularization.

E. Genetics, Gene Expression, and Systems Biology

There is current evidence that most polymorphisms related to asthma determine risk for disease in the context of other genes and the environment (594,595). Position cloning has identified genes such as ADAM 33 (596,597), PHF11, DPP10, HLA-G, and G protein–related receptor for asthma (GPRA) (598,599). Airway epithelium may be important for barrier defense with DPP10, GPRA, and SPINK5 (600,601). Nucleotide-binding oligomerization domain protein 1 (NOD-1) polymorphisms have been associated with asthma (602) and atopic eczema (603). In addition, genetic variants regulating ORMDL3 expression have been found to contribute to the risk of childhood asthma (604). Recently a genome wide association study of global gene expression in asthma has been published (605).

Microarray technology has exciting potential for research into mechanisms of allergy and lung disease. Gene profiling has been performed on nasal cells in allergic rhinitis (606), in skin lesions from atopic dermatitis and psoriasis (607), and in asthma (608,609). Gene expression profiling techniques have identified increased arachidonate 15-lipoxygenase (ALOX 15) and fractalkine receptor (CX3CR1) in asthma (610).

The genetics and genomics of COPD has been moving forward fast (611–613). A recent study of resected peripheral lung tissue from COPD patients showed decreased expression of antioxidant enzymes and increased expression of chemokines (614). The U.S. National Emphysema Treatment Trial (NETT) has performed genome-wide analysis to lead to the identification of two promising candidate genes for COPD, TGFB1 and SERPINE2 (612).

Pharmacogenetics studies have increasing relevance to the practice of medicine (615) and potential utility for clinical studies in patients with asthma (616,617). Multiple single-nucleotide polymorphisms (SNPs) in the β-adrenoceptor of smooth muscle influence responses to β-agonist (618), and the pharmacogenetics of this receptor is now well profiled (619). Abnormalities in the ALOX5 gene for leukotriene metabolism caused decreased responses to a 5-lipoxygenase (5LO) inhibitor (620), and variation in the TNF-α promoter may influence response TNF-α-directed therapy (621).

VI. Conclusion

Translating advances in basic research into the clinic as new therapies is an international priority for respiratory and other diseases (622,623). This is recognized by a U.S. initiative involving the NIH through the Clinical and Translational Science Awards (CTSAs) (624), in Europe there is the Innovative Medicines Initiative (625), and United Kingdom is setting up Biomedical Research Centers (BMRCs) (626). More specifically, GlaxoSmithKline is funding a three-year longitudinal study in 2180 COPD subjects entitled "Evaluation of COPD Longitudinally to Identify Predictive Surrogate Endpoints" (ECLIPSE), and the ATS/ERS Task Force recognizes the complexity of outcomes for COPD patients in pharmacological studies (71). It is a major disappointment that advances in genetics and our understanding of disease processes have resulted in relatively few new therapies being tested in man. The last decade has seen considerable advances in pharmacokinetic and pharmacodynamic evaluation of new drugs, with new clinical pharmacology models, novel biomarkers, and more precise dose range finding. With specific biologics, we can expect clinical studies to involve "niche pharmacology" through assessment of genotypes and phenotypes to identify potential responders to specific therapies. In the future, there are real possibilities for the development of preventive and even curative treatments for allergy, although reversal of airways remodeling and alveolar regeneration are more challenging goals.

References

1. Bateman ED, Hurd SS, Barnes PJ, et al. Global strategy for asthma management and prevention: GINA executive summary. Eur Respir J 2008; 31(1):143–178.
2. Braman SS. The global burden of asthma. Chest 2006; 130(1 suppl):4S–12S.
3. Mannino DM, Buist AS. Global burden of COPD: risk factors, prevalence, and future trends. Lancet 2007; 370(9589):765–773.
4. Poole JA, Matangkasombut P, Rosenwasser LJ. Targeting the IgE molecule in allergic and asthmatic diseases: review of the IgE molecule and clinical efficacy. J Allergy Clin Immunol 2005; 115(3):S376–S385.
5. Holgate ST, Djukanovic R, Casale T, et al. Anti-immunoglobulin E treatment with oma-lizumab in allergic diseases: an update on anti-inflammatory activity and clinical efficacy. Clin Exp Allergy 2005; 35:408–416.
6. Calverley PM, Rennard SI. What have we learned from large drug treatment trials in COPD? Lancet 2007; 370(9589):774–785.
7. Fan CK. Phosphodiesterase inhibitors in airways disease. Eur J Pharmacol 2006; 533(1–3): 110–117.
8. Conti M, Beavo J. Biochemistry and physiology of cyclic nucleotide phosphodiesterases: essential components in cyclic nucleotide signaling. Annu Rev Biochem 2007; 76:481–511.
9. Compton CH, Gubb J, Nieman R, et al. Cilomilast, a selective phosphodiesterase-4 inhibitor for treatment of patients with chronic obstructive pulmonary disease: a randomised, dose-ranging study. Lancet 2001; 358(9278):265–270.
10. Gamble E, Grootendorst DC, Brightling CE, et al. Antiinflammatory effects of the phos-phodiesterase-4 inhibitor cilomilast (ariflo) in chronic obstructive pulmonary disease. Am J Respir Crit Care Med 2003; 168(8):976–982.
11. Rennard SI, Schachter N, Strek M, et al. Cilomilast for COPD: results of a 6-month, placebo-controlled study of a potent, selective inhibitor of phosphodiesterase 4. Chest 2006; 129(1):56–66.
12. Giembycz MA. An update and appraisal of the cilomilast phase III clinical development pro-gramme for chronic obstructive pulmonary disease. Br J Clin Pharmacol 2006; 62(2):138–152.
13. van Schalkwyk EM, van Heerden K, Bredenbroker D, et al. Dose-dependent inhibitory effect of roflumilast, a new, orally active, selective phosphodieterase 4 inhibitor, on allergen-induced early and late asthmatic reaction. Eur Resp J 2002; 20:110S.
14. Louw C, Williams Z, Venter L, et al. Roflumilast, a phosphodiesterase 4 inhibitor, reduces airway hyperresponsiveness after allergen challenge. Respiration 2007; 74(4):411–417.
15. Bousquet J, Aubier M, Sastre J, et al. Comparison of roflumilast, an oral anti-inflammatory, with beclomethasone dipropionate in the treatment of persistent asthma. Allergy 2006; 61(1): 72–78.
16. Bateman ED, Izquierdo JL, Harnest U, et al. Efficacy and safety of roflumilast in the treatment of asthma. Ann Allergy Asthma Immunol 2006; 96(5):679–686.
17. Albrecht A, Leichtl S, Bredenbroker D, et al. Comparison of Roflumilast, a new orally active, selective phosphodiesterase 4 Inhibitor, with beclomethasone diproprionate in asthma control. Eur Resp J 2002; 20:304S.
18. Timmer W, Leclerc V, Birraux G, et al. The new phosphodiesterase 4 inhibitor roflumilast is efficacious in exercise-induced asthma and leads to suppression of LPS-stimulated TNF-alpha ex vivo. J Clin Pharmacol 2002; 42(3):297–303.
19. Bredenbroker D, Syed J, Leichtl S, et al. Roflumilast, a new orally active, selective phosphodiesterase 4 Inhibitor, is effective in the treatment of chronic obstructive pulmonary disease. Eur Resp J 2002; 20:374S.
20. Rabe KF, Bateman ED, O'Donnell D, et al. Roflumilast—an oral anti-inflammatory treatment for chronic obstructive pulmonary disease: a randomised controlled trial. Lancet 2005; 366(9485):563–571.

21. Calverley PM, Sanchez-Toril F, McIvor A, et al. Effect of 1-year treatment with roflumilast in severe chronic obstructive pulmonary disease. Am J Respir Crit Care Med 2007; 176(2): 154–161.

22. Giembycz MA. Can the anti-inflammatory potential of PDE4 inhibitors be realized: guarded optimism or wishful thinking? Br J Pharmacol 2008; 155(3):288–290.

23. Holgate ST, Polosa R. Treatment strategies for allergy and asthma. Nat Rev Immunol 2008; 8(3):218–230.

24. Hughes B. 2007 FDA drug approvals: a year of flux. Nat Rev Drug Discov 2008; 7(2): 107–109.

25. Bailey WC, Tashkin DP. Pharmacologic therapy: novel approaches for chronic obstructive pulmonary disease. Proc Am Thorac Soc 2007; 4(7):543–548.

26. Yasothan U, Kar S. From the analyst's couch: therapies for COPD. Nat Rev Drug Discov 2008; 7:285–286.

27. Hanania NA, Donohue JF. Pharmacologic interventions in chronic obstructive pulmonary disease: bronchodilators. Proc Am Thorac Soc 2007; 4(7):526–534.

28. Barnes PJ. Immunology of asthma and chronic obstructive pulmonary disease. Nat Rev Immunol 2008; 8(3):183–192.

29. Sin DD, Man SF. Why are patients with chronic obstructive pulmonary disease at increased risk of cardiovascular diseases? The potential role of systemic inflammation in chronic obstructive pulmonary disease. Circulation 2003; 107(11):1514–1519.

30. Hanania NA. Targeting airway inflammation in asthma: current and future therapies. Chest 2008; 133(4):989–998.

31. Barnes PJ. Frontrunners in novel pharmacotherapy of COPD. Curr Opin Pharmacol 2008; 8(3): 300–307.

32. Curtis JL, Freeman CM, Hogg JC. The immunopathogenesis of chronic obstructive pulmonary disease: insights from recent research. Proc Am Thorac Soc 2007; 4(7):512–521.

33. Holgate ST. Pathogenesis of asthma. Clin Exp Allergy 2008; 38(6):872–897.

34. Griffin JP, O'Grady J, eds. The Textbook of Pharmaceutical Medicine. 5th ed. Oxford: Blackwell Publisher, 2006.

35. Wang DL, Bakhai A, eds. Clinical Trials: A Practical Guide to Design, Analysis, and Reporting. London: Remedica, 2005.

36. Directive 2001/20/EC of the European Parliament and of the Council of 4 April 2001 on the approximation of the laws, regulations and administrative provisions of the Member States relating to the implementation of good clinical practice in the conduct of clinical trials on medicinal products for human use. Official J Eur Commun 2001; L121:34–44.

37. The European Agency for the Evaluation of Medicinal Products, Committee for Proprietary Medicinal Products (CPMP).Note for guidance on the clinical investigation of medicinal products in the treatment of asthma. CPMP/EWP/2922/01 2002.

38. EMEA CPMP.Points to consider on clinical investigation of medicinal products in the chronic treatment of patients with chronic obstructive pulmonary disease (COPD). Human Medicines Evaluation Unit, European Medicines Evaluation Agency (EMEA). CPMP/EWP 562/98 1999.

39. U.S. Dept of Health and Human Service, Food and Drug Administration, Center for Drug Evaluation and Research (CDER).Draft Guidance for Industry: Chronic Obstructive Pulmonary Disease. Developing Drugs for Treatment. 2007. Available at: http://www.fda.gov/downloads/Drugs/GuidanceComplianceRegulatoryInformation/Guidances/ucm071575.pdf .

40. National Institutes of Health (NIH), National Heart Lung and Blood Institute (NHLBI).Global Initiative for Asthma (GINA): Global Strategy for Asthma Management and Prevention. Available at: http://www.ginasthma.com/Guidelineitem.asp??l1=2&l2=1&intId=1561.

41. National Institutes of Health (NIH), National Heart Lung and Blood Institute (NHLBI), World Health Organisation (WHO).Global Initiative for Chronic Obstructive Lung Disease (GOLD): Global Strategy for the Diagnosis, Management, and Prevention of Chronic

Obstructive Pulmonary Disease. Available at: http://www.goldcopd.com/GuidelinesResources. asp?l1=2&l2=0.

42. Bousquet J, Van Cauwenberge P, Khalttaev N; the WHO Panel. Allergic rhinitis and its impact on asthma. ARIA. In collaboration with the World Health Organization. J Allergy Clin Immunol 2001; 108:S1–S315.

43. Bousquet J, Van CP, Ait KN, et al. Pharmacologic and anti-IgE treatment of allergic rhinitis ARIA update (in collaboration with GA2LEN). Allergy 2006; 61(9):1086–1096.

44. U.S. Dept of Health and Human Service, Food and Drug Administration, Center for Drug Evaluation and Research (CDER).Allergic Rhinitis: Clinical Development Programs for Drug Products. 2000. Available at: http://www.fda.gov/cder/guidance/index htm.

45. Ministry of Health.Release of Draft Guidance Document: Submission Requirements for Subsequent Market Entry Inhaled Corticosteroid Products for Use in the Treatment of Asthma. File Number: 07-118017-24 2007.

46. European Medicines Agency.Guideline on the requirements for clinical documentations for orally inhaled products (OIP) Including the requirements for demonstration of therapeutic equivalence between two inhaled products for use in the treatment of asthma and chronic obstructive pulmonary disease (COPD). CPMP/EWP/4151/00 Rev 1 2007.

47. Day RO, Chalmers DR, Williams KM, et al. The death of a healthy volunteer in a human research project: implications for Australian clinical research. Med J Aust 1998; 168(9): 449–451.

48. Steinbrook R. Protecting research subjects—the crisis at Johns Hopkins. N Engl J Med 2002; 346(9):716–720.

49. Suntharalingam G, Perry MR, Ward S, et al. Cytokine storm in a phase 1 trial of the anti-CD28 monoclonal antibody TGN1412. N Engl J Med 2006; 355(10):1018–1028.

50. Expert Group on Phase One Clinical Trials (Chairman: Professor Gordon W.Duff).Expert Scientific Group on Phase One Clinical Trials: Final Report. The Stationery Office, U.K. 2006; ISBN 10 0 11 703722 2.

51. Committee for Medicinal Products for Human Use (CHMP).Guideline on requirements for first-in-Man clinical trials for potential high-risk medicinal products (Draft). European Medicines Agency 2007; Doc. Ref.EMEA/CHMP/SWP/28367/2007 Corr.

52. Nelson HS, Weiss ST, Bleecker ER, et al. The Salmeterol Multicenter Asthma Research Trial: a comparison of usual pharmacotherapy for asthma or usual pharmacotherapy plus salmeterol. Chest 2006; 129(1):15–26.

53. Juniper EF, Guyatt GH, Ferrie PJ, et al. Measuring quality of life in asthma. Am Rev Respir Dis 1993; 147(4):832–838.

54. Jones PW, Quirk FH, Baveystock CM. The St George's Respiratory Questionnaire. Respir Med 1991; 85(suppl B):25–31.

55. Mahler DA, Mackowiak JI. Evaluation of the short-form 36-item questionnaire to measure health-related quality of life in patients with COPD. Chest 1995; 107(6):1585–1589.

56. Meltzer EO, Hamilos DL, Hadley JA, et al. Rhinosinusitis: developing guidance for clinical trials. J Allergy Clin Immunol 2006; 118(5 suppl):S17–S61.

57. National Institutes of Health (NIH).Biomarkers and surrogate endpoints: preferred definitions and conceptual framework. Clin Pharmacol Ther 2001; 69(3):89–95.

58. Cazzola M, MacNee W, Martinez FJ, et al. Outcomes for COPD pharmacological trials: from lung function to biomarkers. Eur Respir J 2008; 31(2):416–469.

59. Miller MR, Hankinson J, Brusasco V, et al. Standardisation of spirometry. Eur Respir J 2005; 26(2):319–338.

60. Joos GF, O'Connor B, Anderson SD, et al. Indirect airway challenges. Eur Respir J 2003; 21: 1050–1068.

61. American Thoracic Society.ATS statement: guidelines for the six-minute walk test. Am J Respir Crit Care Med 2002; 166(1):111–117.

62. Palange P, Ward SA, Carlsen KH, et al. Recommendations on the use of exercise testing in clinical practice. Eur Respir J 2007; 29(1):185–209.
63. American Thoracic Society, European Respiratory Society.ATS/ERS recommendations for standardized procedures for the online and offline measurement of exhaled lower respiratory nitric oxide and nasal nitric oxide, 2005. Am J Respir Crit Care Med 2005; 171(8):912–930.
64. Horvath I, Hunt J, Barnes PJ. Exhaled breath condensate: methodological recommendations and unresolved questions. Eur Respir J 2005; 26(3):523–548.
65. Djukanovic R, Sterk PJ, Fahy JV, et al., eds. Standardised methodology of sputum induction and processing. European Respiratory Society Task Force. Eur Respir J 2002; 20(suppl 37): 1s–55s.
66. Busse WW, Wanner A, Adams K, et al. Investigative bronchoprovocation and broncho-scopy in airway diseases. Am J Respir Crit Care Med 2005; 172(7):807–816.
67. Jeffery P, Holgate S, Wenzel S. Methods for the assessment of endobronchial biopsies in clinical research: application to studies of pathogenesis and the effects of treatment. Am J Respir Crit Care Med 2003; 168(6 pt 2):S1–S17.
68. Donaldson GC, Wedzicha JA. COPD exacerbations. 1: Epidemiology. Thorax 2006; 61(2): 164–168.
69. Jones P, Higenbottam T. Quantifying of severity of exacerbations in chronic obstructive pulmonary disease: adaptations to the definition to allow quantification. Proc Am Thorac Soc 2007; 4(8):597–601.
70. O'Reilly JF, Williams AE, Holt K, et al. Defining COPD exacerbations: impact on esti-mation of incidence and burden in primary care. Prim Care Respir J 2006; 15:346–353.
71. Cazzola M, MacNee W, Martinez FJ, et al. Outcomes for COPD pharmacological trials: from lung function to biomarkers. Eur Respir J 2008; 31(2):416–469.
72. Scicchitano R, AAlbers R, Ukena D, et al. Efficacy and safety of budesonide/formoterol single inhaler therapy versus a higher dose of budesonide in moderate to severe asthma. Curr Med Res Opin 2004; 20(9):1403–1418.
73. O'Byrne PM, Bisgaard H, Godard PP, et al. Budesonide/formoterol combination therapy as both maintenance and reliever medication in asthma. Am J Respir Crit Care Med 2005; 171(2): 129–136.
74. Rabe KF, Pizzichini E, Stallberg B, et al. Budesonide/formoterol in a single inhaler for maintenance and relief in mild-to-moderate asthma: a randomized, double-blind trial. Chest 2006; 129(2):246–256.
75. Vogelmeier C, D'Urzo A, Pauwels R, et al. Budesonide/formoterol maintenance and reliever therapy: an effective asthma treatment option? Eur Respir J 2005; 26(5):819–828.
76. Rabe KF, Atienza T, Magyar P, et al. Effect of budesonide in combination with formoterol for reliever therapy in asthma exacerbations: a randomised controlled, double-blind study. Lancet 2006; 368(9537):744–753.
77. Kuna P, Peters MJ, Manjra AI, et al. Effect of budesonide/formoterol maintenance and reliever therapy on asthma exacerbations. Int J Clin Pract 2007; 61(5):725–736.
78. Bousquet J, Boulet LP, Peters MJ, et al. Budesonide/formoterol for maintenance and relief in uncontrolled asthma vs. high-dose salmeterol/fluticasone. Respir Med 2007; 101(12): 2437–2446.
79. Bisgaard H, Le Roux P, Bjamer D, et al. Budesonide/formoterol maintenance plus reliever therapy: a new strategy in pediatric asthma. Chest 2006; 130(6):1733–1743.
80. Dahl R, Kapp A, Colombo G, et al. Efficacy and safety of sublingual immunotherapy with grass allergen tablets for seasonal allergic rhinoconjunctivitis. J Allergy Clin Immunol 2006; 118(2):434–440.
81. Durham SR, Yang WH, Pedersen MR, et al. Sublingual immunotherapy with once-daily grass allergen tablets: a randomized controlled trial in seasonal allergic rhinoconjunctivitis. J Allergy Clin Immunol 2006; 117(4):802–809.

82. Dahl R, Stender A, Rak S. Specific immunotherapy with SQ standardized grass allergen tablets in asthmatics with rhinoconjunctivitis. Allergy 2006; 61(2):185–190.
83. Anzueto A, Tashkin D, Menjoge S, et al. One-year analysis of longitudinal changes in spirometry in patients with COPD receiving tiotropium. Pulm Pharmacol Ther 2005; 18(2):75–81.
84. Seemungal T, Stockley R, Calverley P, et al. Investigating new standards for prophylaxis in reduction of exacerbations—the INSPIRE study methodology. COPD 2007; 4(3):177–183.
85. Wedzicha JA, Calverley PM, Seemungal TA, et al. The prevention of COPD exacerbations by salmeterol/fluticasone propionate or tiotropium bromide. Am J Respir Crit Care Med 2007; 177:19–26.
86. Decramer M, Celli B, Tashkin DP, et al. Clinical trial design considerations in assessing long-term functional impacts of tiotropium in COPD: the Uplift trial. J Chronic Obstruct Pulm Dis 2004; 1:303–312.
87. Tashkin DP. The role of patient-centered outcomes in the course of chronic obstructive pulmonary disease: how long-term studies contribute to our understanding. Am J Med 2006; 119(10 suppl 1):63–72.
88. Bateman ED, Boushey HA, Bousquet J, et al. Can guideline-defined asthma control be achieved? The Gaining Optimal Asthma ControL study. Am J Respir Crit Care Med 2004; 170(8):836–844.
89. Bateman ED, Bousquet J, Keech ML, et al. The correlation between asthma control and health status: the GOAL study. Eur Respir J 2007; 29(1):56–62.
90. Bateman ED, Clark TJ, Frith L, et al. Rate of response of individual asthma control measures varies and may overestimate asthma control: an analysis of the goal study. J Asthma 2007; 44(8):667–673.
91. van Noord JA, Aumann JL, Janssens E, et al. Effects of tiotropium with and without formoterol on airflow obstruction and resting hyperinflation in patients with COPD. Chest 2006; 129(3):509–517.
92. Di MF, Verga M, Santus P, et al. Effect of formoterol, tiotropium, and their combination in patients with acute exacerbation of chronic obstructive pulmonary disease: a pilot study. Respir Med 2006; 100(11):1925–1932.
93. Tashkin DP, Littner M, Andrews CP, et al. Concomitant treatment with nebulized formoterol and tiotropium in subjects with COPD: a placebo-controlled trial. Respir Med 2008; 102(4):479–487.
94. Aaron SD, Vandemheen KL, Fergusson D, et al. Tiotropium in combination with placebo, salmeterol, or fluticasone-salmeterol for treatment of chronic obstructive pulmonary disease: a randomized trial. Ann Intern Med 2007; 146(8):545–555.
95. Singh D, Brooks J, Hagan G, et al. Superiority of "triple" therapy with salmeterol/fluticasone propionate and tiotropium bromide versus individual components in moderate to severe COPD. Thorax 2008; 63:592–598.
96. Pauwels RA, Lofdahl CG, Laitinen LA, et al. Long-term treatment with inhaled budesonide in persons with mild chronic obstructive pulmonary disease who continue smoking. European Respiratory Society Study on Chronic Obstructive Pulmonary Disease. N Engl J Med 1999; 340(25):1948–1953.
97. Burge PS, Calverley PM, Jones PW, et al. Randomised, double blind, placebo controlled study of fluticasone propionate in patients with moderate to severe chronic obstructive pulmonary disease: the ISOLDE trial. BMJ 2000; 320(7245):1297–1303.
98. Lung Health Study Research Group.Effect of inhaled triamcinolone on the decline in pulmonary function in chronic obstructive pulmonary disease. N Engl J Med 2000; 343(26): 1902–1909.
99. Vestbo J, Sorensen T, Lange P, et al. Long-term effect of inhaled budesonide in mild and moderate chronic obstructive pulmonary disease: a randomised controlled trial. Lancet 1999; 353(9167):1819–1823.

100. Paggiaro PL, Dahle R, Bakran I, et al. Multicentre randomised in placebo-controlled trial of inhaled fluticasone propionate in patients with chronic obstructive pulmonary disease. Lancet 1998; 351:773–780.

101. Wouters EF, Postma DS, Fokkens B, et al. Withdrawal of fluticasone propionate from combined salmeterol/fluticasone treatment in patients with COPD causes immediate and sustained disease deterioration: a randomised controlled trial. Thorax 2005; 60(6):480–487.

102. Choudhury AB, Dawson CM, Kilvington HE, et al. Withdrawal of inhaled corticosteroids in people with COPD in primary care: a randomised controlled trial. Respir Res 2007; 8:93.

103. Calverley PMA, Pauwels R, Vestbo J, et al. Combined salmeterol and fluticasone in the treatment of chronic obstructive pulmonary disease: a randomised controlled trial. Lancet 2003; 361:449–456.

104. Mahler DA, Wire P, Horstman D, et al. Effectiveness of fluticasone propionate and salmeterol combination delivered via the Diskus device in the treatment of chronic obstructive pulmonary disease. Am J Respir Crit Care Med 2002; 166(8):1084–1091.

105. Hanania NA, Darken P, Horstman D, et al. The efficacy and safety of fluticasone propionate (250mcg)/salmeterol (50mcg) combined in the diskus inhaler for the treatment of COPD. Chest 2003; 124:834–843.

106. Szafranski W, Cukier A, Ramirez A, et al. Efficacy and safety of budesonide/formoterol in the management of chronic obstructive pulmonary disease. Eur Respir J 2003; 21(1):74–81.

107. Calverley PM, Boonsawat W, Cseke Z, et al. Maintenance therapy with budesonide and formoterol in chronic obstructive pulmonary disease. Eur Respir J 2003; 22(6):912–919.

108. Calverley PM, Anderson JA, Celli B, et al. Salmeterol and fluticasone propionate and survival in chronic obstructive pulmonary disease. N Engl J Med 2007; 356(8):775–789.

109. Rabe KF. Treating COPD—the TORCH trial, P values, and the Dodo. N Engl J Med 2007; 356(8):851–854.

110. Celli BR, Thomas NE, Anderson JA, et al. Effect of pharmacotherapy on rate of decline of lung function in chronic obstructive pulmonary disease: results from the TORCH study. Am J Respir Crit Care Med 2008; 178(4):332–338.

111. Barnes NC, Qiu YS, Pavord ID, et al. Antiinflammatory effects of salmeterol/fluticasone propionate in chronic obstructive lung disease. Am J Respir Crit Care Med 2006; 173(7): 736–743.

112. Milgrom H, Fick RB Jr., Su JQ, et al. Treatment of allergic asthma with monoclonal anti-IgE antibody. N Engl J Med 1999; 341(26):1966–1973.

113. Soler M, Matz J, Townley R, et al. The anti-IgE antibody omalizumab reduces exacerbations and steroid requirement in allergic asthmatics. Eur Respir J 2001; 18(2):254–261.

114. Busse W, Corren J, Lanier BQ, et al. Omalizumab, anti-IgE recombinant humanized monoclonal antibody, for the treatment of severe allergic asthma. J Allergy Clin Immunol 2001; 108(2):184–190.

115. Ayres JG, Higgins B, Chilvers ER, et al. Efficacy and tolerability of anti-immunoglobulin E therapy with omalizumab in patients with poorly controlled (moderate-to-severe) allergic asthma. Allergy 2004; 59(7):701–708.

116. Holgate ST, Chuchalin AG, Hebert J, et al. Efficacy and safety of a recombinant anti-immunoglobulin E antibody (omalizumab) in severe allergic asthma. Clin Exp Allergy 2004; 34(4):632–638.

117. Bousquet J, Cabrera P, Berkman N, et al. The effect of treatment with omalizumab, an anti-IgE antibody, on asthma exacerbations and emergency medical visits in patients with severe persistent asthma. Allergy 2005; 60(3):302–308.

118. Humbert M, Beasley R, Ayres J, et al. Benefits of omalizumab as add-on therapy in patients with severe persistent asthma who are inadequately controlled despite best available therapy (GINA 2002 step 4 treatment): INNOVATE. Allergy 2005; 60(3):309–316.

119. Decramer M, Rutten-van Molken M, Dekhuijzen PN, et al. Effects of N-acetylcysteine on outcomes in chronic obstructive pulmonary disease (Bronchitis Randomized on NAC

Cost-Utility Study, BRONCUS): a randomised placebo-controlled trial. Lancet 2005; 365 (9470): 1552–1560.

120. Zheng JP, Kang J, Huang SG, et al. Effect of carbocisteine on acute exacerbation of chronic obstructive pulmonary disease (PEACE Study): a randomised placebo-controlled study. Lancet 2008; 371(9629):2013–2018.

121. Onder RF. The ethics of placebo-controlled trials: the case of asthma. J Allergy Clin Immunol 2005; 115(6):1228–1234.

122. Bielory L, Lupoli K. Herbal interventions in asthma and allergy. J Asthma 1999; 36:1–65.

123. Stebbings R, Findlay L, Edwards C, et al. "Cytokine Storm" in the phase I trial of monoclonal antibody TGN1412: better understanding the causes to improve preclinical testing of immunotherapeutics. J Immunol 2007; 179(5):3325–3331.

124. Ramsay S. Johns Hopkins takes responsibility for volunteer's death. Lancet 2001; 358 (9277):213.

125. Rennard SI, Fogarty C, Kelsen S, et al. The safety and efficacy of infliximab in moderate to severe chronic obstructive pulmonary disease. Am J Respir Crit Care Med 2007; 175(9): 926–934.

126. O'Connor BJ, Towse LJ, Barnes PJ. Prolonged effect of tiotropium bromide on methacholine-induced bronchoconstriction in asthma. Am J Respir Crit Care Med 1996; 154:876–880.

127. Maesen FPV, Smeets JJ, Sledsens TJH, et al. Tiotropium bromide, a new long-acting antimuscarinic bronchodilator:a pharmacodynamic study in patients with chronic obstructive disease (COPD). Eur Respir J 1995; 8:1506–1513.

128. Rees PJ. Bronchodilators in the therapy of chronic obstructive pulmonary disease. Eur Respir Mon 1998; 7:135–149.

129. Nisar M, Earis JE, Pearson MG, et al. Acute bronchodilator trials in chronic obstructive pulmonary disease. Am Rev Respir Dis 1992; 146:555–559.

130. O'Donnell DE. Assessment of bronchodilator efficacy in symptomatic COPD: is spirometry useful? Chest 2000; 117(2 suppl):42S–47S.

131. Inman MD, Watson RM, Cockcroft DW, et al. Reproducibility of allergen-induced early and late asthmatic responses. J Allergy Clin Immunol 1995; 95:1191–1195.

132. Arshad SH. Bronchial allergen challenge: a model for chronic allergic asthma? Clin Exp Allergy 2000; 30(1):12–15.

133. Taylor DA, Harris JG, O'Connor BJ. Comparison of incremental and bolus dose inhaled allergen challenge in asthmatic patients. Clin Exp Allergy 2000; 30(1):56–63.

134. Rasmussen JB. Late airway response increases at repeat allergen challenge. Allergy 1991; 46(6):419–426.

135. Parameswaran K, Inman MD, Watson RM, et al. Protective effects of fluticasone on allergen-induced airway responses and sputum inflammatory markers. Can Respir J 2000; 7(4): 313–319.

136. O'Shaughnessy KM, Wellings R, Gillies B, et al. Differential effects of fluticasone propionate on allergen-evoked bronchoconstriction and increased urinary leukotriene E_4 excretion. Am Rev Respir Dis 1993; 147:1472–1476.

137. Wood LJ, Sehmi R, Gauvreau GM, et al. An inhaled corticosteroid, budesonide, reduces baseline but not allergen-induced increases in bone marrow inflammatory cell progenitors in asthmatic subjects. Am J Respir Crit Care Med 1999; 159(5 pt 1):1457–1463.

138. Liu MC, Proud D, Lichtenstein LM, et al. Effects of prednisone on the cellular responses and release of cytokines and mediators after segmental allergen challenge of asthmatic subjects. J Allergy Clin Immunol 2001; 108(1):29–38.

139. Sullivan P, Bekir S, Jaffar Z, et al. Anti-inflammatory effects of low-dose oral theophylline in atopic asthma. Lancet 1994; 343(8904):1006–1008.

140. Pauwels RA. New aspects of the therapeutic potential of theophylline in asthma. J Allergy Clin Immunol 1989; 83(2 pt 2):548–553.
141. Diamant Z, Grootendorst DC, Veselic-Charvat M, et al. The effect of montelukast (MK-0476), a cysteinyl leukotriene receptor antagonist, on allergen-induced airway responses and sputum cell counts in asthma. Clin Exp Allergy 1999; 29:42–51.
142. Wenzel SE. Inflammation, leukotrienes and the pathogenesis of the late asthmatic response. Clin Exp Allergy 1999; 29:1–3.
143. Pizzichini E, Pizzichini M-MM, Kidney JC, et al. Induced sputum, bronchoalveolar lavage and blood from mild asthmatics: inflammatory cells, lymphocyte subsets and soluble markers compared. Eur Respir J 1998; 11(4):834.
144. Rasmussen JB, Eriksson LO, Margolskee DJ, et al. Leukotriene D4 receptor blockade inhibits the immediate and late bronchoconstrictor responses to inhaled antigen in patients with asthma. J Allergy Clin Immunol 1992; 90(2):193–201.
145. Fuller RW, Black PN, Dollery CT. Effect of the oral leukotriene D4 antagonist LY171883 on inhaled and intradermal challenge with antigen and leukotriene D4 in atopic subjects. J Allergy Clin Immunol 1989; 83(5):939–944.
146. Crimi E, Brusasco V, Crimi P. Effect of nedocromil sodium on the late asthmatic reaction to bronchial antigen challenge. J Allergy Clin Immunol 1989; 83:985–990.
147. Laube BL, Edwards AM, Dalby RN, et al. The efficacy of slow versus faster inhalation of cromolyn sodium in protecting against allergen challenge in patients with asthma. J Allergy Clin Immunol 1998; 101(4 pt 1):475–483.
148. Crimi E, Brusasco V, Crimi P. Effect of nedocromil sodium on the late asthmatic reaction to bronchial antigen challenge. J Allergy Clin Immunol 1989; 83(5):985–990.
149. Twentyman OP, Sams VR, Holgate ST. Albuterol and nedocromil sodium affect airway and leukocyte responses to allergen. Am Rev Respir Dis 1993; 147(6 pt 1):1425–1430.
150. Twentyman OP, Finnerty JP, Holgate ST. The inhibitory effect of nebulized albuterol on the early and late asthmatic reactions and increase in airway responsiveness provoked by inhaled allergen in asthma. Am Rev Respir Dis 1991; 144(4):782–787.
151. Howarth PH, Durham SR, Lee TH, et al. Influence of albuterol, cromolyn sodium and ipratropium bromide on the airway and circulating mediator responses to allergen bronchial provocation in asthma. Am Rev Respir Dis 1985; 132(5):986–992.
152. Wong CS, Wahedna I, Pavord ID, et al. Effect of regular terbutaline and budesonide on bronchial reactivity to allergen challenge. Am J Respir Crit Care Med 1994; 150:1268–1273.
153. Twentyman OP, Finnerty JP, Harris A, et al. Protection against allergen-induced asthma by salmeterol. Lancet 1990; 336(8727):1338–1342.
154. Dente FL, Bancalari L, Bacci E, et al. Effect of a single dose of salmeterol on the increase in airway eosinophils induced by allergen challenge in asthmatic subjects. Thorax 1999; 54(7): 622–624.
155. Taylor IK, O'Shaughnessy KM, Choudry NB, et al. A comparative study in atopic subjects with asthma of the effects of salmeterol and salbutamol on allergen-induced bronchoconstriction, increase in airway reactivity, and increase in urinary leukotriene E4 excretion. J Allergy Clin Immunol 1992; 89(2):575–583.
156. Pedersen B, Dahl R, Larsen BB, et al. The effect of salmeterol on the early- and late-phase reaction to bronchial allergen and postchallenge variation in bronchial reactivity, blood eosinophils, serum eosinophil cationic protein, and serum eosinophil protein X. Allergy 1993; 48(5):377–382.
157. Weersink EJM, AAlbers R, Koeter GH, et al. Partial inhibitor of the early and late asthmatic response by a single dose of salmeterol. Am J Respir Crit Care Med 1994; 150:1262–1267.
158. Giannini D, Bacci E, Dente FL, et al. Inhaled beclomethasone dipropionate reverts tolerance to the protective effect of salmeterol on allergen challenge. Chest 1999; 115(3): 629–634.

159. Weersink EJ, AAlbers R, Koeter GH, et al. Partial inhibition of the early and late asthmatic response by a single dose of salmeterol. Am J Respir Crit Care Med 1994; 150(5 pt 1): 1262–1267.

160. Giannini D, Di Franco A, Bacci E, et al. Tolerance to the protective effect of salmeterol on allergen challenge can be partially restored by the withdrawal of salmeterol regular treatment. Chest 2001; 119(6):1671–1675.

161. Calhoun WJ, Hinton KL, Kratzenberg JJ. The effect of salmeterol on markers of airway inflammation following segmental allergen challenge. Am J Respir Crit Care Med 2001; 163(4):881–886.

162. Palmqvist M, Balder B, Lowhagen O, et al. Late asthmatic reaction decreased after pretreatment with salbutamol and formoterol, a new long-acting beta 2-agonist. J Allergy Clin Immunol 1992; 89(4):844–849.

163. Wong BJ, Dolovich J, Ramsdale EH, et al. Formoterol compared with beclomethasone and placebo on allergen-induced asthmatic responses. Am Rev Respir Dis 1992; 146(5 pt 1): 1156–1160.

164. Sihra BS, Kon OM, Durham SR, et al. Effect of cyclosporin A on the allergen-induced late asthmatic reaction. Thorax 1997; 52:447–452.

165. Khan LN, Kon OM, Macfarlane AJ, et al. Attenuation of the allergen-induced late asthmatic reaction by cyclosporin A is associated with inhibition of bronchial eosinophils, interleukin-5, granulocyte macrophage colony-stimulating factor, and eotaxin. Am J Respir Crit Care Med 2000; 162(4 pt 1):1377–1382.

166. Boulet LP, Chapman KR, Cote J, et al. Inhibitory effects of an anti-IgE antibody E25 on allergen-induced early asthmatic response. Am J Respir Crit Care Med 1997; 155(6):1835–1840.

167. Fahy JV, Cockcroft DW, Boulet L-P, et al. Effects of aerosolized anti-IgE (E25) on airway responses to inhaled allergen in asthmatic subjects. Am J Resp Crit Care Med 1999; 160:1023–1027.

168. Bryan SA, O'Connor BJ, Matti S, et al. Effects of recombinant human interleukin-12 on eosinophils, airway hyperreactivity and the late asthmatic response. Lancet 2000; 356 (2149):2153.

169. Leckie MJ, ten Brinke A, Khan J, et al. Effects of an interleukin-5 blocking monoclonal antibody on eosinophils, airway hyperresponsiveness, and the late asthmatic response. Lancet 2000; 356:2144–2148.

170. Roquet A, Dahlen B, Kumlin M, et al. Combined antagonism of leukotrienes and histamine produces predominant inhibition of allergen-induced early and late phase airway obstruction in asthmatics. Am J Respir Crit Care Med 1997; 155(6):1856–1863.

171. Sestini P, Refini RM, Pieroni MG, et al. Different effects of inhaled aspirin-like drugs on allergen-induced early and late asthmatic responses. Am J Respir Crit Care Med 1999; 159(4 pt 1):1228–1233.

172. Pavord ID, Wong CS, Williams J, et al. Effect of inhaled prostaglandin E$_2$ on allergen-induced asthma. Am Rev Respir Dis 1993; 148:87–90.

173. Gauvreau GM, Watson RM, O'Byrne PM. Protective effects of inhaled PGE$_2$ on allergen-induced airway responses and airway inflammation. Am J Resp Crit Care Med 1999; 159: 31–36.

174. Hartert TV, Dworski RT, Mellen BG, et al. Prostaglandin E(2) decreases allergen-stimulated release of prostaglandin D(2) in airways of subjects with asthma. Am J Respir Crit Care Med 2000; 162(2 pt 1):637–640.

175. Diamant Z, Timmers MC, van der Veen H, et al. Effect of inhaled heparin on allergen-induced early and late asthmatic responses in patients with atopic asthma. Am J Respir Crit Care Med 1996; 153:1790–1795.

176. Bianco S, Pieroni MG, Refini RM, et al. Protective effect of inhaled furosemide on allergen-induced early and late asthmatic reactions. N Engl J Med 1989; 321:1069–1073.

177. Harbinson PL, MacLeod D, Hawksworth R, et al. The effect of a novel orally active selective PDE4 isoenzyme inhibitor (CDP840) on allergen-induced responses in asthmatic subjects. Eur Respir J 1997; 10:1008–1014.
178. Kanehiro A, Ikemura T, Makela MJ, et al. Inhibition of phosphodiesterase 4 attenuates airway hyperresponsiveness and airway inflammation in a model of secondary allergen challenge. Am J Respir Crit Care Med 2001; 163(1):173–184.
179. Krishna MT, Chauhan A, Little L, et al. Inhibition of mast cell tryptase by inhaled APC 366 attenuates allergen-induced late-phase airway obstruction in asthma. J Allergy Clin Immunol 2001; 107(6):1039–1045.
180. Kuitert LM, Hui KP, Uthayarkumar S, et al. Effect of the platelet-activating factor antagonist UK-74,505 on the early and late response to allergen. Am Rev Respir Dis 1993; 147:82–86.
181. Freitag A, Watson RM, Matsos G, et al. Effect of a platelet activating factor antagonist, WEB 2086, on allergen induced asthmatic responses. Thorax 1993; 48:594–598.
182. Evans DJ, Barnes PJ, Cluzel M, et al. Effects of a potent platelet-activating factor antagonist, SR27417A, on allergen-induced asthmatic responses. Am J Respir Crit Care Med 1997; 156(1):11–16.
183. Wenzel S, Wilbraham D, Fuller R, et al. Effect of an interleukin-4 variant on late phase asthmatic response to allergen challenge in asthmatic patients: results of two phase 2a studies. Lancet 2007; 370(9596):1422–1431.
184. Morley J. Strategies for developing novel anti-asthma drugs. In: Barnes PJ, ed. New Drugs for Asthma. London: IBC Technical Services Ltd.; 1992:258–262.
185. Boushey HA, Fahy JV. Targeting cytokines in asthma therapy: round one. Lancet 2000; 356(9248):2114–2116.
186. Yamagata T, Ichinose M. Agents against cytokine synthesis or receptors. Eur J Pharmacol 2006; 533(1–3):289–301.
187. Barnes PJ. New therapies for asthma. Trends Mol Med 2006; 12(11):515–520.
188. Barnes PJ. Corticosteroids: the drugs to beat. Eur J Pharmacol 2006; 533(1–3):2–14.
189. Effros RM, Nagaraj H. Asthma: new developments concerning immune mechanisms, diagnosis and treatment. Curr Opin Pulm Med 2007; 13(1):37–43.
190. Larche M. Update on the current status of peptide immunotherapy. J Allergy Clin Immunol 2007; 119(4):906–909.
191. Gauvreau GM, Hessel EM, Boulet LP, et al. Immunostimulatory sequences regulate interferon-inducible genes but not allergic airway responses. Am J Respir Crit Care Med 2006; 174(1):15–20.
192. Pettipher R, Hansel TT, Armer R. Antagonism of the prostaglandin D2 receptors DP1 and CRTH2 as an approach to treat allergic diseases. Nat Rev Drug Discov 2007; 6(4):313–325.
193. Woodcock A, Forster L, Matthews E, et al. Control of exposure to mite allergen and allergen-impermeable bed covers for adults with asthma. N Engl J Med 2003; 349(3):225–236.
194. Cazzola M, Matera MG, Lotvall J. Ultra long-acting beta2-agonists in development for asthma and chronic obstructive pulmonary disease. Expert Opin Investig Drugs 2005; 14(7):775–783.
195. Buhl R, Farmer SG. Future directions in the pharmacologic therapy of chronic obstructive pulmonary disease. Proc Am Thorac Soc 2005; 2(1):83–93.
196. Hansel TT, Neighbour H, Erin EM, et al. Glycopyrrolate causes prolonged bronchoprotection and bronchodilatation in patients with asthma. Chest 2005; 128(4):1974–1979.
197. Lipworth BJ. Phosphodiesterase-4 inhibitors for asthma and chronic obstructive pulmonary disease. Lancet 2005; 365(9454):167–175.
198. van Schalkwyk E, Strydom K, Williams Z, et al. Roflumilast, an oral, once-daily phosphodiesterase 4 inhibitor, attenuates allergen-induced asthmatic reactions. J Allergy Clin Immunol 2005; 116(2):292–298.

199. Schmidt BM, Kusma M, Feuring M, et al. The phosphodiesterase 4 inhibitor roflumilast is effective in the treatment of allergic rhinitis. J Allergy Clin Immunol 2001; 108(4):530–536.
200. Flood-Page P, Menzies-Gow A, Phipps S, et al. Anti-IL-5 treatment reduces deposition of ECM proteins in the bronchial subepithelial basement membrane of mild atopic asthmatics. J Clin Invest 2003; 112(7):1029–1036.
201. Flood-Page PT, Menzies-Gow AN, Kay AB, et al. Eosinophil's role remains uncertain as anti-Interleukin-5 only partially depletes numbers in asthmatic airway. Am J Respir Crit Care Med 2003; 167(2):199–204.
202. Menzies-Gow AN, Flood-Page PT, Robinson DS. Effect of inhaled interleukin-5 on eosinophil progenitors in the bronchi and bone marrow of asthmatic and non-asthmatic volunteers. Clin Exp Allergy Rev 2007; 37:1023–1032.
203. Menzies-Gow A, Flood-Page PT, Sehmi R, et al. Anti-IL-5 (mepolizumab) therapy induces bone marrow eosinophil maturational arrest and decreases eosinophil progenitors in the bronchial mucosa of atopic asthmatics. J Allergy Clin Immunol 2003; 111(4):714–719.
204. Leonardi CL, Powers JL, Matheson RT, et al. Etanercept as monotherapy in patients with psoriasis. N Engl J Med 2003; 349(21):2014–2022.
205. Flood-Page P, Swenson C, Faiferman I, et al. A study to evaluate safety and efficacy of mepolizumab in patients with moderate persistent asthma. Am J Respir Crit Care Med 2007; 176(11):1062–1071.
206. Phipps S, Flood-Page P, Menzies-Gow A, et al. Intravenous anti-IL-5 monoclonal antibody reduces eosinophils and tenascin deposition in allergen-challenged human atopic skin. J Invest Dermatol 2004; 122(6):1406–1412.
207. Oldhoff JM, Darsow U, Werfel T, et al. Anti-IL-5 recombinant humanized monoclonal antibody (mepolizumab) for the treatment of atopic dermatitis. Allergy 2005; 60(5): 693–696.
208. Braun-Falco M, Fischer S, Plotz S-G RJ. Correspondence: angiolymphoid hyperplasia with eosinophilia treated with anti-interleukin-5 antibody (mepolizumba). J Dermatol 2004; 151: 1103–1113.
209. Stein ML, Collins MH, Villanueva JM, et al. Anti-IL-5 (mepolizumab) therapy for eosinophilic esophagitis. J Allergy Clin Immunol 2006; 118(6):1312–1319.
210. Plotz SG, Simon HU, Darsow U, et al. Use of an anti-interleukin-5 antibody in the hypereosinophilic syndrome with eosinophilic dermatitis. N Engl J Med 2003; 349(24): 2334–2339.
211. Garrett JK, Jameson SC, Thomson B, et al. Anti-interleukin-5 (mepolizumab) therapy for hypereosinophilic syndromes. J Allergy Clin Immunol 2004; 113(1):115–119.
212. Klion AD, Law MA, Noel P, et al. Safety and efficacy of the monoclonal anti-interleukin-5 antibody SCH55700 in the treatment of patients with hypereosinophilic syndrome. Blood 2004; 103(8):2939–2941.
213. Borish LC, Nelson HS, Lanz MJ, et al. Interleukin-4 receptor in moderate atopic asthma: a phase I/II randomized, placebo-controlled trial. Am J Resp Crit Care Med 1999; 160: 1816–1823.
214. Borish LC, Nelson HS, Corren J, et al. Efficacy of soluble IL-4 receptor for the treatment of adults with asthma. J Allergy Clin Immunol 2001; 107(6):963–970.
215. Howarth PH, Babu KS, Arshad HS, et al. Tumour necrosis factor (TNFalpha) as a novel therapeutic target in symptomatic corticosteroid dependent asthma. Thorax 2005; 60(12): 1012–1018.
216. Berry MA, Hargadon B, Shelley M, et al. Evidence of a role of tumor necrosis factor alpha in refractory asthma. N Engl J Med 2006; 354(7):697–708.
217. Morjaria JB, Chauhan AJ, Babu KS, et al. The role of a soluble TNFalpha receptor fusion protein (etanercept) in corticosteroid refractory asthma: a double blind, randomised, placebo controlled trial 1. Thorax 2008; 63(7):584–591.

218. Erin EM, Leaker BR, Nicholson GC, et al. The effects of a monoclonal antibody directed against tumor necrosis factor-alpha in asthma. Am J Respir Crit Care Med 2006; 174: 753–762.

219. van der Vaart H, Koeter GH, Postma DS, et al. First study of infliximab treatment in patients with chronic obstructive pulmonary disease. Am J Respir Crit Care Med 2005; 172(4): 465–469.

220. Baughman RP, Drent M, Kavuru M, et al. Infliximab therapy in patients with chronic sarcoidosis and pulmonary involvement. Am J Respir Crit Care Med 2006; 174(7):795–802.

221. Nielsen BW, Reimert CM, Hammer R, et al. Interferon therapy for atopic dermatitis reduces basophil histamine release, but does not reduce serum IgE or eosinophilic proteins. Allergy 1994; 49(2):120–128.

222. Basaran MM, Barlan IB, Tukenmez F, et al. Effect of interferon-alpha therapy on serum IgE, IL-4, and sCD23 levels in childhood asthma. J Asthma 1995; 32(3):215–220.

223. Li JT, Yunginger JW, Reed CE, et al. Lack of suppression of IgE production by recombinant interferon gamma: a controlled trial in patients with allergic rhinitis. J Allergy Clin Immunol 1990; 85(5):934–940.

224. Boguniewicz M, Jaffe HS, Izu A, et al. Recombinant gamma interferon in treatment of patients with atopic dermatitis and elevated IgE levels. Am J Med 1990; 88(4):365–370.

225. Boguniewicz M, Martin RJ, Martin D, et al. The effects of nebulized recombinant interferon-gamma in asthmatic airways. J Allergy Clin Immunol 1995; 95(1 pt 1):133–135.

226. Ziesche R, Hofbauer E, Wittmann K, et al. A preliminary study of long-term treatment with interferon gamma-1b and low-dose prednisolone in patients with idiopathic pulmonary fibrosis. N Engl J Med 1999; 341(17):1264–1269.

227. Leonard JP, Sherman ML, Fisher GL, et al. Effect of single-dose interleukin-12 exposure on interleukin-12-associated toxicity and interferon-γ production. Blood 1997; 90:2541–2548.

228. Dolgachev V, Berlin AA, Lukacs NW. Eosinophil activation of fibroblasts from chronic allergen-induced disease utilizes stem cell factor for phenotypic changes. Am J Pathol 2008; 172(1):68–76.

229. Gleich GJ, Leiferman KM, Pardanani A, et al. Treatment of hypereosinophilic syndrome with imatinib mesilate. Lancet 2002; 359(9317):1577–1578.

230. Cools J, DeAngelo DJ, Gotlib J, et al. A tyrosine kinase created by fusion of the PDGFRA and FIP1L1 genes as a therapeutic target of imatinib in idiopathic hypereosinophilic syndrome. N Engl J Med 2003; 348(13):1201–1214.

231. Quintas-Cardama A, Aribi A, Cortes J, et al. Novel approaches in the treatment of systemic mastocytosis. Cancer 2006; 107(7):1429–1439.

232. Guyer BJ, Shimamoto SR, Bradhurst AL, et al. Mast cell inhibitor R112 is well tolerated and affects prostaglandin D2 but not other mediators, symptoms, or nasal volumes in a nasal challenge model of allergic rhinitis. Allergy Asthma Proc 2006; 27:208–213.

233. Meltzer EO, Berkowitz RB, Grossbard EB. An intranasal Syk-kinase inhibitor (R112) improves the symptoms of seasonal allergic rhinitis in a park environment. J Allergy Clin Immunol 2005; 115(4):791–796.

234. Trulock EP III. Lung transplantation for COPD. Chest 1998; 113(4 suppl):269S–276S.

235. Kon OM, Sihra BS, Compton CH, et al. Randomised, dose-ranging, placebo-controlled study of chimeric antibody to CD4 (keliximab) in chronic severe asthma. Lancet 1998; 352(9134):1109–1113.

236. Rosenwasser LJ, Busse WW, Lizambri RG, et al. Allergic asthma and an anti-CD23 mAb (IDEC-152): results of a phase I, single-dose, dose-escalating clinical trial. J Allergy Clin Immunol 2003; 112(3):563–570.

237. Poole JA, Meng J, Reff M, et al. Anti-CD23 monoclonal antibody, lumiliximab, inhibited allergen-induced responses in antigen-presenting cells and T cells from atopic subjects. J Allergy Clin Immunol 2005; 116(4):780–788.

238. Norris V, Choong L, Tran D, et al. Effect of IVL745, a VLA-4 antagonist, on allergen-induced bronchoconstriction in patients with asthma. J Allergy Clin Immunol 2005; 116(4): 761–767.

239. Meyer M, Beeh KM, Beier J, et al. Tolerability and pharmacokinetics of inhaled bimosiamose disodium in healthy males. Br J Clin Pharmacol 2007; 63(4):451–458.

240. Meyer M, Jilma B, Zahlten R, et al. Physiochemical properties, safety and pharmacokinetics of bimosiamose disodium after intravenous administration. Int J Clin Pharmacol Ther 2005; 43(10):463–471.

241. Avila PC, Boushey HA, Wong H, et al. Effect of a single dose of the selectin inhibitor TBC1269 on early and late asthmatic responses. Clin Exp Allergy 2004; 34(1):77–84.

242. Beeh KM, Beier J, Meyer M, et al. Bimosiamose, an inhaled small-molecule pan-selectin antagonist, attenuates late asthmatic reactions following allergen challenge in mild asthmatics: a randomized, double-blind, placebo-controlled clinical cross-over-trial. Pulm Pharmacol Ther 2006; 19(4):233–241.

243. Mahler DA, Huang S, Tabrizi M, et al. Efficacy and safety of a monoclonal antibody recognizing interleukin-8 in COPD: a pilot study. Chest 2004; 126(3):926–934.

244. McCusker CT, Wang Y, Shan J, et al. Inhibition of experimental allergic airways disease by local application of a cell-penetrating dominant-negative STAT-6 peptide. J Immunol 2007; 179(4):2556–2564.

245. Hunninghake DB. Cardiovascular disease in chronic obstructive pulmonary disease. Proc Am Thorac Soc 2005; 2(1):44–49.

246. Jain MK, Ridker PM. Anti-inflammatory effects of statins: clinical evidence and basic mechanisms. Nat Rev Drug Discov 2005; 4(12):977–987.

247. Mancini GB, Etminan M, Zhang B, et al. Reduction of morbidity and mortality by statins, angiotensin-converting enzyme inhibitors, and angiotensin receptor blockers in patients with chronic obstructive pulmonary disease. J Am Coll Cardiol 2006; 47(12):2554–2560.

248. Frost FJ, Petersen H, Tollestrup K, et al. Influenza and COPD mortality protection as pleiotropic, dose-dependent effects of statins. Chest 2007; 131(4):1006–1012.

249. Soyseth V, Brekke PH, Smith P, et al. Statin use is associated with reduced mortality in COPD. Eur Respir J 2007; 29(2):279–283.

250. Massaro GD, Massaro D. Retinoic acid treatment abrogates elastase-induced pulmonary emphysema in rats. Nat Med 1997; 3(6):675–677.

251. Fujita M, Ye Q, Ouchi H, et al. Retinoic acid fails to reverse emphysema in adult mouse models. Thorax 2004; 59(3):224–230.

252. Mao JT, Tashkin DP, Belloni PN, et al. All-trans retinoic acid modulates the balance of matrix metalloproteinase-9 and tissue inhibitor of metalloproteinase-1 in patients with emphysema. Chest 2003; 124(5):1724–1732.

253. Roth MD, Connett JE, D'Armiento JM, et al. Feasibility of retinoids for the treatment of emphysema study. Chest 2006; 130(5):1334–1345.

254. Klimanskaya I, Rosenthal N, Lanza R. Derive and conquer: sourcing and differentiating stem cells for therapeutic applications. Nat Rev Drug Discov 2008; 7(2):131–142.

255. Polak JM, Bishop AE. Stem cells and tissue engineering: past, present, and future. Ann N Y Acad Sci 2006; 1068:352–366.

256. Simpson JL, Powell H, Boyle MJ, et al. Clarithromycin targets neutrophilic airway inflammation in refractory asthma. Am J Respir Crit Care Med 2008; 177(2):148–155.

257. Johnston SL, Blasi F, Black PN, et al. The effect of telithromycin in acute exacerbations of asthma. N Engl J Med 2006; 354(15):1589–1600.

258. Rogers DF, Barnes PJ. Treatment of airway mucus hypersecretion. Ann Med 2006; 38(2): 116–125.

259. Hudson TJ. Dornase in treatment of chronic bronchitis. Ann Pharmacother 1996; 30: 674–675.

260. Gauvreau GM, Boulet LP, Cockcroft DW, et al. Antisense therapy against CCR3 and the common beta chain attenuates allergen-induced eosinophilic responses. Am J Respir Crit Care Med 2008; 177(9):952–958.

261. Hamelmann E, Gelfand EW. IL-5-induced airway eosinophilia—the key to asthma? Immunol Rev 2001; 179:182–191.

262. Sampson AP. IL-5 priming of eosinophil function in asthma. Clin Exp Allergy 2001; 31(4): 513–517.

263. O'Byrne PM, Inman MD, Parameswaran K. The trials and tribulations of IL-5, eosinophils, and allergic asthma. J Allergy Clin Immunol 2001; 108(4):503–508.

264. Hansel TT, Sterk PJ, Holgate ST, et al. Letter to Editor. The trials and tribulations of anti-IL5. J Allergy Clin Immunol 2002; 109(3):575.

265. Kips JC, O'Connor BJ, Langley SJ, et al. Effect of SCH55700, a humanized anti-human interleukin-5 antibody, in severe persistent asthma: a pilot study. Am J Respir Crit Care Med 2003; 167(12):1655–1659.

266. Rothenberg ME, Klion AD, Roufosse FE, et al. Treatment of patients with the hypereosinophilic syndrome with mepolizumab. N Engl J Med 2008; 358(12):1215–1228.

267. Passalacqua G, Ciprandi G, Canonica GW. The nose-lung interaction in allergic rhinitis and asthma: united airways disease. Curr Opin Allergy Clin Immunol 2001; 1(1):7–13.

268. de Benedictis FM, del Giudice MM, Severini S, et al. Rhinitis, sinusitis and asthma: one linked airway disease. Paediatr Respir Rev 2001; 2(4):358–364.

269. Passalacqua G, Canonica GW. Impact of rhinitis on airway inflammation: biological and therapeutic implications. Respir Res 2001; 2(6):320–323.

270. Vignola AM, Bresciani M, Demoly P, et al. Allergic inflammation of the upper and lower airways: a continuum of disease? Eur Respir Rev 2001; 11(81):152–156.

271. Barnes PJ. New molecular targets for the treatment of neutrophilic diseases. J Allergy Clin Immunol 2007; 119(5):1055–1062.

272. Cazzola M, Matera MG, Rogliani P, et al. Treating systemic effects of COPD. Trends Pharmacol Sci 2007; 28(10):544–550.

273. Gounni AS, Gregory B, Nutku E, et al. Interleukin-9 enhances interleukin-5 receptor expression, differentiation, and survival of human eosinophils. Blood 2000; 96(6): 2163–2171.

274. Cheng G, Arima M, Honda K, et al. Anti-interleukin-9 antibody treatment inhibits airway inflammation and hyperreactivity in mouse asthma model. Am J Respir Crit Care Med 2002; 166(3):409–416.

275. O'byrne P, Boulet LP, Gaureau G, et al. A single dose of MEDI-528, a monoclonal antibody against interleukin-9, is well tolerated in mild and moderate asthmatics in the phase II trial MI-CP-138. Chest 2007; 132:478S (abstr).

276. Mattes J, Yang M, Siqueira A, et al. IL-13 induces airways hyperreactivity independently of the IL-4R alpha chain in the allergic lung. J Immunol 2001; 167(3):1683–1692.

277. Miyahara S, Miyahara N, Matsubara S, et al. IL-13 is essential to the late-phase response in allergic rhinitis. J Allergy Clin Immunol 2006; 118(5):1110–1116.

278. Malavia NK, Mih JD, Raub CB, et al. IL-13 induces a bronchial epithelial phenotype that is profibrotic. Respir Res 2008; 9:27.

279. Barnes PJ. IL-10: a key regulator of allergic disease. Clin Exp Allergy 2001; 31(5): 667–669.

280. Blaser K, Akdis CA. Interleukin-10, T regulatory cells and specific allergy treatment. Clin Exp Allergy 2004; 34(3):328–331.

281. Kennedy NS, Barnstein B, Brenzovich J, et al. IL-10 Suppresses mast cell IgE receptor expression and signaling in vitro and in vivo. J Immunol 2008; 180(5):2848–2854.

282. Ruckert R, Brandt K, Braun A, et al. Blocking IL-15 prevents the induction of allergen-specific T cells and allergic inflammation in vivo. J Immunol 2005; 174(9):5507–5515.

283. Kawaguchi M, Adachi M, Oda N, et al. IL-17 cytokine family. J Allergy Clin Immunol 2004; 114(6):1265–1273.
284. Iwakura Y, Ishigame H. The IL-23/IL-17 axis in inflammation. J Clin Invest 2006; 116(5): 1218–1222.
285. Bowman EP, Chackerian AA, Cua DJ. Rationale and safety of anti-interleukin-23 and anti-interleukin-17A therapy. Curr Opin Infect Dis 2006; 19(3):245–252.
286. Linden A. Interleukin-17 and airway remodelling. Pulm Pharmacol Ther 2006; 19(1):47–50.
287. Linden A, Laan M, Anderson GP. Neutrophils, interleukin-17A and lung disease. Eur Respir J 2005; 25(1):159–172.
288. Izakovicova HL. Interleukin-18 in asthma and other allergies. Clin Exp Allergy 2003; 33(8): 1023–1025.
289. Sebelova S, Izakovicova-Holla L, Stejskalova A, et al. Interleukin-18 and its three gene polymorphisms relating to allergic rhinitis. J Hum Genet 2007; 52(2):152–158.
290. Tsutsui H, Yoshimoto T, Hayashi N, et al. Induction of allergic inflammation by interleukin-18 in experimental animal models. Immunol Rev 2004; 202:115–138.
291. Hiromura Y, Kishida T, Nakano H, et al. IL-21 administration into the nostril alleviates murine allergic rhinitis. J Immunol 2007; 179(10):7157–7165.
292. Kishida T, Hiromura Y, Shin-Ya M, et al. IL-21 induces inhibitor of differentiation 2 and leads to complete abrogation of anaphylaxis in mice. J Immunol 2007; 179(12):8554–8561.
293. Lei Z, Liu G, Huang Q, et al. SCF and IL-31 rather than IL-17 and BAFF are potential indicators in patients with allergic asthma. Allergy 2008; 63(3):327–332.
294. Hayakawa H, Hayakawa M, Kume A, et al. Soluble ST2 blocks interleukin-33 signaling in allergic airway inflammation. J Biol Chem 2007; 282(36):26369–26380.
295. Scotton CJ, Chambers RC. Molecular targets in pulmonary fibrosis: the myofibroblast in focus. Chest 2007; 132(4):1311–1321.
296. Chambers RC. Procoagulant signalling mechanisms in lung inflammation and fibrosis: novel opportunities for pharmacological intervention? Br J Pharmacol 2008; 153(suppl 1): S367–S378.
297. Ihn H. Pathogenesis of fibrosis: role of TGF-beta and CTGF. Curr Opin Rheumatol 2002; 14(6):681–685.
298. Bartram U, Speer CP. The role of transforming growth factor beta in lung development and disease. Chest 2004; 125(2):754–765.
299. Wilson MS, Elnekave E, Mentink-Kane MM, et al. IL-13Ralpha2 and IL-10 coordinately suppress airway inflammation, airway-hyperreactivity, and fibrosis in mice. J Clin Invest 2007; 117(10):2941–2951.
300. Quintas-Cardama A, Kantarjian H, Cortes J. Flying under the radar: the new wave of BCR-ABL inhibitors. Nat Rev Drug Discov 2007; 6(10):834–848.
301. Donnelly LE, Barnes PJ. Chemokine receptors as therapeutic targets in chronic obstructive pulmonary disease. Trends Pharmacol Sci 2006; 27(10):546–553.
302. O'Neill LA. Targeting signal transduction as a strategy to treat inflammatory diseases. Nat Rev Drug Discov 2006; 5(7):549–563.
303. Cousins DJ, McDonald J, Lee TH. Therapeutic approaches for control of transcription factors in allergic disease. J Allergy Clin Immunol 2008; 121(4):803–809.
304. Chatila TA, Li N, Garcia-Lloret M, et al. T-cell effector pathways in allergic diseases: transcriptional mechanisms and therapeutic targets. J Allergy Clin Immunol 2008; 121(4):812–823.
305. Birrell MA, Wong S, Hardaker EL, et al. IkappaB kinase-2-independent and -dependent inflammation in airway disease models: relevance of IKK-2 inhibition to the clinic. Mol Pharmacol 2006; 69(6):1791–1800.
306. Birrell MA, Hardaker E, Wong S, et al. Ikappa-B kinase-2 inhibitor blocks inflammation in human airway smooth muscle and a rat model of asthma. Am J Respir Crit Care Med 2005; 172(8):962–971.

307. Tanaka A, Konno M, Muto S, et al. A novel NF-kappaB inhibitor, IMD-0354, suppresses neoplastic proliferation of human mast cells with constitutively activated c-kit receptors. Blood 2005; 105(6):2324–2331.
308. D'Acquisto F, Ianaro A. From willow bark to peptides: the ever widening spectrum of NF-kappaB inhibitors. Curr Opin Pharmacol 2006; 6(4):387–392.
309. Holgate ST. The airway epithelium is central to the pathogenesis of asthma. Allergol Int 2008; 57(1):1–10.
310. Liu YJ. Thymic stromal lymphopoietin: master switch for allergic inflammation. J Exp Med 2006; 203(2):269–273.
311. Ito T, Wang YH, Duramad O, et al. TSLP-activated dendritic cells induce an inflammatory T helper type 2 cell response through OX40 ligand. J Exp Med 2005; 202(9):1213–1223.
312. Ebner S, Nguyen VA, Forstner M, et al. Thymic stromal lymphopoietin converts human epidermal Langerhans cells into antigen-presenting cells that induce proallergic T cells. J Allergy Clin Immunol 2007; 119(4):982–990.
313. Al-Shami A, Spolski R, Kelly J, et al. A role for TSLP in the development of inflammation in an asthma model. J Exp Med 2005; 202(6):829–839.
314. Rahman I, Adcock IM. Oxidative stress and redox regulation of lung inflammation in COPD. Eur Respir J 2006; 28(1):219–242.
315. Baur JA, Sinclair DA. Therapeutic potential of resveratrol: the in vivo evidence. Nat Rev Drug Discov 2006; 5(6):493–506.
316. Bumcrot D, Manoharan M, Koteliansky V, et al. RNAi therapeutics: a potential new class of pharmaceutical drugs. Nat Chem Biol 2006; 2(12):711–719.
317. Howarth PH, Persson CG, Meltzer EO, et al. Objective monitoring of nasal airway inflammation in rhinitis. J Allergy Clin Immunol 2005; 115(3 pt 2):S414–S441.
318. Greiff L, Pipkorn U, Alkner U, et al. The 'nasal pool' device applies controlled concentrations of solutes on human nasal airway mucosa and samples its surface exudations/secretions. Clin Exp Allergy 1990; 20(3):253–259.
319. Terada N, Hamano N, Kim WJ, et al. The kinetics of allergen-induced eotaxin level in nasal lavage fluid: its key role in eosinophil recruitment in nasal mucosa. Am J Respir Crit Care Med 2001; 164(4):575–579.
320. Greiff L, Petersen H, Mattsson E, et al. Mucosal output of eotaxin in allergic rhinitis and its attenuation by topical glucocorticosteroid treatment. Clin Exp Allergy 2001; 31(8):1321–1327.
321. Linden M, Svensson C, Andersson E, et al. Immediate effect of topical budesonide on allergen challenge-induced nasal mucosal fluid levels of granulocyte-macrophage colony-stimulating factor and interleukin-5. Am J Respir Crit Care Med 2000; 162(5):1705–1708.
322. Hanazawa T, Antuni J, Kharitonov S, et al. Intranasal administration of eotaxin increases nasal eosinophils and nitric oxide in patients with allergic rhinitis. J Allergy Clin Immunol 2000; 105:58–64.
323. Douglass JA, Dhami D, Gurr CE, et al. Influence of interleukin-8 challenge in the nasal mucosa in atopic and nonatopic subjects. Am J Respir Crit Care Med 1994; 150(4):1108–1113.
324. Juniper EF, Thompson AK, Ferrie PJ, et al. Development and validation of the mini rhinoconjunctivitis quality of life questionnaire. Clin Exp Allergy 2000; 30:132–140.
325. Juniper EF, Guyatt GH. Development and testing of a new measure of health status for clinical trials in rhinoconjunctivitis. Clin Exp Allergy 1991; 21:77–83.
326. Pipkorn U, Proud D, Lichtenstein LM, et al. Inhibition of mediator release in allergic rhinitis by pretreatment with topical glucocorticosteroids. N Engl J Med 1987; 316(24):1506–1510.
327. Ciprandi G, Tosca MA, Passalacqua G, et al. Intranasal mometasone furoate reduces late-phase inflammation after allergen challenge. Ann Allergy Asthma Immunol 2001; 86(4):433–438.
328. Rak S, Jacobson MR, Sudderick RM, et al. Influence of prolonged treatment with topical corticosteroid (fluticasone propionate) on early and late phase nasal responses and cellular

infiltration in the nasal mucosa after allergen challenge. Clin Exp Allergy 1994; 24(10): 930–939.

329. Gronborg H, Bisgaard H, Romeling F, et al. Early and late nasal symptom response to allergen challenge. The effect of pretreatment with a glucocorticosteroid spray. Allergy 1993; 48(2):87–93.

330. Seemungal TA, Harper-Owen R, Bhowmik A, et al. Detection of rhinovirus in induced sputum at exacerbation of chronic obstructive pulmonary disease. Eur Respir J 2000; 16(4): 677–683.

331. Wilkinson TM, Hurst JR, Perera WR, et al. Effect of interactions between lower airway bacterial and rhinoviral infection in exacerbations of COPD. Chest 2006; 129(2):317–324.

332. Hurst JR, Perera WR, Wilkinson TM, et al. Systemic and upper and lower airway inflammation at exacerbation of chronic obstructive pulmonary disease. Am J Respir Crit Care Med 2006; 173(1):71–78.

333. Hurst JR, Wilkinson TM, Perera WR, et al. Relationships Among Bacteria, Upper Airway, Lower Airway, and Systemic Inflammation in COPD. Chest 2005; 127(4):1219–1226.

334. Roberts NJ, Lloyd-Owen SJ, Rapado F, et al. Relationship between chronic nasal and respiratory symptoms in patients with COPD. Respir Med 2003; 97(8):909–914.

335. Sigsgaard T, Bonefeld-Jorgensen EC, Kjaergaard SK, et al. Cytokine release from the nasal mucosa and whole blood after experimental exposures to organic dusts. Eur Respir J 2000; 16(1):140–145.

336. Danuser B, Rebsamen H, Weber C, et al. Lipopolysaccharide-induced nasal cytokine response: a dose-response evaluation. Eur Arch Otorhinolaryngol 2000; 257(10):527–532.

337. Peden DB, Tucker K, Murphy P, et al. Eosinophil influx to the nasal airway after local, low-level LPS challenge in humans. J Allergy Clin Immunol 1999; 104(2 pt 1):388–394.

338. Nita I, Hollander C, Westin U, et al. Prolastin, a pharmaceutical preparation of purified human alpha1-antitrypsin, blocks endotoxin-mediated cytokine release. Respir Res 2005; 6(12): 1–11.

339. Crapo RO, Casaburi R, Coates AL, et al. Guidelines for methacholine and exercise challenge testing-1999. This official statement of the American Thoracic Society was adopted by the ATS Board of Directors, July 1999. Am J Respir Crit Care Med 2000; 161(1):309–329.

340. Manning PJ, Watson RM, Margolskee DJ, et al. Inhibition of exercise-induced broncho-constriction by MK-571, a potent leukotriene D_4-receptor antagonist. N Engl J Med 1990; 323:1736–1739.

341. Kemp JP, Dockhorn RJ, Shapiro GG, et al. Montelukast once daily inhibits exercise-induced bronchoconstriction in 6 to 14 year old children with asthma. J Pediatr 1998; 133:424–428.

342. Leff JA, Busse WW, Pearlman D, et al. Montelukast, a leukotriene-receptor antagonist, for the treatment of mild asthma and exercise-induced bronchoconstriction. N Engl J Med 1998; 339:147–152.

343. Dahlen B, Roquet A, Inman MD, et al. Influence of zafirlukast and loratadine on exercise-induced bronchoconstriction. J Allergy Clin Immunol 2002; 109(5):789–793.

344. Anderson SD, Brannan JD. Exercise-induced asthma: is there still a case for histamine? J Allergy Clin Immunol 2002; 109(5 pt 1):771–773.

345. Haahtela T, Jarvinen M, Kava T, et al. Comparison of a beta 2-agonist, terbutaline, with an inhaled corticosteroid, budesonide, in newly detected asthma. N Engl J Med 1991; 325(6): 388–392.

346. Haahtela T, Jarvinen M, Kava T, et al. Effects of reducing or discontinuing inhaled budesonide in patients with mild asthma. N Engl J Med 1994; 331(11):700–705.

347. Lim S, Jatakanon A, John M, et al. Effect of inhaled budesonide on lung function and airway inflammation. Assessment by various inflammatory markers in mild asthma. Am J Respir Crit Care Med 1999; 159:22–30.

348. Jatakanon A, Kharitonov S, Lim S, et al. Effect of differing doses of inhaled budesonide on markers of airway inflammation in patients with mild asthma. Thorax 1999; 54(2):108–114.

349. Taylor DA, Jensen MW, Kanabar V, et al. A dose-dependent effect of the novel inhaled corticosteroid ciclesonide on airway responsiveness to adenosine-5'-monophosphate in asthmatic patients. Am J Respir Crit Care Med 1999; 160(1):237–243.

350. Kelly HW. Establishing a therapeutic index for the inhaled corticosteroids: Part 1. Pharmacokinetic/pharmacodynamic comparison of the inhaled corticosteroids. J Allergy Clin Immunol 1998; 102:S36–S51.

351. O'Byrne P, Pedersen S. Measuring efficacy and safety of different inhaled corticosteroid preparations. J Allergy Clin Immunol 1998; 102:879–886.

352. Efthimiou J, Barnes PJ. Effect of inhaled corticosteroids on bones and growth. Eur Respir J 1998; 11(5):1167–1177.

353. Gibson PG, Saltos N, Fakes K. Acute anti-inflammatory effects of inhaled budesonide in asthma: a randomized controlled trial. Am J Respir Crit Care Med 2001; 163(1):32–36.

354. Evans DJ, Taylor DA, Zetterstrom O, et al. A comparison of low-dose inhaled budesonide plus theophylline and high- dose inhaled budesonide for moderate asthma. N Engl J Med 1997; 337(20):1412–1418.

355. National Institutes of Health (NIH), National Heart Lung and Blood Institute (NHLBI). Global Initiative for Asthma (GINA): Global Strategy for Asthma Management and Prevention. Available at: www.ginasthma.com. Updated. 2005.

356. Nelson HS. Advair: combination treatment with fluticasone propionate/salmeterol in the treatment of asthma. J Allergy Clin Immunol 2001; 107:397–416.

357. Zetterstrom O, Buhl R, Mellem H, et al. Improved asthma control with budesonide/formoterol in a single inhaler, compared with budesonide alone. Eur Respir J 2001; 18(2):262–268.

358. Drazen JM, Israel E, O'Byrne PM. Treatment of asthma with drugs modifying the leukotriene pathway. N Engl J Med 1999; 340:197–206.

359. Laviolette M, Malmstrom K, Lu S, et al. Montelukast added to inhaled beclomethasone in treatment of asthma. Am J Resp Crit Care Med 1999; 160:1862–1868.

360. Gibson PG, Wong BJO, Hepperle MJE, et al. A research method to induce and examine a mild exacerbation of asthma by withdrawal of inhaled corticosteroid. Clin Exp Allergy 1992; 22:525–532.

361. Veen JC, Smits HH, Hiemstra PS, et al. Lung function and sputum characteristics of patients with severe asthma during and induced exacerbation by double-blind steroid withdrawal. Am J Resp Crit Care Med 1999; 160:93–99.

362. van der Valk P, Monninkhof E, van der Palen J, et al. Effect of discontinuation of inhaled corticosteroids in patients with chronic obstructive pulmonary disease: the COPE study. Am J Respir Crit Care Med 2002; 166(10):1358–1363.

363. Lock SH, Kay AB, Barnes NC. Double-blind, placebo-controlled study of cyclosporin A as a corticosteroid-sparing agent in corticosteroid-dependent asthma. Am J Respir Crit Care Med 1996; 153(2):509–514.

364. Milgrom H, Berger W, Nayak A, et al. Treatment of childhood asthma with anti-immunoglobulin E antibody (omalizumab). Pediatrics 2001; 108(2):E36.

365. Redington AE, Howarth PH. Airway wall remodelling in asthma. Thorax 1997; 52:310–312.

366. Bousquet J, Jeffery PK, Busse WW, et al. Asthma. From bronchoconstriction to airways inflammation and remodeling. Am J Respir Crit Care Med 2000; 161(5):1720–1745.

367. Holgate ST, Davies DE, Lackie PM, et al. Epithelial-mesenchymal interactions in the pathogenesis of asthma. J Allergy Clin Immunol 2000; 105(2 pt 1):193–204.

368. van Essen-Zandvliet EE, Hughes MD, Waalkens HJ, et al. Remission of childhood asthma after long-term treatment with an inhaled corticosteroid (budesonide): can it be achieved? Eur Respir J 1994; 7:63–68.

369. Huang S. Molecular modulation of allergic responses. J Allergy Clin Immunol 1998; 102:887–892.

370. Van Uden J, Raz E. Immunostimulatory DNA and applications to allergic disease. J Allergy Clin Immunol 1999; 104(5):902–910.
371. Hasko G, Szabo C. IL-12 as a therapeutic target for pharmacological modulation in immune- mediated and inflammatory diseases: regulation of T helper 1/T helper 2 responses. Br J Pharmacol 1999; 127(6):1295–1304.
372. Scanlon PD, Connett JE, Waller LA, et al. Smoking cessation and lung function in mild-to-moderate chronic obstructive pulmonary disease. The lung health study. Am J Respir Crit Care Med 2000; 161(2 pt 1):381–390.
373. Burge PS. EUROSCOP, ISOLDE and the Copenhagen city lung study. Thorax 1999; 54(4): 287–288.
374. Wang ML, Gunel E, Petsonk EL. Design strategies for longitudinal spirometry studies: study duration and measurement frequency. Am J Respir Crit Care Med 2000; 162(6):2134–2138.
375. Thomas PS. Tumour necrosis factor-alpha: the role of this multifunctional cytokine in asthma. Immunol Cell Biol 2001; 79(2):132–140.
376. Feldman M, Taylor P, Paleolog E, et al. Anti-TNF alpha therapy is useful in rheumatoid arthritis and Crohn's disease: analysis of the mechanism of action predicts utility in other diseases. Transplant Proc 1998; 30(8):4126–4127.
377. Schols AM, Soeters PB, Mostert R, et al. Physiologic effects of nutritional support and anabolic steroids in patients with chronic obstructive pulmonary disease. A placebo-controlled randomized trial. Am J Respir Crit Care Med 1995; 152(4 pt 1):1268–1274.
378. Schols AM, Slangen J, Volovics L, et al. Weight loss is a reversible factor in the prognosis of chronic obstructive pulmonary disease. Am J Respir Crit Care Med 1998; 157(6 pt 1): 1791–1797.
379. Schols AM, Soeters PB, Dingemans AM, et al. Prevalence and characteristics of nutritional depletion in patients with stable COPD eligible for pulmonary rehabilitation. Am Rev Respir Dis 1993; 147(5):1151–1156.
380. Wouters EF. Nutrition and metabolism in COPD. Chest 2000; 117(5 suppl 1):274S–280S.
381. Tattersfield AE. Limitations of current treatment. Lancet 1997; 350 (suppl II):24–27.
382. Rodriguez-Roisin R. Toward a consensus definition for COPD exacerbations. Chest 2000; 117(5 suppl 2):398S–401S.
383. Pauwels RA, Lofdahl C-G, Postma DS, et al. Effect of inhaled formoterol and budesonide on exacerbations of asthma. N Engl J Med 1997; 337:1405–1411.
384. Kips JC, Pauwels RA. Long-acting inhaled beta(2)-agonist therapy in asthma. Am J Respir Crit Care Med 2001; 164(6):923–932.
385. Chang TW. The pharmacological basis of anti-IgE therapy. Nat Biotechnol 2000; 18(2): 157–162.
386. McFadden ER, Hejal R. Asthma. Lancet 1995; 345(8959):1215–1220.
387. Schuh S, Reisman J, Alshehri M, et al. A comparison of inhaled fluticasone and oral prednisone for children with severe acute asthma. N Engl J Med 2000; 343(10):689–694.
388. Reddel H, Ware S, Marks G, et al. Differences between asthma exacerbations and poor asthma control. Lancet 1999; 353(9150):364–369; Erratum in: Lancet 1999; 353(9154):758.
389. Niewoehner DE, Erbland ML, Deupree RH, et al. Effect of systemic glucocorticoids on exacerbations of chronic obstructive pulmonary disease. Department of Veterans Affairs Cooperative Study Group. N Engl J Med 1999; 340(25):1941–1947.
390. Maltais F, Ostinelli J, Bourbeau J, et al. Comparison of nebulized budesonide and oral pre-dnisolone with placebo in the treatment of acute exacerbations of chronic obstructive pulmonary disease: a randomized controlled trial. Am J Respir Crit Care Med 2002; 165(5):698–703.
391. Crapo RO. Pulmonary function testing. N Engl J Med 1994; 331:25–30.
392. ATS. American Thoracic Society statement: standardization of spirometry. Am J Respir Crit Care Med 1995; 152:1107–1136.

393. Hughes JM, Pride NB, eds. Lung function tests: physiological principles and clinical applications. London: W B Saunders, 1999.

394. Peto R, Speizer FE, Cochrane AL, et al. The relevance in adults of air-flow obstruction, but not of mucus hypersecretion, to mortality from chronic lung disease. Results from 20 years of prospective observation. Am Rev Respir Dis 1983; 128(3):491–500.

395. Anthonisen NR, Wright EC, Hodgkin JE. Prognosis in chronic obstructive pulmonary disease. Am Rev Respir Dis 1986; 133:14–20.

396. Burrows B, Earle RH. Course and prognosis of chronic obstructive lung disease. A prospective study of 200 patients. N Engl J Med 1969; 280(8):397–404.

397. Hansen EF, Phanareth K, Laursen LC, et al. Reversible and irreversible airflow obstruction as predictor of overall mortality in asthma and chronic obstructive pulmonary disease. Am J Respir Crit Care Med 1999; 159(4 pt 1):1267–1271.

398. Niewoehner DE, Kleinerman J, Rice DB. Pathologic changes in the peripheral airways of young cigarette smokers. N Engl J Med 1974; 291(15):755–758.

399. Tattersall SF, Benson MK, Hunter D, et al. The use of tests of peripheral lung function for predicting future disability from airflow obstruction in middle-aged smokers. Am Rev Respir Dis 1978; 118:1035–1050.

400. Stanescu DC, Rodenstein DO, Hoeven C, et al. "Sensitive tests" are poor predictors of the decline in forced expiratory volume in one second in middle-aged smokers. Am Rev Respir Dis 1987; 135:585–590.

401. Stanescu D, Sanna A, Veriter C, et al. Identification of smokers susceptible to development of chronic airflow limitation: a 13-year follow-up. Chest 1998; 114(2):416–425.

402. O'Donnell DE, Webb KA. Exertional breathlessness in patients with chronic airflow limitation. The role of lung hyperinflation. Am Rev Respir Dis 1993; 148(5):1351–1357.

403. Belman MJ, Botnick WC, Shin JW. Inhaled bronchodilators reduce dynamic hyperinflation during exercise in patients with chronic obstructive pulmonary disease. Am J Respir Crit Care Med 1996; 153(3):967–975.

404. Taube C, Lehnigk B, Paasch K, et al. Factor analysis of changes in dyspnea and lung function parameters after bronchodilation in chronic obstructive pulmonary disease. Am J Respir Crit Care Med 2000; 162(1):216–220.

405. Santanello NC, Barber BL, Reiss TF, et al. Measurement characteristics of two asthma symptom diary scales for use in clinical trials. Eur Respir J 1997; 10(3):646–651.

406. Juniper EF, O'Byrne PM, Guyatt GH, et al. Development and validation of a questionnaire to measure asthma control. Eur Respir J 1999; 14(4):902–907.

407. Jones PW, Mahler DA. Key outcomes in COPD: health-related quality of life. Proceedings of an expert round table held July 20–22, 2001 in Boston, Massachusetts, USA. Eur Respir Rev 2002; 12(83):57–107.

408. Jones PW. Health status measurement in chronic obstructive pulmonary disease. Thorax 2001; 56(11):880–887.

409. Rutten-van Molken MP, Roos B, van Noord JA. An empirical comparison of the St George's respiratory questionnaire (SGRQ) and the chronic respiratory disease questionnaire (CRQ) in a clinical trial setting. Thorax 1999; 54(11):995–1003.

410. Engstrom CP, Persson LO, Larsson S, et al. Health-related quality of life in COPD: why both disease-specific and generic measures should be used. Eur Respir J 2001; 18(1):69–76.

411. Juniper EF, Guyatt GH, Epstein RS, et al. Evaluation of impairment of health related quality of life in asthma: development of a questionnaire for use in clinical trials. Thorax 1992; 47(2): 76–83.

412. Barley EA, Jones PW. A comparison of global questions versus health status questionnaires as measures of the severity and impact of asthma. Eur Respir J 1999; 14(3):591–596.

413. Juniper EF, O'Byrne PM, Ferrie PJ, et al. Measuring asthma control. Clinic questionnaire or daily diary? Am J Respir Crit Care Med 2000; 162(4 pt 1):1330–1334.

414. Juniper EF, Buist AS, Cox FM, et al. Validation of a standardized version of the Asthma Quality of Life Questionnaire. Chest 1999; 115(5):1265–1270.
415. Polosa R, Rorke S, Holgate ST. Evolving concepts on the value of adenosine hyperresponsiveness in asthma and chronic obstructive pulmonary disease. Thorax 2002; 57(7):649–654.
416. Polosa R, Holgate S. Adenosine bronchoprovocation:a promising marker of allergic inflammation in asthma? Acta Otolaryngol 1997; 52:919–923.
417. Fozard JR, Hannon P. Species differences in adenosine receptor-mediated bronchoconstrictor responses. Clin Exp Allergy 2000; 30:1213–1214.
418. Van Den BM, Kerstjens HA, Meijer RJ, et al. Corticosteroid-induced improvement in the PC20 of adenosine monophosphate is more closely associated with reduction in airway inflammation than improvement in the PC20 of methacholine. Am J Respir Crit Care Med 2001; 164(7):1127–1132.
419. Holgate ST, Arshad H, Stryszak P, et al. Mometasone furoate antagonizes AMP-induced bronchoconstriction in patients with mild asthma. J Allergy Clin Immunol 2000; 105(5):906–911.
420. Ketchell RI, Jensen MW, Lumley P, et al. Rapid effect of inhaled fluticasone propionate on airway responsiveness to adenosine 5'-monophosphate in mild asthma. J Allergy Clin Immunol 2002; 110(4):603–606.
421. Anderson SD. Provocative challenges to help diagnose and monitor asthma: exercise, methacholine, adenosine, and mannitol. Curr Opin Pulm Med 2008; 14(1):39–45.
422. Koskela HO, Hyvarinen L, Brannan JD, et al. Responsiveness to three bronchial provocation tests in patients with asthma. Chest 2003; 124(6):2171–2177.
423. Koskela HO, Hyvarinen L, Brannan JD, et al. Sensitivity and validity of three bronchial provocation tests to demonstrate the effect of inhaled corticosteroids in asthma. Chest 2003; 124(4):1341–1349.
424. Brannan JD, Koskela HO, Anderson S.D. Monitoring asthma therapy using indirect bronchial provocation tests. Clin Respir J 2007; 1:3–15.
425. Enright PL, Sherrill DL. Reference equations for the six-minute walk in healthy adults. Am J Respir Crit Care Med 1998; 158(5 pt 1):1384–1387.
426. Solway S, Brooks D, Lacasse Y, et al. A qualitative systematic overview of the measurement properties of functional walk tests used in the cardiorespiratory domain. Chest 2001; 119(1):256–270.
427. Singh SJ, Morgan MD, Scott S, et al. Development of a shuttle walking test of disability in patients with chronic airways obstruction. Thorax 1992; 47(12):1019–1024.
428. Dyer CA, Singh SJ, Stockley RA, et al. The incremental shuttle walking test in elderly people with chronic airflow limitation. Thorax 2002; 57(1):34–38.
429. Revill SM, Morgan MD, Singh SJ, et al. The endurance shuttle walk: a new field test for the assessment of endurance capacity in chronic obstructive pulmonary disease. Thorax 1999; 54(3):213–222.
430. Newton MF, O'Donnell DE, Forkert L. Response of lung volumes to inhaled salbutamol in a large population of patients with severe hyperinflation. Chest 2002; 121(4):1042–1050.
431. O'Donnell DE, Lam M, Webb KA. Spirometric correlates of improvement in exercise performance after anticholinergic therapy in chronic obstructive pulmonary disease. Am J Respir Crit Care Med 1999; 160(2):542–549.
432. O'Donnell DE, Lam M, Webb KA. Measurement of symptoms, lung hyperinflation, and endurance during exercise in chronic obstructive pulmonary disease. Am J Respir Crit Care Med 1998; 158(5 pt 1):1557–1565.
433. Muller NL, Coxson H. Chronic obstructive pulmonary disease. 4: Imaging the lungs in patients with chronic obstructive pulmonary disease. Thorax 2002; 57(11):982–985.
434. O'Brien C, Guest PJ, Hill SL, et al. Physiological and radiological characterisation of patients diagnosed with chronic obstructive pulmonary disease in primary care. Thorax 2000; 55(8):635–642.

435. Cosio MG, Snider GL. Chest computed tomography: is it ready for major studies of chronic obstructive pulmonary disease? Eur Respir J 2001; 17(6):1062–1064.

436. Cleverley JR, Muller NL. Advances in radiologic assessment of chronic obstructive pulmonary disease. Clin Chest Med 2000; 21(4):653–663.

437. Ferretti GR, Bricault I, Coulomb M. Virtual tools for imaging of the thorax. Eur Respir J 2001; 18(2):381–392.

438. Soejima K, Yamaguchi K, Kohda E, et al. Longitudinal follow-up study of smoking-induced lung density changes by high-resolution computed tomography. Am J Respir Crit Care Med 2000; 161(4 pt 1):1264–1273.

439. Remy-Jardin M, Remy J, Boulenguez C, et al. Morphologic effects of cigarette smoking on airways and pulmonary parenchyma in healthy adult volunteers: CT evaluation and correlation with pulmonary function tests. Radiology 1993; 186(1):107–115.

440. Remy-Jardin M, Edme JL, Boulenguez C, et al. Longitudinal follow-up study of smoker's lung with thin-section CT in correlation with pulmonary function tests. Radiology 2002; 222(1):261–270.

441. Dowson LJ, Guest PJ, Stockley RA. Longitudinal changes in physiological, radiological, and health status measurements in alpha(1)-antitrypsin deficiency and factors associated with decline. Am J Respir Crit Care Med 2001; 164(10 pt 1):1805–1809.

442. Dowson LJ, Guest PJ, Hill SL, et al. High-resolution computed tomography scanning in alpha1-antitrypsin deficiency: relationship to lung function and health status. Eur Respir J 2001; 17(6):1097–1104.

443. Dirksen A, Friis M, Olesen KP, et al. Progress of emphysema in severe alpha1-antitrypsin deficiency as assessed by annual CT. Acta Radiol 1997; 38:826–832.

444. Dirksen A, Dijkman JH, Madsen F, et al. A randomized clinical trial of alpha-1-antitrypsin augmentation therapy. Am J Resp Crit Care Med 1999; 160:1468–1472.

445. Mao JT, Goldin JG, Dermand J, et al. A pilot study of all-trans-retinoic acid for the treatment of human emphysema. Am J Respir Crit Care Med 2002; 165(5):718–723.

446. Hansell DM. Small airways diseases: detection and insights with computed tomography. Eur Respir J 2001; 17(6):1294–1313.

447. King GG, Muller NL, Pare PD. Evaluation of airways in obstructive pulmonary disease using high-resolution computed tomography. Am J Respir Crit Care Med 1999; 159(3):992–1004.

448. Brown RH, Scichilone N, Mudge B, et al. High-resolution computed tomographic evaluation of airway distensibility and the effects of lung inflation on airway caliber in healthy subjects and individuals with asthma. Am J Respir Crit Care Med 2001; 163(4):994–1001.

449. Mclean AN, Sproule MW, Cowan MD, et al. High resolution computed tomography in asthma. Thorax 1998; 53(4):308–314.

450. American Thoracic Society. ATS/ERS statement on respiratory muscle testing. Am J Respir Crit Care Med 2002; 166(4):518–624.

451. Levine S, Kaiser L, Leferovich J, et al. Cellular adaptations in the diaphragm in chronic obstructive pulmonary disease. N Engl J Med 1997; 337(25):1799–1806.

452. Polkey MI, Kyroussis D, Hamnegard CH, et al. Diaphragm strength in chronic obstructive pulmonary disease. Am J Respir Crit Care Med 1996; 154(5):1310–1317.

453. Reid MB. COPD as a muscle disease. Am J Respir Crit Care Med 2001; 164(7):1101–1102.

454. Agusti AG, Sauleda J, Miralles C, et al. Skeletal muscle apoptosis and weight loss in chronic obstructive pulmonary disease. Am J Respir Crit Care Med 2002; 166(4):485–489.

455. American Thoracic Society. Supplement: American Thoracic Society/European Respiratory Society—Skeletal muscle dysfunction in chronic obstructive pulmonary disease. Am J of Respir Crit Care Med 1999; 159(pt 2):S1–S40.

456. Gosselink R, Troosters T, Decramer M. Peripheral muscle weakness contributes to exercise limitation in COPD. Am J Respir Crit Care Med 1996; 153(3):976–980.

457. Engelen MP, Schols AM, Does JD, et al. Skeletal muscle weakness is associated with wasting of extremity fat-free mass but not with airflow obstruction in patients with chronic obstructive pulmonary disease. Am J Clin Nutr 2000; 71(3):733–738.

458. Marquis K, Debigare R, Lacasse Y, et al. Midthigh muscle cross-sectional area is a better predictor of mortality than body mass index in patients with chronic obstructive pulmonary disease. Am J Respir Crit Care Med 2002; 166(6):809–813.

459. Celli BR, Cote CG, Marin JM, et al. The body-mass index, airflow obstruction, dyspnea, and exercise capacity index in chronic obstructive pulmonary disease. N Engl J Med 2004; 350(10):1005–1012.

460. Martinez FJ, Han MK, Andrei AC, et al. Longitudinal change in the BODE index predicts mortality in severe emphysema. Am J Respir Crit Care Med 2008; 178(5):491–499.

461. Cote CG, Pinto-Plata V, Marin JM, et al. The modified BODE index: validation with mortality in COPD. Eur Respir J 2008; 32(5):1269–1274.

462. Fletcher C, Peto R. The natural history of chronic airflow obstruction. BMJ 1977; 1: 1645–1648.

463. Suissa S, Ernst P, Benayoun S, et al. Low-dose inhaled corticosteroids and the prevention of death from asthma. N Engl J Med 2000; 343(5):332–336.

464. Frank R, Hargreaves R. Clinical biomarkers in drug discovery and development. Nat Rev Drug Discov 2003; 2(7):566–580.

465. Kola I, Hazuda D. Innovation and greater probability of success in drug discovery and development—from target to biomarkers. Curr Opin Biotechnol 2005; 16(6):644–646.

466. Phillips KA, Van BS, Issa AM. Diagnostics and biomarker development: priming the pipeline. Nat Rev Drug Discov 2006; 5(6):463–469.

467. Altar CA. The biomarkers consortium: on the critical path of drug discovery. Clin Pharmacol Ther 2008; 83(2):361–364.

468. Vestbo J, Anderson W, Coxson HO, et al. Evaluation of COPD longitudinally to identify predictive surrogate end-points (ECLIPSE). Eur Respir J 2008; 31(4):869–873.

469. Moore WC, Bleecker ER, Curran-Everett D, et al. Characterization of the severe asthma phenotype by the National Heart, Lung, and Blood Institute's Severe Asthma Research Program. J Allergy Clin Immunol 2007; 119(2):405–413.

470. Munoz NM, Rabe KF, Neeley SP, et al. Eosinophil VLA-4 binding to fibronectin augments bronchial narrowing through 5-lipoxygenase activation. Am J Physiol 1996; 270(4 pt 1): L587–L594.

471. Frew AJ. GA2LEN—the Global Allergy and Asthma European Network. Clin Exp Allergy 2005; 35(2):122–125.

472. Erin EM, Williams TJ, Barnes PJ, et al. Eotaxin receptor (CCR-3) antagonism in asthma and allergic disease. Curr Drug Targets Inflamm Allergy 2002; 1:201–214.

473. Sabroe I, Hartnell A, Jopling LA, et al. Differential regulation of eosinophil chemokine signaling via CCR3 and non-CCR3 pathways. J Immunol 1999; 162:2946–2955.

474. Bryan SA, Jose P, Topping JR, et al. Responses of leukocytes to chemokines in whole blood and their antagonism by novel CCR3 antagonists. Am J Respir Crit Care Med 2002; 165:1602–1609.

475. Zhang L, Soares MP, Guan Y, et al. Functional expression and characterization of macaque C-C chemokine receptor 3 (CCR3) and generation of potent antagonistic anti-macaque CCR3 monoclonal antibodies. J Biol Chem 2002; 277(37):33799–33810.

476. Nicholson GC, Tennant RC, Carpenter DC, et al. Employing flow cytometric assays of human whole blood neutrophil and monocyte CD11b upregulation and shape change to assess pharmacodynamic activity of a chemokine receptor (CXCR2) antagonist. Pulm Pharmacol Ther 2007; 20:52–59.

477. Hogan SP, Rosenberg HF, Moqbel R, et al. Eosinophils: biological properties and role in health and disease. Clin Exp Allergy 2008; 38(5):709–750.

478. Kharitonov S, Alving K, Barnes PJ. Exhaled and nasal nitric oxide measurements: recommendations. The European Respiratory Society Task Force. Eur Respir J 1997; 10(7): 1683–1693.

479. Medoff BD, Thomas SY, Luster AD. T cell trafficking in allergic asthma: the ins and outs. Annu Rev Immunol 2008; 26:205–232.

480. Corrigan CJ, Hartnell A, Kay AB. T lymphocyte activation in acute severe asthma. Lancet 1988; 1(8595):1129–1132.

481. Gemou-Engesaeth V, Fagerhol MK, Toda M, et al. Expression of activation markers and cytokine mRNA by peripheral blood CD4 and CD8 T cells in atopic and nonatopic childhood asthma: effect of inhaled glucocorticoid therapy. Pediatrics 2002; 109(2):E24.

482. Hansel NN, Cheadle C, Diette GB, et al. Analysis of CD4+ T-cell gene expression in allergic subjects using two different microarray platforms. Allergy 2008; 63(3):366–369.

483. Robinson DS, Hamid Q, Ying S, et al. Predominant Th2-like bronchoalveolar T-lymphocyte population in atopic asthma. N Engl J Med 1992; 326:298–304.

484. Syed F, Huang CC, Li K, et al. Identification of interleukin-13 related biomarkers using peripheral blood mononuclear cells. Biomarkers 2007; 12(4):414–423.

485. Akdis M, Verhagen J, Taylor A, et al. Immune responses in healthy and allergic individuals are characterized by a fine balance between allergen-specific T regulatory 1 and T helper 2 cells. J Exp Med 2004; 199(11):1567–1575.

486. Larche M. Regulatory T cells in allergy and asthma. Chest 2007; 132(3):1007–1014.

487. Deniz G, Erten G, Kucuksezer UC, et al. Regulatory NK cells suppress antigen-specific T cell responses. J Immunol 2008; 180(2):850–857.

488. Mamessier E, Nieves A, Lorec AM, et al. T-cell activation during exacerbations: a longitudinal study in refractory asthma. Allergy 2008; 63(9):1202–1210.

489. Hashimoto T, Akiyama K, Kobayashi N, et al. Comparison of IL-17 production by helper T cells among atopic and nonatopic asthmatics and control subjects. Int Arch Allergy Immunol 2005; 137(suppl 1):51–54.

490. Barczyk A, Pierzchala W, Sozanska E. Interleukin-17 in sputum correlates with airway hyperresponsiveness to methacholine. Respir Med 2003; 97(6):726–733.

491. Molet S, Hamid Q, Davoine F, et al. IL-17 is increased in asthmatic airways and induces human bronchial fibroblasts to produce cytokines. J Allergy Clin Immunol 2001; 108(3):430–438.

492. Schmidt-Weber CB, Akdis M, et al. TH17 cells in the big picture of immunology. J Allergy Clin Immunol 2007; 120(2):247–254.

493. Schnyder-Candrian S, Togbe D, Couillin I, et al. Interleukin-17 is a negative regulator of established allergic asthma. J Exp Med 2006; 203(12):2715–2725.

494. Burnett D, Chamba A, Hill SL, et al. Neutrophils from subjects with chronic obstructive lung disease show enhanced chemotaxis and extracellular proteolysis. Lancet 1987; 2 (8567):1043–1046.

495. Noguera A, Batle S, Miralles C, et al. Enhanced neutrophil response in chronic obstructive pulmonary disease. Thorax 2001; 56(6):432–437.

496. Noguera A, Busquets X, Sauleda J, et al. Expression of adhesion molecules and G proteins in circulating neutrophils in chronic obstructive pulmonary disease. Am J Respir Crit Care Med 1998; 158(5 pt 1):1664–1668.

497. de Torres JP, Cordoba-Lanus E, Lopez-Aguilar C, et al. C-reactive protein levels and clinically important predictive outcomes in stable COPD patients. Eur Respir J 2006; 27(5):902–907.

498. Man SF, Sin DD. Effects of corticosteroids on systemic inflammation in chronic obstructive pulmonary disease. Proc Am Thorac Soc 2005; 2(1):78–82.

499. Hurst JR, Donaldson GC, Perera WR, et al. Use of plasma biomarkers at exacerbation of chronic obstructive pulmonary disease. Am J Respir Crit Care Med 2006; 174(8):867–874.

500. Perera WR, Hurst JR, Wilkinson TM, et al. Inflammatory changes, recovery and recurrence at COPD exacerbation. Eur Respir J 2007; 29(3):527–534.

501. Pinto-Plata V, Toso J, Lee K, et al. Profiling serum biomarkers in patients with COPD: associations with clinical parameters. Thorax 2007; 62(7):595–601.
502. Oudijk EJ, Nijhuis EH, Zwank MD, et al. Systemic inflammation in COPD visualised by gene profiling in peripheral blood neutrophils. Thorax 2005; 60(7):538–544.
503. Barcelo B, Pons J, Ferrer JM, et al. Phenotypic characterisation of T-lymphocytes in COPD: abnormal CD4+CD25+ regulatory T-lymphocyte response to tobacco smoking. Eur Respir J 2008; 31(3):555–562.
504. Barcelo B, Pons J, Fuster A, et al. Intracellular cytokine profile of T lymphocytes in patients with chronic obstructive pulmonary disease. Clin Exp Immunol 2006; 145(3):474–479.
505. Kharitonov SA, Yates D, Robbins RA, et al. Increased nitric oxide in exhaled air of asthmatic patients. Lancet 1994; 343(8890):133–135.
506. Kharitonov SA, Barnes PJ. Exhaled biomarkers. Chest 2006; 130(5):1541–1546.
507. ATS. Recommendations for standardized procedures for the on-line and off-line measurement of exhaled lower respiratory nitric oxide and nasal nitric oxide in adults and children-1999. This official statement of the American Thoracic Society was adopted by the ATS Board of Directors, July 1999. Am J Respir Crit Care Med 1999; 160(6):2104–2117.
508. Brindicci C, Ito K, Barnes PJ, et al. Effect of an inducible nitric oxide synthase inhibitor on differential flow-exhaled nitric oxide in asthmatic patients and healthy volunteers. Chest 2007; 132(2):581–588.
509. Berry M, Hargadon B, Morgan A, et al. Alveolar nitric oxide in adults with asthma: evidence of distal lung inflammation in refractory asthma. Eur Respir J 2005; 25(6):986–991.
510. van Veen IH, Sterk PJ, Schot R, et al. Alveolar nitric oxide versus measures of peripheral airway dysfunction in severe asthma. Eur Respir J 2006; 27(5):951–956.
511. Brindicci C, Ito K, Barnes PJ, et al. Differential flow analysis of exhaled nitric oxide in patients with asthma of differing severity. Chest 2007; 131(5):1353–1362.
512. Smith AD, Cowan JO, Brassett KP, et al. Use of exhaled nitric oxide measurements to guide treatment in chronic asthma. N Engl J Med 2005; 352(21):2163–2173.
513. Taylor DR, Pijnenburg MW, Smith AD, et al. Exhaled nitric oxide measurements: clinical application and interpretation. Thorax 2006; 61(9):817–827.
514. Jones SL, Kittelson J, Cowan JO, et al. The predictive value of exhaled nitric oxide measurements in assessing changes in asthma control. Am J Respir Crit Care Med 2001; 164(5):738–743.
515. Kharitonov SA, Yates DH, Barnes PJ. Changes in the dose of inhaled steroid affect exhaled nitric oxide levels in asthmatic patients. Eur Respir J 1996; 9:196–201.
516. Jatakanon A, Lim S, Barnes PJ. Changes in sputum eosinophils predict loss of asthma control. Am J Respir Crit Care Med 2000; 161(1):64–72.
517. Kharitonov SA, Barnes PJ. Exhaled markers of pulmonary disease. Am J Respir Crit Care Med 2001; 163(7):1693–1722.
518. van Den Toorn LM, Prins JB, Overbeek SE, et al. Adolescents in clinical remission of atopic asthma have elevated exhaled nitric oxide levels and bronchial hyperresponsiveness. Am J Respir Crit Care Med 2000; 162(3 pt 1):953–957.
519. Kharitonov SA, Yates DH, Barnes PJ. Inhaled glucocorticosteroids decrease nitric oxide in exhaled air of asthmatic patients. Am J Respir Crit Care Med 1996; 153:454–457.
520. Kharitinov SA, Donnelly LE, Corradi M, et al. Dose-dependent onset and duration of action of 100/400mcg budesonide on exhaled nitric oxide and related changes in other potential markers of airway inflammation in mild asthma. Am J Respir Crit Care Med 2000; 161:A186.
521. Kharitonov SA, Barnes PJ. Does exhaled nitric oxide reflect asthma control? Yes, it does! Am J Respir Crit Care Med 2001; 164(5):727–728.
522. Bayley DL, Abusriwil H, Ahmad A, et al. Validation of assays for inflammatory mediators in exhaled breath condensate. Eur Respir J 2008; 31(5):943–948.
523. Hoffmann HJ, Tabaksblat LM, Enghild JJ, et al. Human skin keratins are the major proteins in exhaled breath condensate. Eur Respir J 2008; 31(2):380–384.

524. Effros RM, Hoagland KW, Bosbous M, et al. Dilution of respiratory solutes in exhaled condensates. Am J Respir Crit Care Med 2002; 165(5):663–669.
525. Effros RM, Peterson B, Casaburi R, et al. Epithelial lining fluid solute concentrations in chronic obstructive lung disease patients and normal subjects. J Appl Physiol 2005; 99(4): 1286–1292.
526. Effros RM, Casaburi R, Su J, et al. The effects of volatile salivary acids and bases on exhaled breath condensate pH. Am J Respir Crit Care Med 2006; 173(4):386–392.
527. Gaber F, Acevedo F, Delin I, et al. Saliva is one likely source of leukotriene B4 in exhaled breath condensate. Eur Respir J 2006; 28(6):1229–1235.
528. Effros RM, Casaburi R, Su J, et al. The effects of volatile salivary acids and bases on exhaled breath condensate pH. Am J Respir Crit Care Med 2006; 173(4):386–392.
529. Marteus H, Tornberg DC, Weitzberg E, et al. Origin of nitrite and nitrate in nasal and exhaled breath condensate and relation to nitric oxide formation. Thorax 2005; 60(3):219–225.
530. Rosias PP, Robroeks CM, Niemarkt HJ, et al. Breath condenser coatings affect measurement of biomarkers in exhaled breath condensate. Eur Respir J 2006; 28(5):1036–1041.
531. Chan HP, Lewis C, Thomas PS. Exhaled breath analysis: novel approach for early detection of lung cancer. Lung Cancer 2009; 63(2):164–168.
532. Mazzone PJ, Hammel J, Dweik R, et al. Diagnosis of lung cancer by the analysis of exhaled breath with a colorimetric sensor array. Thorax 2007; 62(7):565–568.
533. Fahy JV, Boushey HA, Lazarus SC, et al. Safety and reproducibility of sputum induction in asthmatic subjects in a multicenter study. Am J Respir Crit Care Med 2001; 163(6): 1470–1475.
534. Brightling CE, Monterio W, Green RH, et al. Induced sputum and other outcome measures in chronic obstructive pulmonary disease: safety and repeatability. Respir Med 2001; 95: 999–1002.
535. Moodley YP, Dorasamy T, Venketasamy S, et al. Correlation of CD4:CD8 ratio and tumour necrosis factor (TNF)alpha levels in induced sputum with bronchoalveolar lavage fluid in pulmonary sarcoidosis. Thorax 2000; 55(8):696–699.
536. Grootendorst DC, Sont JK, Willems LNA, et al. Comparison of inflammatory cell counts in asthma: induced sputum vs bronchoalveolar lavage and bronchial biopsies. Clin Exp Allergy 1997; 27:769–779.
537. Keatings VM, Evans DJ, O'Connor BJ, et al. Cellular profiles in asthmatic airways: a comparison of induced sputum, bronchial washings, and bronchoalveolar lavage fluid. Thorax 1997; 52(4):372–374.
538. Vignola AM, Rennard SI, Hargreave FE, et al. Report of working group 8: future directions. Eur Respir J 2002; 20(suppl 37):51s–55s.
539. Kips JC, Fahy JV, Hargreave FE, et al. Methods for sputum induction and analysis of induced sputum: a method for assessing airway inflammation in asthma. Eur Respir J 1998; 11(suppl 26):9s–12s.
540. Jayaram L, Parameswaran K, Sears MR, et al. Induced sputum cell counts: their usefulness in clinical practice. Eur Respir J 2000; 16(1):150–158.
541. Green RH, Brightling CE, McKenna S, et al. Asthma exacerbations and sputum eosinophil counts: a randomised controlled trial. Lancet 2002; 360(9347):1715–1721.
542. Lex C, Payne DN, Zacharasiewicz A, et al. Sputum induction in children with difficult asthma: safety, feasibility, and inflammatory cell pattern. Pediatr Pulmonol 2005; 39(4): 318–324.
543. Zacharasiewicz A, Wilson N, Lex C, et al. Clinical use of noninvasive measurements of airway inflammation in steroid reduction in children. Am J Respir Crit Care Med 2005; 171(10): 1077–1082.
544. Lex C, Ferreira F, Zacharasiewicz A, et al. Airway eosinophilia in children with severe asthma: predictive values of noninvasive tests. Am J Respir Crit Care Med 2006; 174(12): 1286–1291.

545. Lex C, Jenkins G, Wilson NM, et al. Does sputum eosinophilia predict the response to systemic corticosteroids in children with difficult asthma? Pediatr Pulmonol 2007; 42(3): 298–303.

546. Sapey E, Bayley D, Ahmad A, et al. Inter-relationships between inflammatory markers in patients with stable COPD with bronchitis: intra-patient and inter-patient variability. Thorax 2008; 63(6):493–499.

547. Beckman JS, Beckman TW, Chen J, et al. Apparent hydroxyl radical production by peroxynitrite: implications for endothelial injury from nitric oxide and superoxide. Proc Natl Acad Sci U S A 1990; 87(4):1620–1624.

548. Keatings VM, Collins PD, Scott DM, et al. Differences in interleukin-8 and tumor necrosis factor-alpha in induced sputum from patients with chronic obstructive pulmonary disease or asthma. Am J Respir Crit Care Med 1996; 153(2):530–534.

549. Gibson PG, Simpson JL, Saltos N. Heterogeneity of airway inflammation in persistent asthma: evidence of neutrophilic inflammation and increased sputum interleukin-8. Chest 2001; 119(5):1329–1336.

550. Simpson JL, Timmins NL, Fakes K, et al. Effect of saliva contamination on induced sputum cell counts, IL-8 and eosinophil cationic protein levels. Eur Respir J 2004; 23(5):759–762.

551. Crooks SW, Bayley DL, Hill SL, et al. Bronchial inflammation in acute bacterial exacerbations of chronic bronchitis: the role of leukotriene B4. Eur Respir J 2000; 15:274–280.

552. Traves SL, Culpitt SV, Russell RE, et al. Increased levels of the chemokines GROalpha and MCP-1 in sputum samples from patients with COPD. Thorax 2002; 57(7):590–595.

553. Vignola AM, Riccobono L, Profita M, et al. Effects of low doses of inhaled fluticasone propionate on inflammation and remodelling in persistent-mild asthma. Allergy 2005; 60(12): 1511–1517.

554. Louis R, Shute J, Goldring K, et al. The effect of processing on inflammatory markers in induced sputum. Eur Respir J 1999; 13(3):660–667.

555. Woolhouse IS, Bayley DL, Stockley RA. Effect of sputum processing with dithiothreitol on the detection of inflammatory mediators in chronic bronchitis and bronchiectasis. Thorax 2002; 57(8):667–671.

556. Kelly MM, Keatings V, Leigh R, et al. European Respiratory Society Task Force. Standardized methodology of sputum induction and processing: analysis of fluid-phase mediators. Eur Respir J 2002; 20:24s–39s.

557. Hansel TT, Braunstein JB, Walker C, et al. Sputum eosinophils from asthmatics express ICAM-1 and HLA-DR. Clin Exp Immunol 1991; 86:271–277.

558. Qiu D, Tan WC. Dithiothreitol has a dose-response effect on cell surface antigen expression. J Allergy Clin Immunol 1999; 103(5 pt 1):873–876.

559. Kelly MM, Leigh R, Horsewood P, et al. Induced sputum: validity of fluid-phase IL-5 measurement. J Allergy Clin Immunol 2000; 105(6 pt 1):1162–1168.

560. Kelly MM, Leigh R, Carruthers S, et al. Increased detection of interleukin-5 in sputum by addition of protease inhibitors. Eur Respir J 2001; 18(4):685–691.

561. Berry MA, Parker D, Neale N, et al. Sputum and bronchial submucosal IL-13 expression in asthma and eosinophilic bronchitis. J Allergy Clin Immunol 2004; 114(5):1106–1109.

562. Saha SK, Berry MA, Parker D, et al. Increased sputum and bronchial biopsy IL-13 expression in severe asthma. J Allergy Clin Immunol 2008; 121(3):685–691.

563. Saha S, Mistry V, Siva R, et al. Induced sputum and bronchial mucosal expression of interleukin-13 is not increased in chronic obstructive pulmonary disease. Allergy 2008; 63(9): 1239–1243.

564. Erin EM, Jenkins GR, Kon OM, et al. Optimised dialysis and protease inhibition of sputum dithiothreitol supernatants. Am J Respir Crit Care Med 2008; 177(2):132–141.

565. Konno S, Gonokami Y, Kurokawa M, et al. Cytokine concentrations in sputum of asthmatic patients. Int Arch Allergy Immunol 1996; 109(1):73–78.

566. Hill AT, Bayley DL, Stockley RA. The interrelationship of sputum inflammatory markers in patients with chronic bronchitis. Am J Respir Crit Care Med 1999; 160:893–898.

567. Stockley RA, Bayley DL. Validation of assays for inflammatory mediators in sputum. Eur Respir J 2000; 15(4):778–781.

568. Grebski E, Peterson C, Medici TC. Effect of physical and chemical methods of homogenization on inflammatory mediators in sputum of asthma patients. Chest 2001; 119(5): 1521–1525.

569. Parr DG, White AJ, Bayley DL, et al. Inflammation in sputum relates to progression of disease in subjects with COPD: a prospective descriptive study. Respir Res 2006; 7:136.

570. Kim JS, Hackley GH, Okamoto K, et al. Sputum processing for evaluation of inflammatory mediators. Pediatr Pulmonol 2001; 32(2):152–158.

571. Gray RD, MacGregor G, Noble D, et al. Sputum proteomics in inflammatory and suppurative respiratory diseases. Am J Respir Crit Care Med 2008; 178(5):444–452.

572. Robinson D. Bronchoalveolar lavage as a tool for studying airway inflammation in asthma. Eur Respir Rev 1998; 8:1072–1074.

573. Haslam PL, Baughman RP, eds. Report of European Respiratory Society (ERS) Task Force: guidelines for measurement of acellular components and recommendations for standardization of bronchoalveolar lavage (BAL). Eur Respir Rev 1999; 9(66):25–157.

574. British Thoracic Society guidelines on diagnostic flexible bronchoscopy. Thorax 2001; 56(suppl 1):i1–i21.

575. Mehta AC, Prakash UB, Garland R, et al. American College of Chest Physicians and American Association for Bronchology [corrected] consensus statement: prevention of flexible bronchoscopy-associated infection. Chest 2005; 128(3):1742–1755.

576. Ouellette DR. The safety of bronchoscopy in a pulmonary fellowship program. Chest 2006; 130(4):1185–1190.

577. Pavord ID, Cox G, Thomson NC, et al. Safety and efficacy of bronchial thermoplasty in symptomatic, severe asthma. Am J Respir Crit Care Med 2007; 176(12):1185–1191.

578. Kavuru MS, Dweik RA, Thomassen MJ. Role of bronchoscopy in asthma research. Clin Chest Med 1999; 20(1):153–189.

579. Krause A, Hohberg B, Heine F, et al. Cytokines derived from alveolar macrophages induce fever after bronchoscopy and bronchoalveolar lavage. Am J Respir Crit Care Med 1997; 155(5):1793–1797.

580. Zhang JY, Wenzel SE. Tissue and BAL based biomarkers in asthma. Immunol Allergy Clin North Am 2007; 27(4):623–632.

581. Faul JL, Demers EA, Burke CM, et al. The reproducibility of repeat measures of airway inflammation in stable atopic asthma. Am J Respir Crit Care Med 1999; 160(5 pt 1):1457–1461.

582. Hattotuwa KL, Gizycki MJ, Ansari TW, et al. The effects of inhaled fluticasone on airway inflammation in chronic obstructive pulmonary disease: a double-blind, placebo-controlled biopsy study. Am J Respir Crit Care Med 2002; 165(12):1592–1596.

583. Faul JL, Leonard CT, Burke CM, et al. Fluticasone propionate induced alterations to lung function and the immunopathology of asthma over time. Thorax 1998; 53:753–761.

584. Ward C, Pais M, Bish R, et al. Airway inflammation, basement membrane thickening and bronchial hyperresponsiveness in asthma. Thorax 2002; 57(4):309–316.

585. Ishizaka A, Watanabe M, Yamashita T, et al. New bronchoscopic microsample probe to measure the biochemical constituents in epithelial lining fluid of patients with acute respiratory distress syndrome. Crit Care Med 2001; 29(4):896–898.

586. Ishizaka A, Matsuda T, Albertine KH, et al. Elevation of KL-6, a lung epithelial cell marker, in plasma and epithelial lining fluid in acute respiratory distress syndrome. Am J Physiol Lung Cell Mol Physiol 2004; 286(6):L1088–L1094.

587. Komaki Y, Sugiura H, Koarai A, et al. Cytokine-mediated xanthine oxidase upregulation in chronic obstructive pulmonary disease's airways. Pulm Pharmacol Ther 2005; 18(4):297–302.

588. Nakano Y, Tasaka S, Saito F, et al. Endothelin-1 level in epithelial lining fluid of patients with acute respiratory distress syndrome. Respirology 2007; 12(5):740–743.

589. Sasabayashi M, Yamazaki Y, Tsushima K, et al. Usefulness of bronchoscopic microsampling to detect the pathogenic bacteria of respiratory infection. Chest 2007; 131(2):474–479.

590. Watanabe M, Ishizaka A, Ikeda E, et al. Contributions of bronchoscopic microsampling in the supplemental diagnosis of small peripheral lung carcinoma. Ann Thorac Surg 2003; 76(5): 1668–1672.

591. Yamazaki K, Ogura S, Ishizaka A, et al. Bronchoscopic microsampling method for measuring drug concentration in epithelial lining fluid. Am J Respir Crit Care Med 2003; 168(11): 1304–1307.

592. Kikuchi J, Yamazaki K, Kikuchi E, et al. Pharmacokinetics of gatifloxacin after a single oral dose in healthy young adult subjects and adult patients with chronic bronchitis, with a comparison of drug concentrations obtained by bronchoscopic microsampling and bronchoalveolar lavage. Clin Ther 2007; 29(1):123–130.

593. Kikuchi J, Yamazaki K, Kikuchi E, et al. Pharmacokinetics of telithromycin using bronchoscopic microsampling after single and multiple oral doses. Pulm Pharmacol Ther 2007; 20(5):549–555.

594. Martinez FD. Genes, environments, development and asthma: a reappraisal. Eur Respir J 2007; 29(1):179–184.

595. Zhang J, Pare PD, Sandford AJ. Recent advances in asthma genetics. Respir Res 2008; 9:4.

596. Holgate ST, Davies DE, Rorke S, et al. Identification and possible functions of ADAM33 asa an asthma susceptibility gene. Clin Exp Allergy Rev 2004; 4:49–55.

597. Shapiro SD, Owen CA. ADAM-33 surfaces as an asthma gene. N Engl J Med 2002; 347(12): 936–938.

598. Kormann MS, Carr D, Klopp N, et al. G-Protein-coupled receptor polymorphisms are associated with asthma in a large German population. Am J Respir Crit Care Med 2005; 171(12): 1358–1362.

599. Postma DS, Koppelman GH. Confirmation of GPRA: a putative drug target for asthma. Am J Respir Crit Care Med 2005; 171(12):1323–1324.

600. Lilly CM, Palmer LJ. The role of prostaglandin D receptor gene in asthma pathogenesis. Am J Respir Cell Mol Biol 2005; 33(3):224–226.

601. Cookson W. The immunogenetics of asthma and eczema: a new focus on the epithelium. Nat Rev Immunol 2004; 4(12):978–988.

602. Hysi P, Kabesch M, Moffatt MF, et al. NOD1 variation, immunoglobulin E and asthma. Hum Mol Genet 2005; 14(7):935–941.

603. Weidinger S, Klopp N, Rummler L, et al. Association of NOD1 polymorphisms with atopic eczema and related phenotypes. J Allergy Clin Immunol 2005; 116(1):177–184.

604. Moffatt MF, Kabesch M, Liang L, et al. Genetic variants regulating ORMDL3 expression contribute to the risk of childhood asthma. Nature 2007; 448(7152):470–473.

605. Dixon AL, Liang L, Moffatt MF, et al. A genome-wide association study of global gene expression. Nat Genet 2007; 39(10):1202–1207.

606. Benson M, Jansson L, Adner M, et al. Gene profiling reveals decreased expression of uterglobin and other anti-inflammatory genes in nasal fluid cells from patients with intermittent allergic rhinitis. Clin Exp Allergy 2005; 35:473–478.

607. Nomura I, Gao B, Boguniewicz M, et al. Distinct patterns of gene expression in the skin lesions of atopic dermatitis and psoriasis: a gene microarray analysis. J Allergy Clin Immunol 2003; 112(6):1195–1202.

608. Zimmermann N, King NE, Laporte J, et al. Dissection of experimental asthma with DNA microarray analysis identifies arginase in asthma pathogenesis. J Clin Invest 2003; 111(12): 1863–1874.

609. Yuyama N, Davies DE, Akaiwa M, et al. Analysis of novel disease-related genes in bronchial asthma. Cytokine 2002; 19(6):287–296.
610. Hansel NN, Diette GB. Gene expression profiling in human asthma. Proc Am Thorac Soc 2007; 4(1):32–36.
611. Cookson WOC. Genetics and genomics of chronic obstructive pulmonary disease. Proc Am Thorac soc 2008; 3:473–477.
612. Hersh CP, DeMeo DL, Silverman EK. National emphysema treatment trial state of the art: genetics of emphysema. Proc Am Thorac Soc 2008; 5(4):486–493.
613. Kalsheker N, Chappell S. The new genetics and chronic obstructive pulmonary disease. COPD 2008; 5(4):257–264.
614. Tomaki M, Sugiura H, Koarai A, et al. Decreased expression of antioxidant enzymes and increased expression of chemokines in COPD lung. Pulm Pharmacol Ther 2007; 20(5):596–605.
615. Brockmoller J, Tzvetkov MV. Pharmacogenetics: data, concepts and tools to improve drug discovery and drug treatment. Eur J Clin Pharmacol 2008; 64(2):133–157.
616. Wechsler ME, Israel E. How pharmacogenomics will play a role in the management of asthma. Am J Respir Crit Care Med 2005; 172(1):12–18.
617. Hall IP. Pharmacogenetics of asthma. Chest 2006; 130(6):1873–1878.
618. Drysdale CM, McGraw DW, Stack CB, et al. Complex promoter and coding region beta2-adrenergic receptor haplotypes alter receptor expression and predict in vivo responsiveness. PNAS 2000; 97:10483–10488.
619. Ortega VE, Hawkins GA, Peters SP, et al. Pharmacogenetics of the beta 2-adrenergic receptor gene. Immunol Allergy Clin North Am 2007; 27(4):665–684.
620. Drazen JM, Yandava CN, Dube L, et al. Pharmacogenetic association between ALOX5 promoter genotype and the response to anti-asthma treatment. Nat Genet 1999; 22(2): 168–170.
621. Witte JS, Palmer LJ, O'Connor RD, et al. Relation between tumour necrosis factor polymorphism TNFalpha-308 and risk of asthma. Eur J Hum Genet 2002; 10(1):82–85.
622. Honey K. Translating medical science around the world. J Clin Invest 2007; 117(10):2737.
623. Farre R, nh-Xuan AT. Translational research in respiratory medicine. Eur Respir J 2007; 30(6): 1041–1042.
624. National Institutes of Health (NIH). NIH launches national consortium to transform clinical research. Available at: http://www.nih.gov/news/pr/oct2006/ncrr-03.htm.
625. Overview of IMI (online). Nat Rev Drug 2007. Available at: http://imi.europa.eu/docs/overview-presentation-of-imi_en.pdf.
626. National Institues of Health (NIH). Biomedical Research Centres. J Clin Invest 2006. Available at: http://www.nihr.ac.uk/infrastructure_biomedical_research_centres.aspx.

3

Assessment of Responses of the Airways to Therapeutic Agents

JOHN D. BRANNAN and PAUL M. O'BYRNE
Firestone Institute for Respiratory Health, St. Joseph's Hospital and McMaster University, Hamilton, Ontario, Canada

I. Introduction

Asthma is a chronic inflammatory disease of the airways, which is characterized by physiological abnormalities of variable airflow obstruction and airway hyperresponsiveness (AHR) to a wide variety of physical and inhaled chemical stimuli and the presence of symptoms, such as dyspnea, cough, chest tightness, and wheezing. Over the past 40 years, very effective medications have been developed to treat asthma, the most effective of which are inhaled β_2-agonists for acute symptom relief and inhaled corticosteroids (ICS) for long-term management (1). Important insights into the optimal management of asthma were made in the early 1980s, when the central role of airway inflammation was identified to be important in asthma pathogenesis, even in very mild disease (2). This resulted in a change of focus from the relief of symptoms with frequent use of inhaled short-acting β_2-agonists (such as salbutamol or terbutaline) to the prevention of symptoms and exacerbations by the regular use of ICS. This approach is extremely effective in the majority of asthmatic patients, and in those who remain symptomatic despite ICS treatment, the combination of ICS and a long-acting inhaled β_2-agonists (such as formoterol or salmeterol) is generally sufficient to control asthma (3).

The concept of asthma control has developed to the point where asthma treatment guidelines have identified that the primary goal of management is to achieve optimal asthma control (1). Control has been defined as the minimization of nighttime and daytime symptoms, activity limitation, rescue bronchodilator use, and airway narrowing. The search for new and effective asthma treatments has persisted, and the approaches developed to assess these new treatment approaches have changed in light of the appreciation of inflammation as central to asthma pathophysiology and the focus on asthma control as the most important treatment outcome. This review will focus on the relevant outcomes that need to be considered when evaluating the efficacy of new therapeutic options for asthma.

II. Activity Vs. Efficacy Vs. Effectiveness

Drug development is usually considered as a four-phase process (Table 1). Phase I is the evaluation of the new entity for safety in normal volunteers, although this phase is sometimes also used to look for some evidence of activity. Phase II is when the "proof of

Table 1 The Four Phases of Drug Development

Phase	Goal	Number of subjects
I	Initial safety and tolerability Determine safe dosage range Identify side effects	20–80
II	Effectiveness/proof of concept Dose response Evaluation of safety Identify side effects	100–300
III	Efficacy Compare to commonly used therapies Collect additional safety information Monitor side effects	1000–5000
IV	Post marketing Efficacy in the general population Optimizing clinical use of therapy Monitor side effects	Real-world population sample

concept" study are done, and in studies for new entities in asthma, this is usually in mildly symptomatic patients with airflow obstruction, or in a clinical model of allergic inflammation. These studies are really examining for activity of the new entity in asthmatic airways and evidence of this activity does not always translate to evidence of efficacy in asthma. Also, these phase II studies are usually small in size and of short duration, which provides little information on the safety of the entity in asthmatic patients. Phase II is sometimes divided into phase IIa, where the proof of concept study is done, and phase IIb, where the entity is evaluated in small studies of more symptomatic patients, to help develop the designs for the efficacy studies. Efficacy is evaluated in phase III studies, which are designed to meet the requirements of regulatory agencies to show both efficacy and safety in the patient population for whom the new drug is to be prescribed. These studies are large (often >1000 patients) and long (usually 1 year of treatment). Evidence of efficacy is required in two such studies to obtain regulatory approval of the new treatment. The requirement for the outcomes to be evaluated in these phase III studies differs in different countries granting regulatory approval.

The final phase of clinical trial development involves phase IV studies, conducted after drug approval has been obtained. These studies are usually used to best position the drug in the marketplace and to collect additional information on safety. However, very few new drugs for asthma have been formally evaluated for effectiveness, which is the usefulness of the drug in the real-world setting.

III. Assessment of Responses of the Airways to Therapeutic Agents

The choice of the outcome variable chosen to assess the activity and efficacy of a therapeutic agent for asthma depends on the class of drug being tested (bronchodilators or controller medications), as well as the phase of drug development. This review will only consider those outcomes commonly used for phase II and III clinical trials.

A. Airway Challenge Testing

AHR is defined as a sensitivity of the airways to a variety of natural or pharmacological stimuli. This is measured by challenging the airways with a variety of constrictor agonists and naturally occurring stimuli, which results in constriction of the airway smooth muscle, leading to airway narrowing and airflow limitation (4). AHR is a key feature of asthma (5). Tests for AHR are useful clinically to identify persons who are suspected of having asthma and who have normal lung function. Traditionally, tests for AHR originated from research in the investigation of mechanisms of airway narrowing and later in the assessment of therapies in the treatment of asthma by protecting against AHR. While most tests for AHR have a role in research, some have use in the clinic for assisting diagnosis of asthma (6), with an emerging role in monitoring therapy (6,7). These procedures have standardized protocols that are available (8–10).

It is imperative that sufficient knowledge of the mechanism of a selected test to induce AHR is understood if the test is to be properly implemented into a research protocol designed to assess a therapeutic agent. Further, prior studies assessing the efficacy of current asthma therapies may assist when considering the design of a protocol for a new therapy. For such trials, inclusion criteria should be well defined to include persons with clinically active disease, as they must be a representative sample of those who will potentially benefit from these therapies in the community. The most appropriate outcome measure when using tests for AHR is assessing changes in airway caliber. This is performed using spirometry and the parameter of forced expiratory volume in one second (FEV_1), which is an accessible, rapid, and reproducible measure of airway caliber (11).

There are two distinct mechanisms by which the airways can narrow to a constrictor stimulus and are defined by the pathways they take to induce AHR. Direct stimuli are pharmacological agents administered exogenously and that act "directly" on specific receptors on the bronchial smooth muscle to cause constriction. These include agents that have a clinical use, such as methacholine (12) and histamine (13), which act on muscarinic and histamine (H_1) receptors, respectively. Furthermore, eicosanoid mediators such as prostaglandins or thromboxane (14) and cysteinyl leukotrienes (15) when inhaled are useful for investigating their receptor-mediated actions on airway smooth muscle, though their role is confined to research. An airway response in persons with asthma is characterized by an increase in airway smooth muscle sensitivity to these individual agents compared with normal healthy persons. The response is defined by a steeper slope of the dose response curve, translating into a greater maximal airway response for a given dose of the stimuli.

Another mechanism of AHR is via the use of indirect stimuli, which includes natural stimuli such as allergen (16) or exercise (17). They also include pharmacological agents such as adenosine monophosphate (AMP) (18) and hyperosmotic agents [e.g., hypertonic saline (17) or dry powder mannitol (19)]. These stimuli induce airway narrowing "indirectly" by causing the endogenous release of mediators of bronchoconstriction from airway inflammatory cells. While the precise mechanism of each stimulus to cause mediator release may differ, they are dependent upon the presence of inflammation, in particular the mast cell and possibly the eosinophils. The response is also determined by the airway smooth muscle sensitivity to these mediators.

There is accumulating evidence linking both direct and indirect AHR to the presence of inflammation in persons with clinically defined asthma (20). However, these correlations to direct measures of AHR are usually not strong, and the airway sensitivity to indirect AHR may better reflect the level of airway inflammation, which appears to be logical when considering the mechanism (20,21).

IV. Direct Bronchial Provocation Tests

Protocols for assessing AHR using direct agents or pharmacological stimuli such as methacholine and histamine have been standardized (9) and used in clinical trials for assessing the efficacy of therapeutic agents (22,23). The airway response is expressed as a provoking concentration (PC) or provoking dose (PD) of the stimuli to cause a 20% reduction in FEV_1. Cutoff values that determine suitable AHR for the evaluation of a therapy in a clinical trial are taken from the clinical cutoff values, which is a PD_{20} of 8 μmol or PC_{20} of 16 mg/mL. Cutoff values may need to be assessed for individual studies, for example, assessing therapy in persons with more active disease may require a lower cutoff value. The reproducibility of the airway sensitivity to direct stimuli also needs to be considered and is reported to be within 1.7 doubling doses (24).

AHR to direct stimuli have been used to assess therapies currently used in the treatment of asthma, for both chronic and long-term uses. The inhibition of AHR by these therapies has in turn provided some explanation as to the mechanisms of direct AHR. Regular use of ICS is well known to attenuate direct AHR (25,26) and they have been proposed as a clinical monitor of ICS (7). However, AHR may remain in many persons with asthma over long-term ICS therapy and can take many months to years to normalize (27). The improvements with ICS on direct AHR suggest that short-term changes are related to reductions in airway inflammation. More long-term improvements may be suggestive of improvements in airway remodeling; however, this is not well defined.

Acutely, $β_2$-agonists are powerful inhibitors at decreasing smooth muscle sensitivity of agents that induce direct AHR (28). The mechanism of action is functional antagonism of the bronchoconstrictor stimulus via $β_2$-receptor-induced airway smooth muscle relaxation. The methacholine challenge is a recognized methodology for assessing efficacy and duration of action of bronchoprotection and the pharmacoequivalence of a $β_2$-agonist (29). It should be noted that persons who regularly use $β_2$-agonists can demonstrate increased airway sensitivity to both direct and indirect AHRs translating to a decreased bronchoprotection (30–32).

The acute use of a leukotriene antagonist (33) and mast cell stabilizing agent such as sodium cromoglycate (34) and nedocromil sodium (35) demonstrate minimal effect to no effect on AHR to direct stimuli. The reasons for this suggest there are limitations in using direct AHR to investigate the bronchoprotective effect of therapies that involve the specific antagonism via individual receptors on the bronchial smooth muscle or for agents that stabilize the mast cell.

V. Indirect Bronchial Provocation Tests

Indirect stimuli may include allergen or stimuli such as dry air hyperpnoea, AMP, or osmotic aerosols. Antigenic stimuli are confined to research while the others have applications clinically, and these differences provide unique opportunities when investigating a specific bronchoprotective or anti-inflammatory action of a pharmacotherapy.

The administration of antigenic stimuli via the aerosol delivery of specific allergens has been well characterized and is useful for understanding the mechanisms of allergic airway inflammation and AHR (36). The administered allergen cross-links antigen-specific IgE that is bound to IgE receptors on mast cells resident in the airway and circulating basophils. This is followed by mast cell degranulation and the upregulation of eicosanoid pathways to release a variety of preformed (e.g., histamine) and newly formed mediators (e.g., leukotrienes and prostaglandins) of bronchoconstriction, which also lead to increasing vascular permeability. The immediate onset of bronchoconstriction by these mediators constitutes the early airway response (EAR) and can reach a maximum at 30 minutes after inhalation of allergen and resolve within three hours. However, in approximately half the individuals who have an EAR, a late airway response (LAR) can generally result between four and eight hours, with some reports of this occurring beyond this period. This response is mechanistically different and results from an increase in the recruitment of cellular inflammation (both metachromatic cells and eosinophils) (37), vascular permeability, and mucous secretion, with a well-characterized increase in AHR to nonallergic stimuli, such as methacholine (16), exercise (38), and AMP (39). This model of bronchoconstriction has been useful at exploring the usefulness of anti-inflammatory therapies in allergic asthma, demonstrating effective attenuation of both the early and late response and airway inflammation of currently used therapies (40,41) (Fig. 1A, B), as well as new therapies (42,43).

The other indirect stimuli differ from allergen in that they are known only to elicit an immediate airway response, and therefore are attractive for clinical use, as well as research (44). Different to direct stimuli, some therapeutic interventions can shift the dose-response curve in some individuals, while inhibiting the stimuli completely in others, which may in some cases be related to an individual's sensitivity to these stimuli.

AMP is a receptor-mediated indirect stimulus that acts by causing airway narrowing via activation of A2b receptors on the mast cell surface, leading to mast cell degranulation and the release of bronchoconstricting mediators (8). AMP is administered in a similar fashion to the administration of direct stimuli such as methacholine and is documented as a PC to cause a 20% fall in FEV_1 (PC_{20}) (8).

Exercise-induced bronchoconstriction (EIB) is a common feature of asthma and a real-life stimulus that can occur in the majority of persons with active asthma. Exercise or dry air hyperpnea causes airway narrowing from the evaporative and cooling effects of respiratory water loss (45). This results in an increase in the osmolarity of the airway surface, which causes the release of bronchoconstricting mediators such as histamine (46), prostaglandins (47), and leukotrienes (48). Thus, the inhalation of hypertonic aerosols has been demonstrated to be effective at identifying persons susceptible of having EIB (49) as well as demonstrating the efficacy of therapies both in the acute and long-term inhibition of EIB and in the treatment of asthma (50).

Protocols for exercise are standardized and have been used in the evaluation of therapies for their acute protective effect on EIB in persons with asthma (51,52). Subjects exercise vigorously breathing a source of dry air, and a sufficient level of ventilation should be reached and sustained by either running or cycling for six to eight minutes to induced adequate airway dehydration. An abnormal response is a 10% to 15% fall in FEV_1 after exercise, measured periodically at least 15 to 20 minutes after exercise. The reproducibility of the airway response to exercise is less variable for persons having at least a 20% fall in FEV_1 and for establishing efficacy of a therapy,

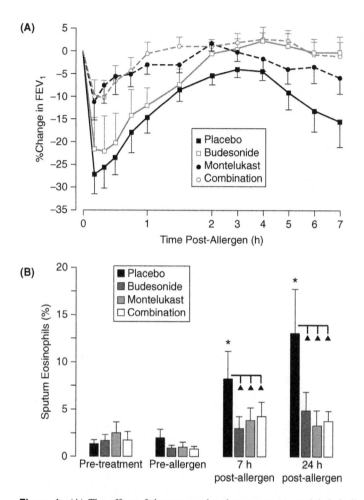

Figure 1 (A) The effect of therapy on the airway response to inhaled allergen; demonstrating time course of the mean (SD) decline in FEV_1 (expressed as percent of prechallenge FEV_1 values) following allergen challenge to assess the efficacy of 10 days of treatment with an inhaled corticosteroid (budesonide; 400 μg daily) and a leukotriene antagonist (montelukast; 10 mg daily) on the early and LAR to inhaled allergen in 10 asthmatic subjects. Significant attenuation of the early response was observed with either montelukast or the combination of budesonide and montelukast when compared with placebo ($p < 0.01$). Significant attenuation of the LAR was observed by all three active treatment regimens when compared with placebo ($p < 0.01$). (B) The mean (SD) percentage of sputum eosinophils before and after an inhaled corticosteroid (budesonide) and a leukotriene antagonist (montelukast) before and following an allergen inhalation challenge in 10 asthmatic subjects in the study of Leigh et al. (40). In association with the attenuation of the LAR to budesonide, montelukast and its combination (A), there was a subsequent reduction in the allergen-induced eosinophilia in the presence of all treatments. * Indicates significant difference from preallergen value in the same treatment group ($p < 0.01$). Filled triangles indicate a significant difference from placebo at the same time point ($p < 0.05$). *Abbreviations*: FEV_1, forced expiratory volume in one second; LAR, late airway response. *Source*: From Ref. 40.

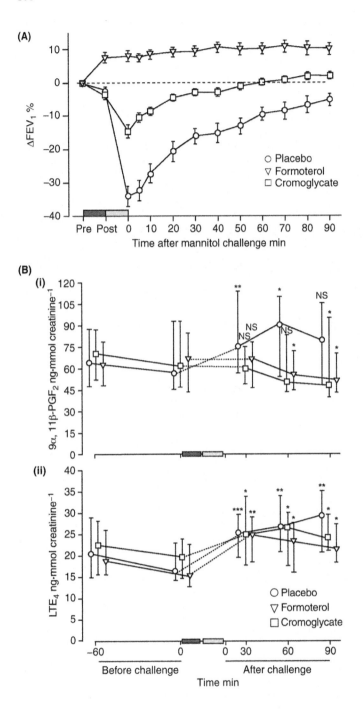

persons with such airway responses are desirable (51). Following an exercise challenge, the reproducibility of the percentage fall in FEV_1 is greater than that of the area under the postexercise FEV_1 versus time curve and the power calculations for sample sizes for these outcomes are available (53).

Surrogate tests for EIB have been developed that have practical and safety advantages for clinical use. These surrogate tests for EIB include eucapnic voluntary hyperventilation (EVH) and osmotic stimuli delivered either as an aerosol of hypertonic saline or mannitol (17). Both of these tests have been derived from the understanding of the mechanism of EIB. EVH testing, first developed by the U.S. Army to screen recruits (54), has a use clinically in persons who have normal lung function and who are suspected of having EIB alone, such as athletes (55). The advantage of this test over exercise is that it can be performed without the need to exercise the patient. Also, higher levels of ventilation can be achieved more rapidly, which is important in an athlete population, who may not demonstrate AHR from a laboratory exercise challenge (55). However, EVH provides a "bolus dose" of hyperventilation and can cause significant bronchoconstriction in known asthmatics, and in this subject group should be used with caution.

Osmotic bronchial provocation tests using nebulized hypertonic saline (using a 4.5% concentration) or dry powder mannitol (Aridol™ or Osmohale™) have been developed to assist in further improving the ease of administration of indirect testing (19) (Fig. 2). Mannitol provides a common operating standard that may be attractive for multicenter studies as well as demonstrate suitable reproducibility, comparable with direct stimuli (56,57). Similar to AMP and direct stimuli, osmotic challenges are dose response challenges that do not induce significant reductions in FEV_1 and have shown adequate safety in large populations (19).

Pharmacotherapy for the treatment of asthma has revealed much about the mechanism of indirect AHR. Acute use of β_2-agonist demonstrates the most potent

---

Figure 2 (A) The acute effect of therapy on the airway response to an osmotic challenge, demonstrating the time course of the mean (SD) decline in FEV_1 (expressed as percent of pre-challenge FEV_1 values) following inhaled mannitol to assess the acute effect of a β_2-agonist (formoterol) and a cromolyn (sodium cromoglycate) on the airway sensitivity and airway recovery in 14 asthmatic subjects. The mannitol challenge commenced 15 minutes following the inhalation of 40 mg of cromoglycate or 24 µg of formoterol or placebo after identifying the cumulative dose of mannitol to cause a 25% fall in FEV_1 on a control day. Formoterol demonstrated greater inhibition of the airway sensitivity compared with cromoglycate, both significant compared with placebo ($p < 0.001$) (90). (B) The change in urinary excretion of mediators of bronchoconstriction in association with the airway response to an osmotic stimulus in 14 asthmatic subjects; the mean (interquartile range) of the urinary concentration of (i) $9\alpha,11\beta$-prostaglandin (PG) F_2 and (ii) leukotriene (LT) E_4 over 60 minutes before and 90 minutes after mannitol challenge in the presence of sodium cromoglycate, formoterol, and placebo in the study of Brannan et al. (90). In association with the inhibition of the airway response to inhaled mannitol by cromoglycate and formoterol (i) there was an inhibition of the urinary excretion of $9\alpha,11\beta$-prostaglandin (PG) F_2, marker of mast cell PGD_2 release. There was no significant reduction in the excretion of LTE4. * Indicates $p < 0.05$; **, $p < 0.01$; and ***, $p < 0.001$ versus mean of the two baseline samples. *Abbreviations*: FEV_1, forced expiratory volume in one second; NS, nonsignificant.

protective effect on indirect stimuli, likely due to a combination of functional antagonism of mediators causing bronchoconstriction, as well as via β_2-receptor-mediated mast cell stabilization (58) (Fig. 2A). Drugs such as sodium cromoglycate and nedocromil sodium are also potent inhibitors of indirect AHR due to their mast cell stabilizing properties (58,59). Leukotriene antagonists are not as protective at inhibiting the initial bronchoconstrictive response to indirect stimuli; however, they have a powerful effect on causing a rapid recovery from indirect induced AHR (60,61). Thus, the airway sensitivity and recovery from an indirect bronchoconstricting stimulus may be important to consider when assessing new pharmacotherapy.

VI. Biomarkers

Airway inflammation is a key feature of airway disease, and thus, it is important to assess the efficacy of anti-inflammatory therapies by demonstrating a decrease in markers of airway inflammation, preferably in association of other markers of airway dysfunction and symptoms. However, the measurement of airway inflammation can be practically difficult to achieve and historically was obtained using invasive techniques; however, there is a general shift to less-invasive or noninvasive methods.

The most direct measurements of airway inflammation are through the use of bronchoscopy, such as bronchoalveolar lavage, endobronchial brushing, or biopsy (62). Such techniques have been important in exploring the pathological features of airway disease, such as the assessment of inflammation and tissue remodeling. Profiles of infiltrating inflammatory cells and inflammatory markers can correlate with clinical markers of airway disease (63). Segmental bronchial challenge can also be performed via instillation through a bronchoscope into an isolated airway, which is more commonly performed using allergen (62). Bronchial biopsy has been performed before and following anti-inflammatory therapies such as ICS to demonstrate a reduction in inflammatory cells such as mast cells and eosinophils as well as epithelial repair and markers of airway remodeling, in association with improvements in symptoms (64,65). While there are concerns over safety of these techniques, particularly in asthmatic patients, studies assessing safety have found that these procedures can be performed with adequate safety (62).

Less direct measures of airway inflammation provide an option for assessing changes in inflammation to therapy in the clinical trial setting. The use of induced sputum has been validated as a test for assessing the presence of airway inflammation through differential cell counting (66). This technique provides a focus on migratory inflammatory cells in the airway such as the eosinophils and neutrophils obtained from selected sputum, following induction with aerosolized hypertonic saline. The level of eosinophils in sputum has been demonstrated to correlate well with those obtained through biopsy (67). The presence of the eosinophils in sputum in persons with asthma has proven to be sensitive to ICS in association with known clinical improvements (68,69). This has created increased interest in its use to assess the efficacy of new anti-inflammatory therapies either alone or following allergen challenge (42). As inhaled hypertonic saline can provoke bronchoconstriction, current protocols using this stimulus for sputum has proven to be safe when patients are premedicated with standard dose of a β_2-agonist (70).

Less is known on the effects of anti-inflammatory therapies on airway neutrophils. There is evidence that the presence of airway neutrophils may be sustained in the presence of ICS (71) and only a small number of studies have found reductions in levels of neutrophils in response to therapy (72,73). It should be noted that airway infections can increase the levels of neutrophils temporarily; thus, studies should consider individuals who have persistent elevated neutrophils in the absence of infection (74).

The measurement of the fractional concentration of exhaled nitric oxide (FeNO) is a noninvasive measure of the presence of airway inflammation (75). Nitric oxide is measured easily in the exhaled breath and is thought to originate from the airways via the cellular synthesis from the amino acid L-arginine by a variety of NO synthase (NOS) enzymes. Exhaled NO is thought to have multiple cellular origins as the NOS enzymes can be expressed in epithelial and endothelial cells as well as in a variety of inflammatory cells (76). FeNO appears to be a nonspecific marker of airway inflammation, and as a result of the sensitivity of this marker to ICS, there has been interest in regard to its potential role in both diagnosis and management of asthma (77). FeNO measurement has been standardized (75) and has a practical advantage of being rapid and simple to perform, with clinical utility in a pediatric population. However, it appears that it may be more reflective of allergic airway inflammation as FeNO levels are raised in atopic but not in nonatopic asthma (78,79). FeNO has been positively correlated to the level of eosinophils in sputum (80,81) and AHR to direct (82,83) and indirect stimuli (20,21). However, there are data demonstrating a poor relationship to other markers of inflammation and AHR (79,84). It is important to note that as a result of the attenuation of eNO values by acute doses of ICS, this should be considered when interpreting the effects of new therapies in patients taking ICS. Further, there are other factors that may have an acute influence eNO values such as nitrate-rich diet (85) and increased exposure to air pollution containing oxides of nitrogen (86).

Biomarkers in body fluids such as blood and urine are gaining interest with the increasing range of analytical assay's becoming available, with increasing analytical sensitivity. However, these markers often represent whole-body production and thus may be the reason that it can be difficult to correlate these markers with disease severity, end organ responsiveness, or other physiological hallmarks of airway disease. Thus, considering the preexisting published data on a particular biomarker and its reproducibility is important when choosing one or more to understand the efficacy of a particular therapy. Markers of eicosanoid metabolism in blood are difficult to measure due to potential modification of their levels following blood taking and can be assessed in cells in the blood ex vivo. However, an interesting marker of mast cell activation, a metabolite of PGD_2, $9\alpha,11\beta$-PGF_2 has been successfully measured in the blood (87).

Urinary markers of inflammatory pathways have been a recent focus of interest in understanding disease mechanisms and likely require more validation with regard to understanding mechanisms of therapy. The most common inflammatory markers in urine are the measurement of eicosanoid, measuring the presence of the stable end metabolite of the leukotriene pathway, LTE_4 (Fig. 2B). Urinary LTE_4 is raised at baseline levels in persons with asthma, though this is more prominent in persons with aspirin-sensitive asthma. The marker of mast cell activation $9\alpha,11\beta$-PGF2 can also be measured in urine (88). Both mediators are raised following indirect stimuli such as allergen, exercise, and osmotic stimuli (88–90), with urinary $9\alpha,11\beta$-PGF_2

effectively inhibited with β_2-agonists and cromolyn, both known to stabilize mast cells in the presence of stimulus that causes mast cell degranulation (Fig. 2B) (90). Measurements of urinary metabolites of histamine have proven less useful due to the extensive whole-body metabolism of histamine, as well as the uncertainty of a precise cellular source (88).

VII. Lung Function: Acute Responses and Preventing Decline

Measuring acute improvements in lung function, within minutes to hours, has been well established as an outcome variable to evaluate inhaled bronchodilators. The most commonly used outcome measurement has been the FEV_1 because of its ease of measurement and reproducibility. Measurements of FEV_1 and the forced vital capacity (FVC) are made during a forced expiratory maneuver using a spirometer. The degree of reversibility in FEV_1, which indicates a diagnosis of asthma, is generally accepted as $\geq 12\%$ and ≥ 200 mL from the prebronchodilator value. The methods of measurements have been standardized (91). Rapid-onset bronchodilators, which are inhaled β_2-agonists, begin to improve FEV_1 in asthmatic patients with airflow obstruction within two to five minutes (92). The longer-acting inhaled β_2-agonists have a duration of bronchodilating activity of at least 12 hours (93).

Regulatory agencies have often mandated longer-term studies demonstrating improvements in FEV_1 as a requirement for approval of a new treatment for asthma. These studies, particularly of controller therapies for asthma, vary in duration from 12 weeks to 1 year [e.g., (94–96)]. The FEV_1 measurements are typically made at clinic visits during the study and are usually powered to find a 10% to 15% improvement in the prebronchodilator FEV_1. Only relatively recently has a drug (omalizumab, a humanized monoclonal antibody against IgE), which did not demonstrate a significant improvement in FEV_1 during its clinical trial development program, been approved for use in the United States and Europe (97).

Another commonly used measurement of lung function in clinical trials in asthma is measurements of peak expired flows (PEF) (98). These measurements have the potential advantage that they can be made daily and recorded on a paper record, or, more recently, electronically. They are, however, a more variable measurement than FEV_1. Careful instruction is required to reliably measure PEF because PEF measurements are effort dependent. Most commonly, PEF is measured first thing in the morning before treatment is taken, when values are often close to their lowest, and last thing at night when values are usually higher. Studies are often powered to find at least a 20 to 30 L/min improvement in PEF.

VIII. Measurements of Asthma Control

The term "asthma control" refers to a spectrum of characteristics that describe the extent to which the clinical manifestations of asthma have been reduced or removed by treatment. The level of asthma control is gauged from the level of symptoms and the extent to which the patient is enabled to carry out activities of daily living and achieve optimum quality of life. Asthma control has been defined as the minimization of nighttime and daytime symptoms, activity limitation, rescue bronchodilator use, and

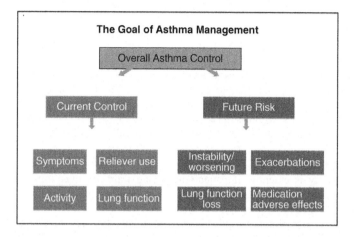

Figure 3 The objective of asthma management is obtaining overall asthma control, which consists of two domains, current (day-to-day) control and minimizing future risk.

airway narrowing. In addition, the assessment of asthma control encompasses both the patient's current clinical status and the risk of future adverse events including loss of control and asthma exacerbations (Fig. 3).

Many asthma treatment guidelines have now moved to an approach that focuses on asthma control as the outcome around which treatment decisions are made (1). There are now a range of questionnaires and diaries that have been developed to measure asthma control, and each one has its strengths and weaknesses. Among the most commonly used are the Asthma Control Questionnaire (99), Asthma Control Test (100), Asthma Therapy Assessment Questionnaire (101), Royal College of Physicians Asthma Questionnaire (102), and Asthma Control Diary (103). There are important features that are necessary to consider when making a choice between them.

A. Content Validity

Does the questionnaire contain all the components of asthma control? The questionnaire must include daytime symptoms (including daily bronchodilator use), activity limitations, nighttime symptoms, and airway caliber. If the questionnaire does not include measurements of airway caliber, inadequate control may be missed in patients with poor perception of airway narrowing.

B. Construct Validity

This is evidence that the instrument measures what it purports to measure. In the absence of a "gold standard" for asthma control, validity is usually established by showing that the questionnaire correlates with other asthma outcomes in a predictable manner (construct validation). These outcomes might include an asthma-specific quality-of-life questionnaire, a generic health status questionnaire (e.g., SF-36), an asthma symptom diary, daily peak flow measurements, or eNO, etc.

C. Reliability

Is the questionnaire able to detect different levels of asthma control? If the questionnaire includes all the components of asthma control, if each question has a good range of response choices, and if patients, whose asthma is stable, give very consistent responses when they respond a second time to the questionnaire (about a week later), it is highly likely that the questionnaire will be able to detect differences in level of control (reliability). The test statistic that will provide this information is the intraclass correlation coefficient (ICC), which relates within-subject variance (noise) to between-subject variance (signal). Ideally the ICC should be at least 0.90 and ideally above 0.95.

D. Responsiveness

This measurement property is essential if patients are being followed over time to evaluate improvements and deteriorations in asthma control. The responsiveness of a questionnaire is usually assessed by giving patients an intervention of known therapeutic efficacy and checking that the instrument is able to detect small, but clinically important, improvements. If this information is not available, the number of response choices that the patient is given for each question needs to be checked. If there is a wide range (e.g., a seven-point scale or a 10-cm visual analog scale), the questionnaire is likely to be able to pick up small, but clinically important changes. If the response choices are few or just yes/no, the questionnaire is likely to miss important changes.

IX. Asthma Exacerbations

Severe asthma exacerbations are events that require urgent action on the part of the patient and physician to prevent a serious outcome, such as hospitalization or death from asthma. Severe exacerbations are an important outcome variable in clinical trials of new drugs for asthma. In some respects, exacerbations are the most important outcome to improve in asthmatics. This is because they are the time of greatest risk for asthmatic patients; the cause of most stress for the patient and their families; and the cause of greatest cost to health care systems. However, adequately powering a study to evaluate severe asthma exacerbations requires a large and long-term study (usually at least 1 year).

The first study to use a reduction in severe asthma exacerbations as the primary outcome variable was the Formoterol and Corticosteroids Establishing Therapy (FACET) trial (104). This study included more than 800 patients randomly allocated to treatment with low or high doses of the ICS budesonide, with or without the addition of the long-acting inhaled β_2-agonist, formoterol. This study described severe exacerbations as (*i*) the use of oral/systemic corticosteroids as determined by the managing physician; or (*ii*) a hospitalization or ER visit because of asthma, requiring oral/systemic corticosteroids; or a 30% decline in PEF from baseline for at least two days. The study demonstrated a 50% reduction in severe exacerbations by a fourfold increase in ICS dose and a further significant decline with the addition of formoterol. However, there was a poor association between the specific PEF criteria and clinician prescription of corticosteroids, which called into question the clinical relevance of PEF in defining severe exacerbations. Many "severe exacerbations" were identified from retrospective analysis of paper PEF diaries, without the episode having been clinically serious enough to lead to use of systemic corticosteroids or an ER visit. For this reason, this component of the definition is no longer recommended. Subsequently many studies have used severe asthma exacerbations as a primary outcome variable (105–109) and shown that it is responsive to asthma treatments. As a result of a review of these and other studies, the ERS/ATS Committee on Asthma Control Outcomes has recommended that the definition of a severe asthma exacerbation should include, at a minimum, at least (*i*) the need for oral/systemic corticosteroids at the investigators discretion and (*ii*) a hospitalization/ ER visit because of asthma requiring systemic corticosteroids (106). The definition of a moderate asthma exacerbation should include deterioration in symptoms, rescue bronchodilator use, and/or lung function that lasts at least two days, but which is not severe enough to warrant oral corticosteroid use and/or a hospital visit. The FACET study also included mild asthma exacerbations as an outcome variable (106). However, a definition of a "mild asthma exacerbation" is not justifiable with present methods of analysis, because these episodes are only just outside the normal range of variation for the individual patient and may reflect transient loss of asthma control.

X. Conclusions

When embarking on the clinical development of therapeutic agents in airway disease, designing effective studies to investigate the airway response requires an understanding of the available outcomes that are clinically relevant, such as asthma exacerbations and asthma control. These should also be considered in association with the appropriate standardized physiological and biochemical markers to validate efficacy, such as markers for inflammation and AHR, the hallmarks of dysfunction in airway disease that are likely the targets of a new therapeutic agent. All outcome measures, whether chosen as primary or secondary outcomes, may have certain limitations that need to be understood before they are applied in an effort to maximize their usefulness in establishing efficacy of a therapeutic agent.

The practical and safety considerations of a chosen outcome measure, in particular those that are more invasive, should be well understood and carefully considered. When designing a clinical trial, prior studies that demonstrate the success of known therapies in airway disease should also be considered in an effort to demonstrate equivalent or superior efficacy and safety compared with existing therapies. Finally, and with no less importance, the most appropriate patient population at each stage of development of a therapeutic agent needs to be selected that reflects the broadest applicable patient population that will translate to benefits in the real-world population with airway disease.

References

1. Bateman ED, Hurd SS, Barnes PJ, et al. Global strategy for asthma management and prevention: GINA executive summary. Eur Respir J 2008; 31:143–178.
2. Kirby JG, Hargreave FE, Gleich GJ, et al. Bronchoalveolar cell profiles of asthmatic and nonasthmatic subjects. Am Rev Respir Dis 1987; 136:379–383.
3. Bateman ED, Boushey HA, Bousquet J, et al. Can guideline-defined asthma control be achieved? The Gaining Optimal Asthma ControL study. Am J Respir Crit Care Med 2004; 170:836–844.
4. Hargreave FE, Ryan G, Thomson NC, et al. Bronchial responsiveness to histamine or methacholine in asthma: measurement and clinical significance. J Allergy Clin Immunol 1981; 68:347–355.

5. Cockcroft DW, Hargreave FE. Airway hyperresponsiveness: relevance of random population data to clinical usefulness. Am Rev Respir Dis 1990; 142:497–500.

6. Anderson SD. Provocative challenges to help diagnose and monitor asthma: exercise, methacholine, adenosine, and mannitol. Curr Opin Pulm Med 2008; 14:39–45.

7. Sont JK, Willems LN, Bel EH, et al. Clinical control and histopathologic outcome of asthma when using airway hyperresponsiveness as an additional guide to long-term treatment. The AMPUL Study Group. Am J Respir Crit Care Med 1999; 159:1043–1051.

8. Sterk PJ, Fabbri LM, Quanjer PH, et al. Airway responsiveness. Standardized challenge testing with pharmacological, physical and sensitizing stimuli in adults. Report Working Party Standardization of Lung Function Tests, European Community for Steel and Coal. Official Statement of the European Respiratory Society. Eur Respir J Suppl 1993; 16:53–83.

9. Crapo RO, Casaburi R, Coates AL, et al. Guidelines for methacholine and exercise challenge testing-1999. This official statement of the American Thoracic Society was adopted by the ATS Board of Directors, July 1999. Am J Respir Crit Care Med 2000; 161:309–329.

10. Anderson SD. Drugs and the control of exercise-induced asthma. Eur Respir J 1993; 6:1090–1092.

11. Miller MR, Crapo R, Hankinson J, et al. General considerations for lung function testing. Eur Respir J 2005; 26:153–161.

12. Juniper EF, Frith PA, Dunnett C, et al. Reproducibility and comparison of responses to inhaled histamine and methacholine. Thorax 1978; 33:705–710.

13. Cockcroft DW, Killian DN, Mellon JJ, et al. Bronchial reactivity to inhaled histamine: a method and clinical survey. Clin Allergy 1977; 7:235–243.

14. Jones GL, Saroea HG, Watson RM, et al. Effect of an inhaled thromboxane mimetic (U46619) on airway function in human subjects. Am Rev Respir Dis 1992; 145:1270–1274.

15. Adelroth E, Morris MM, Hargreave FE, et al. Airway responsiveness to leukotrienes C4 and D4 and to methacholine in patients with asthma and normal controls. N Engl J Med 1986; 315:480–484.

16. O'Byrne PM, Dolovich J, Hargreave FE. Late asthmatic responses. Am Rev Respir Dis 1987; 136:740–751.

17. Anderson SD, Brannan JD. Methods for "indirect" challenge tests including exercise, eucapnic voluntary hyperpnea, and hypertonic aerosols. Clin Rev Allergy Immunol 2003; 24:27–54.

18. de Meer G, Heederik DJ, Brunekreef B, et al. Repeatability of bronchial hyperresponsiveness to adenosine-5'-monophosphate (AMP) by a short dosimeter protocol. Thorax 2001; 56:362–365.

19. Brannan JD, Anderson SD, Perry CP, et al. The safety and efficacy of inhaled dry powder mannitol as a bronchial provocation test for airway hyperresponsiveness: a phase 3 comparison study with hypertonic (4.5%) saline. Respir Res 2005; 6:144.

20. Porsbjerg C, Brannan JD, Anderson SD, et al. Relationship between airway responsiveness to mannitol and to methacholine and markers of airway inflammation, peak flow variability and quality of life in asthma patients. Clin Exp Allergy 2008; 38:43–50.

21. van den Berge M, Meijer RJ, Kerstjens HA, et al. PC(20) adenosine 5'-monophosphate is more closely associated with airway inflammation in asthma than PC(20) methacholine. Am J Respir Crit Care Med 2001; 163:1546–1550.

22. Parameswaran KN, Inman MD, Ekholm BP, et al. Protection against methacholine bronchoconstriction to assess relative potency of inhaled beta2-agonist. Am J Respir Crit Care Med 1999; 160:354–357.

23. Juniper EF, Kline PA, Vanzieleghem MA, et al. Effect of long-term treatment with an inhaled corticosteroid (budesonide) on airway hyperresponsiveness and clinical asthma in nonsteroid-dependent asthmatics. Am Rev Respir Dis 1990; 142:832–836.

24. Chinn S, Britton JR, Burney PG, et al. Estimation and repeatability of the response to inhaled histamine in a community survey. Thorax 1987; 42:45–52.
25. Juniper EF, Kline PA, Vanzieleghem MA, et al. Long-term effects of budesonide on airway responsiveness and clinical asthma severity in inhaled steroid-dependent asthmatics. Eur Respir J 1990; 3:1122–1127.
26. Reddel HK, Jenkins CR, Marks GB, et al. Optimal asthma control, starting with high doses of inhaled budesonide. Eur Respir J 2000; 16:226–235.
27. van Grunsven PM, van Schayck CP, Molema J, et al. Effect of inhaled corticosteroids on bronchial responsiveness in patients with "corticosteroid naive" mild asthma: a meta-analysis. Thorax 1999; 54:316–322.
28. Page CP, Spina D. Beta2-agonists and bronchial hyperresponsiveness. Clin Rev Allergy Immunol 2006; 31:143–162.
29. Parameswaran K. Concepts of establishing clinical bioequivalence of chlorofluorocarbon and hydrofluoroalkane beta-agonists. J Allergy Clin Immunol 1999; 104:S243–S245.
30. Cheung D, Timmers MC, Zwinderman AH, et al. Long-term effects of a long-acting beta 2-adrenoceptor agonist, salmeterol, on airway hyperresponsiveness in patients with mild asthma. N Engl J Med 1992; 327:1198–1203.
31. Kalra S, Swystun VA, Bhagat R, et al. Inhaled corticosteroids do not prevent the development of tolerance to the bronchoprotective effect of salmeterol. Chest 1996; 109:953–956.
32. Swystun VA, Gordon JR, Davis EB, et al. Mast cell tryptase release and asthmatic responses to allergen increase with regular use of salbutamol. J Allergy Clin Immunol 2000; 106:57–64.
33. Davis BE, Cockcroft DW. Effect of a single dose of montelukast sodium on methacholine chloride PC20. Can Respir J 2005; 12:26–28.
34. Boner AL, Vallone G, Andreoli A, et al. Nebulised sodium cromoglycate and verapamil in methacholine induced asthma. Arch Dis Child 1987; 62:264–268.
35. Crimi E, Brusasco V, Brancatisano M, et al. Effect of nedocromil sodium on adenosine- and methacholine-induced bronchospasm in asthma. Clin Allergy 1987; 17:135–141.
36. Boulet LP, Gauvreau G, Boulay ME, et al. The allergen bronchoprovocation model: an important tool for the investigation of new asthma anti-inflammatory therapies. Allergy 2007; 62:1101–1110.
37. Gauvreau GM, Watson RM, O'Byrne PM. Kinetics of allergen-induced airway eosinophilic cytokine production and airway inflammation. Am J Respir Crit Care Med 1999; 160:640–647.
38. Mussaffi H, Springer C, Godfrey S. Increased bronchial responsiveness to exercise and histamine after allergen challenge in children with asthma. J Allergy Clin Immunol 1986; 77:48–52.
39. Aalbers R, Kauffman HF, Koeter GH, et al. Dissimilarity in methacholine and adenosine 5'-monophosphate responsiveness 3 and 24 h after allergen challenge. Am Rev Respir Dis 1991; 144:352–357.
40. Leigh R, Vethanayagam D, Yoshida M, et al. Effects of montelukast and budesonide on airway responses and airway inflammation in asthma. Am J Respir Crit Care Med 2002; 166:1212–1217.
41. Subbarao P, Dorman SC, Rerecich T, et al. Protection by budesonide and fluticasone on allergen-induced airway responses after discontinuation of therapy. J Allergy Clin Immunol 2005; 115:745–750.
42. Gauvreau GM, Boulet LP, Cockcroft DW, et al. Antisense therapy against CCR3 and the common beta chain attenuates allergen-induced eosinophilic responses. Am J Respir Crit Care Med 2008; 177:952–958.
43. Gauvreau GM, Becker AB, Boulet LP, et al. The effects of an anti-CD11a mAb, efalizumab, on allergen-induced airway responses and airway inflammation in subjects with atopic asthma. J Allergy Clin Immunol 2003; 112:331–338.

44. van Schoor J, Joos GF, Pauwels RA. Indirect bronchial hyperresponsiveness in asthma: mechanisms, pharmacology and implications for clinical research. Eur Respir J 2000; 16:514–533.

45. Anderson SD, Daviskas E. The mechanism of exercise-induced asthma is. J Allergy Clin Immunol 2000; 106:453–459.

46. Finnerty JP, Holgate ST. Evidence for the roles of histamine and prostaglandins as mediators in exercise-induced asthma: the inhibitory effect of terfenadine and flurbiprofen alone and in combination. Eur Respir J 1990; 3:540–547.

47. O'Sullivan S, Roquet A, Dahlen B, et al. Evidence for mast cell activation during exercise-induced bronchoconstriction. Eur Respir J 1998; 12:345–350.

48. Manning PJ, Watson RM, Margolskee DJ, et al. Inhibition of exercise-induced bronchoconstriction by MK-571, a potent leukotriene D4-receptor antagonist. N Engl J Med 1990; 323:1736–1739.

49. Brannan JD, Koskela H, Anderson SD, et al. Responsiveness to mannitol in asthmatic subjects with exercise- and hyperventilation-induced asthma. Am J Respir Crit Care Med 1998; 158:1120–1126.

50. Brannan JD, Koskela H, Anderson SD. Monitoring asthma therapy using indirect bronchial provocation tests. Clin Respir J 2007; 1:3–15.

51. Anderson SD, Lambert S, Brannan JD, et al. Laboratory protocol for exercise asthma to evaluate salbutamol given by two devices. Med Sci Sports Exerc 2001; 33:893–900.

52. Subbarao P, Duong M, Adelroth E, et al. Effect of ciclesonide dose and duration of therapy on exercise-induced bronchoconstriction in patients with asthma. J Allergy Clin Immunol 2006; 117:1008–1013.

53. Dahlen B, O'Byrne PM, Watson RM, et al. The reproducibility and sample size requirements of exercise-induced bronchoconstriction measurements. Eur Respir J 2001; 17:581–588.

54. Argyros GJ, Roach JM, Hurwitz KM, et al. Eucapnic voluntary hyperventilation as a bronchoprovocation technique: development of a standardized dosing schedule in asthmatics. Chest 1996; 109:1520–1524.

55. Rundell KW, Anderson SD, Spiering BA, et al. Field exercise vs laboratory eucapnic voluntary hyperventilation to identify airway hyperresponsiveness in elite cold weather athletes. Chest 2004; 125:909–915.

56. Anderson SD, Brannan J, Spring J, et al. A new method for bronchial-provocation testing in asthmatic subjects using a dry powder of mannitol. Am J Respir Crit Care Med 1997; 156:758–765.

57. Barben J, Roberts M, Chew N, et al. Repeatability of bronchial responsiveness to mannitol dry powder in children with asthma. Pediatr Pulmonol 2003; 36:490–494.

58. Brannan JD, Gulliksson M, Anderson SD, et al. Inhibition of mast cell PGD2 release protects against mannitol-induced airway narrowing. Eur Respir J 2006; 27:944–950.

59. Kelly KD, Spooner CH, Rowe BH. Nedocromil sodium versus sodium cromoglycate in treatment of exercise-induced bronchoconstriction: a systematic review. Eur Respir J 2001; 17:39–45.

60. Brannan JD, Anderson SD, Gomes K, et al. Fexofenadine decreases sensitivity to and montelukast improves recovery from inhaled mannitol. Am J Respir Crit Care Med 2001; 163:1420–1425.

61. Reiss TF, Hill JB, Harman E, et al. Increased urinary excretion of LTE4 after exercise and attenuation of exercise-induced bronchospasm by montelukast, a cysteinyl leukotriene receptor antagonist. Thorax 1997; 52:1030–1035.

62. Busse WW, Wanner A, Adams K, et al. Investigative bronchoprovocation and bronchoscopy in airway diseases. Am J Respir Crit Care Med 2005; 172:807–816.

63. O'Byrne PM, Postma DS. The many faces of airway inflammation. Asthma and chronic obstructive pulmonary disease. Am J Respir Crit Care Med 1999; 159:S41–S63.

64. Djukanovic R, Homeyard S, Gratziou C, et al. The effect of treatment with oral cortico-steroids on asthma symptoms and airway inflammation. Am J Respir Crit Care Med 1997; 155:826–832.
65. Laitinen LA, Laitinen A, Haahtela T. A comparative study of the effects of an inhaled corticosteroid, budesonide, and a beta 2-agonist, terbutaline, on airway inflammation in newly diagnosed asthma: a randomized, double-blind, parallel-group controlled trial. J Allergy Clin Immunol 1992; 90:32–42.
66. Pizzichini MM, Popov TA, Efthimiadis A, et al. Spontaneous and induced sputum to measure indices of airway inflammation in asthma. Am J Respir Crit Care Med 1996; 154:866–869.
67. Fahy JV, Wong H, Liu J, et al. Comparison of samples collected by sputum induction and bronchoscopy from asthmatic and healthy subjects. Am J Respir Crit Care Med 1995; 152:53–58.
68. Green RH, Brightling CE, McKenna S, et al. Asthma exacerbations and sputum eosinophil counts: a randomised controlled trial. Lancet 2002; 360:1715–1721.
69. Jayaram L, Pizzichini MM, Cook RJ, et al. Determining asthma treatment by monitoring sputum cell counts: effect on exacerbations. Eur Respir J 2006; 27:483–494.
70. Vlachos-Mayer H, Leigh R, Sharon RF, et al. Success and safety of sputum induction in the clinical setting. Eur Respir J 2000; 16:997–1000.
71. Cox G. Glucocorticoid treatment inhibits apoptosis in human neutrophils. Separation of survival and activation outcomes. J Immunol 1995; 154:4719–4725.
72. Maneechotesuwan K, Essilfie-Quaye S, Meah S, et al. Formoterol attenuates neutrophilic airway inflammation in asthma. Chest 2005; 128:1936–1942.
73. Simpson JL, Powell H, Boyle MJ, et al. Clarithromycin targets neutrophilic airway inflammation in refractory asthma. Am J Respir Crit Care Med 2008; 177:148–155.
74. D'silva L, Allen CJ, Hargreave FE, et al. Sputum neutrophilia can mask eosinophilic bronchitis during exacerbations. Can Respir J 2007; 14:281–284.
75. Kharitonov S, Alving K, Barnes PJ. Exhaled and nasal nitric oxide measurements: recom-mendations. The European Respiratory Society Task Force. Eur Respir J 1997; 10:1683–1693.
76. Kharitonov SA, Barnes PJ. Clinical aspects of exhaled nitric oxide. Eur Respir J 2000; 16:781–792.
77. Smith AD, Cowan JO, Brassett KP, et al. Use of exhaled nitric oxide measurements to guide treatment in chronic asthma. N Engl J Med 2005; 352:2163–2173.
78. Ludviksdottir D, Janson C, Hogman M, et al. Exhaled nitric oxide and its relationship to airway responsiveness and atopy in asthma. BHR-Study Group. Respir Med 1999; 93:552–556.
79. Ho LP, Wood FT, Robson A, et al. Atopy influences exhaled nitric oxide levels in adult asthmatics. Chest 2000; 118:1327–1331.
80. Jatakanon A, Lim S, Kharitonov SA, et al. Correlation between exhaled nitric oxide, sputum eosinophils, and methacholine responsiveness in patients with mild asthma. Thorax 1998; 53:91–95.
81. Piacentini GL, Bodini A, Costella S, et al. Exhaled nitric oxide and sputum eosinophil markers of inflammation in asthmatic children. Eur Respir J 1999; 13:1386–1390.
82. Dupont LJ, Rochette F, Demedts MG, et al. Exhaled nitric oxide correlates with airway hyperresponsiveness in steroid-naive patients with mild asthma. Am J Respir Crit Care Med 1998; 157:894–898.
83. Henriksen AH, Lingaas-Holmen T, Sue-Chu M, et al. Combined use of exhaled nitric oxide and airway hyperresponsiveness in characterizing asthma in a large population survey. Eur Respir J 2000; 15:849–855.
84. Lim S, Jatakanon A, Meah S, et al. Relationship between exhaled nitric oxide and mucosal eosinophilic inflammation in mild to moderately severe asthma. Thorax 2000; 55:184–188.

85. Olin AC, Aldenbratt A, Ekman A, et al. Increased nitric oxide in exhaled air after intake of a nitrate-rich meal. Respir Med 2001; 95:153–158.

86. Baraldi E, Azzolin NM, Dario C, et al. Effect of atmospheric nitric oxide (NO) on measurements of exhaled NO in asthmatic children. Pediatr Pulmonol 1998; 26:30–34.

87. Bochenek G, Nagraba K, Nizankowska E, et al. A controlled study of 9alpha,11beta-PGF2 (a prostaglandin D2 metabolite) in plasma and urine of patients with bronchial asthma and healthy controls after aspirin challenge. J Allergy Clin Immunol 2003; 111:743–749.

88. O'Sullivan S, Dahlen B, Dahlen SE, et al. Increased urinary excretion of the prostaglandin D2 metabolite 9 alpha, 11 beta-prostaglandin F2 after aspirin challenge supports mast cell activation in aspirin-induced airway obstruction. J Allergy Clin Immunol 1996; 98: 421–432.

89. O'Sullivan S, Dahlen B, Roquet A, et al. Urinary 9 alpha, 11 beta-PGF2 as a marker of mast cell activation in allergic and aspirin-intolerant asthma. Adv Exp Med Biol 1997; 433:159–162.

90. Brannan JD, Gulliksson M, Anderson SD, et al. Evidence of mast cell activation and leukotriene release after mannitol inhalation. Eur Respir J 2003; 22:491–496.

91. Standardization of Spirometry, 1994 Update. American Thoracic Society. Am J Respir Crit Care Med 1995; 152:1107–1136.

92. Sykes AP, Ayres JG. A study of the duration of the bronchodilator effect of 12 micrograms and 24 micrograms of inhaled formoterol and 200 micrograms inhaled salbutamol in asthma. Respir Med 1990; 84:135–138.

93. Lofdahl CG, Svedmyr N. Formoterol fumarate, a new beta 2-adrenoceptor agonist. Acute studies of selectivity and duration of effect after inhaled and oral administration. Allergy 1989; 44:264–271.

94. Busse WW, Chervinsky P, Condemi J, et al. Budesonide delivered by Turbuhaler is effective in a dose-dependent fashion when used in the treatment of adult patients with chronic asthma. J Allergy Clin Immunol 1998; 101:457–463.

95. Israel E, Rubin P, Kemp JP, et al. The effect of inhibition of 5-lipoxygenase by zileuton in mild-to-moderate asthma. Ann Intern Med 1993; 119:1059–1066.

96. Chapman KR, Patel P, D'Urzo AD, et al. Maintenance of asthma control by once-daily inhaled ciclesonide in adults with persistent asthma. Allergy 2005; 60:330–337.

97. Busse W, Corren J, Lanier BQ, et al. Omalizumab, anti-IgE recombinant humanized monoclonal antibody, for the treatment of severe allergic asthma. J Allergy Clin Immunol 2001; 108:184–190.

98. Reddel HK, Ware SI, Salome CM, et al. Standardization of ambulatory peak flow monitoring: the importance of recent beta2-agonist inhalation. Eur Respir J 1998; 12:309–314.

99. Juniper EF, O'Byrne PM, Ferrie PJ, et al. Measuring asthma control. Clinic questionnaire or daily diary? Am J Respir Crit Care Med 2000; 162:1330–1334.

100. Nathan RA, Sorkness CA, Kosinski M, et al. Development of the asthma control test: a survey for assessing asthma control. J Allergy Clin Immunol 2004; 113:59–65.

101. Skinner EA, Diette GB, gatt-Bergstrom PJ, et al. The Asthma Therapy Assessment Questionnaire (ATAQ) for children and adolescents. Dis Manag 2004; 7:305–313.

102. Pearson MG, Bucknall CE. Measuring Clinical Outcomes in Asthma—A Patient Focussed Approach. London: Royal College of Physicians, 1999.

103. Bateman ED. Measuring asthma control. Curr Opin Allergy Clin Immunol 2001; 1:211–216.

104. Pauwels RA, Lofdahl CG, Postma DS, et al. Effect of inhaled formoterol and budesonide on exacerbations of asthma. Formoterol and Corticosteroids Establishing Therapy (FACET) International Study Group. N Engl J Med 1997; 337:1405–1411.

105. O'Byrne PM, Barnes PJ, Rodriguez-Roisin R, et al. Low dose inhaled budesonide and formoterol in mild persistent asthma: the OPTIMA randomized trial. Am J Respir Crit Care Med 2001; 164:1392–1397.

106. O'Byrne PM, Bisgaard H, Godard PP, et al. Budesonide/formoterol combination therapy as both maintenance and reliever medication in asthma. Am J Respir Crit Care Med 2005; 171:129–136.
107. Rabe KF, Atienza T, Magyar P, et al. Effect of budesonide in combination with formoterol for reliever therapy in asthma exacerbations: a randomised controlled, double-blind study. Lancet 2006; 368:744–753.
108. Bousquet J, Boulet LP, Peters MJ, et al. Budesonide/formoterol for maintenance and relief in uncontrolled asthmas vs. high-dose salmeterol/fluticasone. Respir Med 2007; 101:2437–2446.
109. Busse WW, Massanari M, Kianifard F, et al. Effect of omalizumab on the need for rescue systemic corticosteroid treatment in patients with moderate-to-severe persistent IgE-mediated allergic asthma: a pooled analysis. Curr Med Res Opin 2007; 23:2379–2386.

4

Pharmacogenetics and Pharmacogenomics of Airway Diseases

YOUMING ZHANG, WILLIAM COOKSON, and MIRIAM MOFFATT
National Heart and Lung Institute, Imperial College, London, U.K.

I. Introduction

Asthma and chronic obstructive pulmonary disease (COPD) are complex syndromes of airway inflammation. Asthma is a disease of the small airways of the lung. Intermittent narrowing of the respiratory bronchioles produces airway limitation and the symptoms of wheezing, chest tightness, and breathlessness. By contrast, in COPD the limitation of airflow is poorly reversible and usually gets progressively worse over time. The disease is primarily, but not exclusively, seen in smokers and former smokers. Environmental and genetic factors contribute to the etiology of both diseases. Cigarette smoking is the main risk factor for COPD, although less than 20% of chronic heavy smokers will develop symptoms of airway obstruction (1). Bronchodilators and corticosteroids are currently the most common medications used in the treatment of asthma and COPD.

The term "pharmacogenetics" was originally used to describe clinical observations of inherited differences in drug effects in the 1950s (2). It is now defined as the study of interindividual variations in DNA sequence (polymorphisms) related to drug response (3,4). It is the ambition of pharmacogenetic studies that the analysis of variation of a specific gene or group of genes may be used to predict responses to a specific drug or class of drugs. Genetic variation in a population is detected by assays of individual genotypes. Traits such as drug responses may be determined by environmental as well as genetic influences. Genetic variation also underlies the differential susceptibility of organisms to diseases and sensitivity to toxins.

Most drug effects are determined by the interplay of several gene products that influence the pharmacokinetics and pharmacodynamics of medications, including inherited differences in drug targets (e.g., receptors), drug disposition (e.g., metabolizing enzymes and transporters) (5), drug metabolism (3), and drug adverse reaction (6). It is estimated that genetic polymorphisms can account for 20% to 95% of variability in drug disposition and effects (5).

Although the terms pharmacogenetics and pharmacogenomics are synonymous for all practical purposes, pharmacogenomics uses genome-wide approaches to study all the genes that influence drug responses (5) while pharmacogenetics involves the study of a single gene's interactions with drugs. The pharmacogenomics approach tends to be applied to identify genes in the search for novel drug targets. This is in contrast to traditional drug design that depends on a prior knowledge of the target and is based on high-throughput screening of such targets to identify small-molecule antagonists or agonists.

The successful completion of the Human Genome Project was regarded as one of the greatest scientific achievements in the last 50 years. The project identified thousands of protein-coding genes in the human genome, many of which could be important targets for drug development. On the basis of the project, a second generation human haplotype map of over 3.1 million single nucleotide polymorphisms (SNPs) was finished in 2007 (7). The public databases of these findings together with genome sequence of other species such as the mouse provide extremely useful resources for pharmacogenetics and pharmacogenomics of clinical practice.

In this chapter, we review how pharmacogenetic and pharmacogenomic approaches have developed in the search for novel drug treatments for airway diseases. In addition, we summarize the current progress for investigating genetic variations to common drugs that are used in asthma and COPD.

II. Approaches for Studying Pharmacogenetics and Pharmacogenomics

The human genome has about 20,000 to 25,000 genes (8). The identification of all human genes and their regulatory regions provides the essential framework for understanding the molecular basis of diseases. It also provides a foundation for the future of pharmacogenomics studies. Rapid developments in global gene analysis, gene product analysis, siRNA, targeted molecular genetic testing, and medical bioinformatics are already changing the practice of medicine (9). The study of genetic variation has the potential to understand individual variation in mechanisms of airway diseases and the response of patients to treatment. However, no single variant interrogated in airway diseases has yet been found to explain more than 10% of the total phenotypic variance of treatment response of any drug (10).

The forced expiratory volume in one second (FEV_1) and peak expiratory flow (PEF) are the measures of airflow usually studied for drug response in airway diseases. These parameters can be used to measure the response to inhaled bronchodilators, corticosteroids, and other treatments. Other traits that are worthy of study by pharmacogenetics include drug metabolism [e.g., clearance of theophylline (TP) in serum] and drug adverse effects. Since the mid-1990s genes involved in most airway drug targets have been successfully screened. The polymorphisms within these genes have been identified, and the associations between these polymorphisms and response to airway drugs have been intensively investigated.

A. Human Genome Variation and Pharmacogenetics Research

Common genetic variants are observed between humans at both the individual and the population levels. SNPs are the most frequent variants found in the genome, accounting for 90% of human genetic variation. Recent whole genome sequencing has revealed approximately 10 million SNPs in the human genome (11,12). SNPs have been found within coding sequences of genes (exons), noncoding regions of genes (introns), as well as within intergenic regions. Examples of exonic SNPs are those found within the β2-adrenergic receptor gene (*ADRB2*) that have been linked to altered response to β2-agonists.

Insertion and deletion of short segments of DNA (INDEL) is another type of common polymorphism. More than 500,000 INDELs are distributed throughout the human genome, with approximately 36% of them being located within promoters, introns, and exons of known genes (11). INDELs can have a significant impact on gene function not only when present in exonic coding sequence but also when within a gene intron. For example, an INDEL polymorphism of a 287 bp Alu sequence in intron 16 of the angiotensin-I converting enzyme accounts for 50% of the variance of serum enzyme levels. Homozygosity for the insertion allele (II genotype) results in individuals having significantly lower serum enzyme levels than carriers of the deletion allele (ID and DD genotypes) (13).

VNTRs (variable number of tandem repeats) polymorphisms are widespread in the genome and contain variable numbers of repeated nucleotide sequences that result in alleles of varying lengths. Because of their large numbers of alleles, VNTR loci therefore typically have high levels of heterozygosity that make them very informative for genetics research. A VNTR mutation in the promoter of the arachidonate 5-lip-oxygenase (*ALOX5*) gene has been shown to have an effect on the efficiency of both inhibitors and antagonists of its receptor (14).

Inversions may involve larger regions of the genome in which a segment of a chromosome is reversed end to end and occur when a chromosome breaks in two places. Interestingly, a 900-kb inversion has been identified within a large region of conserved linkage disequilibrium (LD) on human chromosome 17, and contained within the inversion region is the corticotrophin-releasing hormone receptor 1 gene (*CRHR1*). Polymorphisms within *CRHR1* have been shown to be associated with inhaled corti-costeroid (ICS) response in asthma (15).

A copy number variant (CNV) is a segment of DNA for which there are more or less than two copies in the genome. The genetic segment involved may range from one kilobase to several megabases in size (16). Copy number variation is not only about quantity but also about quality. A variety of techniques can allow the detection and discovery of CNVs including cytogenetic techniques such as fluorescent in situ hybridization, comparative genomic hybridization, and by large-scale SNP genotyping.

A further type of variation involves RNA rather than DNA. RNA alternative splicing occurs when the exons of a primary gene transcript, the pre-mRNA, are sep-arated and reconnected so as to produce alternative ribonucleotide arrangements. These linear combinations then undergo the process of translation where unique sequences of amino acids are specified, resulting in different protein isoforms. Alternative splicing includes intron retaining mode, exon cassette mode, and alternative donor/acceptor site mode.

B. Methods for Identification of Gene Variation Underlying Drug Responses

There are a variety of approaches that can be applied to identify potential genes underlying drug responses. These include candidate genes analysis and positional cloning, genome-wide association (GWA) studies, gene expression profiling, and microRNA targeting.

The candidate gene approach examines particular genes known to have specific roles in targeting, metabolism, and disposition of drugs. Variations in these genes can be compared between cases exhibiting particular drug responses and appropriate controls. An excellent example of this type of study in the case of airway diseases is the examination of mutations of the glucocorticoid receptor (*GR*) gene and their effect on the response to corticosteroid therapy.

Positional cloning involves the detection of genetic linkage between chromosome region and drug response traits through the study of families. Subsequent fine mapping of the genetically linked region leads eventually to identification of the gene underlying drug responses. The vast number of SNPs identified throughout the genome and developments in microarray technology mean that positional cloning has now been superseded by GWA studies.

GWA studies involve genotyping thousands of samples, either as case control cohorts or in family trios, for hundreds of thousands of SNPs distributed throughout the genome. Genotyping is followed by the comparison of the frequencies of either single SNP alleles, genotypes, or multimarker haplotypes between drug response traits and controls. GWA studies allow the identification of trait susceptibility genes with only modest increases in risk. A recent example of a GWA in pharmacogenetics was the study of myopathy in myocardial infarction patients receiving simvastin treatment. A GWA scan of only 90 patents with myopathy and 90 controls identified a single strongly associated SNP, *rs4363657*. This initial result led on to the identification of a common mutation in *SLCOB1B1* that was strongly associated with an increased risk of statin-induced myopathy. It is likely that genotyping of the *SLCOB1B1* variants will help to achieve the benefits of statin therapy more safely and effectively (17).

Gene expression profiling is the measurement of the expression (transcript abundance) of thousands of genes simultaneously and (ideally) genome wide, to create a global picture of cellular function. These gene expression profiles can, for example, distinguish between cells that are actively dividing, or show how cells react to a particular drug treatment. The data generated from such genome-wide expression experiments provides enormous information about the genetic pathways involved in regulation of cell cycle, RNA processing, DNA repair, immune responses, and apoptosis (18).

The discovery of small "noncoding" or "nonmessenger" RNA molecules that are repressors of translation (microRNAs) has provided the opportunity to specifically suppress a gene or clusters of genes. The recent employment of synthetic analogs of these small RNA molecules termed "antagomirs" has shown that microRNAs of interest can be specifically targeted. Understanding the role of microRNAs, in fundamental processes associated with complex diseases, has the potential of being of assistance in disease diagnosis, prognosis, and may also result in the identification of new therapeutic targets (19).

Many, if not all, of the above techniques rely heavily on bioinformatics, that is, the application of information technology to the field of molecular biology. Bioinformatics entails the creation and advancement of databases, algorithms, computational and statistical techniques, and theory to solve formal and practical problems arising from the management and analysis of genomic data. The size of the task is exemplified by the completion of whole genome sequencing for more than 40 species. Major research efforts in bioinformatics include sequence alignment, gene finding, genome assembly, protein structure alignment, protein structure prediction, prediction of gene expression and protein-protein interactions, and the modeling of evolution.

For airway diseases, application of bioinformatics to expression quantitative trait loci (eQTL) has the potential for discovery of novel loci that contribute to heterogeneity in response to asthma and COPD pharmacotherapy. Additionally, the development of statistical models that predict the genomics of response to airway drugs will complement SNP discovery in moving toward personalized medicine.

C. Molecular Tools for Pharmacogenetics

When polymorphisms of genes that have suspected pharmacogenetic effects have been identified, it is possible to study their functional roles by applying molecular biologic approaches. Short interfering/silencing RNA (siRNA), transfection, electrophoretic mobility shift assay (EMSA), and mouse models are at present the most commonly utilized methods to try and establish the functional consequences of gene variants.

siRNA is a class of 20 to 25 nucleotide-long double-stranded RNA molecules that play a variety of roles in biology. Most notably, siRNA is involved in the RNA interference (RNAi) pathway, where it alters the expression of specific genes. Although just one decade has passed since the discovery of RNAi, human clinical trials of RNAi therapy are currently occurring for diseases such as macular degeneration, respiratory syncytial virus infection, hepatitis, pachyonychia congenita, and solid tumors (20).

Transfection is a technique that allows one to study gene function by artificially introducing the foreign DNA into cultured eukaryotic cells. Stable integration of the DNA into the recipient genome and subsequent examination of both RNA and protein expression of the gene allows ascertainment of the pharmacogenomic effect of gene polymorphisms. An EMSA, also referred to as a gel shift assay, band shift assay, or gel retardation assay, is a common technique used to study protein-DNA or protein-RNA interactions. It is particularly useful to study the polymorphisms within regulatory sequences and introns of a gene. This procedure can determine if a protein or mixture of proteins is capable of binding to a given DNA or RNA sequence thereby effecting its expression, and can sometimes indicate if more than one protein molecule is involved in the binding complex.

The most important issue in pharmacogenetics is the testing of identified functional polymorphisms in the range of populations who may receive the drug. Retrospective, prospective studies, and finally, the study of random samples by way of clinical trials are all required to validate potential pharmacogenetic loci. Only then can personalization of medication in clinical care be feasible (Fig. 1).

Difficulties in obtaining direct access to human tissues means that direct determination of the mechanism of action of polymorphisms may be almost impossible. Mouse models can, however, bridge the gap between in vitro cell-based studies and human clinical traits. They provide a unique platform for investigation of altered drug response as well as being a tool for potential drug discovery (21). A large degree of syntenic homology exists between the mouse and the human genomes. Nearly all human genes have counterparts in the mouse, which can usually be recognized by cross-species hybridization. The cloning of a human gene usually leads directly to the cloning of a mouse homolog, and this can then be used for pharmacogenomic studies. Application of both in vitro and in silico approaches successfully resulted in the rapid identification of the basis for genetic variability in irinotecan, a chemotherapeutic agent. The drug's metabolism in mice was found to mirror genetic variability in humans that contributes to interindividual differences in response to the medication (22).

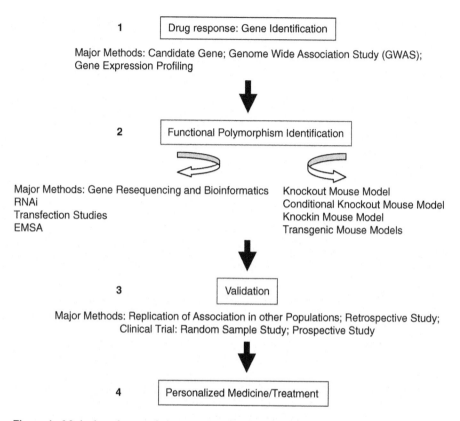

Figure 1 Methods and steps of pharmacogenetics and pharmacogenomics study.

III. Mouse Pharmacogenetic Approaches for Airway Diseases

Many mouse models are widely used in respiratory experiments. Inbred strains and genetic modified mice can also have important roles in pharmacogenetic and pharmacogenomic approaches for airway diseases (Table 1).

Genetic mapping in inbred strains can identify loci that are associated with phenotypic traits of interest. This strategy requires two strains of mice in which the phenotypic trait or traits of interest are significantly different, for example, at opposite ends of the distribution. Two studies have used this methodology to successfully localize the QTLs of bronchial hyperresponsiveness in mice (23,24). Susceptibility to acute lung injury by ozone has also been assessed, and the key loci identified (25). Inbred mouse strains with different drug response characteristics could also be used to apply an inbred gene mapping approach to pharmacogenomics (21).

Like inbred mice, genetically modified mice are also of great utility, including gene knockout, gene knockin, and transgenic mouse models. A knockout mouse is a genetically engineered mouse in which one or more genes have been made inoperative.

Table 1   Types of Mouse Model for Use in Pharmacogenetics and Pharmacogenomics Studies

Mouse model	Genotypes	Characteristics and usages
Knockout	−/−	Loss of function, allowing dissection of unknown gene function
Conditional knockout	−/−	Loss of function, allowing dissection of unknown gene function in time and space
Transgenic:		
Transgenic overexpression of human gene	m/m, H/H	Gain of function, allowing dissection of human gene function
Transgenic overexpression of both human alleles	m/m, H/h	Gain of function, allowing dissection of function of human SNP allele
Knockout/knockin	m^-/m^-, H/H	Gain of function, allowing dissection of human gene function without the mouse homolog of the gene being present

m/m and m^-/m^- represent mouse genotypes
H/H and H/h represent human genotypes or alleles
Abbreviation: SNP, single nucleotide polymorphism.

Knockout mice are important animal models for studying the role of genes that have unknown functions.

The disadvantage of gene knockout is that it can cause potential lethal or developmental effects. For example, knockout of the *GR* gene was found to result in mouse death at the embryonic stage (26). To avoid this problem, a conditional knockout approach allows researchers to delete the gene of interest in a time- and space-dependent manner. Site-specific recombinase systems Cre-loxP and Flip-FRT are used to excise a critical part of the gene. Timing and tissue-dependence are achieved by the choice of promoter used to drive the Cre gene. The recombineering technique uses homologous recombination mediated by the lambda phage Red proteins to rapidly introduce loxP or FRT sites into the subcloned DNA to achieve conditional knockout (27).

An example of a drug target developed by knockout comes from the study of T-bet, a TH1-specific T-box transcription factor. T-bet transactivates the IFN-γ gene in TH1 cells and has the unique ability to redirect fully polarized TH2 cells into TH1 cells. *T-bet* knockout mice demonstrated a physiological and inflammatory phenotype in murine airways similar to that created by allergen exposure in sensitized mice, in the absence of an induced inflammatory response. This phenotype existed in naive mice spontaneously and was similar to that observed in mice following allergen sensitization and challenge. It suggested that T-bet might be an attractive target for the development of anti-asthmatic drugs (28).

A knockin mouse model is when the normal mouse gene is replaced by a mutant version of the mouse gene using homologous recombination allowing study of the variant gene. A transgenic overexpression model is when an allele of a human polymorphism is put into a mouse either with or without the mouse background. This technique enables the dissection of the pharmacogenetic effect of human polymorphisms. The transgenic overexpression model can also be made tissue-specific by the use of different promoters.

The overexpression of human allelic variants in separate lines of mice is a very useful tool to study human pharmacogenomic variants. An excellent example of this are the transgenic FVB/N mice containing human *ADRB2*. A threonine to isoleucine polymorphism at amino acid 164 in the fourth transmembrane spanning domain of the β2-adrenergic receptor (β2AR) is known to occur in the human population (29). To explore potential differences between the two receptors, transgenic mice were created that either overexpressed wild-type β2AR or the mutant Ile-164 receptor in a targeted manner in the heart using a murine α-myosin heavy chain promoter. The functional properties of the two receptors were then assessed at the level of in vitro cardiac myocyte signaling and in vivo cardiac responses in intact animals. Comparison of the expression levels of these receptors in the two mouse lines revealed an approximately 45-fold increase in β2AR expression in the mutant Ile-164 receptor transgenic mice in comparison to the wild-type overexpression mice. Myocyte membrane adenylyl cyclase activity in the basal state was significantly lower in the Ile-164 mice compared to wild-type β2AR mice. The Ile-164 polymorphism was substantially dysfunctional therefore in the relevant target tissue (30).

The opportunities with mouse models are expanding as new and relevant techniques are being developed such as vectors that allow knockin genes to be exchanged more readily—so-called gene-swapping. A knockout/knockin approach may be used to create mouse lines that express human allelic variants that can then be evaluated for their pharmacologic relevance. In these experiments, the mouse gene is removed and replaced with human major and minor allelic variants. This technique of "zygotic injection" means that mouse lines carrying numerous human alleles could be a reality in the very near future (31).

IV. Pharmacogenetics and Pharmacogenomics Research into Airway Diseases

To date, progress in pharmacogenetics and pharmacogenomics of airway diseases has predominantly focused on the targets of commonly used drugs such as β2-adrenergic agonists, corticosteroids, and leukotriene (LT) modifiers. However, only a limited number of polymorphisms with pharmacogenetic roles have been identified and prospective clinical trials are on the way to validate the effects of these genetic variations in clinical practice.

A. β2-Adrenergic Agonists

β2-Adrenoceptor agonists (β-agonists) have been used for at least 5000 years to relieve bronchoconstriction (32). There are two general classes of β-adrenergic agonists. Short-acting β-agonists are used in the management of mild asthma to relax airway smooth muscle. Long-acting β-agonists are usually prescribed for moderate to severe persistent asthma or patients with COPD.

The β2AR is the target molecule of β2-agonists. The gene for the receptor, *ADRB2*, is located on chromosome 5q31. It is a small, intronless gene with 413 amino acid residues (33). The pharmacogenetic screen of *ADRB2* began with the work of Liggett and his colleagues (34). It is a highly polymorphic gene with more than 50 SNPs within it and in close proximity to it (35). Three coding (nonsynonymous) polymorphisms have been identified in *ADRB2*: Arg16Gly, Gln27Glu, and Thr164Ille. The two SNPs at amino acid positions 16 and 27 have been well characterized. Thr164Ille is a rare polymorphism with a minor allele frequency of 3% in the Caucasian population (36). Most clinical studies have therefore focused on the Arg16Gly SNP. Arg16 homozygotes had been found to have greater initial bronchodilator responses to β2-agonists than Gly16 homozygotes in response to short-acting β-agnoists (37,38). However, following prolonged exposure to the short-acting β-agnoists, greater downregulation was observed (39). There have been many other small retrospective reports of this particular polymorphism that have either confirmed the original findings or contradicted the original results with either opposite observations or no associations seen at all (40). In two randomized studies to test the Gly16Arg polymorphism and its effect on the response to long-acting β2-agonist therapy, no pharmacogenetic effect of *ADRB2* variation on therapeutic response in asthma patients, irrespective of their Arg16Gly genotype, was observed (41). The Gln27Glu polymorphism has been found to be associated with the response to β2-agonist treatment in children during an asthma exacerbation. Homozygous Gln27 patients responded less effectively to treatment with inhaled β2-agonists during an acute asthma exacerbation (42).

The fundamental question of the pharmacogenetic role of the *ADRBR2* locus, in particular the nonsynonymous amino acid changes, remains somewhat uncertain. LD is strong across the region, indicating that other variants nearby may be involved. The next pharmacogenetic approach for the *ADRB2* locus would be the implementation of carefully designed prospective studies of asthmatic patients with short-acting or long-acting β2-agnoists treatments.

Arginase I (ARG1) is another gene that has recently been identified as a potential novel bronchodilator response gene (43). The gene is located on chromosome 6q23 and has 8 exons that through alternative exon splicing result in 10 splice variant transcripts. Three of these splice variants translate into proteins. The transcript length of the gene is 1532 bps and it encodes 322 amino acids. The ARG1 protein targets L-arginine. L-arginine is a substrate of nitric oxide synthases (NOSs) and its catalysis by NOSs results in the formation of the endogenous dilator nitric oxide (NO) (44). Arginase (ARG1) is postulated to be involved in asthma by deleting stores of L-arginine, which leads to decreased production of NO. This process results in inhibition of smooth muscle relaxation (45).

In a study of 844 SNPs from 111 candidate genes selected from β-agonist and corticosteroids pathways, three *ARG1* SNPs were associated with inhaled bronchodilator after long-acting β2-agonist treatment. One SNP *rs2781659* was significantly associated with bronchodilator in the four population association study. Homozygote A/A individuals of *rs2781659* were found to have a greater response to β2-adrenergic agonists than homozygote G/G individuals (43). The functions of the variant remain unknown, but all three associated *ARG1* SNPs were in the promoter region of the gene and were in tight LD with each other. Genotyping of all known SNPs in the gene or resequencing of the gene will need to be performed to determine if these three promoter SNPs are in LD with any of the four nonsynonymous SNPs previously identified in the gene. Studies of human asthma bronchoalveolar lavage cells have shown elevation of the ARG1 protein (45) while mouse studies have shown that *ARG1* expression is increased in the murine asthma lung. Further studies in mice in which RNAi for arginase 1 in the lungs has been performed resulted in a loss of airway hyperresponsiveness to methacholine (46).

B. Corticosteroids

Corticosteroids are the most effective and commonly used drugs for the treatment of asthma and COPD. They bind to the intracellular GR after which the complex translocates to the nucleus where it is involved in the regulation of gene expression (47). The response to ICSs in patients with asthma or COPD is highly variable. Some subjects are deemed unresponsive since they fail to react to high doses of inhaled or even oral glucocorticoids (GCs) (48,49). GC-resistant patients have been shown to have abnormalities in the activity of proinflammatory transcription factors AP1 and NF-κB. These two factors are important for the induction of transcription of a number of chemoattractants, cytokines, cytokine receptors, and cell adhesion molecules (50).

To evaluate the gene expression profiling of GC-sensitive and GC-resistant asthmatic patients, Hakonarson et al. applied gene microarrays, allowing expression measurement of 11,812 genes, using as substrate blood mononuclear cells at baseline and poststimulation with IL-1β/TNF-α with or without dexamethasone. The expression profile of 923 genes was significantly reversed in GC responders in the presence of GC. Fifteen genes were found to predict GC response on extreme phenotypes (51). The results, although not definitive, provide an interesting resource for the future pharmacogenetic investigations.

A few candidate genes have been implicated in the response to corticosteroids. The *GR* gene (also known as *NR3C1*) belongs to a large family of nuclear receptors. The *GR* gene is located on chromosome 5q31 and contains nine exons that encode for a 778 amino acid peptide of which there are five splice variants. There are two naturally occurring isoforms of the *GR* gene: GRα (functional) and GRβ (no hormone-binding ability). A total of 15 missense, 3 nonsense, 3 frameshift, 1 splice site, and 2 alternative spliced mutations have been reported in the *GR* gene as well as 16 SNPs in noncoding regions, and many have shown association with GC resistance (52). One polymorphism Asp363Ser, although rare, may nonetheless be of importance. In a study of 216 elderly patients, 13 heterozygotes for the Asp363Ser site were identified. Individuals carrying 363Ser polymorphism seemed healthy at clinical examination but had a higher sensitivity to exogenously administered GCs, with respect to both cortisol suppression and insulin response (53).

CRHR1 is a major regulator of GC synthesis. It plays a key role in the stress response through its regulation of endogenous GC and catecholamine production. In the absence of the CRHR1 ligand, it was found that endogenous GC and catecholamine production decreased, resulting in allergen-induced airway inflammation and lung mechanical dysfunction (54). The *CRHR1* gene is located on human chromosome 17q21.3 and it has 14 exons that encode 447 amino acids. Two splicing variants of *CRHR1* have been identified. Three haplotype-tagging SNPs (*rs1876828, rs242939, rs242941*) in *CRHR1* were found to be associated with lung function improvement after eight weeks' treatment with ICSs in patients with asthma. Individuals homozygous for the haplotype GAT/GAT had an enhanced response to glucocorticoids (55,56). However, association of the three *CRHR1* SNPs variants with long-acting β2-agonists response was not observed in an asthma cohort study that spanned 22 years (57).

The genome structure of the chromosome 17q21.3 region is interesting since within it there is a 900-kb inversion contained within a large region of conserved LD and also containing the *CRHR1*gene. It is therefore conceivable that the CRHR1 response to

ICSs may be as a result of natural selection resulting from inversion status or by long-range LD with another gene (15) and is certainly worthy of further investigation.

T-box 21 (*TBX21*) encodes T-bet, a transcription factor crucial for naive T-lymphocyte production that influences naive T-lymphocyte development and has been implicated in asthma pathogenesis. The T-bet knockout mouse spontaneously develops airways inflammation and hyperresponsiveness suggestive of asthma (28). *TBX21* is located on chromosome 17q21.32 and it has six exons encoding 535 amino acids. In a large clinical trial spanning over four years, a nonsynonymous variation in *TBX21*, coding for replacement of histidine with glutamine at aa position 33, has showed association with significant improvement in the PC(20) of asthmatic children. This increase enhanced the overall improvement in PC(20) that was associated with ICS usage (58). TBX21 may therefore be an important pharmacogenetic determinant of response to the therapy of asthma with ICSs.

A novel variant in *FCER2*, which encodes for the low-affinity immunoglobulin E (IgE) receptor, has recently been associated with asthma exacerbation and ICSs. The gene is located on chromosome 19p13 and has 11 exons that encode 321 amino acids. In a study of the relationship between polymorphisms of *FCER2* and severe exacerbations in children with asthma, three *FCER2* SNPs were significantly associated with elevated IgE levels at year 4 follow up. Each SNP was also found to be associated with increased severe exacerbations. Using multivariable models, associations between one novel mutation T2206C and severe exacerbations in both white and African-American children were seen. The T2206C SNP was associated with increased risk of exacerbations in asthmatic children taking ICSs despite the protective nature of this medication with regard to exacerbations (59). The novel variant was also associated with higher IgE levels, suggesting that differential expression in *FCER2* can adversely affect normal negative feedback in the control of IgE synthesis and action (40).

C. LT Modifiers

LT modifiers inhibit the action of LTs, which are a family of lipoxygenated eicosatetraenoic acids derived from the metabolism of arachidonic acid. They have been shown to be produced in the airways where they act as potent bronchoconstrictors. Many enzymes are involved in the processing of the LTs. Two classes of LT modifier are available for use in the management of asthma: 5 lipoxygenases (5-LO) inhibitors and LT receptor antagonists, for example, montelukast and zafirlukast.

The polymorphisms of several genes have been associated with altered responses to LT modifiers and inhibitors. The *ALOX5* gene is located on chromosome 10q11. It contains 14 exons and encodes 674 amino acids. To date, 14 SNPs have been identified in the transcript. In a study of the 5-lipoxygeanses inhibitor ABT-761, response to treatment was shown to be related to genotypes of a VNTR in the promoter region of the *ALOX5* gene (14). Further studies however did not confirm these initial findings.

Another 5-lipoxygenase inhibitor called montelukast was associated with a 73% reduced risk of an asthma exacerbation in carriers of mutant allele as compared with homozygous wild type (5/5 repeats) (60), which was not consistent with the original report (14). In another somewhat smaller study, montelukast treatment decreased the number of asthma exacerbations in patients with 5/5 or 4/5 repeats but not in participants who were 4/4 homozygotes for the VNTR (61). In a study of the VNTR polymorphism and asthma severity, asthmatics with non5/non5 genotype expressed less ALOX5 mRNA and produced less LTC4 into culture supernatants than 5/5 individuals while asthmatic children bearing non5/non5 genotype had more moderate-severe asthma than children with the 5/5 genotype. Multivariate logistic regression identified *ALOX5* promoter genotype as a significant predictor of disease severity. Children bearing the non5/non5 genotype had a greater response to exercise as measured by the maximum fall after exercise and the area under the exercise curve (62). These confusing results indicate that the VNTR variant in the promoter of *ALOX5* needs to be studied in larger and more diverse populations with asthma to validate its functional role in LT modifiers treatment.

LT C4 synthase (LTC4S) and LT A4 hydrolase (LTA4H) are enzymes of the LT pathway. The gene *LTC4S* is located on human chromosome 5q35.3 and has five exons that encode 150 amino acids. Five splice variants of the gene exist, and to date three SNPs have been identified in the gene. A promoter SNP -444A/C has been reported to be associated with severe asthma (63). Three independent reports suggested an association between the response to long-acting β-agonists and the C allele of the same promoter polymorphism (64–66). The gene *LTA4H* is located on 12q23 and has 19 exons and encodes 611 amino acids. Individuals homozygote for the G allele of the SNP *rs2660845* in *LTA4H* exhibit a four- to fivefold increased probability of having an asthma exacerbation while receiving montelukast treatment comparing with individuals homozygous for the A allele (60).

SLCO2B1 (solute carrier organic anion transporter family, member 2B1) codes OATP2B1, a transporter of montelukast. This gene is located on chromosome 11q13. It has four exons that encode 709 amino acids. A nonsynonymous SNP (*rs12422149*, Arg312Gly) within the gene has been shown to be associated with symptom improvement scores after montelukast treatment. Patients with the Arg/Arg genotype significantly exhibited a reduced plasma concentration on the morning after an evening dose of montelukast as well as the observation of a significant improvement in symptoms (67). The relatively small sample size is however a limitation of this study. Consequently, more studies involving larger sample sizes will be needed to accurately access the associations between the Arg312Gly polymorphism and responsiveness to montelukast treatment.

CYSLTR2 encodes the CysLT2 receptor, which is involved in the LT pathway, has a greater response to LT modifiers, and plays an important role in smooth muscle cell proliferation. The gene is located on chromosome 13q14 and has a single exon that encodes a protein 346 amino acids in length. Two SNPs (*rs912278*, *rs912277*) within the gene have been reported to be associated with montelukast treatment. The common *CYSLTR2* TT and TC haplotypes of SNPs *rs912278* and *rs912277* have both been shown to have a significantly lower mean change in morning PEF observations and this is consistent with the single-marker results (68).

D. Theophylline

TP and other methylxanthine derivatives have weak bronchodilator and anti-inflammatory effects that have been used in both COPD and asthma management. TP has a narrow therapeutic range because of its dose-related toxicities. The plasma concentrations of some patients have been shown to have the potential to reach the toxic range (over 20 μg/mL) despite the fact that patients were only prescribed 400 mg/day of a slow-release TP and were administered no other medications and had no disease complications. Cytochrome P450 (CYP) 1A2 is the major metabolic enzyme of TP. The gene (*CYP1A2*) is located on chromosome 15q24.1 and has 7 exons encoding 516 amino acids. A common promoter polymorphism –2964G/A of the gene is associated with altered clearance of TP. The clearance of TP in patients with the A/A genotype was markedly reduced when compared with patients possessing the G/G genotype. This genetic variation could be helpful in predetermining individuals (A/A homozygotes for –2964G/A) who may be sensitive to TP toxicity despite being described standard routine doses of slow-release TP (69).

Most of the pharmacogenetic loci for airway diseases detailed above (Table 2) were identified in studies involving relatively small sample sizes. A consistent theme from all of these studies is that the next key pharmacogenetic approach would be to verify these potentially functional polymorphisms in larger population sets.

E. Other Treatments

Antihistamine, anticholinergic, and anticytokine treatments are all further types of management implemented in the treatment of airway diseases.

Histamine is a bronchoconstrictor that is involved in the pathogenesis of airway disease. In the bronchial epithelium, histamine *N*-methyltransferases (HNMTs) play an important role in histamine biotransformation by catalyzing the methylation of histamine. The levels of HNMT activity in human tissues are controlled, in part, by genetic variation. A common C314T polymorphism within the *HNMT* gene results in a Thr105Ile change in the encoded amino acid at position 105 (nucleotide position 314), and the T314 allele is associated with decreased levels of both HNMT enzymatic activity and immunoreactive protein. Presence of the T314 allele would therefore be anticipated to result in reduced histamine metabolism and increased bronchoconstriction. In an association study of this polymorphism with asthma patients, T-allele frequency was found to be significantly higher in asthma patients. This suggests that individual variation in histamine metabolism might contribute to the pathophysiology and/or response to therapy of this disease (70).

Anticholinergic agents are substances that block the neurotransmitter acetylcholine in the central and the peripheral nervous system. The majority of anticholinergic drugs are antimuscarinics. Antimuscarinic agents are effective as bronchodilators in treatment of both COPD and asthma. Ipratropium bromide is a nonselective antimuscarinic agent that acts as an antagonist at M1, M2, and M3 receptors. The genes encoding the receptors are therefore potential targets for a pharmacogenetic study. The coding regions for the M2 and M3 receptor genes (*CHRM2* and *CHRM3*) have already been screened for polymorphic variants, and while both aa coding regions of the two genes contain SNPs, the level of expression of the M2 and M3 receptors in the airways is partly driven by a transcriptional controlling mechanism. Both *CHRM2* and *CHRM3* promoters have been defined and are known to contain a range of polymorphic variants, but until now no evidence has been found for any association between the promoter polymorphisms and drug response (34).

Anticytokines are quite new and novel therapies for asthma and COPD. TH2 cytokines are recognized to play an important role in airway inflammation. IL-4 and IL-13 are critical cytokines in the expression of atopy and allergic disease. IL-4 triggers B lymphocytes to produce IgE, induces the expression of adhesion molecules on endothelium that specifically attract eosinophils, and triggers T cells to become TH2 cells,

Table 2 Potential Pharmacogenetic Loci for Airway Diseases

Gene	Name	Chromosome location	Pharmacogenetic polymorphism allele	Drug target	Associated phenotypes
ADRB2	β2-Adrenergic receptor	5q31.32	Arg16Gly	β2-Adrenergic agonists	Arg/Arg homozygotes have greater response to β2-agonists
ARG1	Arginase I	6q23	*rs2278I659*	β2-Adrenergic agonists	A/A homozygotes have greater response to β2-agonists
GR	Glucocorticoid receptor	5q31	Asp363 Ser	Corticosteroid	363Ser have an enhanced response to glucocorticoids
CRHR1	Corticotropin-releasing hormone receptor 1	7q21.3	Haplotype	Corticosteroid	GAT/GAT homozygotes have an enhanced response to glucocorticoids
TBX21	T-box 21	17q21.32	His33Gln	Corticosteroid	33Gln have an enhanced response to glucocorticoids
FCER2	Fc fragment of IgE, low affinity II, receptor	19p13.2	T2206C	Corticosteroid	T/T homozygotes have an enhanced response to glucocorticoids
ALOX5	Arachidonate 5-lipoxygenase	10q11.2	Promoter VNTR	Leukotriene modifiers	Mutant homozygotes have decreased 5-lipoxygenease inhibitor
LTC4S	Leukotriene C4 synthase	5q35.3	Promoter A-444C	Leukotriene modifiers	-444C has greater response to leukotriene modifiers
LTA4H	Leukotriene A4 hydrolase	12q23	*rs2660845*	Leukotriene modifiers	A/A homozygotes have greater response to leukotriene modifiers
CYSLTR2	Cysteinyl leukotriene receptor 2	13q14	*rs91227/rs912278*	Leukotriene modifiers	Haplotype CC has greater response to leukotriene modifiers
SLCO2B1	Solute carrier organic anion transporter family, member 2B1	11q13	Arg312Gly	Leukotriene modifiers	Arg312 homozygotes have greater response to leukotriene modifiers
CYP1A2	Cytochrome P450, family 1, subfamily A, polypeptide 2	15q24.1	-2964G/A	Theophylline	Heterozygotes G/A and homozygotes A/A reduce clearance of theophylline

which in turn further release IL-4 and mediate allergic diseases. IL-13 is a cytokine closely related to IL-4 that binds to IL-4R and is also expressed by TH2 cells from asthma patients (71). Genetic regulation of IL-4 and IL-13 is an important pivot in the genetic predisposition to allergy. Administration of either IL-13 or IL-4 confers an asthma-like phenotype, by an IL-4 receptor chain-dependent pathway, in nonimmunized T cell–deficient mice (72).

For IL-4 blockade, two vaccines have been tried in mice. One is limpet hemocyanin (73), an IL-4 derivative immunogen. The other is a 14–amino acid peptide from IL-4 inserted into the variant hepatitis B core antigen (74). Both vaccines induced high antibody titers in mice and inhibited antigen-induced lung inflammation. IL-13 not only binds to the low-affinity IL-13α1 subunit but also binds to the high-affinity complex formed by the IL-13α1 and IL-4α1 subunits. Binding of the latter leads to the activation of Janus kinase1 (JAK1) and JAK2, and the signal transducer and activator of transcription STAT6 (75). A nonsignaling high affinity IL-13Rα2 was shown to strongly inhibit the activity of IL-13 in mice and in humans (76). In humans, an IL-13-specific mAb CAT-354 in mild asthma has been used in phase 2 studies (75). STAT6 is the transcription factor for both IL-4 and IL-13. In humans, the polymorphisms of the gene are associated with asthma (77,78). A study involving local application of cell-penetrating peptide inhibitors (a dominant-negative novel chimeric peptide) of STAT-6 showed significant promise with regard to the treatment of allergic rhinitis and asthma (79).

In addition to IL-4 and IL-13, other cytokines play crucial roles in airway diseases. IL-5 and IL-9 are the major cytokines that drive eosinophil differentiation while IL-10 and IFN-γ inhibit multiple inflammatory cytokines. IL-12 induces naive T cells into the Th1 pathway. TNF-α is another Th2 pathway simulator. There is strong evidence that polymorphisms of many of the genes encoding these cytokines as well as those encoding *IL-15* and *IL-17F* are associated with human airway diseases traits. Inhibition of single cytokines may not be sufficient in the treatment of airway disease, and there needs to be elucidation of the function of the variants underlying the associations that have been seen. Nonetheless, these cytokines are potential therapeutic targets in airway disease and some clinical trials are already in progress (Table 3).

V. The Future of Pharmacogenetics and Pharmacogenomics of Airway Diseases

Although there are already a number of genetic studies that have identified functional polymorphisms of relevance to drug targets and drug responses, prospective clinical studies of these polymorphisms and the genes they are in have been relatively small. Most studies have been retrospective and have involved small numbers of patients, and have been focused on specific polymorphisms without systematic representation of the variation in the genes that are under study (4).

The field of genetics has the opportunity of identifying new associations in novel genes for airway diseases. To date there have been more than 500 papers published of disease-gene studies (predominantly candidate gene studies) for asthma, with over 100 genes reportedly being associated with asthma phenotypes (113). Whole genome linkage screens have identified new loci for asthma (114) and COPD (115) that following fine mapping and positional cloning has ultimately resulted in disease gene identification.

Table 3 Major Cytokines That Are Potential Therapeutic Targets for Airway Diseases

Gene	Chromosome location	Traits gene polymorphisms associated with humans	Animal models established for the purpose of drug development	Clinical trial approaches	Predicted effects of novel therapeutic targets
IL-4	5q31	Asthma (80); IgE (81)	Vaccines in mice (73,82), mAb in monkey (83)	Inhaled IL-4 receptor (84)	Blocking IL-4 Th2 phenotype
IL-13	5q31	Asthma (85); IgE (86)	IL-13 Rα chain (72) in mice, mAb in monkey (87)	mAb: CAT-354 (75); inhaled pitrakinra (88)	Blocking IL-13, IL-4 Th2 phenotype
IL-5	5q31	Eosinophil counts (89)		mAb: Sch-55700 (90); mepolizumab (91)	Blocking eosinophil differentiation
IL-10	1q32	Asthma (92); COPD (93)	Administration of IL-10 in mice (94)	Administration of IL-10 (95)	Inhibiting inflammatory cytokines
IL-12A/B	3q25/5q33	Asthma (96)	Overexpressing IL-12-in mice dendritic cell (97)	Administration of rhIL-12 (98)	Boosting Th1 pathway
IFN-γ	12q14	Asthma (99)	Administration of IFN-γ in mice (100)	Administration of rhIFN-γ (101)	Suppression of Th2 inflammation
TNF-α	6p21	Asthma (102); IgE (103); COPD (104)	Administration of infliximab in mice (105)	Etanercept (106), mAb (107)	Anti-inflammatory
IL-15	4q31.21	Asthma (108)	Soluble IL-15α in mice (109)	Mikbeta1 in leukemia (110)	Suppression of Th2 inflammation
IL-17F	6p12.2	Asthma (111)	Pravastatin in mice (112)		Anti-IL-17 mediating inflammation

Pitrakinra, an IL-4 mutant protein; mepolizumab, humanized blocking IgG mAb; infliximab, anti-tumour necrosis factor (TNF)-α mAb; etanercept, TNF receptor fusion protein; Mikbeta1, monoclonal antibody identifies CD122, the β-subunit shared by the IL-2 and IL-15 receptor.
Abbreviation: mAb, monoclonal antibody.

These genes include *ADAM33* (a disintegrin and metalloproteinase-33) on chromosome 20p13 (49), *DPP10* (dipeptidyl peptidase-10) on chromosome 2q14 (116), *PHF11* (plant homeodomain finger protein 11) on chromosome 13q14 (117), *GPRA* (G protein–coupled receptor for asthma) on chromsome7p14 (118), *HLA-G* on chromosome 6p21, and *CYFLP* on chromosome 5q33 (119). Both candidate and positional cloning approaches have in some instances identified genes that could be useful targets for pharmaceutical intervention.

To date there has only been one GWA study for asthma, which has resulted in the gene *ORMDL3* (and potentially the neighboring *GSDML1* gene) being identified as an important risk factor for the development of childhood asthma (120). Disease gene identification was aided by analyses of *ORMDL3* transcript levels through genome-wide gene expression data from Epstein-Barr virus-transformed lymphoblastoid cells from children in the genotyped family samples (121). Little is known about the function of *ORMDL3*, which is a member of a conserved family of endoplasmic reticulum membrane proteins. It remains to be established whether *ORMDL3* is a suitable target for drug development, although the protein contains four transmembrane regions and has the potential to act as a druggable transporter (122).

α1-Antitrypsin deficiency remains a paradigm for COPD and is still the most important known genetic risk factor for COPD (123). Mutations in the serpin peptidase inhibitor, clade A (α-1 antiproteinase, antitrypsin), member 1 (*SERPINA1*) gene cause α-1 antitrypsin deficiency. Numerous other candidate genes could also be linked to disease pathogenesis. However, the candidate gene approach is often limited by inconsistent results in other study populations. The association of the following genes with COPD were confirmed by different studies: transforming growth factor-β1 (*TGFB1*), surfactant protein B (*SFTPB*), serpin peptidase inhibitor clade E member 2 (*SERPINE2*), and microsomal epoxide hydrolase (*EPHX1*) (124). Interestingly, many of the genes identified by genome-wide linkage and/or association studies for asthma and COPD are expressed in the mucosa and respiratory epithelium, for example, *DPP10* and *GPRA*, indicating that events at epithelial-cell surfaces might be driving disease processes. Understanding events at the epithelial-cell surface might provide new insights for the development of new treatments for inflammatory epithelial disease (125).

VI. Conclusions

In recent years, considerable progress has been made in the identification of pharmacogenetic and pharmacogenomic loci for airway diseases, but nonetheless we are still in the early stages of our understanding of the genetic effects on drug targets, metabolism, and disposition. With the available sequence information, including the intragenic noncoding regions of the human genome, the increasingly recognized regulatory microRNA profiles, the completion of sequences of human, mouse, and other species genomes, the establishment of different animal models and with advances in bioinformatics and methods to allow rapid genome-wide sequencing, genotyping, and expression studies, it is possible that more pharmacogenetic and pharmacogenomic loci for asthma and COPD genes will emerge soon. Translation of these findings into therapeutics for airway diseases will take time, but it is conceivable that improved patient care will be possible in the not too distant future (126).

References

1. Fletcher C, Peto R. The natural history of chronic airflow obstruction. Br Med J 1977; 1(6077):1645–1648.
2. Motulsky AG. Drug reactions enzymes, and biochemical genetics. JAMA 1957; 165(7): 835–837.
3. Weinshilboum R. Inheritance and drug response. N Engl J Med 2003; 348(6):529–537.
4. Goldstein DB, Tate SK, Sisodiya SM. Pharmacogenetics goes genomic. Nat Rev Genet 2003; 4(12):937–947.
5. Evans WE, McLeod HL. Pharmacogenomics—drug disposition, drug targets, and side effects. N Engl J Med 2003; 348(6):538–549.
6. Meyer UA. Pharmacogenetics and adverse drug reactions. Lancet 2000; 356(9242): 1667–1671.
7. Frazer KA, Ballinger DG, Cox DR, et al. A second generation human haplotype map of over 3.1 million SNPs. Nature 2007; 449(7164):851–861.
8. Stein LD. Human genome: end of the beginning. Nature 2004; 431(7011):915–916.
9. Kumar D. Genomic medicine: a new frontier of medicine in the twenty first century. Genomic Med 2007; 1(1–2):3–7.
10. Drazen JM, Silverman EK, Lee TH. Heterogeneity of therapeutic responses in asthma. Br Med Bull 2000; 56(4):1054–1070.
11. Mills RE, Luttig CT, Larkins CE, et al. An initial map of insertion and deletion (INDEL) variation in the human genome. Genome Res 2006; 16(9):1182–1190.
12. Bentley DR, Balasubramanian S, Swerdlow HP, et al. Accurate whole human genome sequencing using reversible terminator chemistry. Nature 2008; 456(7218):53–59.
13. Rigat B, Hubert C, Alhenc-Gelas F, et al. An insertion/deletion polymorphism in the angiotensin I-converting enzyme gene accounting for half the variance of serum enzyme levels. J Clin Invest 1990; 86(4):1343–1346.
14. Drazen JM, Yandava CN, Dube L, et al. Pharmacogenetic association between ALOX5 promoter genotype and the response to anti-asthma treatment. Nat Genet 1999; 22(2):168–170.
15. Tantisira KG, Lazarus R, Litonjua AA, et al. Chromosome 17: association of a large inversion polymorphism with corticosteroid response in asthma. Pharmacogenet Genomics 2008; 18(8):733–737.
16. Cook EH Jr., Scherer SW. Copy-number variations associated with neuropsychiatric conditions. Nature 2008; 455(7215):919–923.
17. Link E, Parish S, Armitage J, et al. SLCO1B1 variants and statin-induced myopathy—a genomewide study. N Engl J Med 2008; 359(8):789–799.
18. Dixon AL, Liang L, Moffatt MF, et al. A genome-wide association study of global gene expression. Nat Genet 2007; 39(10):1202–1207.
19. Mattes J, Yang M, Foster PS. Regulation of microRNA by antagomirs: a new class of pharmacological antagonists for the specific regulation of gene function? Am J Respir Cell Mol Biol 2007; 36(1):8–12.
20. Castanotto D, Rossi JJ. The promises and pitfalls of RNA-interference-based therapeutics. Nature 2009; 457(7228):426–433.
21. Liggett SB. Genetically modified mouse models for pharmacogenomic research. Nat Rev Genet 2004; 5(9):657–663.
22. Guo Y, Lu P, Farrell E, et al. In silico and in vitro pharmacogenetic analysis in mice. Proc Natl Acad Sci U S A 2007; 104(45):17735–17740.
23. De Sanctis GT, Merchant M, Beier DR, et al. Quantitative locus analysis of airway hyperresponsiveness in A/J and C57BL/6J mice. Nat Genet 1995; 11(2):150–154.
24. Zhang Y, Lefort J, Kearsey V, et al. A genome-wide screen for asthma-associated quantitative trait loci in a mouse model of allergic asthma. Hum Mol Genet 1999; 8(4): 601–605.

25. Prows DR, Shertzer HG, Daly MJ, et al. Genetic analysis of ozone-induced acute lung injury in sensitive and resistant strains of mice. Nat Genet 1997; 17(4):471–474.
26. Cole TJ, Blendy JA, Monaghan AP, et al. Targeted disruption of the glucocorticoid receptor gene blocks adrenergic chromaffin cell development and severely retards lung maturation. Genes Dev 1995; 9(13):1608–1621.
27. Liu P, Jenkins NA, Copeland NG. A highly efficient recombineering-based method for generating conditional knockout mutations. Genome Res 2003; 13(3):476–484.
28. Finotto S, Neurath MF, Glickman JN, et al. Development of spontaneous airway changes consistent with human asthma in mice lacking T-bet. Science 2002; 295(5553):336–338.
29. Hall IP. Pharmacogenetics, pharmacogenomics and airway disease. Respir Res 2002; 3:10.
30. Turki J, Lorenz JN, Green SA, et al. Myocardial signaling defects and impaired cardiac function of a human beta 2-adrenergic receptor polymorphism expressed in transgenic mice. Proc Natl Acad Sci U S A 1996; 93(19):10483–10488.
31. Nebert DW, Dalton TP, Stuart GW, et al. "Gene-swap knock-in" cassette in mice to study allelic differences in human genes. Ann N Y Acad Sci 2000; 919:148–170.
32. Sears MR, Lotvall J. Past, present and future—beta2-adrenoceptor agonists in asthma management. Respir Med 2005; 99(2):152–170.
33. Ensemble. Browse a Genome. Available at: http://www.ensembl.org.
34. Reihsaus E, Innis M, MacIntyre N, et al. Mutations in the gene encoding for the beta 2-adrenergic receptor in normal and asthmatic subjects. Am J Respir Cell Mol Biol 1993; 8(3): 334–339.
35. Hall IP. Pharmacogenetics of asthma. Chest 2006; 130(6):1873–1878.
36. Hall IP, Sayers I. Pharmacogenetics and asthma: false hope or new dawn? Eur Respir J 2007; 29(6):1239–1245.
37. Choudhry S, Ung N, Avila PC, et al. Pharmacogenetic differences in response to albuterol between Puerto Ricans and Mexicans with asthma. Am J Respir Crit Care Med 2005; 171(6): 563–570.
38. Martinez FD, Graves PE, Baldini M, et al. Association between genetic polymorphisms of the beta2-adrenoceptor and response to albuterol in children with and without a history of wheezing. J Clin Invest 1997; 100(12):3184–3188.
39. Israel E, Drazen JM, Liggett SB, et al. The effect of polymorphisms of the beta(2)-adrenergic receptor on the response to regular use of albuterol in asthma. Am J Respir Crit Care Med 2000; 162(1):75–80.
40. Lima JJ, Blake KV, Tantisira KG, et al. Pharmacogenetics of asthma. Cur Opin Pulm Med 2009; 15(1):57–62.
41. Bleecker ER, Postma DS, Lawrance RM, et al. Effect of ADRB2 polymorphisms on response to long-acting beta2-agonist therapy: a pharmacogenetic analysis of two randomised studies. Lancet 2007; 370(9605):2118–2125.
42. Martin AC, Zhang G, Rueter K, et al. Beta2-adrenoceptor polymorphisms predict response to beta2-agonists in children with acute asthma. J Asthma 2008; 45(5):383–388.
43. Litonjua AA, Lasky-Su J, Schneiter K, et al. ARG1 is a novel bronchodilator response gene: screening and replication in four asthma cohorts. Am J Respir Crit Care Med 2008; 178(7): 688–694.
44. Ricciardolo FL, Sterk PJ, Gaston B, et al. Nitric oxide in health and disease of the respiratory system. Physiol Rev 2004; 84(3):731–765.
45. Zimmermann N, King NE, Laporte J, et al. Dissection of experimental asthma with DNA microarray analysis identifies arginase in asthma pathogenesis. J Clin Invest 2003; 111(12): 1863–1874.
46. Yang M, Rangasamy D, Matthaei KI, et al. Inhibition of arginase I activity by RNA interference attenuates IL-13-induced airways hyperresponsiveness. J Immunol 2006; 177:5595–5603.

47. Adcock IM, Barnes PJ. Molecular mechanisms of corticosteroid resistance. Chest 2008; 134(2): 394–401.
48. Ito K, Chung KF, Adcock IM. Update on glucocorticoid action and resistance. J Allergy Clin Immunol 2006; 117(3):522–543.
49. Van Eerdewegh P, Little RD, Dupuis J, et al. Association of the ADAM33 gene with asthma and bronchial hyperresponsiveness. Nature 2002; 418(6896):426–430.
50. Umland SP, Schleimer RP, Johnston SL. Review of the molecular and cellular mechanisms of action of glucocorticoids for use in asthma. Pulm Pharmacol Ther 2002; 15(1):35–50.
51. Hakonarson H, Bjornsdottir US, Halapi E, et al. Profiling of genes expressed in peripheral blood mononuclear cells predicts glucocorticoid sensitivity in asthma patients. Proc Natl Acad Sci U S A 2005; 102(41):14789–14794.
52. Bray PJ, Cotton RG. Variations of the human glucocorticoid receptor gene (NR3C1): pathological and in vitro mutations and polymorphisms. Hum Mutat 2003; 21(6):557–568.
53. Huizenga NA, Koper JW, De Lange P, et al. A polymorphism in the glucocorticoid receptor gene may be associated with and increased sensitivity to glucocorticoids in vivo. J Clin Endocrinol Metab 1998; 83(1):144–151.
54. Silverman ES, Breault DT, Vallone J, et al. Corticotropin-releasing hormone deficiency increases allergen-induced airway inflammation in a mouse model of asthma. J Allergy Clin Immunol 2004; 114(4):747–754.
55. Tantisira KG, Lake S, Silverman ES, et al. Corticosteroid pharmacogenetics: association of sequence variants in CRHR1 with improved lung function in asthmatics treated with inhaled corticosteroids. Hum Mol Genet 2004; 13(13):1353–1359.
56. Weiss ST, Lake SL, Silverman ES, et al. Asthma steroid pharmacogenetics: a study strategy to identify replicated treatment responses. Proc Am Thorac Soc 2004; 1(4):364–367.
57. Dijkstra A, Koppelman GH, Vonk JM, et al. Pharmacogenomics and outcome of asthma: no clinical application for long-term steroid effects by CRHR1 polymorphisms. J Allergy Clin Immunol 2008; 121(6):1510–1513.
58. Tantisira KG, Hwang ES, Raby BA, et al. TBX21: a functional variant predicts improvement in asthma with the use of inhaled corticosteroids. Proc Natl Acad Sci U S A 2004; 101(52): 18099–18104.
59. Tantisira KG, Silverman ES, Mariani TJ, et al. FCER2: a pharmacogenetic basis for severe exacerbations in children with asthma. J Allergy Clin Immunol 2007; 120(6):1285–1291.
60. Lima JJ, Zhang S, Grant A, et al. Influence of leukotriene pathway polymorphisms on response to montelukast in asthma. Am J Respir Crit Care Med 2006; 173(4):379–385.
61. Telleria JJ, Blanco-Quiros A, Varillas D, et al. ALOX5 promoter genotype and response to montelukast in moderate persistent asthma. Respir Med 2008; 102(6):857–861.
62. Kalayci O, Birben E, Sackesen C, et al. ALOX5 promoter genotype, asthma severity and LTC production by eosinophils. Allergy 2006; 61(1):97–103.
63. Sayers I, Barton S, Rorke S, et al. Allelic association and functional studies of promoter polymorphism in the leukotriene C4 synthase gene (LTC4S) in asthma. Thorax 2003; 58(5): 417–424.
64. Sampson AP, Siddiqui S, Buchanan D, et al. Variant LTC(4) synthase allele modifies cysteinyl leukotriene synthesis in eosinophils and predicts clinical response to zafirlukast. Thorax 2000; 55(suppl 2):S28–S31.
65. Asano K, Shiomi T, Hasegawa N, et al. Leukotriene C4 synthase gene A(-444)C polymorphism and clinical response to a CYS-LT(1) antagonist, pranlukast, in Japanese patients with moderate asthma. Pharmacogenetics 2002; 12(7):565–570.
66. Whelan GJ, Blake K, Kissoon N, et al. Effect of montelukast on time-course of exhaled nitric oxide in asthma: influence of LTC4 synthase A(-444)C polymorphism. Pediatr Pulmonol 2003; 36(5):413–420.

67. Mougey EB, Feng H, Castro M, et al. Absorption of montelukast is transporter mediated: a common variant of OATP2B1 is associated with reduced plasma concentrations and poor response. Pharmacogenet Genomics 2009; 19(2):129–138.

68. Klotsman M, York TP, Pillai SG, et al. Pharmacogenetics of the 5-lipoxygenase biosynthetic pathway and variable clinical response to montelukast. Pharmacogenet Genomics 2007; 17(3):189–196.

69. Obase Y, Shimoda T, Kawano T, et al. Polymorphisms in the CYP1A2 gene and theophylline metabolism in patients with asthma. Clin Pharmacol Ther 2003; 73(5):468–474.

70. Yan L, Galinsky RE, Bernstein JA, et al. Histamine N-methyltransferase pharmacogenetics: association of a common functional polymorphism with asthma. Pharmacogenetics 2000; 10(3):261–266.

71. Minty A, Chalon P, Derocq JM, et al. Interleukin-13 is a new human lymphokine regulating inflammatory and immune responses. Nature 1993; 362(6417):248–250.

72. Grunig G, Warnock M, Wakil AE, et al. Requirement for IL-13 independently of IL-4 in experimental asthma. Science 1998; 282(5397):2261–2263.

73. Le Buanec H, Paturance S, Couillin I, et al. Control of allergic reactions in mice by an active anti-murine IL-4 immunization. Vaccine 2007; 25(41):7206–7216.

74. Ma Y, HayGlass KT, Becker AB, et al. Novel recombinant interleukin-13 peptide-based vaccine reduces airway allergic inflammatory responses in mice. Am J Respir Crit Care Med 2007; 176(5):439–445.

75. Holgate ST. Novel targets of therapy in asthma. Curr Opin Pulm Med 2009; 15(1):63–71.

76. Andrews AL, Nasir T, Bucchieri F, et al. IL-13 receptor alpha 2: a regulator of IL-13 and IL-4 signal transduction in primary human fibroblasts. J Allergy Clin Immunol 2006; 118(4): 858–865.

77. Duetsch G, Illig T, Loesgen S, et al. STAT6 as an asthma candidate gene: polymorphism-screening, association and haplotype analysis in a Caucasian sib-pair study. Hum Mol Genet 2002; 11(6):613–621.

78. Pykalainen M, Kinos R, Valkonen S, et al. Association analysis of common variants of STAT6, GATA3, and STAT4 to asthma and high serum IgE phenotypes. J Allergy Clin Immunol 2005; 115(1):80–87.

79. McCusker CT, Wang Y, Shan J, et al. Inhibition of experimental allergic airways disease by local application of a cell-penetrating dominant-negative STAT-6 peptide. J Immunol 2007; 179(4):2556–2564.

80. Sandford AJ, Chagani T, Zhu S, et al. Polymorphisms in the IL4, IL4RA, and FCERIB genes and asthma severity. J Allergy Clin Immunol 2000; 106(1 pt 1):135–140.

81. Marsh DG, Neely JD, Breazeale DR, et al. Linkage analysis of IL4 and other chromosome 5q31.1 markers and total serum immunoglobulin E concentrations. Science 1994; 264(5162): 1152–1156.

82. Linhart B, Bigenzahn S, Hartl A, et al. Costimulation blockade inhibits allergic sensitization but does not affect established allergy in a murine model of grass pollen allergy. J Immunol 2007; 178(6):3924–3931.

83. Hart TK, Blackburn MN, Brigham-Burke M, et al. Preclinical efficacy and safety of pascolizumab (SB 240683): a humanized anti-interleukin-4 antibody with therapeutic potential in asthma. Clin Exp Immunol 2002; 130(1):93–100.

84. Borish LC, Nelson HS, Corren J, et al. Efficacy of soluble IL-4 receptor for the treatment of adults with asthma. J Allergy Clin Immunol 2001; 107(6):963–970.

85. Heinzmann A, Mao XQ, Akaiwa M, et al. Genetic variants of IL-13 signalling and human asthma and atopy. Hum Mol Genet 2000; 9(4):549–559.

86. Liu X, Nickel R, Beyer K, et al. An IL13 coding region variant is associated with a high total serum IgE level and atopic dermatitis in the German multicenter atopy study (MAS-90). J Allergy Clin Immunol 2000; 106(1 pt 1):167–170.

87. Bree A, Schlerman FJ, Wadanoli M, et al. IL-13 blockade reduces lung inflammation after Ascaris suum challenge in cynomolgus monkeys. J Allergy Clin Immunol 2007; 119(5): 1251–1257.

88. Wenzel S, Wilbraham D, Fuller R, et al. Effect of an interleukin-4 variant on late phase asthmatic response to allergen challenge in asthmatic patients: results of two phase 2a studies. Lancet 2007; 370(9596):1422–1431.

89. Yamamoto N, Sugiura H, Tanaka K, et al. Heterogeneity of interleukin 5 genetic background in atopic dermatitis patients: significant difference between those with blood eosinophilia and normal eosinophil levels. J Dermatol Sci 2003; 33(2):121–126.

90. Kips JC, O'Connor BJ, Langley SJ, et al. Effect of SCH55700, a humanized anti-human interleukin-5 antibody, in severe persistent asthma: a pilot study. Am J Respir Crit Care Med 2003; 167(12):1655–1659.

91. Flood-Page P, Swenson C, Faiferman I, et al. A study to evaluate safety and efficacy of mepolizumab in patients with moderate persistent asthma. Am J Respir Crit Care Med 2007; 176(11):1062–1071.

92. Hunninghake GM, Soto-Quiros ME, Lasky-Su J, et al. Dust mite exposure modifies the effect of functional IL10 polymorphisms on allergy and asthma exacerbations. J Allergy Clin Immunol 2008; 122(1):93–98, 98 e1–e5.

93. He JQ, Shumansky K, Zhang X, et al. Polymorphisms of interleukin-10 and its receptor and lung function in COPD. Eur Respir J 2007; 29(6):1120–1126.

94. Fu CL, Chuang YH, Chau LY, et al. Effects of adenovirus-expressing IL-10 in alleviating airway inflammation in asthma. J Gene Med 2006; 8(12):1393–1399.

95. Chernoff AE, Granowitz EV, Shapiro L, et al. A randomized, controlled trial of IL-10 in humans. Inhibition of inflammatory cytokine production and immune responses. J Immunol 1995; 154(10):5492–5499.

96. Khoo SK, Hayden CM, Roberts M, et al. Associations of the IL12B promoter polymorphism in longitudinal data from asthmatic patients 7 to 42 years of age. J Allergy Clin Immunol 2004; 113(3):475–481.

97. Kuipers H, Heirman C, Hijdra D, et al. Dendritic cells retrovirally overexpressing IL-12 induce strong Th1 responses to inhaled antigen in the lung but fail to revert established Th2 sensitization. J Leukoc Biol 2004; 76(5):1028–1038.

98. Bryan SA, O'Connor BJ, Matti S, et al. Effects of recombinant human interleukin-12 on eosinophils, airway hyper-responsiveness, and the late asthmatic response. Lancet 2000; 356(9248):2149–2153.

99. Nakao F, Ihara K, Kusuhara K, et al. Association of IFN-gamma and IFN regulatory factor 1 polymorphisms with childhood atopic asthma. J Allergy Clin Immunol 2001; 107(3): 499–504.

100. Reisinger J, Triendl A, Kuchler E, et al. IFN-gamma-enhanced allergen penetration across respiratory epithelium augments allergic inflammation. J Allergy Clin Immunol 2005; 115(5): 973–981.

101. Boguniewicz M, Martin RJ, Martin D, et al. The effects of nebulized recombinant interferon-gamma in asthmatic airways. J Allergy Clin Immunol 1995; 95(1 pt 1):133–135.

102. Moffatt MF, Cookson WO. Tumour necrosis factor haplotypes and asthma. Hum Mol Genet 1997; 6(4):551–554.

103. Shin HD, Park BL, Kim LH, et al. Association of tumor necrosis factor polymorphisms with asthma and serum total IgE. Hum Mol Genet 2004; 13(4):397–403.

104. Sakao S, Tatsumi K, Igari H, et al. Association of tumor necrosis factor alpha gene promoter polymorphism with the presence of chronic obstructive pulmonary disease. Am J Respir Crit Care Med 2001; 163(2):420–422.

105. Deveci F, Muz MH, Ilhan N, et al. Evaluation of the anti-inflammatory effect of infliximab in a mouse model of acute asthma. Respirology 2008; 13(4):488–497.

106. Berry MA, Hargadon B, Shelley M, et al. Evidence of a role of tumor necrosis factor alpha in refractory asthma. N Engl J Med 2006; 354(7):697–708.
107. Erin EM, Leaker BR, Nicholson GC, et al. The effects of a monoclonal antibody directed against tumor necrosis factor-alpha in asthma. Am J Respir Crit Care Med 2006; 174(7): 753–762.
108. Kurz T, Strauch K, Dietrich H, et al. Multilocus haplotype analyses reveal association between 5 novel IL-15 polymorphisms and asthma. J Allergy Clin Immunol 2004; 113(5): 896–901.
109. Ruckert R, Brandt K, Braun A, et al. Blocking IL-15 prevents the induction of allergen-specific T cells and allergic inflammation in vivo. J Immunol 2005; 174(9):5507–5515.
110. Morris JC, Janik JE, White JD, et al. Preclinical and phase I clinical trial of blockade of IL-15 using Mikbeta1 monoclonal antibody in T cell large granular lymphocyte leukemia. Proc Natl Acad Sci U S A 2006; 103(2):401–406.
111. Ramsey CD, Lazarus R, Camargo CA Jr., et al. Polymorphisms in the interleukin 17F gene (IL17F) and asthma. Genes Immun 2005; 6(3):236–241.
112. Imamura M, Okunishi K, Ohtsu H, et al. Pravastatin attenuates allergic airway inflammation by suppressing antigen sensitisation, interleukin 17 production and antigen presentation in the lung. Thorax 2009; 64(1):44–49.
113. Ober C, Hoffjan S. Asthma genetics 2006: the long and winding road to gene discovery. Genes Immun 2006; 7(2):95–100.
114. Daniels SE, Bhattacharrya S, James A, et al. A genome-wide search for quantitative trait loci underlying asthma. Nature 1996; 383(6597):247–250.
115. Demeo DL, Campbell EJ, Barker AF, et al. IL10 polymorphisms are associated with airflow obstruction in severe alpha1-antitrypsin deficiency. Am J Respir Cell Mol Biol 2008; 38(1): 114–120.
116. Allen M, Heinzmann A, Noguchi E, et al. Positional cloning of a novel gene influencing asthma from chromosome 2q14. Nat Genet 2003; 35(3):258–263.
117. Zhang Y, Leaves NI, Anderson GG, et al. Positional cloning of a quantitative trait locus on chromosome 13q14 that influences immunoglobulin E levels and asthma. Nat Genet 2003; 34(2):181–186.
118. Laitinen T, Polvi A, Rydman P, et al. Characterization of a common susceptibility locus for asthma-related traits. Science 2004; 304(5668):300–304.
119. Ober C, Tan Z, Sun Y, et al. Effect of variation in CHI3L1 on serum YKL-40 level, risk of asthma, and lung function. N Engl J Med 2008; 358(16):1682–1691.
120. Moffatt MF, Kabesch M, Liang L, et al. Genetic variants regulating ORMDL3 expression contribute to the risk of childhood asthma. Nature 2007; 448(7152):470–473.
121. Moffatt MF. Genes in asthma: new genes and new ways. Curr Opin Allergy Clin Immunol 2008; 8(5):411–417.
122. Hjelmqvist L, Tuson M, Marfany G, et al. ORMDL proteins are a conserved new family of endoplasmic reticulum membrane proteins. Genome Biol 2002; 3(6):Research0027.
123. Kalsheker N, Chappell S. The new genetics and chronic obstructive pulmonary disease. COPD 2008; 5(4):257–264.
124. Seifart C, Plagens A. Genetics of chronic obstructive pulmonary disease. Int J Chron Obstruct Pulmon Dis 2007; 2(4):541–550.
125. Cookson W. The immunogenetics of asthma and eczema: a new focus on the epithelium. Nat Rev Immunol 2004; 4(12):978–988.
126. Avila PC, Kishiyama JL, Adelman DC. Pharmacological approaches. Clin Allergy Immunol 2002; 16:469–494.

5

Delivery of Drugs to the Airways

OMAR S. USMANI
National Heart and Lung Institute, Imperial College, and Royal Brompton Hospital,
London, U.K.

I. Introduction

The delivery of drug to the lungs via the inhaled route has long been established as a successful and effective approach in the management of respiratory disorders (1). Inhalation therapy confers distinct therapeutic benefits by targeting drug directly to the lungs, which allows a more rapid onset of action, the use of smaller drug doses, and a better efficacy to safety ratio, compared with systemic therapy. Increasingly, the respiratory tract is also being used as a conduit for the systemic administration of drug. This chapter reviews the existing inhalation devices in clinical use, new and emerging inhaler technologies, the factors controlling the deposition of inhaled drug within the airways, and aerosols for systemic delivery of drug.

II. Inhalation Systems

The inhalation systems used to generate therapeutic aerosols for delivery of drugs to the airways are pressurized metered-dose inhalers, dry powder inhalers (DPIs), and nebulizers. There are numerous devices available within each group and this, combined with the array of inhaled respiratory drugs available for prescription, often leads to a confusing choice for physicians in selecting the most suitable device-drug combination for their patients. This choice has been further complicated by the recent proliferation of devices based on new inhaler technologies. To address issues relating to inhaler selection in the common respiratory disorders of asthma and chronic obstructive pulmonary disease, evidence-based guidelines have recently been published by the American College of Chest Physicians (2). Their recommendations suggest the following points should be considered when choosing an inhaler: the clinical condition and disease severity, availability of the inhaler device for the drug prescription, the patient's ability to use the selected device correctly, consideration given to using the same inhaler type for all drugs, the setting and convenience of outpatient and inpatient use, the time required for drug administration, cost and reimbursement, and the inhaler preference of the patient and physician. The advantages and disadvantages of the different inhalation systems are summarized in Table 1.

A. Pressurized Metered-Dose Inhalers

The development of the pressurized metered-dose inhaler (pMDI) in 1956 was a significant technological milestone that heralded the advent of modern inhalation therapy

Table 1   Advantages and Disadvantages of Inhalation Systems

Inhalation system	Advantages	Disadvantages
Pressurized metered-dose inhaler (pMDI)	• Compact and portable • Quick treatment time • Multidose • Drug in sealed canister • Inexpensive	• Difficulty in coordination • Propellants affect climate change • High oral deposition • Difficult to assess empty canister
Dry powder inhaler (DPI)	• Compact and portable • Quick treatment time • Breath actuated, removes need for hand-mouth coordination • No propellants, no "cold Freon" effect	• Reliant on sufficient inspiratory flow to disperse drug • High oral deposition can occur • Older devices not multidose • Contain additives, e.g., lactose intolerance • Humidity can lead to drug degradation
Conventional nebulizers (ultrasonic, jet)	• Relaxed tidal breathing technique • Large drug doses can be given • Aerosolize many drug solutions • No propellants • Suitable for young, old and acutely ill patients	• Bulky and cumbersome • Long treatment time • Expensive • Wasted drug in nebulizer reservoir • Need for power source • Contamination risk • Variation in aerosol output performance between models

(3). The Medihaler came into pharmaceutical production within a year following the suggestion of the asthmatic daughter of the president of Riker Laboratories, and initial devices were manufactured with salts of isoproterenol and adrenaline. Fifty years on, the pMDI remains the most commonly used inhalation device for drug delivery to the lungs. It is a convenient multidose device, quick to use, compact, portable, and relatively cheap (4). Following international agreement on the Montreal Protocol Treaty to eradicate the global use of chlorofluorocarbons (CFCs) to protect the ozone layer in the stratosphere (5), pMDIs are being reformulated (6).

The essential design of pMDIs consists of a sealed high-pressure canister in which medication is suspended, or dissolved in solution, with liquid gaseous propellant, surfactants, and excipients. In addition, other formulation ingredients may be present such as chemical preservatives and flavoring agents (4). When the canister is depressed against the actuator seat, a trigger mechanism opens a one-way metering valve that ensures an exact dose of drug-propellant mixture is released through the atomizing nozzle. The liquid propellants rapidly expand and vaporize during actuation, and this provides the required force to aerosolize the medication and propel it at high velocity through the opening of the mouthpiece. The vaporization of the propellant causes cooling of the aerosol and this can give rise to the "cold Freon effect" experienced by some patients as the cold aerosol hits the back of the oropharynx, which causes them to stop inhaling (7). The surfactants and dispersing agents prevent agglomeration of the solid drug particles and lubricate the metering valve to allow it to function accurately; however, some of these agents have been shown to cause bronchospasm, wheeze, and cough in asthmatic patients (8).

The emitted aerosol spray consists of droplets of varying diameters in size. The size of the particles in the aerosol cloud and the speed at which they are expelled from the device determine the quantity of drug reaching the lungs. The design of the actuator seat and nozzle together with the vapor pressure of the propellant are the key factors controlling the characteristics of the aerosol output from a pMDI (9). Aerosol particle size is reduced as the vapor pressure increases and the atomizing nozzle diameter decreases. As the aerosol spray leaves the pMDI it slows down quickly from a starting velocity of around 30 m/sec and, as the propellant evaporates, aerosol particle size decreases rapidly from an initial droplet size of 30 μm (10). Because of the ballistic nature of the high-velocity aerosol spray, a large proportion of the emitted drug particles impact in the oropharynx and less than 20% reaches the lungs (11). Depending on the pharmacokinetic behavior and metabolism of the drug, oropharyngeal deposition may potentially give rise to unwanted local and systemic adverse effects as a result of absorption either from the buccal cavity or from the gastrointestinal tract after swallowing.

The storage and handling of pMDIs may have an effect on the output of the aerosol dose. Storing the pMDI canister with the valve in the downright position between uses may lead to a marked reduction in the delivered drug dose (12). Thoroughly shaking the canister before use helps reduce propellant loss from the metering valve as, without propellant, minimal drug is discharged on actuation (13). Following these observations, discharge of an initial "waste" dose from a pMDI has been suggested before use, particularly with inhalers that are infrequently used. The storage of CFC-pMDIs at extreme temperatures can result in a reduction of the drug dose (14).

The mandatory requirement to reformulate pMDIs with non-CFC propellant has led to new developments in drug chemistry and device design technology (6). The damaging CFCs are being replaced with environmental friendly non-ozone depleting propellants such as hydrofluoroalkanes (HFAs) (15). Novel surfactants and cosolvent excipients such as ethanol have been added to improve the solubility of the HFA drug formulation. The different drug chemistry has led to alterations in the intrinsic design of pMDIs to ensure reproducible drug delivery to the lungs. Some of the features have included new compatible elastomeric valve components and changes in the actuator and orifice geometry (16). Particle size distributions of the aerosol output as well as toxicity data on the new drug formulation and device combinations have been undertaken in clinical studies to ensure they compare favorably to existing CFC preparations (17). Although HFAs have no ozone depletion potential compared with CFCs, they do have an impact on climate change, yet current consensus suggests no safe alternative for patients. It can be envisaged that in the future, alternatives to HFAs may be needed.

Studies investigating the optimal use of pMDIs suggest that more favorable clinical responses are achieved when, after removing the device cap, the inhaler canister is thoroughly shaken, the mouthpiece is placed in the mouth between the lips, and, following normal exhalation to functional residual capacity, the pMDI is actuated at the beginning of a deep-slow inhalation followed by a breath-hold pause of 10 seconds at the end of inspiration (18,19). However, many patients are unable to use pMDIs correctly and effectively (20–22). An inability to properly carry out one or more of the steps outlined may lead to the suboptimal use of the inhalation device and an improper technique, which can ultimately affect clinical efficacy (23,24). The most common problem with pMDI devices is the failure to coordinate inhalation and actuation of the inhaler and, as discussed later, these errors may be a result of failure to understand the technique or poor instruction in use. To overcome the difficulties related to pMDI use, other inhalation delivery devices have been developed that include breath-actuated pMDIs, breath-coordinated inhalers, and add-on accessory spacer attachments (4).

B. Breath-Actuated Metered-Dose Inhalers

Breath-actuated metered-dose inhalers (BA-MDIs) require the patient's inspiratory effort to actuate the valve on the inhaler and include devices such as Autohaler (3M Health Care, Minnesota, U.S.) and Easi-Breathe (Baker Norton, Florida, U.S.). Though these inhalation devices are more expensive compared with pMDIs, they respond to low inspiratory flows, require less training on their correct use, are easier to learn, and have been used with many drug formulations. In a controlled study, BA-MDI use did not offer added advantage over patients with good pMDI inhaler technique, although they were beneficial in those with bad pMDI coordination (24). However, in the primary care setting the use of a BA-MDI was shown to achieve better asthma control compared with pMDI use (25). The Spacehaler (Evans Medical, Surrey, U.K.) is a compact BA-MDI that has an integrated vortex chamber causing release of a low-velocity aerosol for inhalation. The creation of a slower plume velocity can decrease oropharyngeal impaction and alleviate the cold Freon effect (26). The SmartMist (Aradigm, California, U.S.) inhaler has an integral microprocessor unit that automatically actuates the device after inhalation of a predefined volume at a specific inspiratory flow and provides visual feedback to the patient on inhalation technique (27).

C. Breath-Coordinated Devices

Breath-coordinated devices are different from BA-MDIs as they do not depend on the patient's inspiratory flow for actuation (28). Rather, these inhalers help patients achieve coordination with aerosol inhalation. Devices such as the Breath-Coordinated Inhaler (Aeropharm, Germany) and Easidose (Bespak, Hertfordshire, U.K.) carefully control the inspiratory flow through the actuator and inhaler such that the patient has enough time to comfortably actuate the pMDI and coordinate the aerosol delivery with the start of their inhalation. The Tempo (MAP Pharmaceuticals, California, U.S.) device is a breath-synchronized plume controlled inhaler that automatically coordinates drug discharge with the patient's breathing cycle. The device features an aerosol flow controller that ensures consistent drug delivery to the lungs to reduce dose variation.

D. Spacer Devices

Spacer devices were developed in the late 1970s to be used in conjunction with pMDIs to assist in the delivery of inhaled drug to the lungs (29). Spacers include valved-holding chambers that have a one-way inspiratory valve in the mouthpiece and only allow airflow through the chamber when the patient inhales, simple extension devices that are nonvalved add-on products, and reverse-flow devices in which the aerosol spray is actuated away from the patient into a collapsible bag or a chamber through which outside air is entrained. The central principle on which spacers work is to provide a "standing" aerosol cloud reservoir within the device, from which patients can breathe tidally, to overcome the difficulties of pMDI coordination.

Spacers are attached to pMDIs and form an extension to the mouthpiece of the inhaler device. By increasing the distance the aerosol cloud has to travel, spacers slow down the high velocity of the emitted aerosol, which has a twofold effect. First, it allows time for evaporation of the aerosol propellants, which leads to smaller drug particles that have the potential to reach the lower respiratory tract, and second, there is a reduction in the ballistic impact of the aerosol against the oropharynx. In addition, spacers allow large drug particles to deposit on the walls of the device, which further assists in reducing oropharyngeal deposition. This may lead to decreased local unwanted side effects particularly with inhaled corticosteroids, and allows a reduction in the amount of inhaled drug being absorbed into the systemic circulation via the gastrointestinal tract that could, otherwise, give rise to adverse effects. As with pMDIs, slow inspiration with spacer devices is preferable and some spacers have audible inspiratory flow alarms that inform the patient if their inhalation is too fast. Spacer attachments with pMDIs have also been shown to be as effective as nebulizers in the management of patients with asthma exacerbations (30).

There are a variety of available spacer devices that have different design characteristics. Large-volume spacers tend to have less particle deposition on their walls and deliver a higher fine-particle dose compared with small-volume devices. Spacers should be prescribed with pMDIs they are compatible with, as each combination is distinct in its aerosol output characteristics and airways drug delivery (31). Patient-related factors of improper use can lead to inconsistent delivery of medication (32). One dose actuation at a time from a pMDI into the spacer device should be employed, as simultaneous multiple dose administration may cause a considerable reduction in the drug delivered (33). In addition, electrostatic charge attraction of drug particles onto the walls of plastic spacer devices also decreases drug delivery to the lungs (34), and therefore, spacers should be primed with the pMDI prior to use or washed with ionic detergent and air-dried (35). Antistatic wall linings improve the efficiency of a spacer and nonelectrostatic materials are being developed for use in future devices.

E. Dry Powder Inhalers

DPIs contain no propellant gases and do not require the coordination of inhaler actuation with breathing, which is necessary with pMDIs. DPIs contain micronized powdered drug particles bound into loose aggregates or drug particles associated with larger carrier molecules such as lactose (36). DPI delivery systems are breath-actuated devices that rely on the patient's inspiratory effort to operate.

Since the introduction of DPIs in 1970, there has been a considerable increase in the number of devices available, particularly in the last decade (37). Early devices were single-dose systems that dispensed individual drug measures from punctured gelatine capsules, such as Rotahaler (Allen and Hanburys, Middlesex, U.K.) and Spinhaler (Fisons, Ipswich, U.K.). Examples of more recent devices include Handihaler (Boehringer-Ingelheim, Germany), Eclipse (Sanofi-Aventis, France), and Aerolizer (Novartis, Switzerland). All single-dose delivery systems require drug to be individually loaded into the inhaler prior to use. In contrast, multiple-dosing delivery DPIs avoid the inconvenience associated with repeated drug loading and can be divided into "multidose" or "multi-unit-dose" systems.

Multidose systems deliver drug that is metered from a powder reservoir and include devices such as Clickhaler (Innovata Biomed, Hertfordshire, U.K.), Turbuhaler (AstraZeneca, Sweden), Easyhaler (Orion, Finland), Ultrahaler (Sanofi-Aventis), Taifun (Leiras, Finland), and Pulvinal (Chiesi, Italy). Although multidose reservoir inhalers have added desiccant to protect them from moisture exposure, it has been shown that damp and humid conditions can cause drug to deteriorate and these devices should be stored in a dry environment (38). Multiple-unit-dose DPIs such as Diskhaler/Rotadisk (Allen and Hanburys) contain drug sealed in individual foil blisters or, as in Diskus/Accuhaler (Allen and Hanburys), drug sealed in pockets on a moving strip.

DPI devices are critically dependent on the generation of a sufficient and sustained inspiratory flow by patients for therapeutic success. An adequate and controlled inspiratory flow is required to deaggregate the drug particles from the carrier molecules and disperse the aerosol into particles of appropriate size to allow delivery to the lungs (39). It has been shown that inhalation flow has a significant effect on the drug dose emitted, which is related to clinical efficacy (40). In addition, some DPI devices are more dependent than others on inhalation flow, resulting in variable dosage emissions that may give rise to unpredictable clinical control (41). Inhalation delivery systems such as Acu-Breathe DPI (Respirics, North Carolina, U.S.) have been developed that minimize dose variability using technology that triggers the drug dose only after a predetermined inspiratory flow and preliminary in vitro data have used flows of 45 to 90 L/min. Devices with a high inspiratory resistance, such as Turbuhaler, require inhalation flows of 60 L/min or greater throughout the inspiratory cycle to achieve optimal drug deposition to the lungs (42). However, patients with asthma and chronic obstructive airways disease have been shown to inhale from DPI delivery systems using suboptimal inspiratory flows, leading to poor drug release and low pulmonary deposition (40). Also, patients in acute respiratory distress and young children may not be able to generate the necessary inspiratory flows required (43). It has been shown that training and counselling patients in their inhalation technique can increase the peak inspiratory flows generated through DPIs (44,45) and this may be achieved by using portable handheld meters that assess the suitability of different DPIs to various patient groups (40).

New DPI device systems have been developed that reduce the dependence of aerosol generation on the patient's inspiratory effort, and there are a number of formulation technologies and devices undergoing clinical development (37,46). The Novolizer (MEDA, Sweden) is a multidose, refillable DPI that has a unique feedback and control mechanism which guides the patient through the correct inhalation maneuver. It requires an inspiratory flow of around 35 L/min and has a dose counter that only advances after a correct inhalation. The FlowCaps (Hovione, Portugal) and Spiros S2 (Elan Pharmaceuticals, Ireland) delivery systems need inhalations flows of as little as 15 to 30 L/min to effectively aerosolize drug powder from the device. The Nektar Pulmonary Inhaler (Nektar Therapeutics, California, U.S.) is entirely independent of the patient's breathing maneuver. It uses a bolus of compressed air to disperse powdered aerosol from a blister into a holding chamber, ready for the patient to inhale.

F. Conventional Nebulizers

Liquid nebulizers are commonly used in clinical practice and fall into two main categories: ultrasonic nebulizer and jet nebulizer (47). Ultrasonic nebulizers utilize the energy of sound waves generated by vibration of a piezoelectric crystal at high frequency. The sound waves pass through the drug solution, which leads to the separation of liquid droplets to form aerosol sprays for inhalation. The frequency of the ultrasonic vibrations determines the size of the aerosol particles generated. Although ultrasonic nebulizers are smaller and less noisy, they are usually more fragile, expensive, and not as effective in nebulizing drug suspensions compared with jet nebulizers. Jet nebulizers utilize either compressed gas or an electrical compressor to produce aerosolized particles. A high-velocity airstream is directed through a narrow Venturi opening creating a low-pressure zone, which draws up the liquid drug from the nebulizer reservoir. The drug is drawn into the air stream through a capillary system resulting in fragmented aerosol droplets of different size within the chamber. Large particles impact onto baffles that return any formed liquid back into the nebulizer reservoir, whereas small particles are carried into the patient's airstream.

Nebulizers do not need much patient coordination and require relaxed tidal breathing for effective use. A significant amount of medication may be lost to the surrounds during exhalation because of the constant aerosol generation throughout the respiratory cycle. Lung deposition can be markedly reduced with shallow rapid inspirations or crying that may occur with children. Care needs to be taken with any facemask/nebulizer combination, especially when delivering drug to children, as an inappropriate mask design and incorrect mask insertion into the nebulizer may give rise to unwanted deposition of drug onto the face and eyes (48). The main disadvantage of the conventional nebulizer devices is the size of the equipment, length of treatment time, and lack of portability. There is great variation in the efficiency of aerosol output and the particle size distributions between different models (49). Some of these variations may be addressed by matching the correct compressor and gas flow rate with the nebulizer model (50).

G. New Nebulizer Devices

Modifications to the design of the constant-output conventional nebulizer system have resulted in a newer generation of nebulizers that offer a noticeable improvement in the efficiency and precision of pulmonary drug delivery (51,52). The devices are more costly, although they may be cost-effective particularly with expensive drugs that have a narrow therapeutic index, by utilizing a reduced drug dose and chamber volume than is currently employed in older systems.

Breath-enhanced "open vent" nebulizer devices, such as Ventstream (Respironics, Pittsburgh, U.S.) and LC Plus and LCD (PARI GmbH, Germany), direct the patient's inspiratory flow through the nebulizer chamber. The Sidestream (Respironics) entrains additional air through the nebulizer. These nebulizer systems create a continuous output of aerosol like the conventional nebulizers, but allow an increased generation of aerosolized drug during the inspiratory phase of breathing and reduce aerosol exhalation during the expiratory phase, so more drug reaches the lungs (53).

Breath-actuated dosimetric nebulizers deliver aerosol only during inspiration. The AeroEclipse (Monaghan Medical, New York, U.S.) has a sensing valve that monitors tidal breathing and generates "on-demand" aerosol only during the inspiratory phase. The Circulaire nebulizer (Westmed, Arizona, U.S.) is an adaptation of the conventional jet nebulizer. It has a one-way exhalation valve in the mouthpiece that directs the aerosol output into a storage reservoir bag, which allows for an increase in drug available for inhalation during the following inspiratory cycle (54). Similar to the constant-output nebulizers, the breath-enhanced and breath-actuated systems also differ significantly in their technical performance (55).

A number of novel aerosol delivery systems have been developed that force liquid through nozzles either under pressure or by using ultrasonic principles. The AERx (Aradigm) is a liquid aerosol generator that forces the drug solution under pressure through an array of small holes to produce a controlled spray. The drug is supplied as multiple-unit-dose blisters on a strip. The aerosol dose is timed with each breath and the device provides feedback to the patient to guide their inhalation technique. The Respimat Soft-Mist Inhaler (Boehringer-Ingelheim) is a handheld, multidose device that uses mechanical power from a spring, which pushes drug solution through narrow channels in a nozzle to generate an aerosol spray. The aerosol spray contains a higher fraction of fine particles and exits the inhaler more slowly and for a longer duration compared with pMDIs, offering the patient more time between device actuation and inhalation (56).

Nebulizer technologies have utilized the energy generated from a ceramic element or piezoelectric crystal to produce vibration of a plate or mesh that has been perforated with multiple micron-sized holes. Medication is extruded through the numerous apertures in the vibrating mesh/plate, which leads to the controlled generation of a fine mist aerosol with consistent aerosol droplet particle size (57,58). These systems include devices such as Aeroneb and Aerodose (Aerogen, Ireland), the e-flow nebulizer device (PARI GmbH), and MicroAir (Omron Healthcare, Illinois, U.S.), which are all battery operated, portable, and lightweight. The devices all share similar advantages over conventional nebulizers in that they can nebulize suspensions and solutions, the residual volume remaining in the device is minimal, and they have shorter nebulization times. The main limitation is that drug particles may build up and block the small mesh apertures, which can lead to altered characteristics of the aerosol spray, rather than a failure to generate aerosol. Consequently, this could have clinical implications and so these inhalation devices must be regularly and carefully cleaned.

Device systems have been developed that control the inhalation maneuver to minimize the variability in dose delivery that occurs during tidal breathing. The AKITA system (Activaero GmbH, Germany) is designed to maximize inhaled drug deposition to the lungs by controlling breathing patterns and tailoring drug delivery to each individual patient (59). The device uses personalized smart-card technology that stores optimized predetermined respiratory parameters tailored to each patient's breathing pattern; these are inhalation flow, inhaled volume, and breath-hold pause. The system does not allow the patient to breathe tidally but takes control over the breathing maneuver and provides slow, deep, and prolonged inhalation using an inspiratory resistance. Aerosolized drug may be pulsed during any period in the inspiratory cycle. These features promote the targeting and deposition of drug to the peripheral airways and decrease drug loss on exhalation. The computer-controlled system displays feedback on the remaining number of breaths and allows an integral assessment of patient compliance, by recording the actual inhaled volumes and number of breaths taken. The device has recently been combined with vibrating mesh technology to create a new nebulizer combination that allows enhanced inhalation therapy by optimizing both patient breathing patterns and drug particle size distributions, to provide more selective and regional airways targeting of drug deposition within the lungs (59).

The I-neb (Respironics) device is a handheld adaptive aerosol delivery system that is battery powered and computer controlled. It is a third-generation device that incorporates vibrating mesh technology to generate aerosolized drug and adds further refinement to nebulized aerosol delivery compared with earlier models of this nebuliser (60).

This system analyzes the pattern of the patient's spontaneous tidal breathing. By continually monitoring pressure changes in the patient's preceding three respiratory cycles, the device automatically adapts to deliver a controlled and precise drug dose constantly during the first-half of the inspiratory phase, thereby compensating for intrapatient variability in breathing patterns. The device also has breathing mode features that can be adapted to the patient's preference in that the delivery of aerosolized drug to the patient can occur during spontaneous tidal breathing, or, in patients who can manage, vibratory feedback at the mouthpiece can be used to guide patients to perform slow and deep inhalation. This can increase lung deposition and shorten nebulization times. The aerosol delivery system provides an accurate assessment of the volume of drug delivered per breath, such that the total preprogrammed dose is correctly received by the patient. The device is able to give audible and visual feedback to the patient informing them that their treatment is complete and records information on patient's use of the device and compliance with treatment.

These "smart" nebulizers achieve greater control and intrapulmonary targeting of aerosolized drug delivery. Such requirements may be needed for newer and more expensive respiratory drugs in development that have a narrow therapeutic index and may only be safely delivered to the lungs via the inhaled route (61).

III. Drug Deposition Within the Respiratory Tract

To achieve successful delivery of inhaled drug to the lungs an appreciation of the basic aerosol mechanisms and factors affecting drug deposition is required, together with an understanding of the in vitro and in vivo methods used to assess intrapulmonary deposition.

A. Mechanisms of Deposition

Deposition is the process that determines the fraction of the inspired particles that will be caught within the airways and therefore, fail to exit with exhaled air. The main mechanisms that contribute to the deposition of inhaled therapeutic medical aerosols within the human respiratory tract are inertial impaction, sedimentation, and diffusion (62,63). *Inertial impaction* occurs when the momentum of a drug particle leads it to continue in its original direction of flow, impacting on an airway wall, in a region where there is a change in the bulk direction of the airstream. This happens particularly at airway bifurcations in larger airways, where airflow velocities are high and rapid changes in the direction of the airstream occur. *Sedimentation* describes particle deposition under the action of gravity and results when the gravitational force acting on a drug particle overcomes the total force of air resistance. Sedimentation is most efficient within the small airways where airflow velocities are low and there is increased time available for particles to settle within the airway (residence time). *Diffusion* refers to the random collision of gas molecules with very small particles that push these particles about in an irregular fashion. Thus, a particle in stationary air moves about in a random manner even in the absence of gravity and this can result in contact onto airway surfaces. Deposition occurs mainly in the small airways, where airflow velocities are lowest, residence time is long, and the distance a particle has to travel before it hits an airway wall is short.

Inertial impaction and gravitational sedimentation are most important for the deposition of large, fast-moving particles between 1 and 10 μm, whereas diffusion is the main deposition determinant of smaller, slow-moving submicron particles. These mechanisms act simultaneously and collectively contribute to the deposition of inhaled drug particles within the respiratory tract. The relative extent to which each mechanism predominates depends on the physical characteristics of the drug particle, local airways' geometry, airstream parameters, and breathing patterns.

B.   Factors Affecting Deposition

The factors that may affect the deposition of inhaled drug particles within the respiratory tract can be divided into aerosol characteristics and patient variables. These are summarized in Table 2.

Aerosol Characteristics

Of the physical aerosol characteristics, particle size is the most important factor determining the extent and site of inhaled drug deposition within the airways. The human respiratory tract has evolved to act as a series of filters that remove airborne particulate matter from the inspired air. In general, particles >100 μm in size are usually trapped in the nasal cavity, those >10 μm deposit in the oropharynx, particles between 2 and 6 μm deposit in the conducting airways, and those <1 μm are directed to peripheral lung regions or are exhaled. As previously discussed aerosol particle size affects the probabilities of impaction, sedimentation, and diffusion.

Recent data suggest it may be important to generate different particle sizes for different classes of inhaled drug to optimize clinical benefit, and this will depend on the pharmacology of the drug and in which particular lung region it is thought best to target the drug. For example, it has been shown in studies using short-acting β-agonist that

Table 2 Factors Affecting Airways Deposition of Inhaled Medical Aerosols

Aerosol factors	Patient factors
Drug particle characteristics	Inhalation maneuver
• Size	• Inspiratory flow
• Density	• Inhaled aerosol volume
• Shape	• Breath-hold pause
	• Degree of lung inflation
	• Breathing frequency
	• Nose vs. mouth breathing
Drug formulation	Airway features
• Hygroscopicity	• Diameter and obstruction
• Surfactant	• Airway disease type
• Molecule charge	• Disease severity
	• Paediatric vs. adult
Aerosol generation system	Healthcare features
• Device type (see Table 1)	• Training and instruction
• Maintenance	• Patient technique
	• Patient compliance

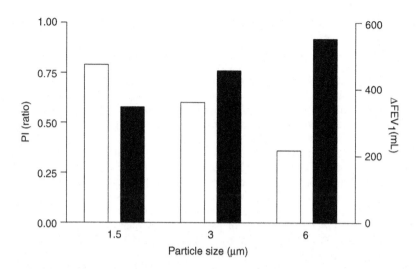

Figure 1 Relationship between monodisperse salbutamol particle size, drug penetration into the lung, and clinical response. Smaller particles achieve less bronchodilation and more peripheral lung penetration compared with larger particles, which are more proximally deposited and attain better clinical responses. *Abbreviations*: PI, penetration index (*blank columns*); ΔFEV_1, change in forced expiratory volume in one second (*shaded columns*). *Source:* Adapted from Ref. 65.

precise aerosol particles of 6- and 3-μm diameter achieved the greatest clinical benefit by targeting the inhaled drug to the main site of drug action in the proximal airways (64,65). However, drug that was targeted to more peripheral regions using smaller particles of 1.5-μm diameter gave much poorer airways bronchodilation (Fig. 1). Studies are needed to determine the optimal particle size using other inhaled drugs, as they may provide critical information in the development of new device technologies to achieve better airways targeting (66).

Drug deposition in the lungs may also be enhanced using low-density gases such as helium and with large porous particles of low density (67,68). The humid environment of the lungs may cause water-soluble drug particles to enlarge in size and this will cause drug particles to deposit more proximally than nonhygroscopic particles. However, the phenomenon of hygroscopic growth has only been demonstrated using non-pharmacological aerosols experimentally in vitro and in healthy subjects in vivo, but not with active drug compounds (69,70).

Patient Variables

The breathing maneuver influences the efficiency and efficacy of the drug delivery system. A slow and deep inhalation is optimal for pMDIs, whereas rapid inhalation decreases lung deposition and increases oropharyngeal impaction (18). Actuation from pMDIs at the beginning of inspiration during low lung volumes results in enhanced deposition of drug throughout the lungs (19). In contrast, DPIs require faster inspiratory flows so that the powdered drug is deaggregated from its carrier molecule and aerosolized, which will greatly improve lung deposition compared with slow inhalation (41).

As discussed, most conventional nebulizers require relaxed tidal breathing, although some of the newer devices take charge of the patient's breathing maneuver. A breath-hold pause at the end of inhalation augments the peripheral lung deposition of inhaled drug, by allowing the required airway residence time for particles to deposit by sedimentation or diffusion (19). A greater inhaled aerosol volume also allows more particles to be carried and deposited within the peripheral airways (71). Airways caliber also affects the lung deposition of inhaled drug. Greater lung deposition has been observed in healthy subjects compared with asthmatics (11) and lower lung deposition occurs following induced bronchoconstriction (72).

Inadequate device demonstration and instruction from healthcare professionals can lead to improper patient use and, as a consequence, this may result in poor clinical control. Patient demonstration is the single most valuable method of evaluating inhaler technique (73). However, studies have shown that healthcare professionals are uncertain about the correct use of inhalers and should themselves undergo formal training in the use of inhaler devices (74,75). Retraining of patients is important, as good technique declines over time and this may be assisted by training aids that help patients maintain their recommended inhaler technique (40,44,76). In elderly patients, decreased cognition (77) and poor hand strength (78) lead to incorrect inhaler technique despite retraining, but age per se is not a predictor.

C. Assessing Airways Deposition
Predictive Models
Experimental models of particle deposition are mainly based on the physics of fluid flowing through simple tubes and have been applied to estimate therapeutic aerosol dosimetry and predict the deposition behavior of inhaled medical aerosols within the human airways (79,80). These models incorporate idealized assumptions and conditions of particle characteristics, airways morphology, and inhalation patterns, to derive simple predictive equations that approximate the complexity of therapeutic particle deposition in vivo.

In Vitro Methods
In vitro test instruments are primarily intended to examine the performance output and monitor quality control of inhaler device systems. These instruments analyze the emitted aerosol spray from the device to determine aerodynamic diameters, particle size distributions, and drug dose. Inertial multistage cascade impactors and optical light-scattering techniques are the methods used to establish aerosol characteristics (81,82). In vitro sizing measurements may allow an estimation of drug delivery in vivo, using a prespecified particle size range to indicate the potential for delivery of drug to the lower respiratory tract. However, in vitro methods remain limited in reliably predicting aerosol deposition and there will remain a need for concurrent in vivo data (83).

Pharmacokinetic Methods
Pharmacokinetic quantification of inhaled drug and its metabolites in plasma, or that excreted in the urine, may allow an indirect assessment of total lung deposition in vivo. The lung deposition (pulmonary bioavailability) of an inhaled drug not metabolized within the airways may be determined by blocking gastrointestinal absorption of the oropharyngeal (swallowed) fraction of drug. Charcoal block has been the method used to assess pulmonary bioavailability for salbutamol (84) and terbutaline (85). Where oral

bioavailability of the drug is known, such as budesonide, the unpleasant charcoal block technique may be avoided to calculate total lung dose (86). Swallowed drug that undergoes complete first-pass hepatic metabolism such as fluticasone propionate (87), or does not get absorbed from the gastrointestinal tract such as sodium cromoglycate (88), has negligible oral bioavailability, and it can be assumed that plasma drug levels represent the inhaled fraction or pulmonary bioavailability.

A urinary excretion method has been shown to indirectly evaluate the pulmonary bioavailability of inhaled salbutamol (89). Collection of urine in the first 30 minutes after dosing can estimate the lung deposition of inhaled salbutamol, as the contribution of the swallowed fraction to systemic bioavailability is negligible during this time. This pharmacokinetic method has also been used to compare lung bioavailability of different inhaler devices (90), assess effects of inspiratory flow on lung deposition (91), and investigate optimal inhaler technique (92). The same collection principle has been applied to plasma samples, although higher salbutamol doses are required to assess the pharmacodynamic response (93).

Radionuclide Imaging

Radionuclide imaging, in addition to total lung deposition, allows visualization of the intrapulmonary distribution of inhaled radiolabeled drug particles and a quantitative assessment of regional airway deposition patterns (94). Two-dimensional (2D) planar γ scintigraphy has been the main technique employed, where drug is radiolabeled with a γ-emitting isotope such as technetium-99m. Following inhalation, images of the oropharynx, lung fields, and stomach are obtained. Lung ventilation images are used to delineate the lung borders and obtained by tidal breathing of radioactive gases such as krypton-81m or xenon-133. Superimposition of the lung outline from the ventilation scan onto the images of radiolabeled drug deposition within the airways allows the lungs to be divided into a series of zones or regions of interest for deposition analysis. Regions of interest have been defined ranging from two- (11) and three-compartment areas (95) to more complex six-compartment concentric lung sections (96).

Three-dimensional imaging techniques such as single-photon emission tomography (SPECT) and positron emission tomography (PET) enable better precision in the spatial resolution of the airways. The lung images are divided into a series of concentric shells so that it is easier to relate regional aerosol deposition patterns to lung anatomy (97). SPECT detects γ ray intensities of radionuclides such as technetium-99m or iodine-123 using a 360° rotation of the γ-camera and has been used to study the intrapulmonary deposition of terbutaline (98) and nedocromil sodium (99). Radionuclides that emit positrons such as carbon-11, nitrogen-13, oxygen-15 and fluorine-18 can interact with tissue electrons to release γ rays, which may be detected by PET scanners (100). The large amounts of radionuclide, high machine costs, the need for long image acquisition times with SPECT, and the very short half-life of positron-emitting radionuclides have limited the use of these 3D imaging modalities for assessing inhaled drug deposition.

IV. Aerosols for Systemic Delivery, Gene Therapy, and Vaccination

The respiratory tract is increasingly being used as a conduit for the systemic administration of drug (101). The lungs have an advantage of a vast alveolar surface from which inhaled drug may be absorbed. Drugs, large molecule peptides, and proteins that cannot be absorbed in the gastrointestinal tract or undergo metabolic breakdown may also benefit from inhaled delivery to achieve a systemic effect. For the patient, the avoidance of needles is an obvious benefit. Interest in systemic drug delivery via the respiratory tract has been stimulated from innovative developments in inhaler and device technologies coupled with advances in pharmaceutical chemistry and formulations that have allowed more selective and regional airways targeting of aerosol deposition within the lungs. A variety of aerosolized drugs have been utilized and some examples include prostanoids for pulmonary hypertension (102), narcotics for analgesia (103), antimigraine drugs (104), as well as many different peptides, proteins, and hormones (105).

Aerosolized insulin to treat diabetes has been the most prominent development in systemic drug delivery (106). An inhaled formulation was available in the United States in the middle of 2006; however, the product Exubera, a powdered form of recombinant human insulin, manufactured by Pfizer in collaboration with Nektar Therapeutics Pulmonary Inhaler system, was withdrawn in late 2007. Concerns related to dosing errors, the continued need for a daily long-acting insulin injection, and difficulties in device coordination led to a poor reception by patients and physicians. Several companies are currently developing inhaled insulin using drug formulations to improve bioavailability and devices to improve the efficiency of pulmonary delivery (107).

Aerosol delivery to the upper respiratory tract may also accomplish the desired aim of drug to reach the systemic circulation (108). The nasal passages are highly vascular and drug may be quickly absorbed to reach the right side of the heart and bypass first-pass hepatic metabolism. The intranasal route also allows for the potential of peptide, hormone, and drug delivery to the central nervous system (109).

The use of inhaled complementary DNA in patients with cystic fibrosis (CF) has undergone the most development in the area of aerosolized gene therapy (110). Difficulties remain centered around a low transfer of the CF transmembrane conductance regulator gene to the target epithelial cells in the airways with the available adenovirus and liposome gene-transfer vector agents. The challenges include achieving adequate lung penetration of the gene-vector beyond obstructed airways, delivering a sufficient enough dose to the airways, overcoming the mucosal and membrane barriers to the epithelial cells, transporting the DNA to the nucleus of the cell, and the need for repeat dosing studies to assess adverse effects as epithelial cell turnover occurs every six weeks. The use of inhaled DNA in the treatment of lung cancer is also being studied in animal models (110).

Interest has recently focused on the use of aerosols for vaccine delivery as a successful alternative to the parenteral route of immunization (111). Clinical trials with vaccines against influenza using intranasal delivery (112) and measles virus using pulmonary delivery (113) have been undertaken, and there is also attention directed on the use of vaccination against inhaled bioterrorism agents (110). Further improvements in inhaler delivery systems and advances in formulation stability and safety profiling may make aerosol inhalation the ideal choice for vaccination programs.

V. Future Directions

Since the advent of the pMDI, the first 50 years of modern inhalation therapy have seen significant progress in aerosol science, growth of sophisticated device technologies, and advances in therapeutic delivery by inhalation. Inhaled drug delivery in the 21st century presents it own unique challenges. There is a pressing need for innovative delivery systems that are able to keep up with the rapid developments in drug discovery, especially those arising from the disciplines of biopharmaceutics and pharmacogenomics. Future inhalation systems need to be designed to achieve greater control of aerosolized drug delivery to the airways for the management of local pathology and for the treatment of systemic disease.

References

1. Yernault JC. Inhalation therapy: an historical perspective. Eur Respir Rev 1994; 4:65–67.
2. Dolovich MB, Ahrens RC, Hess DR, et al. Device selection and outcomes of aerosol therapy: evidence-based guidelines. American College of Chest Physicians/American College of Asthma, Allergy, and Immunology. Chest 2005; 127:335–371.
3. Freedman T. Medihaler therapy for bronchial asthma. A new type of aerosol therapy. Postgrad Med 1956; 20:667–673.
4. Newman SP. Principles of metered-dose inhaler design. Resp Care 2005; 50:1177–1190.
5. Molina MJ, Rowland FS. Stratospheric sink for chlorofluoromethanes: chlorine atom catalysed destruction of ozone. Nature 1974; 249:810–812.
6. Dolovich M. New delivery systems and propellants. Can Respir J 1999; 6:290–295.
7. Crompton GK. Problems patients have using pressurized aerosol inhalers. Eur J Respir Dis Suppl 1982; 119:101–104.
8. Selroos O, Löfroos AB, Pietinalho A, et al. Comparison of terbutaline and placebo from a pressurised metered dose inhaler and a dry powder inhaler in a subgroup of patients with asthma. Thorax 1994; 49:1228–1230.
9. Dunbar CA, Watkins AP, Miller JF. An experimental investigation of the spray issued from a pMDI using laser diagnostic techniques. J Aerosol Med 1997; 10:351–368.
10. Dhand R, Malik SK, Balakrishnan M, et al. High speed photographic analysis of aerosols produced by metered dose inhalers. J Pharm Pharmacol 1988; 40:429–430.
11. Melchor R, Biddiscombe MF, Mak VH, et al. Lung deposition patterns of directly labelled salbutamol in normal subjects and in patients with reversible airflow obstruction. Thorax 1993; 48:506–511.
12. Everard ML, Devadason SG, Summers QA, et al. Factors affecting total and "respirable" dose delivered by a salbutamol metered dose inhaler. Thorax 1995; 50:746–749.
13. Schultz RK. Drug delivery characteristics of metered-dose inhalers. J Allergy Clin Immunol 1995; 96:284–287.
14. Ross DL, Gabrio BJ. Advances in metered dose inhaler technology with the development of a chlorofluorocarbon-free drug delivery system. J Aerosol Med 1999; 12:151–160.
15. Zeidler M, Corren J. Hydrofluoroalkane formulations of inhaled corticosteroids for the treatment of asthma. Treat Respir Med 2004; 3:35–44.
16. Lewis D. Metered-dose inhalers: actuators old and new. Expert Opin Drug Deliv 2007; 4:235–245.
17. Acerbi D, Brambilla G, Kottakis I. Advances in asthma and COPD management: delivering CFC-free inhaled therapy using Modulite technology. Pulm Pharmacol Ther 2007; 20:290–303.
18. Newman SP, Pavia D, Clarke SW. How should a pressurized beta-adrenergic bronchodilator be inhaled? Eur J Resp Dis 1981; 62:3–21.
19. Newman SP, Pavia D, Clarke SW. Improving the bronchial deposition of pressurized aerosols. Chest 1981; 80:909–911.
20. Larsen JS, Hahn M, Ekholm B, et al. Evaluation of conventional press-and-breathe metered-dose inhaler technique in 501 patients. J Asthma 1994; 31:193–199.
21. Khassawneh BY, Al-Ali MK, Alzoubi KH, et al. Handling of inhaler devices in actual pulmonary practice: metered-dose inhaler versus dry powder inhalers. Respir Care 2008; 53:323–328.
22. Giraud V, Roche N. Misuse of corticosteroid metered-dose inhaler is associated with decreased asthma stability. Eur Respir J 2002; 19:246–251.

23. McFadden ER Jr. Improper patient techniques with metered dose inhalers: clinical consequences and solutions to misuse. J Allergy Clin Immunol 1995; 96:278–283.
24. Newman SP, Weisz AW, Talaee N, et al. Improvement of drug delivery with a breath actuated pressurised aerosol for patients with poor inhaler technique. Thorax 1991; 46:712–716.
25. Price D, Thomas M, Mitchell G, et al. Improvement of asthma control with a breath-actuated pressurised metred dose inhaler (BAI): a prescribing claims study of 5556 patients using a traditional pressurised metred dose inhaler (MDI) or a breath-actuated device. Respir Med 2003; 97:12–19.
26. Newman SP, Clarke SW. Bronchodilator delivery from Gentlehaler, a new low-velocity pressurized aerosol inhaler. Chest 1993; 103:1442–1446.
27. Farr SJ, Rowe AM, Rubsamen R, et al. Aerosol deposition in the human lung following administration from a microprocessor controlled pressurized metered dose inhaler. Thorax 1995; 50:639–644.
28. Bell J, Newman S. The rejuvenated pressurised metered dose inhaler. Expert Opin Drug Deliv 2007; 4:215–234.
29. Newman SP. Spacer devices for metered dose inhalers. Clin Pharmacokinet 2004; 43:349–360.
30. Cates CJ, Crilly JA, Rowe BH. Holding chambers (spacers) versus nebulisers for β-agonist treatment of acute asthma. Cochrane Database Syst Rev 2006; 2:CD000052.
31. Wilkes W, Fink J, Dhand R. Selecting an accessory device with a metered-dose inhaler: variable influence of accessory devices on fine particle dose, throat deposition, and drug delivery with asynchronous actuation from a metered-dose inhaler. J Aerosol Med 2001; 14:351–360.
32. Mitchell JP, Nagel MW. Valved holding chambers (VHCs) for use with pressurised metered-dose inhalers (pMDIs): a review of causes of inconsistent medication delivery. Prim Care Respir J 2007; 16:207–214.
33. Barry PW, O'Callaghan C. Multiple actuations of salbutamol MDI into a spacer device reduce the amount of drug recovered in the respirable range. Eur Respir J 1994; 7:1707–1709.
34. Wildhaber JH, Devadason SG, Hayden MJ, et al. Electrostatic charge on a plastic spacer device influences the delivery of salbutamol. Eur Respir J 1996; 9:1943–1946.
35. Piérart F, Wildhaber JH, Vrancken I, et al. Washing plastic spacers in household detergent reduces electrostatic charge and greatly improves delivery. Eur Respir J 1999; 13:673–678.
36. Frijlink HW, De Boer AH. Dry powder inhalers for pulmonary drug delivery. Expert Opin Drug Deliv 2004; 1:67–86.
37. Ashurst II, Malton A, Prime D, et al. Latest advances in the development of dry powder inhalers. Pharm Sci Technol Today 2000; 3:246–256.
38. Meakin BJ, Cainey J, Woodcock PM. Effect of exposure to humidity on terbutaline delivery from turbuhaler dry power inhalation devices. Eur Respir J 1993; 6:760–761.
39. Hindle M, Byron PR. Dose emissions from marketed dry powder inhalers. Int J Pharm 1995; 116:169–177.
40. Chrystyn H. Is inhalation rate important for a dry powder inhaler? Using the In-Check Dial to identify these rates. Respir Med 2003; 97:181–187.
41. Tarsin WY, Pearson SB, Assi KH, et al. Emitted dose estimates from Seretide Diskus and Symbicort Turbuhaler following inhalation by severe asthmatics. Int J Pharm 2006; 316:131–137.
42. Assi K, Chrystyn H. The device resistance of recently introduced dry-powder inhalers. J Pharm Pharmacol 2000; 52:58.
43. Pedersen S. How to use a rotahaler. Arch Dis Child 1986; 61:11–14.
44. Al-Showair RA, Tarsin WY, Assi KH, et al. Can all patients with COPD use the correct inhalation flow with all inhalers and does training help? Respir Med 2007; 101:2395–2401.
45. Hawksworth GM, James L, Chrystyn H. Characterization of the inspiratory manoeuvre when asthmatics inhale through a Turbohaler pre- and post-counselling in a community pharmacy. Respir Med 2000; 94:501–504.

46. Chan HK, Chew NY. Novel alternative methods for the delivery of drugs for the treatment of asthma. Adv Drug Deliv Rev 2003; 55:793–805.
47. Muers MF. Overview of nebuliser treatment. Thorax 1997; 52:S25–S30.
48. Harris KW, Smaldone GC. Facial and ocular deposition of nebulised budesonide: effects of face mask design. Chest 2008; 133:482–488.
49. Loffert DT, Ikle D, Nelson HS. A comparison of commercial jet nebulizers. Chest 1994; 106:1788–1792.
50. Reisner C, Katial RK, Bartelson BB, et al. Characterization of aerosol output from various nebulizer/compressor combinations. Ann Allergy Asthma Immunol 2001; 86: 566–574.
51. Geller DE. New liquid aerosol generation devices: systems that force pressurized liquids through nozzles. Respir Care 2002; 47:1392–1404.
52. Smaldone GC. Smart nebulizers. Respir Care 2002; 47:1434–1441.
53. Leung K, Louca E, Coates AL. Comparison of breath-enhanced to breath-actuated nebulizers for rate, consistency, and efficiency. Chest 2004; 126:1619–1627.
54. Piper SD. In vitro comparison of the circulaire and AeroTee to a traditional nebulizer T-piece with corrugated tubing. Respir Care 2000; 45:313–319.
55. Rau JL, Ari A, Restrepo RD. Performance comparison of nebulizer designs: constant-output, breath-enhanced, and dosimetric. Respir Care 2004; 49:174–179.
56. Hochrainer D, Hölz H, Kreher C, et al. Comparison of the aerosol velocity and spray duration of Respimat Soft Mist inhaler and pressurized metered dose inhalers. J Aerosol Med 2005; 18:273–282.
57. Dhand R. Nebulisers that use a vibrating mesh or plate with mutiple apertures to generate aerosol. Respir Care 2002; 47: 1406–1416.
58. Knoch M, Keller M. The customised electronic nebuliser: a new category of liquid aerosol drug delivery systems. Expert Opin Drug Deliv 2005; 2:377–390.
59. Bennett WD. Controlled inhalation of aerosolised therapeutics. Expert Opin Drug Deliv 2005; 2:763–767.
60. Denyer J, Nikander K, Smith NJ. Adaptive Aerosol Delivery (AAD) technology. Expert Opin Drug Deliv 2004; 1:165–176.
61. Brand P, Beckmann H, Maas Enriquez M, et al. Peripheral deposition of α-1-protease inhibitor using commercial inhalation devices. Eur Respir J 2003; 22:263–267.
62. Agnew JE. Physical properties and mechanisms of deposition of aerosols. In: Clarke SW, Pavia D, eds. Aerosols and the Lung. London: Butterworths, 1994:49–70.
63. Yu J, Chien YW. Pulmonary drug delivery: physiologic and mechanistic aspects. Crit Rev Ther Drug Carrier Syst 1997; 14:395–453.
64. Usmani OS, Biddiscombe MF, Nightingale JA, et al. The effects of bronchodilator particle size in asthmatics using monodisperse aerosols. J Appl Physiol 2003; 95:2106–2112.
65. Usmani OS, Biddiscombe MF, Barnes PJ. Regional lung deposition and bronchodilator response as a function of β2-agonist particle size. Am J Respir Crit Care Med 2005; 172:1497–1504.
66. Biddiscombe MF, Barnes PJ, Usmani OS. Generating monodisperse pharmacological aerosols using a spinning top aerosol generator. J Aerosol Med 2006; 19:245–253.
67. Peterson JB, Prisk GK, Darquenne C. Aerosol deposition in the human lung periphery is increased by reduced-density gas breathing. J Aerosol Med Pulm Drug Deliv 2008; 21(2):159–168.
68. Edwards DA, Ben-Jebria A, Langer R. Recent advances in pulmonary drug delivery using large, porous inhaled particles. J Appl Physiol 1998; 85:379–385.
69. Finlay WH, Stapleton KW, Chan HK, et al. Regional deposition of inhaled hygroscopic aerosols: in vivo SPECT compared with mathematical modeling. J Appl Physiol 1996; 81:374–383.

70. Chan HK, Eberl S, Daviskas E, et al. Changes in lung deposition of aerosols due to hygroscopic growth: a fast SPECT study. J Aerosol Med 2002; 15:307–311.

71. Pavia D, Thomson M, Shannon HS. Aerosol inhalation and depth of deposition in the human lung. The effect of airway obstruction and tidal volume inhaled. Arch Environ Health 1977; 32:131–137.

72. Svartengren M, Anderson M, Philipson K, et al. Individual differences in regional deposition of 6-micron particles in humans with induced bronchoconstriction. Exp Lung Res 1989; 15:139–149.

73. van Beerendonk I, Mesters I, Mudde AN, et al. Assessment of the inhalation technique in outpatients with asthma or chronic obstructive pulmonary disease using a metered-dose inhaler or dry powder device. J Asthma 1998; 35:273–279.

74. Guidry GG, Brown WD, Stogner SW, et al. Incorrect use of metered dose inhalers by medical personnel. Chest 1992; 101:31–33.

75. Hanania NA, Wittman R, Kesten S, et al. Medical personnel's knowledge of and ability to use inhaling devices. Metered-dose inhalers, spacing chambers, and breath-actuated dry powder inhalers. Chest 1994; 105:111–116.

76. Al-Showair RA, Pearson SB, Chrystyn H. The potential of a 2Tone Trainer to help patients use their metered-dose inhalers. Chest 2007; 131:1776–1782.

77. Allen SC. Competence thresholds for the use of inhalers in people with dementia. Age Ageing 1997; 26:83–86.

78. Armitage JM, Williams SJ. Inhaler technique in the elderly. Age Ageing 1988; 17:275–278.

79. Ferron GA. Comparison of experimental and calculated data for total and regional lung deposition in the human lung. J Aerosol Sci 1985; 16:133–143.

80. Martonen TB, Schroeter JD, Hwang D, et al. Human lung morphology models for particle deposition studies. Inhal Toxicol 2000; 12:109–121.

81. Ziegler J, Wachtel H. Comparison of cascade impaction and laser diffraction for particle size distribution measurements. J Aerosol Med 2005; 18:311–324.

82. Mitchell JP, Nagel MW. Time-of-flight aerodynamic particle size analyzers: their use and limitations for the evaluation of medical aerosols. J Aerosol Med 1999; 12:217–240.

83. Thiel CG. Can in vitro particle size measurements be used to predict pulmonary deposition of aerosol from inhalers? J Aerosol Med 1998; 11:S43–S52.

84. Olsson B, Asking L, Borgstrom L, et al. Effect of inlet throat on the correlation between the fine particle dose and lung deposition. In: Dalby RN, Byron PR, Farr SJ, eds. Respiratory Drug Delivery, Vol. V. Illinois: Interpharm Press, 1996:273–281.

85. Borgstrom L, Nilsson M. A method for determination of the absolute pulmonary bioavailability of inhaled drugs: terbutaline. Pharm Res 1990; 7:1068–1070.

86. Thorsson L, Edsbacker S, Conradson TB. Lung deposition of budesonide from Turbuhaler is twice that from a pressurized metered-dose inhaler. Eur Respir J 1994; 7:1839–1844.

87. Mollmann H, Wagner M, Meibohm B, et al. Pharmacokinetic and pharmacodynamic evaluation of fluticasone propionate after inhaled administration. Eur J Clin Pharmacol 1998; 53:459–467.

88. Richards R, Dickson CR, Renwick AG, et al. Absorption and disposition kinetics of cromolyn sodium and the influence of inhalation technique. J Pharmacol Exp Ther 1987; 241:1028–1032.

89. Hindle M, Chrystyn H. Determination of the relative bioavailability of salbutamol to the lung following inhalation. Br J Clin Pharmacol 1992; 34:311–315.

90. Silkstone VL, Dennis JH, Pieron CA, et al. An investigation of in vitro/in vivo correlations for salbutamol nebulised by 8 systems. J Aerosol Med 2002; 15:251–259.

91. Chege JK, Chrystyn H. The relative bioavailability of salbutamol to the lung using urinary excretion following inhalation from a novel dry powder inhaler: the effect of inhalation rate and formulation. Respir Med 2000; 94:51–56.

92. Hindle M, Newton DA, Chrystyn H. Investigations of an optimal inhaler technique with the use of urinary salbutamol excretion as a measure of relative bioavailability to the lung. Thorax 1993; 48:607–610.
93. Newnham DM, McDevitt DG, Lipworth BJ. Comparison of the extrapulmonary beta2-adrenoceptor responses and pharmacokinetics of salbutamol given by standard metered dose-inhaler and modified actuator device. Br J Clin Pharmacol 1993; 36:445–450.
94. Dolovich MB. Measuring total and regional lung deposition using inhaled radiotracers. J Aerosol Med 2001; 14:S35–S44.
95. Newman SP, Hirst PH, Pitcairn GR, et al. Understanding regional lung deposition in γ scintigraphy. In: Dalby RN, Byron PR, Farr SJ, eds. Respiratory Drug Delivery. Vol. VI. Illinois: Interpharm Press, 1998:9–15.
96. Pitcairn GR, Joyson A, Hirst PH, et al. Lung penetration profiles: a new method for analysing regional lung deposition data in scintigraphic studies. In: Dalby RN, Byron PR, Farr SJ, Peart J, eds. Respiratory Drug Delivery. Vol. VIII. Colorado: Davis Horwood, 2002:549–552.
97. Fleming JS, Conway JH, Bolt L, et al. A comparison of planar scintigraphy and SPECT measurement of total lung deposition of inhaled aerosol. J Aerosol Med 2003; 16:9–19.
98. Conway JH, Walker P, Fleming JS, et al. Three-dimensional description of the deposition of inhaled terbutaline sulphate administered via Turbuhaler. In: Dalby RN, Byron PR, Farr SJ, Peart J, eds. Respiratory Drug Delivery. Vol. VII. Raleigh: Serentec Press, 2000:607–609.
99. Perring S, Summers Q, Fleming JS, et al. A new method of quantification of the pulmonary regional distribution of aerosols using combined CT and SPECT and its application to nedocromil sodium administered by metered dose inhaler. Br J Radiol 1994; 67:46–53.
100. Jones T. New opportunities in molecular imaging using PET. Drug Inf J 1997; 31:991–995.
101. Gonda I. Systemic delivery of drugs to humans via inhalation. J Aerosol Med 2006; 19:47–53.
102. Gessler T, Seeger W, Schmehl T. Inhaled prostanoids in the therapy of pulmonary hypertension. J Aerosol Med Pulm Drug Deliv 2008; 21(1):1–12.
103. Dershwitz M, Walsh JL, Morishige RJ, et al. Pharmacokinetics and pharmacodynamics of inhaled versus intravenous morphine in healthy volunteers. Anesthesiology 2000; 93:619–628.
104. Crooks J, Stephen SA, Brass W. Clinical trial of inhaled ergotamine tartrate in migraine. Br Med J 1964; 1:221–224.
105. Patton JS, Tricnchera P, Paltz RM. Bioavailability of pulmonary delivery of peptides and proteins: alpha-interferon, calcitonins and parathyroid hormone. J Control Release 1994; 28:79–85.
106. Owens DR. New horizons—alternative routes for insulin therapy. Nat Rev Drug Discov 2002; 1:529–540.
107. Fuso L, Pitocco D, Incaizi RA. Inhaled insulin and the lung. Curr Med Chem 2007; 14:1335–1347.
108. Costantino HR, Illum L, Brandt G, et al. Intranasal delivery: physicochemical and therapeutic aspects. Int J Pharm 2007; 337:1–24.
109. Graff CL, Pollack GM. Nasal drug administration: potential for targeted central nervous system delivery. J Pharm Sci 2005; 94:1187–1195.
110. Laube BL. The expanding role of aerosols in systemic drug delivery, gene therapy, and vaccination. Respir Care 2005; 50:1161–1176.
111. Lu D, Hickey AJ. Pulmonary vaccine delivery. Expert Rev Vaccines 2007; 6:213–226.
112. McCarthy MW, Kockler DR. Trivalent intranasal influenza vaccine, live. Ann Pharmacother 2004; 38:2086–2093.
113. Dilraj A, Cutts FT, de Castro JF, et al. Response to different measles vaccine strains given by aerosol and subcutaneous routes to schoolchildren: a randomised trial. Lancet 2000; 355:798–803.

6

Inhaled Corticosteroids in Airways Disease

IAN M. ADCOCK and KIAN FAN CHUNG
National Heart and Lung Institute, Imperial College, and Royal Brompton Hospital, London, U.K.

GAETANO CARAMORI
Research Centre for Asthma and COPD, University of Ferrara, Ferrara, Italy

I. Introduction

Asthma therapy was revolutionized in the early 1970s by the introduction of inhaled corticosteroid (ICS) therapy. ICS therapy has subsequently proved to be the most effective anti-inflammatory treatments for asthma control. Because of the success of ICS for asthma and the realization that chronic obstructive pulmonary disease (COPD) is also a chronic inflammatory disease, ICS therapy has been introduced for the treatment of COPD. However, its effectiveness is less evident than its effect in asthma. The use of ICS monotherapy as the gold standard in airways disease has been superseded by the discovery that in combination with long-acting β-agonist (LABA) the effects of ICS can be improved. It is expected that the combination of ICS and LABA will remain the cornerstone of treatment for the next 10 years. Greater understanding of the molecular mechanisms of ICS suggests that new CS molecules will be developed that could provide greater efficacy with a reduced risk of systemic side effects. Further, understanding the mechanisms underlying relative CS insensitivity in asthma and COPD may lead to novel combinations that will restore CS sensitivity in these patients. This chapter will review the mechanisms of CS actions, the effect and optimal use of ICS in asthma and COPD, and the issue of CS insensitivity in airways disease.

II. Molecular Mechanisms of Corticosteroids

A. Glucocorticoid Receptor Translocation

Corticosteroids belong to the family of 21-carbon steroid nuclear hormones (1) and act by binding to the ubiquitously expressed glucocorticoid receptor (GR, NC3R), which is predominantly localized to the cytoplasm of target cells (Fig. 1). Corticosteroids freely diffuse from the circulation across the cell membrane into cells and bind to the cytoplasmic GR inducing a conformational change in the receptor and loss of its chaperone proteins and its nuclear localization. However, it is likely that continual shuttling between the cytoplasm and the nucleus occurs even in the absence of ligand as leptomycin, an inhibitor of nuclear export, results in a predominant nuclear expression (2). GR contains a classical basic nuclear localization sequence (NLS1, residing in the hinge region) and a second, only poorly characterized NLS (NSL2) residing across the ligand-binding domain (LBD), NLS2 (2), both of which can mediate active nuclear import (3). Nuclear import of

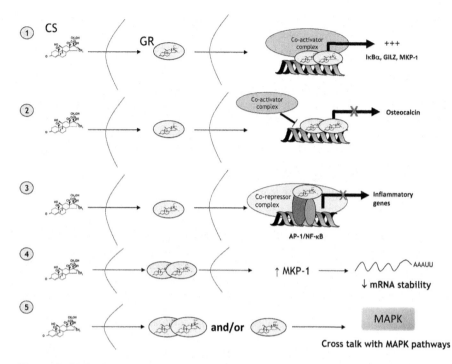

Figure 1 Molecular mechanism of action of CSs. CSs can freely diffuse across the plasma membrane where they associate with the inactivate cytosolic GR. Upon ligand binding GR is activated and can translocate to the nucleus where it binds to a GRE within the controlling region of some glucocorticoid responsive target genes to modulate gene transcription. (1) Two DNA-bound GR monomers can recruit a transcriptional coactivator complex containing basal transcription factors, coactivators chromatin modifiers, and RNA polymerase II, which together induce histone modifications, chromatin remodeling, and subsequent production of mRNAs encoding various genes including the NF-κB inhibitor IκBα, the AP-1 inhibitor GILZ, and the MAPK phosphatase MKP-1. (2) The activated GR dimer can bind to GREs located across the transcription start site of various genes including that of osteocalcin to prevent gene induction. (3) Activated GR acting as a homodimer can repress AP-1/NF-κB-mediated gene expression by recruiting a corepressor complex or altering its activity. (4) GR can also reduce the levels of mRNA by either inducing the dual-specificity MPK-1 that in turn regulates p38 MAPK-mediated mRNA stability or increasing the levels of cell ribonucleases and mRNA destabilizing proteins. (5) GR, acting as either a monomer of dimer, can directly interact with members of the MAPK family to prevent their activity. *Abbreviations*: CS, corticosteroid; GR, glucocorticoid receptor; GRE, glucocorticoid response element; GILZ, glucocorticoid-inducible leucine zipper; MAPK, mitogen-activated protein kinase; MPK-1, MAPK phosphatase-1; AP-1, activator protein 1; NF-κB, nuclear factor kappa B.

GR is mediated through its NLS and interaction with importins, with importin α selectively binding to NLS1 (4) and importins 7 and 8 binding to both NLS1 and NLS2 (4). In addition, the novel importin, importin 13, has been reported to mediate GR nuclear import (5). GR is a phosphoprotein (3) and, as with many other transcription factors, the ability of GR to associate with the importin machinery is regulated by its phosphorylation status (3). As evidenced by the effect of leptomycin, GR nuclear export must also be under tight control; however, as yet, the role of the exportin 1 [chromosome maintenance region 1 (CRM-1)] pathway in GR nuclear export has not been clearly defined (6,7).

B. Chromatin Modifications and Gene Transcription

The molecule mechanisms underlying the actions of GR in regulating the expression of inflammatory genes has been an intense area of research over the past 15 to 20 years. Classically, two GR proteins combine together and bind to DNA at consensus glucocorticoid response elements (GREs) in the regulatory regions of corticosteroid-responsive genes to induce anti-inflammatory or some innate immune genes (8). Once DNA bound, the active GR dimer recruits a number of transcriptional coactivator proteins, including steroid receptor coactivator (SRC-1) and cyclic AMP response element–binding protein (CREB)-binding protein (CBP), and basic transcription factors to form a preinitiation complex. These coactivators have intrinsic histone acetyltransferase (HAT) activity, which tag N-terminal lysine residues in the local histones (H3 and H4) allowing recruitment of chromatin remodeling complexes including the switch/sucrose nonfermentable (SWI/SNF) complex (8). These ATP-dependent processes result in the correct DNA-protein structure that allows enhanced gene transcription (8,9).

In general, the "histone code" refers to these modifications that are set and maintained by histone-modifying enzymes and contribute to coactivator recruitment and subsequent increases in transcription (10). Histone acetylation induced by transcriptional coactivators, such as CBP and p300/CBP-associated factor (9), is associated with increased gene transcription, whereas, in contrast, hypoacetylation induced by histone deacetylases (HDACs) is correlated with reduced transcription or gene silencing (9). Because of the size and the complexity of the transcriptional activator complexes, it is likely that nuclear hormone receptors do not in themselves recruit all the cofactors required at target promoters at the same time (9,11), but steroid receptor coactivators, recruited by GR, can in turn recruit other coactivators and chromatin remodeling complexes that aid in the formation of the transcription initiation complex and result in local chromatin remodeling (9,11).

The magnitude and direction of the transcriptional response to glucocorticoids are dependent on the particular ligand, the number of GREs, and the position of the GREs relative to the transcriptional start site (1,12,13). The consensus GRE and its flanking sequences vary between genes but are conserved for individual genes across species and can lie both upstream and downstream of the transcriptional start site (12,13). Indeed, 63% of GREs lie >10 kbp from the transcriptional start site (13).

In contrast, the expression of some genes, such as prolactin and osteocalcin, is decreased on GR-GRE binding due to the fact that the GRE lies across the transcriptional start site preventing correct formation of the transcriptional initiation complex (1,14). In lung epithelial A549 cells, there are 548 potential GR-GRE responsive genes (13) although many of these genes are indirectly regulated through an interaction with other transcription factors and coactivators (1,14). Indeed, it is now clear that GRs can bind to DNA as heterodimers with many other transcription factors, such as members of the signal transducer and activator of transcription family; the ETS transcription factors and the vitamin D3 receptor (13,15) leading to the recruitment of distinct coactivator (e.g., GRIP-1) or corepressor (e.g., RIP140 or HDAC) complexes (1,14).

It seems highly unlikely that all the widespread anti-inflammatory actions of glucocorticoids could be explained by increased transcription of small numbers of anti-inflammatory genes, such as annexin 1, IL-10, glucocorticoid-inducible leucine zipper (GILZ) that prevents activator protein 1 (AP-1) DNA binding, and the inhibitor of NF-κB (1,14,16). In addition, it is likely that glucocorticoid side effects, such as osteoporosis, cataracts, growth retardation in children, skin fragility, and metabolic effects, are due to gene activation (17).

C. Gene Repression by GRs

In spite of the ability of glucocorticoids to induce gene transcription, the major anti-inflammatory effects of glucocorticoids are probably through repression of inflammatory and immune genes since most GR-repressible genes do not posses negative GREs (1,14). The activated monomeric form of GR can interact directly with other transcription factors, particularly NF-κB and AP-1, which mediate the expression of inflammatory genes (1,14) as exemplified by the anti-inflammatory effects seen in GR dimerization–deficient mice (18,19). As indicated above, maximal inflammatory gene expression probably requires that a number of transcription factors act together in a coordinated manner, and glucocorticoids, by targeting several transcription factors, might have greater effects than if only a single factor was targeted (1,14). The precise mechanism for this repression is still unclear and might include binding and recruiting nuclear receptor corepressors such as NCoR and HDACs, direct repression of coactivator complexes, or effects on RNA polymerase II phosphorylation (1,14,20). For example, in primary airway smooth muscle cells, fluticasone attenuates tumor necrosis factor α (TNF-α)–induced histone H4 acetylation leading to a reduction in p65 association with the native CCL11 promoter and suppression of CCL11 expression (21).

In addition, glucocorticoids might play a role in repressing the action of mitogen-activated protein kinases (MAPKs), such as the extracellular signal-regulated kinase (ERK), p38 MAPK, and c-Jun N-terminal kinase (JNK) (1,3,14). These actions are mutually inhibitory (1,3,14) and, in the case of p38 and JNK, might relate to induction of the dual-specificity MAPK phosphatase 1 (MKP-1), which thereby attenuates MAPK activation (16). Importantly, p38 MAPK-mediated GR phosphorylation can attenuate GR function (1,22).

The mechanistic effects described above are context and gene dependent in that the precise way GR controls gene expression may depend on the exact cell stimulus. Furthermore, not all GR-NF-κB interactions lead to gene repression particularly in the context of control of the innate immune response where the initial reaction of the body is to enhance the beneficial inflammatory response prior to subsequent downregulation (23). Thus, GRs can combine with NF-κB to induce the expression of toll-like receptor 2 and stem cell factor (24,25).

D. Regulation of mRNA Stability

Glucocorticoids can also regulate the stability of proinflammatory gene mRNAs, which contain adenylate uridylate–rich elements (AREs) within their 3′ untranslated regions (16,26). ARE-binding proteins such as tristetraprolin (TTP), which promotes mRNA decay, and Hu antigen R (HuR) family members, which are associated with mRNA stability, interact with AREs to form messenger ribonucleoprotein complexes, which modulate mRNA decay (26). HuR binding to AREs is dependent on p38 MAPK (16,26) and evidence suggests that dexamethasone can control the levels of HuR and TTP, thereby reducing the levels of inflammatory gene mRNAs such as COX-2 and CCL11, through a p38 MAPK-mediated pathway subsequent to induction of MKP-1 (16). However, this is likely to be important for only a subset of inflammatory genes in specific cell types (27).

E. Nongenomic Actions of Glucocorticoids

The traditional genomic theory of steroid action, whether directly interacting with DNA or involving cross talk with other transcription factors, does not fully explain the rapid effects of hormonal steroids. Alternative explanations have been invoked to explain this rapid effect. GR is associated with a number of kinases and phosphatases within the inactive GR-hsp90 complex (1,14), and these are released upon ligand binding. It is possible that these might account for the rapid changes in cell function induced in some cells by glucocorticoids (1,14). In addition, a distinct membrane localized GR has been described (28). Initially reported in amphibians, these receptors have distinctive hormone-binding properties compared with the well-characterized cytoplasmic GR and are probably linked to a number of intracellular signaling pathways acting through G protein–coupled receptors and a number of kinase pathways (29). An important effect seen in asthma that occurs through this mechanism is change in bronchial blood flow induced by ICSs (30).

III. Effects of Corticosteroids in Asthma

A. Effects on Inflammation

Inhaled glucocorticoids are effective anti-asthma agents that can reverse the specific chronic airway inflammation present in asthma (31–34). Inhaled glucocorticoids markedly reduce the number of mast cells, macrophages, T lymphocytes, and eosinophils in the sputum, bronchoalveolar lavage, and bronchial wall (35,36). Furthermore, glucocorticoids reverse the shedding of epithelial cells, the goblet-cell hyperplasia, and the basement-membrane thickening characteristically seen in biopsy specimens of bronchial epithelium from patients with asthma (33,37). There is an increase in vascularity in the bronchial mucosa of asthmatics (38), and high doses of inhaled glucocorticoids may reduce airway wall vascularity in asthmatic patients (38). Inhaled glucocorticoids decrease also the increased airway mucosal blood flow present in asthmatic patients (39). The inflammatory component of asthmatic airways, which is most responsive to glucocorticoid treatment, seems to be eosinophilic inflammation. Importantly, in patients with persistent asthma, well-controlled tapering of inhaled glucocorticoids induces an exacerbation within a few months. This is usually associated with a reversible increase of eosinophilic airway inflammation (40,41). These observations indicate that glucocorticoids suppress the inflammatory response only while being actively taken and the effects wear off with time.

B. Cellular Effects

Glucocorticoids may have direct inhibitory effects on many of the cells involved in airway inflammation in asthma, including macrophages, T lymphocytes, eosinophils, mast cells, and airway smooth muscle and epithelial cells (35,42). In culture, glucocorticoids decrease cytokine mediated survival of eosinophils by stimulating apoptosis (43). This process may explain the reduction in the number of eosinophils in the circulation and airways of patients with asthma during glucocorticoid therapy (33,35).

Glucocorticoids may not inhibit the release of mediators from mast cells (44,45), but they reduce the number of mast cells within the airway (46). In addition, inhaled glucocorticoids reduce the expression of the activation markers CD25 and HLA-DR in both CD_4^+ and CD_8^+ T-cell subsets in peripheral blood and bronchoalveolar lavage fluid of patients with asthma (47,48). Part of the anti-inflammatory activity of glucocorticoids in asthma may involve also a reduction of macrophage eicosanoid (leukotriene B_4 and thromboxane B_2) and cytokine [i.e., interleukin (IL) 1β] synthesis (49,50). In contrast, glucocorticoids either have no effect on, or may even augment, neutrophil-mediated inflammation (51). Glucocorticoids enhance neutrophil function through increased leukotriene and superoxide production, as well as inhibition of apoptosis (52,53).

C. Antimediator Effects

In vivo and in vitro studies suggest that glucocorticoids produce minimal suppression of leukotriene production and in some cases may enhance their production (51). However, levels of exhaled nitric oxide, a marker of asthmatic airway inflammation, are consistently decreased by treatment with inhaled glucocorticoids (36,54). Glucocorticoids also block the generation of several proinflammatory cytokines and chemokines, including IL-1β, IL-4, IL-5, IL-8, granulocyte-macrophage colony-stimulating factor (GM-CSF), TNF-α, RANTES, and macrophage inflammatory protein-1α (55) in the asthmatic lung. In contrast, glucocorticoids can increase the production of the anti-inflammatory cytokine IL-10 from BAL alveolar macrophages (56), but not of IL-1Rα in the bronchial mucosa of asthmatic patients (57).

Airway hyperresponsiveness (AHR) may be directly caused by inflammatory mechanisms (58). Glucocorticoids consistently lessen AHR in asthma (35,59–62), and long-term treatment with glucocorticoids reduced airway responsiveness to both direct and indirect challenges including histamine, cholinergic agonists, allergens (affecting both early and late responses), exercise, fog, cold air, bradykinin, adenosine, and irritants such as sulfur dioxide and metabisulfites (59,63). Glucocorticoid therapy not only makes the airways less sensitive to spasmogens, but also limits the maximal narrowing of the airway in response to a spasmogen (64). The reduction in AHR may not be maximal until treatment has been given for several months, although improvements may occur fairly quickly within a few hours. The magnitude of the reduction varies, but often airway responsiveness remains abnormally increased (59). When therapy is discontinued, airway responsiveness usually returns to pretreatment levels (65–67).

IV. Properties of Topical ICS

The topical corticosteroids have a very high binding affinity for the GR and a high first-pass hepatic metabolism. Many topical corticosteroids are available for asthma and include beclomethasone dipropionate (BDP), budesonide, fluticasone propionate (FP), ciclesonide, flunisolide, triamcinolone acetate, and mometasone furoate (MF). Some pharmacokinetic parameters of ICS are shown in Table 1, while the clinical equivalent doses divided as low, moderate, and high doses are shown in Table 2. The potency of

Table 1 Pharmacokinetic Properties of ICSs

ICS	Receptor affinity	Oral bioavailability (%)	Clearance (L/hr)	$T_{1/2}$ (hr)
Beclomethasone propionate	53	15–20	150	0.5
17-Beclomethasone monopropionate	1345	26	120	2.7
Budesonide	935	11	84	2.8
Ciclesonide	12	<1	152	0.36
Des-ciclesonide	1200	<1	228	3.4
Fluticasone propionate	1800	<1	66–90	7–8
Mometasone furoate	2300	<1	54	5.8
Triamcinolone acetate	233	23	37	2.0

Source: From Ref. 71.

Table 2 Equipotent Daily Doses of ICSs for Adults

ICS	Low daily dose (μg)	Medium daily dose (μg)	High daily dose (μg)
Beclomethasone propionate	200–500	>500–1000	>1000–2000
Budesonide	200–400	>400–800	>800–1600
Ciclesonide	80–160	>160–320	>320–1280
Flunisolide	500–1000	>1000–2000	>2000
Fluticasone propionate	100–250	>250–500	>500–1000
Mometasone furoate	200–400	>400–800	>800–1200
Triamcinolone acetonide	400–1000	>1000–2000	>2000

corticosteroids has been measured in vitro in terms of their binding affinity to GRs in lung tissues and in terms of their ability to induce cutaneous vasoconstriction. For example, FP is twice more potent in terms of binding affinity and cutaneous vaso-constrictor test than budesonide and BDP/BMP, while MF is as potent as fluticasone. In vitro anti-inflammatory assays such as the repression of the activity of proinflammatory transcription factor, NF-κB in A549 lung epithelial cells show the equipotency of BDP, ciclesonide, and budesonide, while FP and MF are 5- to 10-fold more potent (68).

When it comes to assessing the potency of ICS in clinical practice, many factors other than in vitro potencies need to be taken into account, and this is often the subject of dispute and debate because of lack of appropriate data. Efficacy of ICS is affected by the delivery device or by their mechanism of action (e.g., prodrugs like BDP and cicleso-nide). Using the data available in the literature, it is possible to say that BDP and budesonide are nearly equiactive, whereas fluticasone is equally active at half the microgram dosage (69). Mometasone is nearly equipotent as FP and ciclesonide prob-ably falls somewhere between the potency of BDP and fluticasone.

The overall effect of ICS is not only dependent on its potency as a corticosteroid, but also on its deposition in the airways. A large proportion of the dose (60–90% depending on the inhaler device used and on the inhalation technique) is deposited in the upper airways (mouth, larynx, and pharynx) and enters the gastrointestinal tract. The level of systemic absorption of the corticosteroid determines the systemic bioavailability and potential for systemic side effects, and is dependent on the efficiency of absorption of the dose deposited in the lower airways (direct absorption into systemic circulation) and upon the efficiency of first-pass liver metabolism of the portion absorbed from the gastrointestinal tract (70,71).

Most of the drugs that are absorbed through the gastrointestinal tract undergo first-pass metabolism, with maximal breakdown of up to 99% for fluticasone, compared to only 20% for prednisolone (70). The remainder of the bioavailability of ICS is dependent on the absorption through the lower respiratory tract, and if fluticasone and budesonide undergo first-pass metabolism in the liver, then their absorptions though the lower airways determine their bioavailability. The oral bioavailability of ICS has improved considerably with the newer ICS. Values for BDP and budesonide are quoted as 41% and 11%, respectively, and those for the newer ones such as FP, ciclesonide, and MF being less than 1% (71).

Another property of ICS that is important in consideration of systemic availability is its retention in the lungs dependent on lipophilicity. For example, FP is more lipophilic than budesonide, and this increases the affinity of FP for lung tissue, increasing the retention time of FP in the lung. On the other hand, budesonide forms highly lipophilic fatty acid ester conjugation in the lung, which can serve as a depot from which the active moiety can be regenerated. These are not absorbed from the lung into the systemic circulation and are not active. The more lipophilic the ICS, the more slowly it is released into and from the lung lipid layer and the longer the latency between inhalation and its appearance in the plasma. Thus, the rate of dissolution of budesonide in human bronchial fluid is quoted as only six minutes, while it is over eight hours for fluticasone (70). Some topical steroids are only activated in the lungs. BDP is metabolized to BMP in the airways and is a more active steroid than BDP, while budesonide is stable within the airways. Fluticasone furoate has a binding affinity to the human lung GR that is highest of all topical CS together with the most pronounced lung retention in lung tissue (72), properties that may contribute to a prolonged and potent effect in the lungs.

Ciclesonide is a prodrug that is converted into an active moiety in the airways and has a high binding to plasma proteins; it has a pharmacokinetic profile that is associated with a lesser risk of systemic and local side effects. Absorption of ICS, particularly of FP, from the lungs is higher in normal nonasthmatic individuals than in asthmatics with airflow obstruction, probably due to the reduced penetration of aerosols in an obstructed airway (73–75). This differential absorption between normal and asthmatic individuals appear to be less marked for budesonide and ciclesonide (74,75). Another interesting property of ciclesonide is its very high protein binding to plasma proteins of 99%, similar for MF (98–99%) and higher than FP (90%) and budesonide (88%). This property allows the ICS to be kept in the blood stream preventing its diffusion into tissues, hence the propensity of causing systemic side effects.

V. Dose-Response Relationships

The dose range of various ICS in clinical use is shown in Table 2, and the dose range used to treat an asthmatic patient may be determined by the severity of the disease. All ICSs demonstrate a dose-response relationship for efficacy measures for asthma; however, most of the benefit of ICS may be obtained in the low to moderate dose range of each ICS (76). In some patients, higher doses of ICS may lead to further improvement in asthma control, but at the expense of a greater increase in the potential of side effects. For FP, there were no statistically significant differences between 4 to 500 μg and 800 to 1000 μg, and between 50 to 100 μg and 800 to 1000 μg, but 800 to 1000 μg daily favored a greater improvement of FEV_1 (forced expiratory volume in one second) and symptoms compared with the 200 μg, although the gain is relatively small (77). However, very high doses of FP may allow for a reduction in maintenance oral prednisolone in some patients with severe asthma. In terms of prevention of exacerbations the dose-response of ICS in COPD is unclear. It appears that as far as response to symptoms is concerned, there is little difference in effect between 500 and 1000 μg per day dosage (78,79), but there is only one study on the effect of Seretide on exacerbations using 1000 μg daily dose (80). The dose-response effect on reduction of exacerbations in COPD needs to be clarified.

VI. Effects of Corticosteroids on Asthma Control

Control of asthma may be obtained in most asthmatics with inhaled glucocorticoids (81,82) with improvement in asthma symptoms, in lung function, and in a reduction in exacerbations of disease. This applies throughout the severity spectrum of asthma.

A. Mild Persistent Asthma

Recent studies have focused on the use of ICS particularly at the early and at the moderate-to-severe stages of the disease. The early intervention of mild persistent asthma at the time of diagnosis has been conclusively examined in the START study of 7241 patients aged 5 to 66 years in 32 countries who had less than two years of mild intermittent asthma and had not been previously treated with corticosteroids (83). Patients treated with low-dose budesonide had fewer courses of systemic corticosteroids and more symptom-free days than those with placebo. Postbronchodilator FEV_1 improved significantly by 1.48% after one year and by 0.88% after three years. In the first year of the START trial, 34% of asthmatics on placebo needed additional treatment with ICS and 4% had a severe exacerbation. In those treated with ICS, only 20% needed additional ICS and 2% had a severe exacerbation. During the third year, 50% of patients on placebo were being treated with ICS and 6% had a severe exacerbation; correspondingly, in the budesonide arm, 30% were being given additional ICS and 3% had a severe exacerbation. There were small but significant improvements in both prebronchodilator and postbronchodilator FEV_1 at the end of three years. Thus, this study indicated benefits of ICS even in the mildest of asthma patients (Fig. 2).

In the Childhood Asthma Management Plan study, 1041 children aged 5 to 12 years with mild-to-moderate asthma were studied and randomly allocated to budesonide (200 μg/day), nedocromil sodium (8 mg), or placebo twice daily for 4 to 6 years. The active treatments did not change the primary outcome of change in FEV_1 after bronchodilator. However, children who received budesonide had significantly a smaller decline in FEV_1/FVC ratio and improved airway responsiveness to methacholine, fewer hospital admissions, greater reduction in the need for rescue medication, and fewer courses of prednisolone compared to nedocromil (84).

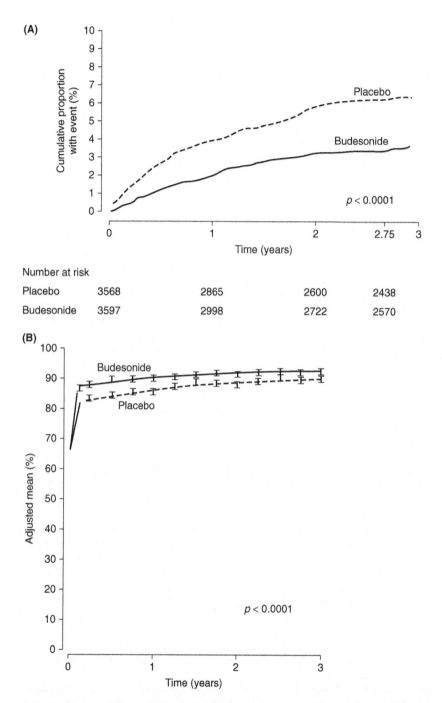

Figure 2 Panel A: Effect of budesonide or placebo inhaler in mild persistent asthma in 3568 and 3597 patients, respectively. Panel A shows Kaplan–Meier curve of time to first severe asthma-related event. Panel B shows mean proportion of symptom-free days. Bars show SEM. *Source*: From Ref. 83.

In a study of mild persistent asthma, budesonide alone (200 µg/day) reduced the rate of severe asthma exacerbations from 0.77 per patient per year to 0.29 per patient per year, with improvement in days with asthma symptoms and nights with nocturnal symptoms (85). In this study, the addition of formoterol to budesonide did not confer any additional benefit in this group of mild persistent asthma.

Because the use of ICS for long periods of time is not a popular option chosen by asthma patients likely because of unreasonable fear of CS adverse effects and poor compliance to inhaled therapies, other possibilities have been looked into such as the use of oral leukotriene receptor antagonist (LTRA). However, LTRA do not provide as good a benefit as low-dose inhaled CS therapy (86,87) but remain an alternative therapy, particularly in pediatric patients. One study indicated that the intermittent use of ICS combined with a short-acting β-agonist (SABA) as needed was as effective as the regular use of ICS twice daily with SABA as needed (88). This is an interesting concept that could be considered further. In addition, the use of intermittent courses of oral corticosteroids to treat exacerbations without any maintenance treatment appears to be as effective as using ICS regularly (89); however, the size of cohort used was probably not big enough to show any differential effect. Another issue with the response of ICS is that at least the bronchodilator response as measured by FEV_1 is not uniform across a population of patients with mild to moderate asthma, and a percentage of patients do not respond to ICS (87,90). In the study of Martin et al. 46% of patients with mild-to-moderate asthma did not respond to low-dose ICS defined as an FEV_1 response of less than 5% of baseline, and the nonresponders were associated with a lesser bronchodilator response to salbutamol but without any greater inflammatory index as measured by sputum eosinophils or exhaled nitric oxide levels (90). Whether this population is more responsive to other treatments such as LTRA is not known.

The other issue is the use of ICS in patients with mild-to-moderate asthma who continue to smoke. The therapeutic response of these patients to ICS is attenuated (91,92), and whether they should be treated with higher doses of ICS or with combination therapy of ICS and LABA or LTRA is unclear.

B. Moderate Persistent Asthma

Moderate persistent asthmatics are patients whose asthma is inadequately controlled on low-dose ICS of <500 µg BDP or equivalent ICS. The additional benefits of adding a LABA to ICS compared to increasing the dose of ICS alone in this group include enhanced effects on lung function parameters and exacerbation rates, and a decrease in the use of rescue inhaled rapid-acting β_2 agonists is seen in all types of asthma from moderate to severe and resulted in similar clinical control at a lower dose of ICS (93). Indeed, even a single dose of combination formoterol/budesonide gave a greater protection against allergen-induced late asthmatic response and bronchial hyperresponsiveness than either component alone (94). In a recent meta-analysis, the addition of a LABA to ICS lowered exacerbation rates by ~14% compared with that observed when ICS doses were doubled (95), resulted in fewer withdrawals from clinical trials, and, apart from increased rates of tremor, was safe (96). The current recommendation is to add LABA to ICS as supported by studies that show no further benefit of doubling the low dose of ICS and the benefit of adding LABA to low-dose ICS. The benefits of combination therapy therefore include a reduction of the rate of asthma exacerbations and prevention of exacerbations with improvement in most indicators of asthma control (85,97–101). In the FACET study, a fourfold increase in the dose of ICS (budesonide 200–800 µg/day) improved all asthma outcomes; addition of LABA to 800 µg/day budesonide provided the greatest benefit, with a maximal fourfold reduction in exacerbation rate compared with budesonide 200 µg/day treatment arm (102).

In the GOAL study, in a group of asthmatics with a wide range of severity, three groups of patients were identified at entry taking no ICS (steroid naive), low-dose ICS, or moderate dose ICS with not well-controlled asthma (101). The patients were allocated to either increasing doses of ICS (flixotide) alone or with or without LABA, salmeterol, for one year. Total asthma control, defined as patients with no symptoms, normal lung function, and no limitation of activities, could be achieved in <50% of the population and <30% of patients already taking moderate doses of ICS at randomization. Well-controlled asthma with only occasional symptoms was reported in 78% of patients not receiving ICS before entry to study and in 62% of these already on moderate doses of ICS. Combination of ICS and LABA was significantly better than ICS alone. Thus, with individualized incremental treatment, comprehensive asthma control can be achieved in the majority of patients (Fig. 3).

Short-term (12-week) studies have shown that these improvements in clinical parameters were associated with reduced tissue and sputum inflammatory markers (93); however, this was not seen in biopsies following 16 weeks of formoterol/budesonide treatment (103). Moreover, improvements in lung function, symptom scores, and bronchial hyperresponsiveness following inhaled fluticasone (500 µg daily) in combination with salmeterol (100 µg daily) treatment were associated with changes in sputum α2 macroglobulin and albumin rather than in sputum cell counts (104) and also reduced serum IL-5 and peripheral blood eosinophil numbers (105).

O'Byrne and colleagues examined in a population of asthmatics with moderate to severe disease the use of the combination formoterol/budesonide (Symbicort) as both maintenance and reliever medication (Symbicort maintenance and relief therapy, SMART) (97). This was associated with a 54% reduction in the annual rate of severe exacerbations compared with ICS alone and a 60% reduction in the mean daily dose of ICS compared with ICS monotherapy. Similar benefits were obtained when formoterol and budesonide combination was used as maintenance and reliever medication when compared with the use of this combination as maintenance, with either as-needed terbutaline or as-needed formoterol (106) (Fig. 4).

These studies also suggest that at least part of the benefit of this approach is due to increasing the glucocorticoid dose in patients at the onset of symptoms. However, this study did not address whether control could be maintained if treatment was reduced. More recent work has suggested that when treatment reduction is indicated it is best to reduce the glucocorticoid dose rather than remove the LABA (107). Currently, overall, there is no clear clinical evidence that suggests that one drug combination is better than the other in the short term (108), although differences in the device may be important in lung deposition in asthmatic patients with poor inspiratory flow (109) and treatment regimes may benefit some patients over others (97,106,110,111). Indeed, the recent demonstration that the combination of formoterol/beclomethasone in a single inhaler is equivalent to formoterol/budesonide with respect to rates of asthma exacerbations and frequency of adverse events emphasizes this point (112).

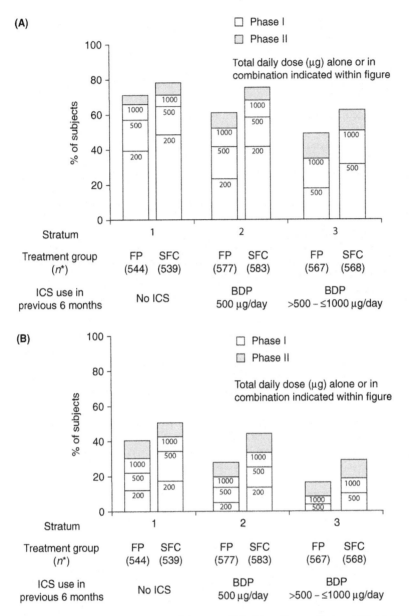

Figure 3 Proportion of patients and dose at which (**A**) well-controlled and (**B**) totally controlled asthma was achieved by treatment with SFC or FP across all three strata according to the use of ICS such as BDP or equivalent in the previous six months. (**A**) Well-controlled asthma. For SFC versus FP: phase I: stratum 1, $p = 0.039$, strata 2 and 3, $p < 0.001$; cumulative phase I and phase II: stratum 1, $p = 0.003$, strata 2 and 3, $p < 0.001$. (**B**) Totally controlled asthma. Phase I: all strata, $p < 0.001$; cumulative phase I and phase II: all strata $p < 0.001$. *Excludes patients with missing baseline FEV$_1$. The definitions of strata are: stratum 1, no ICS; stratum 2, 500 μg or less of BDP daily or equivalent; or stratum 3, more than 500 to 1000 μg or less of BDP daily or equivalent. *Abbreviations*: SFC, salmeterol/fluticasone; FP, fluticasone propionate; ICS, inhaled corticosteroid; FEV$_1$, forced expiratory volume in one second; BDP, beclomethasone dipropionate. *Source*: From Ref. 101.

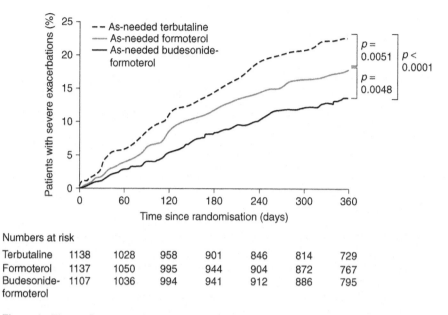

Figure 4 Time to first severe asthma exacerbation defined as a deterioration in asthma resulting in hospitalization, emergency room treatment, or the need for oral steroids for three days or more because of asthma (as judged by investigator). Patients received maintenance budesonide-formoterol 160/4·5 µg, one inhalation twice daily, plus one of the following for as-needed relief: additional inhalations of budesonide-formoterol 160/4·5 µg; formoterol 4·5 µg; or terbutaline 0·4 mg. Significant between-group differences were derived from a log-rank test. *Source*: From Ref. 106.

VII. Effects of ICSs in COPD

COPD has been increasingly recognized as a chronic inflammatory disease of the lower airways, which is enhanced during exacerbations (113). The GOLD guidelines now define COPD as a preventable and treatable disease with some significant extrapulmonary effects that may contribute to its severity (114). The airflow limitation is usually progressive and associated with an inflammatory response of the lung to noxious particles and gases. The pathological hallmarks of COPD are destruction of the lung parenchyma (pulmonary emphysema), inflammation of the peripheral airways (respiratory bronchiolitis), and inflammation of the central airways (115). The inflammation in COPD occurs in the central and peripheral airways (bronchioles) and lung parenchyma, and there is a marked increase in macrophages and neutrophils in bronchoalveolar lavage fluid and induced sputum (116). Patients with COPD have infiltration of T cells (with an increased ratio between CD_8^+ and CD_4^+ T cells), macrophages, and an increased number of neutrophils within the airways mucosa and lung parenchyma (115). The bronchioles are obstructed by fibrosis and infiltrated with macrophages and T lymphocytes. In contrast to the situation with asthma, eosinophils are not prominent except in patients with concomitant asthma or in some patients during exacerbations (115). The mechanisms underlying COPD can be diverse involving local and systemic inflammation, metabolism, immunity, and tissue remodeling (117).

ICSs are now widely prescribed for COPD and are often used as frequently in patients with COPD as in those with asthma. However, long-term clinical trials with high doses of ICS in the treatment of stable COPD have been disappointing, as they do not appear to arrest the progressive decline in lung function even when treatment was started before the disease became symptomatic. Regular long-term treatment of stable COPD patients with ICS has only small and inconsistent effects on symptoms, quality of life, or exacerbations. At the same time this treatment can produce systemic adverse effects, including skin bruising, adrenal suppression, or loss of bone density (118–120). Not surprisingly, the inflammation in COPD is scarcely suppressed by inhaled or oral glucocorticoids, even at high doses (121–123).

A. Effect of ICS Alone

The long-term effects of ICS have been studied over the last 15 years. First, because of its anti-inflammatory effect, it was hoped that long-term ICS could alter the natural course of COPD such as the long-term decline in FEV_1. However, no significant effects of ICS alone on slope have been shown (118,124–126). However, in two subsequent meta-analyses published, one concluded that ICS reduced FEV_1 decline by a small statistical mean rate of 7.7 mL/yr (127) while another meta-analysis showed a nonsignificant 5.0 mL/yr reduction (128). However, in the three-year multicenter double-blind placebo-controlled randomized clinical trial involving 6112 patients with COPD (mean postbronchodilator FEV_1 of 44%) TORCH study, fluticasone showed a significant improvement of FEV_1 decline of −42 mL/yr compared with placebo of −55 mL/yr (129). This effect was not significantly different from that of salmeterol or of the combination of salmeterol and fluticasone together. This definite effect of treatments on lung function decline was likely to have been observed because of the adequate size of the COPD cohort in this study.

What has been shown from these studies is that ICS can induce a small degree of sustained improvement in baseline FEV_1, which averages 50 to 75 mL, and which occurs fairly rapidly after ICS initiation (118,125,130,131). Mean improvements in St George's Respiratory Questionnaire (SGRQ) of between 1 and 3 units are reported (80,118,130,132). In one of the largest studies, the improvement observed with fluticasone over a three-year period by −2.0 units with 95% CI of −1.0 to −2.9 units compared with placebo arm (131) (Fig. 5). These changes were within the 4-unit change in SGRQ that is not considered clinically important. Small improvements in cough and dyspnea have also been reported (78,79,133), which are probably reflected in the improvements in SGRQ. Similar results have been obtained with MF (800 µg/day) taken either once daily or twice daily (134).

In a systematic analysis of 10 trials that included 3724 patients (135), a relative reduction of 22% is observed in the number of subjects who experienced one or more exacerbations. In the TORCH study, fluticasone compared with placebo reduced moderate to severe exacerbations by 18%, but with no significant effect on hospitalization because of exacerbations of COPD (136). Most studies indicate that the greatest benefit in terms of exacerbations appears to be those with the most advanced COPD, as measured by the baseline FEV_1 (132,137,138). Withdrawal studies also led to an increase in the rate of mild exacerbations and symptoms, and a decrease in health status, with decreases in FEV_1 (132,139,140).

Although ICSs do not have an effect on the rate of decline of FEV_1, observational studies of COPD databases have suggested that ICSs either alone or in combination with

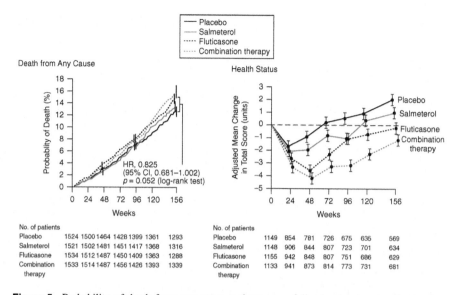

Figure 5 Probability of death from any cause at three years following treatment with placebo, salmeterol, fluticasone, and the combination of salmeterol and fluticasone. The risk of death in the placebo group was 15.2%, as compared with 12.6% in the combination therapy group. The salmeterol and FP group reduced the risk of death at any time during the three-year study by 17.5% (*p* = 0.052). The adjacent panel shows the effect of each study medication on health status as measured by changes in patients' total scores on the St George's respiratory Questionnaire during the three-year period study. *Source*: From Ref. 131.

LABAs may reduce mortality rates in COPD (141–143). Another study did not show this advantage when data were analyzed as per an according-to-treat approach, and the survival benefit of the previous studies was attributed to bias from unaccounted immortal time in the cohort design and analysis (144). In a review of seven randomized controlled trials comparing ICS with placebo that lasted 12 months or longer involving 5058 patients, a significant 27% relative reduction in all-cause mortality was observed, but because the overall rate of mortality was only 4%, the absolute risk reduction works out to be ~1% (145). This data may be biased because of incomplete ascertainment of mortality in those patients who did not complete the study. However, in the TORCH study, there was no effect of ICS alone on mortality compared with placebo (HR 1.06; 95% CI 0.891.27).

B. Combination of ICS with LABA

ICS and LABA combinations are now widely recommended for prescription for COPD as combination formulations such as salmeterol and fluticasone or formoterol and budesonide since, in general, the addition of LABA to ICS provides additional benefits. An additive bronchodilator response from ICS is observed, and most studies show a mean improvement in FEV_1 of 50 to 75 mL (78–80,118,131,133,146). The same studies also demonstrate an additive effect on the SGRQ score, with an average increase below the 4-unit change that is regarded as clinically significant improvement (147). The

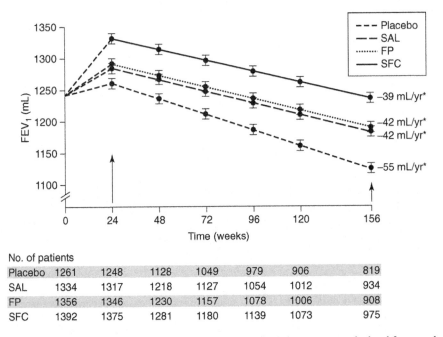

Figure 6 Rate of decline (mL/yr) in postbronchodilator FEV₁ by treatment calculated from week 24 to week 156, as indicated by the arrows, and was steeper in the patients receiving placebo versus those receiving active therapies. *$p \leq 0.003$ compared with placebo. Vertical bars represent standard errors of the adjusted means at each visit. The number of patients at each clinic visit with FEV₁ measurements is shown below the graph. *Abbreviations*: FEV₁, forced expiratory volume in one second; FP, fluticasone propionate; SAL, salmeterol; SFC, salmeterol/FP combination. *Source*: From Ref. 129.

TORCH study is likely to be the best one to demonstrate the effect of the combination of LABA and ICS in reducing the annualized COPD exacerbation rate, which was significantly lower than for ICS alone (131). In the TORCH study, the combination of ICS and LABA reduced the rate of decline in FEV₁ in patients with moderate-to-severe COPD by 16 mL/yr compared with placebo (Fig. 6). This improvement was also observed in the LABA only and in the ICS only group (129).

Combination of LABA with ICS reduced the number of exacerbations over a one-year period, while ICS alone had no effect (130,146). The TORCH study found that there was a 25% reduction in exacerbations with a combination therapy compared with placebo, which was significantly better than ICS alone (131). This study also reported that the combination of salmeterol-fluticasone decreased the risk of all-cause mortality over a three-year period by 17.5% compared with placebo at a *p* value of 0.052 (Fig. 5).

VIII.   Systematic Meta-analysis Reviews

Systematic review of combination therapy with fluticasone and salmeterol combination and budesonide and formoterol combination has been reported by Sin et al. (3 studies, 2951 patients) (137) and by Nannini et al. (6 studies, 4118 patients) (148). Nannini et al.

concluded that combination therapy was better than placebo, with clinically important improvement in lung function, mean exacerbation rate, and quality-of-life scores. Regarding lung function, there were significant differences of combination therapy versus ICSs alone, with the combination of Seretide better than salmeterol alone, but with the combination of Symbicort equal to formoterol alone. Analysis of all studies showed that there were less frequent exacerbations with combination therapy than with placebo or LABA alone, but not when compared with the ICS alone. Nannini et al. found that in comparison with LABAs, there was no significant difference between budesonide and formoterol, and fluticasone and salmeterol. However, compared with their constituent LABA, there was a significant reduction in exacerbation rate for the combination of budesonide and formoterol but not for the combination of fluticasone and salmeterol. The rate ratio of exacerbation rates for the combination of fluticasone and salmeterol compared to salmeterol was 0.93 (0.81–1.08, 95% confidence interval), and for the combination of budesonide and formoterol compared with formoterol alone was 0.76 (0.64–0.90). In COPD patients with a history of one or more exacerbations in the previous year, the difference of 24% could translate to one exacerbation less every four years.

IX. Mechanisms for the Interactions Between Glucocorticoids and LABA

Molecular interactions between glucocorticoids and β_2-adrenoceptors may underlie the clinical-added benefits of combination therapy. Glucocorticoids may increase the number of β_2-adrenoceptors and their coupling with Gs proteins, while β_2-agonists may induce GR nuclear translocation, activate CAAT/enhancer binding protein (C/EBP)α together with corticosteroids, or alter GR phosphorylation (149,150). In cultured cells, the combination of glucocorticoids and LABA potentiates inhibition of CXCL8 (IL-8) and CCL11 (eotaxin) release from human airway smooth muscle cells and their proliferation, and has additive effects on GM-CSF release from epithelial cells (93,151).

Treatment with salmeterol/fluticasone has anti-inflammatory effects on sputum and bronchial biopsies from both current and former smokers with COPD, and this may contribute to its clinical efficacy. Thus, salmeterol/fluticasone reduces sputum differential (but not total) cell counts; sputum neutrophils and eosinophils; bronchial CD_{45}^+, CD_8^+, and CD_4^+ cells; and cells expressing genes for TNF-α and IFN-γ. These anti-inflammatory effects were accompanied by improvements in prebronchodilator FEV_1 (152).

X. Using ICS for Treating Exacerbations of Asthma and COPD
A. Asthma Exacerbations

Three randomized placebo-controlled studies have failed to demonstrate a benefit from doubling the dose of ICS to treat exacerbations of asthma (153–155). Several studies have shown that high-dose ICS can improve symptoms and lung function during exacerbation to the same extent as a standard course of oral corticosteroids (156–162). Single, high ICS doses, as well as high doses delivered in the emergency room over a three- to eight-hour period, also produced improvement in symptoms and/or lung function similar to those achieved by intravenous or oral corticosteroids. Thus, increasing ICS to high doses as alternative to oral corticosteroids to treat exacerbations is supported by evidence in adults. Studies that used ICS doses equivalent to 2400 to 4000 µg of BDP for one to two weeks during mild-to-moderate exacerbations demonstrated improved symptoms and lung function with effects similar to those of oral corticosteroids. It would be reasonable to consider using daily doses of up to 2000 μg of fluticasone or 3200 μg budesonide or equivalent for 7 to 14 days (163). Oral corticosteroids remain the treatment of choice for severe exacerbations or for exacerbations that do not respond to high-dose ICS.

B. COPD Exacerbations

Successful use of nebulized budesonide has been reported in the treatment of acute exacerbations of COPD (164). In this study, nebulized budesonide (2 mg) provided statistically significant improvements in postbronchodilator FEV_1 compared with placebo treatment, and the improvement found was similar to that caused by using prednisolone 30 mg every 12 hours. The treatment with nebulized budesonide was safer than that provided by oral prednisolone, which increased the prevalence of hyperglycemic episodes. One of the major limitations with nebulized treatment in acute exacerbations of COPD is the penetration and deposition of aerosol into the small airways; clearly, any further progress in this area will depend on the development of efficacious methods of aerosol delivery in face of severe airflow obstruction.

XI. Side Effects of ICS

The major local side effects of ICS include oral candidiasis, hoarseness, and dysphonia. Cough is also a potential side effect induced by the inhaler and not dependent on the constituent of the inhaled drug. It can usually be overcome by changing the delivery device (e.g., changing dry powder inhaler to a metered dose inhaler, or adding a spacer device to an MDI). In all studies in COPD, there was greater incidence of candidiasis in the fluticasone only or the combined fluticasone and salmeterol treated groups compared with the placebo and salmeterol groups. In the one-year Tristan study, the frequency of candidiasis in the fluticasone group was 7%, and in the combination group 8% compared with 2% in both placebo and salmeterol groups (10). Oral candidiasis can be prevented by gargling, washing with water, and then spitting out after using the inhaler. Local antifungal agents may be needed. Hoarseness and dysphonia are caused by the myopathy of the arytenoid muscles caused by the deposition of ICS on the vocal cords; these effects are also dose-related and are more of a problem in those who use their voice a lot. Ciclesonide may cause less local side effects since it is not metabolized into active ciclesonide in the upper airways. Use of high-dose ICS is particularly associated with an increased incidence of oral thrush and dysphonia in COPD (137).

Systemic side effects result from the portion of steroids that is absorbed from the bronchial submucosa, with most of the steroids absorbed from the gastrointestinal tract being metabolized by the liver. The degree of systemic side effects also depends on the amount deposited in the lower airways, and this in turn depends on the efficiency of the inhaler device (71). An ideal corticosteroid that would have minimal potential for systemic side effects should stay in the airways for a sufficient period of time to have its anti-inflammatory actions in the airways (2–3 hours), and then be metabolized in inactive metabolites before absorption into the systemic circulation. High protein binding may also be of interest (71).

Systemic side effects of inhaled steroids may be assessed by surrogate markers such as blood cortisols or serum osteocalcin. A progressive reduction in adrenal function can be observed with increasing doses of ICS over relatively shorter periods (73,165,166). For example, five days treatment with high doses of fluticasone and budesonide caused near-complete reduction of the 24-hour plasma cortisol profile (166). Morning cortisols decreased during fluticasone and during combination therapy, while they increased in the placebo and salmeterol groups, after 52 weeks of treatment, but these changes were small and levels remained within the normal reference values. However, cases of adrenal crises have been reported with ICS and in the 33 patients reported 28 were children and most were taking doses of ICS within the recommended doses by U.K. guidelines at that time. There is potential for ICS to cause adrenal suppression but this is not a common event, and clinicians need always to be aware of this potentiality (167,168).

Of the randomized prospective studies of the side effects of ICS when compared with placebo, about twofold increase in patients report easy bruising (125,126) and reduction in growth velocity (83,84) and in bone mineral density (126). There has been no comparable data for the onset of cataract or fractures because such studies would need longer duration of observation, but case-control and cross-sectional studies have found associations between ICS and cataract (169), glaucoma (170), and BMD (171). In children, dose-related inhibition of growth has been seen in some short- and intermediate-term studies, but long-term studies have found no detrimental effect on final height. There was some evidence of a small decrease in statural growth during the initial period of ICS therapy, an effect that was more marked at daily doses of >200 µg and did not apply to all treatment regimens. Studies examining final attained adult height found no difference between children treated with ICS and those receiving nonsteroidal therapy (172).

Of more relevance to COPD, an increase in pneumonia has been reported in patients with moderate-to-severe COPD treated with high-dose ICS (131). In the TORCH study, patients in all fluticasone treatment arms experienced an excess in the rate of nonfatal pneumonia of $\sim 3/100$ per year compared with treatments arms not containing fluticasone. This may be related to the immunosuppressive effect of corticosteroids and the decreased immune responses of advanced COPD.

A. Bone and Risk of Fractures

Long-term studies are needed to assess the risk of osteoporosis. Measurement of morning cortisols and of plasma levels of osteocalcin or markers of bone activity indicates that inhaled steroids at doses above 800 to 1000 µg/day of BDP or budesonide equivalent may have systemic effects. ICSs have minimal systemic effects in most patients when taken at recommended doses and the benefits of ICS therapy outweigh the risks of uncontrolled asthma.

Two studies have now shown a relationship between the doses of ICS taken during a two- to three-year period and a reduction in BMD at one or more than one site, after allowing for other factors that affect BMD (119,173). In COPD patients, triamcinolone 600 µg twice daily was associated with a greater reduction in BMD over three years than those allocated to placebo and with a reduction of femoral neck BMD by 2% over a four-year period (126). However, in a similar study with budesonide (800 µg/day), there was no difference observed against placebo (125), perhaps reflecting the differences between triamcinolone and budesonide. In a study of patients aged 20 to 40 years old with 80% taking beclomethasone, a relationship between BMD measurements and total life cumulative doses of ICS has been reported (171). In this study, it has been calculated that a patient taking 1000 µg/day ICSs for 14 years would expect a reduction in BMD of one SD over that time as a result of ICS. Another study in postmenopausal women performed cross-sectionally did not show any effect of ICS on BMD (174). Cumulative ICS use was associated with a small decrease in bone mineral accretion in boys but not in girls, but no increased risk for osteopenia (175). There is no data on whether any particular ICS is more likely to be associated with a reduction in BMD.

The risk of hip fracture is associated with the use of ICS (84% were taking BDP) with an overall odds ratio of 1.19 after adjustment for the use of oral steroids, with a dose response such that with taking more than 1600 µg ICs per day, the odds ratio increased to 1.84 (176). In a Canadian case-control study there was a dose-response relationship between ICS use and fractures, but there were concurrent contributions by both oral CS exposure and inhaled bronchodilators (177). In COPD patients, an increase in fracture risk is reported among those taking 700 µg ICS or more daily (178). A meta-analysis of 13 studies reported no association between use of ICS and fractures in older adults, although a slight increase in risk was seen in those on high-dose ICS (179).

In all the reported studies, it is difficult to disentangle the potential contribution of confounding factors such as oral steroid use, cigarette smoking, sedentariness, and dietary factors. It is likely that at doses under 800 µg of BDP daily or equivalent the risk of reduced BMD or of fracture is probably not increased but above 1000 µg/day, there is increased risk.

XII. Corticosteroid Insensitivity in Airways Disease

Most patients with asthma can be controlled on low doses of ICSs, which have revolutionized asthma therapy and have now become first-line treatment for the majority of patients (180). However, approximately 5% to 10% of patients require the maximal inhaled dose, and approximately 1% require regular oral corticosteroids (termed steroid-dependent asthma), whereas a very small number of patients are steroid-resistant (SR) defined by no clinical improvement after high-dose oral corticosteroid (prednisolone 40 mg daily) for two weeks (181). Steroid insensitivity in severe asthma has huge health care costs and these 5% to 10% of asthmatic patients account for >50% of total health care costs. Incorrect diagnosis, noncompliance with therapy, and psychological problems are all confounding issues in these subjects and can account for a failure to respond to steroids in many of these patients (182). Patients with severe asthma experience continuing asthma symptoms, exacerbations of asthma, and often present with persistent airflow obstruction despite taking high-dose ICS often with oral prednisolone (182–185).

It now seems likely that steroid resistance represents the end of a spectrum of corticosteroid responsiveness (186). These SR asthmatics differed clinically from steroid-sensitive (SS) patients in having a longer duration of symptoms, lower morning lung function, a greater degree of AHR, and a more frequent family history of asthma. These patients are not cortisol-deficient (Addisonian) and do not suffer from the abnormalities in sex hormones described in familial glucocorticoid resistance (187). Plasma cortisol and adrenal suppression in response to exogenous cortisol are within the normal range in these patients and they unfortunately develop the typical Cushingoid side effects of corticosteroids (188). The lack of response to oral steroids cannot be explained by reduced gastrointestinal absorption of other pharmacokinetic mechanisms (189). This suggests that there is a defect on the anti-inflammatory effects of steroids rather than their metabolic or endocrine effects.

Bronchial biopsies from patients with SR asthma show a similar pattern of inflammation, with increased eosinophils and lymphocytes, compared with SS asthma, despite treatment with high doses of corticosteroids and there is a failure to suppress the T-helper-2 (Th2) cytokines IL-4 and IL-5 (190). There is an increase in the ratio of matrix metalloproteinase (MMP)-9 to tissue inhibitor of MMP (TIMP)-1 in bronchoalveolar lavage from patients with SR asthma compared with SS asthma and macrophages from SR asthmatics fail to show the normal increase TIMP-1 after corticosteroid treatment in vitro (191). There is altered expression of markers of epithelial proliferation, for example, increased expression of Ki67, reduced expression of retinoblastoma, and reduced expression of Bcl-2, a negative regulator of epithelial cell death (192). These changes may result in abnormal tissue remodeling in the airways of SR asthma, which may underlie the reduced bronchodilator (reversibility) response in these patients. An important observation that has led to several subsequent mechanistic studies is that circulating blood mononuclear cells or alveolar macrophages from patients with severe asthma show reduced responses to steroids (22,193).

XIII. COPD

In COPD, the effects of corticosteroids are very limited and compared with asthma, airflow obstruction of COPD responds very little to either inhaled or oral CS therapy. The beneficial effects of ICS have been reviewed earlier, and particularly in combination with LABA, there is a reduction in the number of exacerbations in patients with advanced disease. Accompanying these effects are the small responses of airway inflammation to ICS therapy (194). Dexamethasone is less efficient in inhibiting the induced release of IL-8 by IL-1β or cigarette smoke extracts from AMs of COPD patients compared with non-COPD smokers (195). The ratio of HAT:HDAC activity regulates chromatin structure and transcription factor activity (see previous sections). HDAC2 activity is reduced in the lungs, and in lung macrophages of patients with COPD, the degree of reduction being related to severity of COPD (1), this may result in CS insensitivity through lack of repression of NF-κB-mediated gene expression (1). Since HDAC2 is important for deacetylation of histone H3 (196), the increase in histone H3 acetylation in COPD (197) may result from a reduction in HDAC2 activity.

Theophylline which has been used for the treatment of asthma and COPD as a bronchodilator and as a potential anti-inflammatory agent can recruit HDAC and restore CS sensitivity of macrophages in vitro (198,199). Clinical trials to examine this action of restoring CS insensitivity in COPD are currently under way.

XIV. Mechanisms of Corticosteroid Insensitivity

Several distinct molecular mechanisms contributing to decreased anti-inflammatory effects of corticosteroids have now been identified, so that there is heterogeneity of mechanisms even within a single disease. The early descriptions of SR asthma suggested that it was more commonly found within families (200), indicating that there may genetic factors may determine steroid responsiveness which are outside the GR itself (201). Microarray studies of PBMCs from SS and SR asthma patients identified 11 genes that discriminated between these patients (202), indicating that it may be possible to develop a genomic test for steroid resistance. However, in normal subjects differential gene expression between the 10% with the greatest and least steroid responsiveness of circulating genes identified 24 genes, of which the most discriminant was bone morphogenetic protein receptor type II, which enhanced steroid responsiveness when transfected into cells (203).

IL-2 and IL-4 are overexpressed in the airways of patients with SR asthma (190), and in vitro these cytokines in combination reduce GR nuclear translocation and binding affinity within the nucleus of T cells (1). IL-13 alone mimics this effect in monocytes (1). The mechanism whereby these cytokines reduce GR function may be mediated via phosphorylation of GR by p38 MAPK and their effect is blocked by a p38 MAPK inhibitor (204). In support of this, p38 MAPK shows a greater degree of activation in alveolar macrophages from asthmatics with a poor response to steroids than patients who show a normal response (22). Similar effects are seen with JNK, ERK, and JAK3 depending on the specific stimulus driving steroid insensitivity in vitro (1). Interestingly, in asthmatic patients with poor steroid responses there is a significant reduction in MKP-1 expression in alveolar macrophages after steroid exposure and this is correlated with increased p38 MAPK activity (22).

Increased expression of GRβ has been reported in SR patients of several diseases, including asthma (1). GRβ is induced by proinflammatory cytokines and has the capacity to compete for the binding of GRα to GRE, thus acting as a dominant-negative inhibitor (205). Another mechanism may be through interference with GRα nuclear translocation, since knockdown of GRβ in alveolar macrophages from SR asthma patients results in increased GRα nuclear localization and increased steroid responsiveness (206).

Excessive activation of AP-1 has been identified as a mechanism of steroid resistance in asthma as AP-1 binds GR and thus prevents its interaction with GRE and other transcription factors (1). AP-1 is a heterodimer of Fos and Jun proteins, and there is increased expression of c-Fos in PBMCs and bronchial biopsies of SR compared with SS asthma, with no reduction of JNK activity or c-Jun after high doses of oral steroids (207). This may explain why the increased inflammation found in severe inflammatory disease results in secondary steroid resistance and is a mechanism for perpetuating steroid resistance whatever the initial mechanism.

HDAC2 activity and expression are reduced in severe asthma and particularly in patients with COPD (1,208). Importantly, the steroid resistance of COPD bronchoalveolar macrophages is completely reversed by overexpressing HDAC2 to the level seen in control subjects (199). The mechanism of HDAC2 reduction in COPD may involve oxidative stress, which is increased in most severe and SR inflammatory diseases (209).

IL-10 is an important anti-inflammatory and immunoregulatory cytokine and secreted by regulatory T cells (Treg) in response to steroids (210). In patients with SR asthma, there is a failure of Th cells to secrete IL-10, but this is restored to normal by vitamin D3 (calcitriol) in vitro (15). Furthermore, administration of vitamin D3 to three SR asthmatics also restored the T-cell IL-10 response to steroids, suggesting that this might be a useful therapeutic approach in the future. Vitamin D is now recognized to be an important regulator of the immune system, particularly in the regulation of Tregs so that low dietary intake or lack of sunlight may be contributory to reduced steroid responses in inflammatory diseases.

XV. Reversing Steroid Resistance

The most attractive option for treating steroid resistance is to reverse the cause of resistance if it can be identified. This might be possible for some patients with SR asthma with p38 MAPK, JNK inhibitors, and vitamin D3 in the future (15,204,211).

JAK3 is activated by IL-2 and JAK3 inhibitors may be useful in SR asthma (212). Selective activation of HDAC2 can be achieved with theophylline, which restores HDAC2 activity in COPD macrophages back to normal and reverses steroid resistance (213). In mice exposed to cigarette smoke that develops SR inflammation, oral theophylline is also effective in reversing steroid resistance (214), and clinical trials to test this in COPD patients are currently underway. The molecular mechanism of action of theophylline in restoring HDAC2 is now being elucidated and appears to be via selective inhibition of PI3Kδ, which is activated by oxidative stress in COPD patients (215). This suggests that selective PI3K-δ inhibitors may also be effective and these drugs are currently in clinical development for other diseases (216). Since oxidative stress appears to be an important mechanism in reducing HDAC2 and leads to steroid resistance, antioxidants should also be effective. Unfortunately, currently available antioxidants are not very effective and several more potent antioxidants are in clinical development (209). In the future, novel drugs that increase HDAC2 may be developed when the molecular signaling pathways that regulate HDAC2 are better understood (217).

XVI. Future Aspects of ICS Development

Use of a once-daily ICS may have profound effects on patient compliance and improve control of the disease particularly if combined with an ultra-LABA (218,219). Increasing the potency of corticosteroids by adapting the steroid side chains may also improve clinical efficacy, albeit with an increased risk of side effects (218), and these are in clinical development. Also, addition of an NO-donating group to prednisolone (NCX1015) and budesonide (NCX1020) has resulted in improved corticosteroid efficacy compared with the parent compounds in animal models possibly by donation of the NO moiety to specific residues within the GR LBD (220,221).

Several approaches have been taken to reduce the problem of side effects including systemic or local inactivation or administration of an inactive prodrug that is only converted to active drug in the airways. This is exemplified by ciclesonide (222), which is esterified only in the lung to produce the active form des-ciclesonide, and further advances in producing topical drugs with reduced systemic effects are likely.

Many, but not all, of the side effects of corticosteroids are due to the DNA binding (GRE) effects of the drugs whereas the anti-inflammatory effects are related predominantly to targeting of proinflammatory transcription factors such as NF-κB and AP-1 (1,223,224). The development of dissociated corticosteroids that can interact with NF-κB, but not with GREs, thereby preserving therapeutic anti-inflammatory effects with reduced side-effect profiles has been explored (218). It is hoped that these dissociated corticosteroids may be just as effective as conventional ICS, have a better safety profile, and perhaps even lead to safer oral corticosteroids (17). One of the problems with conventional corticosteroids is that the steroid backbone can also bind to other nuclear hormone receptors such as MR and PR which also cause side effects. The development of dissociated corticosteroids with a nonsteroidal backbone such as AL-438 and ZK 216348 may further improve the therapeutic index as these drugs (17,225).

Other nuclear hormone receptors, for example, LXR, PPARγ, and RXR have distinct anti-inflammatory patterns in murine macrophages (226), which may be complimentary to that seen with corticosteroids. Combinations of steroids or possibly more promiscuous drugs that bind to two or more of these receptors may result in an enhanced anti-inflammatory profile than that seen with current corticosteroids particularly in patients with severe disease (227). Several key signaling pathways play an important role in the inflammatory response (228,229) and also in the modulation of corticosteroid responsiveness in asthma and COPD (22,204,218,230). This raises the potential of novel combination therapies utilizing selective p38 MAPK or PI3K pathway inhibitors and new corticosteroids that reduce the dose of each component necessary to produce a clinically effective response. The future may see the development of multicombination therapies involving corticosteroids and bronchodilators, pathway inhibitors, and other nuclear hormone receptor ligands as seen in other therapeutic areas such as rheumatoid arthritis (231).

Summary

The introduction of inhaled corticosteroid (ICS) therapy represented a revolution in the treatment of asthma, and ICS therapy forms the basis of treatment of asthma of all severities. More recently and usually in combination with a long-acting β-agonist (LABA), ICS use has been established in the treatment of chronic obstructive pulmonary disease (COPD). In asthma, ICS improves asthma control and lung function and prevents exacerbations; in COPD, there are similar improvements albeit to a lesser degree, but useful gains in quality of life likely from an improvement in symptoms such as breathlessness and reduction in exacerbations particularly in more advanced disease. Chronic inflammation is a feature of both asthma and COPD, although there are differences in the characteristics of the inflammatory response and in its site. ICS targets this inflammation although ICS has proven to be less effective in patients with severe asthma and with COPD. ICS acts by binding to and activating specific cytosolic receptors [glucocorticoid receptor (GR)], which then translocate to the nucleus where they regulate gene expression by either binding to DNA and inducing anti-inflammatory genes or by repressing the induction of proinflammatory mediators. GR is able to selectively repress specific inflammatory genes by differing actions on specific intracellular signaling pathways and transcription factors such as nuclear factor kappa B (NF-κB) and on mitogen-activated protein kinase (MAPK) pathways. Abnormal activation of these pathways may result in glucocorticoid refractoriness. ICS taken together with LABA will remain the main focus of treatment of airways diseases; improvements in treatment may be obtained with more potent corticosteroids that have less systemic effects. Drugs that improve the efficacy of corticosteroid actions may be added.

References

1. Ito K, Chung KF, Adcock IM. Update on glucocorticoid action and resistance. J Allergy Clin Immunol 2006; 117:522–543.
2. Savory JG, Hsu B, Laquian IR, et al. Discrimination between NL1- and NL2-mediated nuclear localization of the glucocorticoid receptor. Mol Cell Biol 1999; 19:1025–10237.
3. Weigel NL, Moore NL. Steroid receptor phosphorylation: a key modulator of multiple receptor functions. Mol Endocrinol 2007; 21:2311–2319.
4. Freedman ND, Yamamoto KR. Importin 7 and importin alpha/importin beta are nuclear import receptors for the glucocorticoid receptor. Mol Biol Cell 2004; 15:2276–2286.
5. Tao T, Lan J, Lukacs GL, et al. Importin 13 regulates nuclear import of the glucocorticoid receptor in airway epithelial cells. Am J Respir Cell Mol Biol 2006; 35:668–680.

6. Kumar S, Chaturvedi NK, Nishi M, et al. Shuttling components of nuclear import machinery involved in nuclear translocation of steroid receptors exit nucleus via exportin-1/CRM-1* independent pathway. Biochim Biophys Acta 2004; 1691:73–77.

7. Carrigan A, Walther RF, Salem HA, et al. An active nuclear retention signal in the glucocorticoid receptor functions as a strong inducer of transcriptional activation. J Biol Chem 2007; 282(15):10963–10971.

8. Adcock IM, Barnes PJ. Molecular mechanisms of corticosteroid resistance. Chest 2008; 134:394–401.

9. Li B, Carey M, Workman JL. The role of chromatin during transcription. Cell 2007; 128: 707–719.

10. O'Malley BW, Qin J, Lanz RB. Cracking the coregulator codes. Curr Opin Cell Biol 2008; 20:310–315.

11. Wu RC, Smith CL, O'Malley BW. Transcriptional regulation by steroid receptor coactivator phosphorylation. Endocr Rev 2005; 26:393–399.

12. So AY, Cooper SB, Feldman BJ, et al. Conservation analysis predicts in vivo occupancy of glucocorticoid receptor-binding sequences at glucocorticoid-induced genes. Proc Natl Acad Sci U S A 2008; 105:5745–5749.

13. So AY, Chaivorapol C, Bolton EC, et al. Determinants of cell- and gene-specific transcriptional regulation by the glucocorticoid receptor. PLoS Genet 2007; 3:e94.

14. De Bosscher K, Van Craenenbroeck K, Meijer OC, et al. Selective transrepression versus transactivation mechanisms by glucocorticoid receptor modulators in stress and immune systems. Eur J Pharmacol 2008; 583:290–302.

15. Xystrakis E, Kusumakar S, Boswell S, et al. Reversing the defective induction of IL-10-secreting regulatory T cells in glucocorticoid-resistant asthma patients. J Clin Invest 2006; 116:146–155.

16. Clark AR, Martins JR, Tchen CR. Role of dual specificity phosphatases in biological responses to glucocorticoids. J Biol Chem 2008; 283:25765–25769.

17. Schacke H, Berger M, Rehwinkel H, et al. Selective glucocorticoid receptor agonists (SEGRAs): novel ligands with an improved therapeutic index. Mol Cell Endocrinol 2007; 275(1–2):109–117.

18. Reichardt HM, Tuckermann JP, Gottlicher M, et al. Repression of inflammatory responses in the absence of DNA binding by the glucocorticoid receptor. EMBO J 2001; 20:7168–7173.

19. Reichardt HM, Kaestner KH, Tuckermann J, et al. DNA binding of the glucocorticoid receptor is not essential for survival. Cell 1998; 93:531–541.

20. Luecke HF, Yamamoto KR. The glucocorticoid receptor blocks P-TEFb recruitment by NFkappaB to effect promoter-specific transcriptional repression. Genes Dev 2005; 19: 1116–1127.

21. Nie M, Knox AJ, Pang L. Beta2-Adrenoceptor agonists, like glucocorticoids, repress eotaxin gene transcription by selective inhibition of histone H4 acetylation. J Immunol 2005; 175:478–486.

22. Bhavsar P, Hew M, Khorasani N, et al. Relative corticosteroid insensitivity of alveolar macrophages in severe asthma compared to non-severe asthma. Thorax 2008; 63:784–790.

23. Schleimer RP, Kato A, Kern R, et al. Epithelium: at the interface of innate and adaptive immune responses. J Allergy Clin Immunol 2007; 120:1279–1284.

24. Hermoso MA, Matsuguchi T, Smoak K, et al. Glucocorticoids and tumor necrosis factor alpha cooperatively regulate toll-like receptor 2 gene expression. Mol Cell Biol 2004; 24:4743–4756.

25. Da Silva CA, Kassel O, Lebouquin R, et al. Paradoxical early glucocorticoid induction of stem cell factor (SCF) expression in inflammatory conditions. Br J Pharmacol 2004; 141:75–84.

26. Meyer S, Temme C, Wahle E. Messenger RNA turnover in eukaryotes: pathways and enzymes. Crit Rev Biochem Mol Biol 2004; 39:197–216.

27. Jalonen U, Lahti A, Korhonen R, et al. Inhibition of tristetraprolin expression by dexamethasone in activated macrophages. Biochem Pharmacol 2005; 69:733–740.

28. Norman AW, Mizwicki MT, Norman DP. Steroid-hormone rapid actions, membrane receptors and a conformational ensemble model. Nat Rev Drug Discov 2004; 3:27–41.

29. Croxtall JD, Choudhury Q, Flower RJ. Glucocorticoids act within minutes to inhibit recruitment of signalling factors to activated EGF receptors through a receptor-dependent, transcription-independent mechanism. Br J Pharmacol 2000; 130:289–298.

30. Horvath G, Wanner A. Inhaled corticosteroids: effects on the airway vasculature in bronchial asthma. Eur Respir J 2006; 27:172–187.

31. Jeffery PK, Godfrey RW, Adelroth E, et al. Effects of treatment on airway inflammation and thickening of basement membrane reticular collagen in asthma. A quantitative light and electron microscopic study. Am Rev Respir Dis 1992; 145:890–899.

32. Adelroth E, Rosenhall L, Johansson SA, et al. Inflammatory cells and eosinophilic activity in asthmatics investigated by bronchoalveolar lavage. The effects of anti-asthmatic treatment with budesonide or terbutaline. Am Rev Respir Dis 1990; 142:91–99.

33. Laitinen LA, Laitinen A, Haahtela T. A comparative study of the effects of an inhaled corticosteroid, budesonide, and a beta 2-agonist, terbutaline, on airway inflammation in newly diagnosed asthma: a randomized, double- blind, parallel-group controlled trial. J Allergy Clin Immunol 1992; 90:32–42.

34. Laursen LC, Taudorf E, Borgeskov S, et al. Fiberoptic bronchoscopy and bronchial mucosal biopsies in asthmatics undergoing long-term high-dose budesonide aerosol treatment. Allergy 1988; 43:284–288.

35. Barnes PJ. Inhaled glucocorticoids for asthma. N Engl J Med 1995; 332:868–875.

36. van Rensen EL, Straathof KC, Veselic-Charvat MA, et al. Effect of inhaled steroids on airway hyperresponsiveness, sputum eosinophils, and exhaled nitric oxide levels in patients with asthma. Thorax 1999; 54:403–408.

37. Olivieri D, Chetta A, Del Donno M, et al. Effect of short-term treatment with low-dose inhaled fluticasone propionate on airway inflammation and remodeling in mild asthma: a placebo-controlled study. Am J Respir Crit Care Med 1997; 155:1864–1871.

38. Orsida BE, Li X, Hickey B, et al. Vascularity in asthmatic airways: relation to inhaled steroid dose. Thorax 1999; 54:289–295.

39. Brieva JL, Danta I, Wanner A. Effect of an inhaled glucocorticosteroid on airway mucosal blood flow in mild asthma. Am J Respir Crit Care Med 2000; 161:293–296.

40. Gibson PG, Wong BJ, Hepperle MJ, et al. A research method to induce and examine a mild exacerbation of asthma by withdrawal of inhaled corticosteroid. Clin Exp Allergy 1992; 22:525–532.

41. in't Veen JC, Smits HH, Hiemstra PS, et al. Lung function and sputum characteristics of patients with severe asthma during an induced exacerbation by double-blind steroid withdrawal. Am J Respir Crit Care Med 1999; 160:93–99.

42. Umland SP, Schleimer RP, Johnston SL. Review of the molecular and cellular mechanisms of action of glucocorticoids for use in asthma. Pulm Pharmacol Ther 2002; 15:35–50.

43. Schleimer RP, Bochner BS. The effects of glucocorticoids on human eosinophils. J Allergy Clin Immunol 1994; 94:1202–1213.

44. Schleimer RP. An overview of glucocorticoid anti-inflammatory actions. Eur J Clin Pharmacol 1993; 45(suppl 1):S3–S7.

45. Peters SP, Naclerio RM, Schleimer RP, et al. The pharmacologic control of mediator release from human basophils and mast cells. Respiration 1986; 50(suppl 2):116–122.

46. Djukanovic R, Wilson JW, Britten KM, et al. Effect of an inhaled corticosteroid on airway inflammation and symptoms in asthma. Am Rev Respir Dis 1992; 145:669–674.

47. Majori M, Piccoli ML, Bertacco S, et al. Inhaled beclomethasone dipropionate down-regulates CD4 and CD8 T-lymphocyte activation in peripheral blood of patients with asthma. J Allergy Clin Immunol 1997; 100:379–382.

48. Wilson JW, Djukanovic R, Howarth PH, et al. Inhaled beclomethasone dipropionate downregulates airway lymphocyte activation in atopic asthma. Am J Respir Crit Care Med 1994; 149:86–90.

49. Borish L, Mascali JJ, Dishuck J, et al. Detection of alveolar macrophage-derived IL-1 beta in asthma. Inhibition with corticosteroids. J Immunol. 1992; 149:3078–3082.

50. Dworski R, Fitzgerald GA, Oates JA, et al. Effect of oral prednisone on airway inflammatory mediators in atopic asthma. Am J Respir Crit Care Med 1994; 149:953–959.

51. Wenzel SE, Szefler SJ, Leung DY, et al. Bronchoscopic evaluation of severe asthma. Persistent inflammation associated with high dose glucocorticoids. Am J Respir Crit Care Med 1997; 156:737–743.

52. Cox G. Glucocorticoid treatment inhibits apoptosis in human neutrophils. Separation of survival and activation outcomes. J Immunol 1995; 154:4719–4725.

53. Schleimer RP, Freeland HS, Peters SP, et al. An assessment of the effects of glucocorticoids on degranulation, chemotaxis, binding to vascular endothelium and formation of leukotriene B4 by purified human neutrophils. J Pharmacol Exp Ther 1989; 250:598–605.

54. Kharitonov SA, Yates DH, Barnes PJ. Inhaled glucocorticoids decrease nitric oxide in exhaled air of asthmatic patients. Am J Respir Crit Care Med 1996; 153:454–457.

55. Chung KF, Barnes PJ. Cytokines in asthma. Thorax 1999; 54:825–857.

56. John M, Lim S, Seybold J, et al. Inhaled corticosteroids increase interleukin-10 but reduce macrophage inflammatory protein-1alpha, granulocyte-macrophage colony-stimulating factor, and interferon-gamma release from alveolar macrophages in asthma. Am J Respir Crit Care Med 1998; 157:256–262.

57. Sousa AR, Trigg CJ, Lane SJ, et al. Effect of inhaled glucocorticoids on IL-1 beta and IL-1 receptor antagonist (IL-1 ra) expression in asthmatic bronchial epithelium. Thorax 1997; 52:407–410.

58. Chung KF. Role played by inflammation in the hyperreactivity of the airways in asthma. Thorax 1986; 41:657–662.

59. Barnes PJ. Effect of corticosteroids on airway hyperresponsiveness. Am Rev Respir Dis 1990; 141:S70—S76.

60. Juniper EF, Kline PA, Vanzieleghem MA, et al. Long-term effects of budesonide on airway responsiveness and clinical asthma severity in inhaled steroid-dependent asthmatics. Eur Respir J 1990; 3:1122–1127.

61. Juniper EF, Kline PA, Vanzieleghem MA, et al. Effect of long-term treatment with an inhaled corticosteroid (budesonide) on airway hyperresponsiveness and clinical asthma in nonsteroid-dependent asthmatics. Am Rev Respir Dis 1990; 142:832–8326.

62. Ward C, Pais M, Bish R, et al. Airway inflammation, basement membrane thickening and bronchial hyperresponsiveness in asthma. Thorax 2002; 57:309–316.

63. van den Berge M, Kerstjens HA, Meijer RJ, et al. Corticosteroid-induced improvement in the PC20 of adenosine monophosphate is more closely associated with reduction in airway inflammation than improvement in the PC20 of methacholine. Am J Respir Crit Care Med 2001; 164:1127–1132.

64. Bel EH, Timmers MC, Zwinderman AH, et al. The effect of inhaled corticosteroids on the maximal degree of airway narrowing to methacholine in asthmatic subjects. Am Rev Respir Dis 1991; 143:109–113.

65. Vathenen AS, Knox AJ, Wisniewski A, et al. Time course of change in bronchial reactivity with an inhaled corticosteroid in asthma. Am Rev Respir Dis 1991; 143:1317–1321.

66. Haahtela T, Jarvinen M, Kava T, et al. Effects of reducing or discontinuing inhaled budesonide in patients with mild asthma. N Engl J Med 1994; 331:700–705.

67. Juniper EF, Kline PA, Vanzieleghem MA, et al. Reduction of budesonide after a year of increased use: a randomized controlled trial to evaluate whether improvements in airway responsiveness and clinical asthma are maintained. J Allergy Clin Immunol 1991; 87:483–489.
68. Biggadike K, Uings I, Farrow SN. Designing corticosteroid drugs for pulmonary selectivity. Proc Am Thorac Soc 2004; 1:352–355.
69. British Thoracic Society, Scottish Intercollegiate Guidelines Network. British guideline on the management of asthma. Thorax 2003; 58(suppl 1):i1–i94.
70. Johnson M. Pharmacodynamics and pharmacokinetics of inhaled glucocorticoids. J Allergy Clin Immunol 1996; 97:169–176.
71. Winkler J, Hochhaus G, Derendorf H. How the lung handles drugs: pharmacokinetics and pharmacodynamics of inhaled corticosteroids. Proc Am Thorac Soc 2004; 1:356–363.
72. Valotis A, Hogger P. Human receptor kinetics and lung tissue retention of the enhanced-affinity glucocorticoid fluticasone furoate. Respir Res 2007; 8:54.
73. Harrison TW, Wisniewski A, Honour J, et al. Comparison of the systemic effects of fluticasone propionate and budesonide given by dry powder inhaler in healthy and asthmatic subjects. Thorax 2001; 56:186–191.
74. Harrison TW. Systemic availability of inhaled budesonide and fluticasone propionate: healthy versus asthmatic lungs. BioDrugs 2001; 15:405–11.
75. Harrison TW, Tattersfield AE. Plasma concentrations of fluticasone propionate and budesonide following inhalation from dry powder inhalers by healthy and asthmatic subjects. Thorax 2003; 58:258–260.
76. Adams NP, Jones PW. The dose-response characteristics of inhaled corticosteroids when used to treat asthma: an overview of Cochrane systematic reviews. Respir Med 2006; 100:1297–1306.
77. Adams NP, Bestall JC, Jones P, et al. Fluticasone at different doses for chronic asthma in adults and children. Cochrane Database Syst Rev 2008; CD003534.
78. Mahler DA, Wire P, Horstman D, et al. Effectiveness of fluticasone propionate and salmeterol combination delivered via the Diskus device in the treatment of chronic obstructive pulmonary disease. Am J Respir Crit Care Med 2002; 166:1084–1091.
79. Hanania NA, Darken P, Horstman D, et al. The efficacy and safety of fluticasone propionate (250 microg)/salmeterol (50 microg) combined in the Diskus inhaler for the treatment of COPD. Chest 2003; 124:834–843.
80. Calverley P, Pauwels R, Vestbo J, et al. Combined salmeterol and fluticasone in the treatment of chronic obstructive pulmonary disease: a randomised controlled trial. Lancet 2003; 361:449–456.
81. Salmeron S, Guerin JC, Godard P, et al. High doses of inhaled corticosteroids in unstable chronic asthma. A multicenter, double-blind, placebo-controlled study. Am Rev Respir Dis 1989; 140:167–171.
82. Haahtela T, Jarvinen M, Kava T, et al. Comparison of a beta 2-agonist, terbutaline, with an inhaled corticosteroid, budesonide, in newly detected asthma [see comments]. N Engl J Med 1991; 325:388–392.
83. Pauwels RA, Pedersen S, Busse WW, et al. Early intervention with budesonide in mild persistent asthma: a randomised, double-blind trial. Lancet 2003; 361:1071–1076.
84. Long-term effects of budesonide or nedocromil in children with asthma. The Childhood Asthma Management Program Research Group. N Engl J Med 2000; 343:1054–1063.
85. O'Byrne PM, Barnes PJ, Rodriguez-Roisin R, et al. Low dose inhaled budesonide and formoterol in mild persistent asthma: the OPTIMA randomized trial. Am J Respir Crit Care Med 2001; 164:1392–1397.
86. Israel E, Chervinsky PS, Friedman B, et al. Effects of montelukast and beclomethasone on airway function and asthma control. J Allergy Clin Immunol 2002; 110:847–854.

87. Baumgartner RA, Martinez G, Edelman JM, et al. Distribution of therapeutic response in asthma control between oral montelukast and inhaled beclomethasone. Eur Respir J 2003; 21:123–128.

88. Papi A, Canonica GW, Maestrelli P, et al. Rescue use of beclomethasone and albuterol in a single inhaler for mild asthma. N Engl J Med 2007; 356:2040–2052.

89. Boushey HA, Sorkness CA, King TS, et al. Daily versus as-needed corticosteroids for mild persistent asthma. N Engl J Med 2005; 352:1519–1528.

90. Martin RJ, Szefler SJ, King TS, et al. The predicting response to inhaled corticosteroid efficacy (PRICE) trial. J Allergy Clin Immunol 2007; 119:73–80.

91. Lazarus SC, Chinchilli VM, Rollings NJ, et al. Smoking affects response to inhaled corticosteroids or leukotriene receptor antagonists in asthma. Am J Respir Crit Care Med 2007; 175:783–790.

92. Chalmers GW, MacLeod KJ, Little SA, et al. Influence of cigarette smoking on inhaled corticosteroid treatment in mild asthma. Thorax 2002; 57:226–230.

93. Sin DD, Man SF. Corticosteroids and adrenoceptor agonists: the compliments for combination therapy in chronic airways diseases. Eur J Pharmacol 2006; 533:28–35.

94. Duong M, Gauvreau G, Watson R, et al. The effects of inhaled budesonide and formoterol in combination and alone when given directly after allergen challenge. J Allergy Clin Immunol 2007; 119:322–327.

95. Sin DD, Man J, Sharpe H, et al. Pharmacological management to reduce exacerbations in adults with asthma: a systematic review and meta-analysis. JAMA 2004; 292:367–376.

96. Greenstone IR, Ni Chroinin MN, Masse V, et al. Combination of inhaled long-acting beta2-agonists and inhaled steroids versus higher dose of inhaled steroids in children and adults with persistent asthma. Cochrane Database Syst Rev 2005; CD005533.

97. O'Byrne PM, Bisgaard H, Godard PP, et al. Budesonide/formoterol combination therapy as both maintenance and reliever medication in asthma. Am J Respir Crit Care Med 2005; 171:129–136.

98. Pauwels RA, Lofdahl C, Postma D, et al. Effect of inhaled formoterol and budesonide on exacerbations of asthma. New Engl J Med 1997; 337:1405–1411.

99. Woolcock A, Lundback B, Ringdal N, et al. Comparison of addition of salmeterol to inhaled steroids with doubling of the dose of inhaled steroids. Am J Respir Crit Care Med 1996; 153:1481–1488.

100. Zetterstrom O, Buhl R, Mellem H, et al. Improved asthma control with budesonide/formoterol in a single inhaler, compared with budesonide alone. Eur Respir J 2001; 18:262–268.

101. Bateman ED, Boushey HA, Bousquet J, et al. Can guideline-defined asthma control be achieved? The Gaining Optimal Asthma ControL study. Am J Respir Crit Care Med 2004; 170:836–844.

102. Pauwels RA, Lofdahl CG, Postma DS, et al. Effect of inhaled formoterol and budesonide on exacerbations of asthma. Formoterol and Corticosteroids Establishing Therapy (FACET) International Study Group [see comments]. N Engl J Med 1997; 337:1405–1411. Erratum in: N Engl J Med 1998; 338(2):139.

103. Overbeek SE, Mulder PG, Baelemans SM, et al. Formoterol added to low-dose budesonide has no additional antiinflammatory effect in asthmatic patients. Chest 2005; 128:1121–1127.

104. Koopmans JG, Lutter R, Jansen HM, et al. Adding salmeterol to an inhaled corticosteroid: long term effects on bronchial inflammation in asthma. Thorax 2006; 61:306–312.

105. Koopmans JG, Lutter R, Jansen HM, et al. Adding salmeterol to an inhaled corticosteroid reduces allergen-induced serum IL-5 and peripheral blood eosinophils. J Allergy Clin Immunol 2005; 116:1007–1013.

106. Rabe KF, Atienza T, Magyar P, et al. Effect of budesonide in combination with formoterol for reliever therapy in asthma exacerbations: a randomised controlled, double-blind study. Lancet 2006; 368:744–753.

107. Bateman ED, Jacques L, Goldfrad C, et al. Asthma control can be maintained when flu-ticasone propionate/salmeterol in a single inhaler is stepped down. J Allergy Clin Immunol 2006; 117:563–570.

108. Lotvall J, Langley S, Woodcock A. Inhaled steroid/long-acting beta 2 agonist combination products provide 24 hours improvement in lung function in adult asthmatic patients. Respir Res 2006; 7:110.

109. Tarsin WY, Pearson SB, Assi KH, et al. Emitted dose estimates from Seretide Diskus and Symbicort Turbuhaler following inhalation by severe asthmatics. Int J Pharm 2006; 316:131–137.

110. Vogelmeier C, D'Urzo A, Pauwels R, et al. Budesonide/formoterol maintenance and reliever therapy: an effective asthma treatment option? Eur Respir J 2005; 26:819–828.

111. Fitzgerald JM, Boulet LP, Follows RM. The CONCEPT trial: a 1-year, multicenter, randomized, double-blind, double-dummy comparison of a stable dosing regimen of sal-meterol/fluticasone propionate with an adjustable maintenance dosing regimen of for-moterol/budesonide in adults with persistent asthma. Clin Ther 2005; 27:393–406.

112. Papi A, Paggiaro PL, Nicolini G, et al. Beclomethasone/formoterol versus budesonide/ formoterol combination therapy in asthma. Eur Respir J 2007; 29:682–689.

113. Barnes PJ. Chronic obstructive pulmonary disease. N Engl J Med 2000; 343:269–280.

114. Rabe KF, Hurd S, Anzueto A, et al. Global strategy for the diagnosis, management, and prevention of chronic obstructive pulmonary disease: GOLD executive summary. Am J Respir Crit Care Med 2007; 176:532–555.

115. Hogg JC, Chu F, Utokaparch S, et al. The nature of small-airway obstruction in chronic obstructive pulmonary disease. N Engl J Med 2004; 350:2645–2653.

116. Saetta M, Turato G, Maestrelli P, et al. Cellular and structural bases of chronic obstructive pulmonary disease. Am J Respir Crit Care Med 2001; 163:1304–1309.

117. Chung KF, Adcock IM. Multi-faceted mechanism in COPD: inflammation, immunity & tissue repair and destruction. Eur Respir J 2008; 31:1334–1356.

118. Burge PS, Calverley PM, Jones PW, et al. Randomised, double blind, placebo-controlled study of fluticasone propionate in patients with moderate to severe chronic obstructive pulmonary disease: the ISOLDE trial. BMJ 2000; 320:1297–1303.

119. Israel E, Banerjee TR, Fitzmaurice GM, et al. Effects of inhaled glucocorticoids on bone density in premenopausal women. N Engl J Med 2001; 345:941–947.

120. Pauwels RA, Buist AS, Ma P, et al. Global strategy for the diagnosis, management, and prevention of chronic obstructive pulmonary disease: National Heart, Lung, and Blood Institute and World Health Organization Global Initiative for Chronic Obstructive Lung Disease (GOLD): executive summary. Respir Care 2001; 46:798–825.

121. Culpitt SV, Maziak W, Loukidis S, et al. Effect of high dose inhaled steroid on cells, cytokines, and proteases in induced sputum in chronic obstructive pulmonary disease. Am J Respir Crit Care Med 1999; 160:1635–1639.

122. Keatings VM, Jatakanon A, Worsdell YM, et al. Effects of inhaled and oral glucocorticoids on inflammatory indices in asthma and COPD. Am J Respir Crit Care Med 1997; 155:542–548.

123. Gizycki MJ, Hattotuwa KL, Barnes N, et al. Effects of fluticasone propionate on inflam-matory cells in COPD: an ultrastructural examination of endobronchial biopsy tissue. Thorax 2002; 57:799–803.

124. Vestbo J, Sorensen T, Lange P, et al. Long-term effect of inhaled budesonide in mild and moderate chronic obstructive pulmonary disease: a randomised controlled trial. Lancet 1999; 353:1819–1823.

125. Pauwels RA, Lofdahl CG, Laitinen LA, et al. Long-term treatment with inhaled budesonide in persons with mild chronic obstructive pulmonary disease who continue smoking. European Respiratory Society Study on Chronic Obstructive Pulmonary Disease. N Engl J Med 1999; 340:1948–1953.

126. Lung Health Study Research Group. Effect of inhaled triamcinolone on the decline in pulmonary function in chronic obstructive pulmonary disease. N Engl J Med 2000; 343:1902–1909.

127. Sutherland ER. Inhaled corticosteroids in chronic obstructive pulmonary disease. Ann Intern Med 2003; 139:864–865.

128. Highland KB, Strange C, Heffner JE. Long-term effects of inhaled corticosteroids on FEV1 in patients with chronic obstructive pulmonary disease. A meta-analysis. Ann Intern Med 2003; 138:969–973.

129. Celli BR, Thomas NE, Anderson JA, et al. Effect of pharmacotherapy on rate of decline of lung function in chronic obstructive pulmonary disease: results from the TORCH study. Am J Respir Crit Care Med 2008; 178:332–338.

130. Szafranski W, Cukier A, Ramirez A, et al. Efficacy and safety of budesonide/formoterol in the management of chronic obstructive pulmonary disease. Eur Respir J 2003; 21:74–81.

131. Calverley PM, Anderson JA, Celli B, et al. Salmeterol and fluticasone propionate and survival in chronic obstructive pulmonary disease. N Engl J Med 2007; 356:775–789.

132. van der Valk P, Monninkhof E, van der Palen J, et al. Effect of discontinuation of inhaled corticosteroids in patients with chronic obstructive pulmonary disease: the COPE study. Am J Respir Crit Care Med 2002; 166:1358–1363.

133. Paggiaro PL, Dahle R, Bakran I, et al. Multicentre randomised placebo-controlled trial of inhaled fluticasone propionate in patients with chronic obstructive pulmonary disease. International COPD Study Group. Lancet 1998; 351:773–780.

134. Calverley PM, Rennard S, Nelson HS, et al. One-Year treatment with mometasone furoate in chronic obstructive pulmonary disease. Respir Res 2008; 9:73.

135. Wilt TJ, Niewoehner D, MacDonald R, et al. Management of stable chronic obstructive pulmonary disease: a systematic review for a clinical practice guideline. Ann Intern Med 2007; 147:639–653.

136. Calverley PM, Sanchez-Toril F, McIvor A, et al. Effect of 1-year treatment with roflumilast in severe chronic obstructive pulmonary disease. Am J Respir Crit Care Med 2007; 176:154–161.

137. Sin DD, McAlister FA, Man SF, et al. Contemporary management of chronic obstructive pulmonary disease: scientific review. JAMA 2003; 290:2301–2312.

138. Jones PW, Willits LR, Burge PS, et al. Disease severity and the effect of fluticasone propionate on chronic obstructive pulmonary disease exacerbations. Eur Respir J 2003; 21:68–73.

139. Wouters EF, Postma DS, Fokkens B, et al. Withdrawal of fluticasone propionate from combined salmeterol/fluticasone treatment in patients with COPD causes immediate and sustained disease deterioration: a randomised controlled trial. Thorax 2005; 60:480–487.

140. O'Brien A, Russo-Magno P, Karki A, et al. Effects of withdrawal of inhaled steroids in men with severe irreversible airflow obstruction. Am J Respir Crit Care Med 2001; 164:365–371.

141. Sin DD, Tu JV. Inhaled corticosteroids and the risk of mortality and readmission in elderly patients with chronic obstructive pulmonary disease. Am J Respir Crit Care Med 2001; 164:580–584.

142. Soriano JB, Kiri VA, Pride NB, et al. Inhaled corticosteroids with/without long-acting beta-agonists reduce the risk of rehospitalization and death in COPD patients. Am J Respir Med 2003; 2:67–74.

143. Soriano JB, Vestbo J, Pride NB, et al. Survival in COPD patients after regular use of fluticasone propionate and salmeterol in general practice. Eur Respir J 2002; 20:819–825.

144. Suissa S. Inhaled steroids and mortality in COPD: bias from unaccounted immortal time. Eur Respir J 2004; 23:391–395.

145. Sin DD, Man SF. Systemic inflammation and mortality in chronic obstructive pulmonary disease. Can J Physiol Pharmacol 2007; 85:141–147.

146. Calverley PM, Boonsawat W, Cseke Z, et al. Maintenance therapy with budesonide and formoterol in chronic obstructive pulmonary disease. Eur Respir J 2003; 22:912–919.

147. Jones PW. Measurement of quality of life in chronic obstructive lung disease. Eur Respir Rev 1991; 1:445–453.

148. Nannini L, Cates CJ, Lasserson TJ, et al. Combined corticosteroid and long acting beta-agonist in one inhaler for chronic obstructive pulmonary disease. Cochrane Database Syst Rev 2004; CD003794.

149. Usmani OS, Ito K, Maneechotesuwan K, et al. Glucocorticoid receptor nuclear translocation in airway cells after inhaled combination therapy. Am J Respir Crit Care Med 2005; 172:704–712.

150. Roth M, Johnson PR, Rudiger JJ, et al. Interaction between glucocorticoids and beta2 agonists on bronchial airway smooth muscle cells through synchronised cellular signalling. Lancet 2002; 360:1293–1299.

151. Chung KF, Adcock IM. Combination therapy of long-acting beta2-adrenoceptor agonists and corticosteroids for asthma. Treat Respir Med 2004; 3:279–289.

152. Barnes NC, Qiu YS, Pavord ID, et al. Antiinflammatory effects of salmeterol/fluticasone propionate in chronic obstructive lung disease. Am J Respir Crit Care Med 2006; 173:736–743.

153. Fitzgerald JM, Becker A, Sears MR, et al. Doubling the dose of budesonide versus maintenance treatment in asthma exacerbations. Thorax 2004; 59:550–556.

154. Harrison TW, Oborne J, Newton S, et al. Doubling the dose of inhaled corticosteroid to prevent asthma exacerbations: randomised controlled trial. Lancet 2004; 363:271–275.

155. Rice-McDonald G, Bowler S, Staines G, et al. Doubling daily inhaled corticosteroid dose is ineffective in mild to moderately severe attacks of asthma in adults. Intern Med J 2005; 35:693–698.

156. Gibson PG, Saltos N, Fakes K. Acute anti-inflammatory effects of inhaled budesonide in asthma: a randomized controlled trial. Am J Respir Crit Care Med 2001; 163:32–36.

157. Rodrigo G, Rodrigo C. Inhaled flunisolide for acute severe asthma. Am J Respir Crit Care Med 1998; 157:698–703.

158. Rodrigo GJ, Rodrigo C. Rapid-onset asthma attack: a prospective cohort study about characteristics and response to emergency department treatment. Chest 2000; 118:1547–1552.

159. Edmonds ML, Camargo CA Jr., Pollack CV Jr., et al. Early use of inhaled corticosteroids in the emergency department treatment of acute asthma. Cochrane Database Syst Rev 2003; CD002308.

160. Di Franco A, Bacci E, Bartoli ML, et al. Inhaled fluticasone propionate is effective as well as oral prednisone in reducing sputum eosinophilia during exacerbations of asthma which do not require hospitalization. Pulm Pharmacol Ther 2006; 19:353–360.

161. Levy ML, Stevenson C, Maslen T. Comparison of short courses of oral prednisolone and fluticasone propionate in the treatment of adults with acute exacerbations of asthma in primary care. Thorax 1996; 51:1087–1092.

162. Foresi A, Morelli MC, Catena E. Low-dose budesonide with the addition of an increased dose during exacerbations is effective in long-term asthma control. On behalf of the Italian Study Group. Chest 2000; 117:440–446.

163. Reddel HK, Barnes DJ. Pharmacological strategies for self-management of asthma exacerbations. Eur Respir J 2006; 28:182–199.

164. Maltais F, Ostinelli J, Bourbeau J, et al. Comparison of nebulized budesonide and oral prednisolone with placebo in the treatment of acute exacerbations of chronic obstructive pulmonary disease: a randomized controlled trial. Am J Respir Crit Care Med 2002; 165:698–703.

165. Donnelly R, Williams KM, Baker AB, et al. Effects of budesonide and fluticasone on 24-hour plasma cortisol. A dose-response study. Am J Respir Crit Care Med 1997; 156:1746–1751.

166. Clark DJ, Grove A, Cargill RI, et al. Comparative adrenal suppression with inhaled budesonide and fluticasone propionate in adult asthmatic patients. Thorax 1996; 51:262–266.

167. Todd GR. Adrenal crisis due to inhaled steroids is underestimated. Arch Dis Child 2003; 88:554–555.

168. Todd GR, Acerini CL, Ross-Russell R, et al. Survey of adrenal crisis associated with inhaled corticosteroids in the United Kingdom. Arch Dis Child 2002; 87:457–461.

169. Cumming RG, Mitchell P, Leeder SR. Use of inhaled corticosteroids and the risk of cataracts. N Engl J Med 1997; 337:8–14.

170. Garbe E, LeLorier J, Boivin JF, et al. Inhaled and nasal glucocorticoids and the risks of ocular hypertension or open-angle glaucoma. JAMA 1997; 277:722–727.

171. Wong CA, Walsh LJ, Smith CJ, et al. Inhaled corticosteroid use and bone-mineral density in patients with asthma. Lancet 2000; 355:1399–1403.

172. Pedersen S. Clinical safety of inhaled corticosteroids for asthma in children: an update of long-term trials. Drug Saf 2006; 29:599–612.

173. Tattersfield AE, Town GI, Johnell O, et al. Bone mineral density in subjects with mild asthma randomised to treatment with inhaled corticosteroids or non-corticosteroid treatment for two years. Thorax 2001; 56:272–278.

174. Elmstahl S, Ekstrom H, Galvard H, et al. Is there an association between inhaled corticosteroids and bone density in postmenopausal women? J Allergy Clin Immunol 2003; 111:91–96.

175. Kelly HW, Van Natta ML, Covar RA, et al. Effect of long-term corticosteroid use on bone mineral density in children: a prospective longitudinal assessment in the childhood Asthma Management Program (CAMP) study. Pediatrics 2008; 122:e53–e61.

176. van Staa TP, Leufkens HG, Cooper C. Use of inhaled corticosteroids and risk of fractures. J Bone Miner Res 2001; 16:581–588.

177. Suissa S, Baltzan M, Kremer R, et al. Inhaled and nasal corticosteroid use and the risk of fracture. Am J Respir Crit Care Med 2004; 169:83–88.

178. Lee TA, Weiss KB, Sullivan SD. Cost-effectiveness of inhaled corticosteroids in chronic obstructive pulmonary disease. Am J Med 2004; 117:618–619.

179. Etminan M, Sadatsafavi M, Ganjizadeh ZS, et al. Inhaled corticosteroids and the risk of fractures in older adults: a systematic review and meta-analysis. Drug Saf 2008; 31:409–414.

180. Bateman ED, Hurd SS, Barnes PJ, et al. Global strategy for asthma management and prevention: GINA executive summary. Eur Respir J 2008; 31:143–178.

181. Barnes PJ, Greening AP, Crompton GK. Glucocorticoid resistance in asthma. Am J Respir Crit Care Med 1995; 152:S125–S140.

182. Robinson DS, Campbell DA, Durham SR, et al. Systematic assessment of difficult-to-treat asthma. Eur Respir J 2003; 22:478–483.

183. The ENFUMOSA cross-sectional European multicentre study of the clinical phenotype of chronic severe asthma. Eur Respir J 2003; 22:470–477.

184. Moore WC, Bleecker ER, Curran-Everett D, et al. Characterisation of the severe asthma phenotype by the NHLBI severe asthma reserach program. J Allergy Clin Immunol 2007; 119:405–413.

185. Bumbacea D, Campbell D, Nguyen L, et al. Parameters associated with persistent airflow obstruction in chronic severe asthma. Eur Respir J 2004; 24:122–128.

186. Chung KF. Corticosteroid responsiveness in asthma: clinical aspects. In: Adcock IM, Chung KF, eds. Overcoming Steroid Insensitivity in Respiratory Disease. Chichester: John Wiley & Sons Ltd, 2007:89–108.

187. Charmandari E, Kino T. Novel causes of generalized glucocorticoid resistance. Horm Metab Res 2007; 39:445–450.

188. Lane SJ, Atkinson BA, Swaminathan R, et al. Hypothalamic-pituitary-adrenal axis in corticosteroid-resistant bronchial asthma. Am J Respir Crit Care Med 1996; 153:557–560.

189. Lane SJ, Palmer JB, Skidmore IF, et al. Corticosteroid pharmacokinetics in asthma. Lancet 1990; 336:1265.

190. Leung DY, Martin RJ, Szefler SJ, et al. Dysregulation of interleukin 4, interleukin 5, and interferon gamma gene expression in steroid-resistant asthma. J Exp Med 1995; 181:33–40.

191. Goleva E, Hauk PJ, Boguniewicz J, et al. Airway remodeling and lack of bronchodilator response in steroid-resistant asthma. J Allergy Clin Immunol 2007; 120(5):1065–1072.

192. Cohen L, Xueping E, Tarsi J, et al. Epithelial cell proliferation contributes to airway remodeling in severe asthma. Am J Respir Crit Care Med 2007; 176:138–145.

193. Hew M, Bhavsar P, Torrego A, et al. Relative corticosteroid insensitivity of peripheral blood mononuclear cells in severe asthma. Am J Respir Crit Care Med 2006; 174:134–141.

194. Gan WQ, Man P, Sin DD. Effects of inhaled corticosteroids on sputum cell counts in stable chronic obstructive pulmonary disease: a systematic review and a meta-analysis. BMC Pulm Med 2005; 5:3.

195. Culpitt SV, Rogers DF, Shah P, et al. Impaired Inhibition by dexamethasone of cytokine release by alveolar macrophages from patients with chronic obstructive pulmonary disease. Am J Respir Crit Care Med 2003; 167:24–31.

196. Marban C, Suzanne S, Dequiedt F, et al. Recruitment of chromatin-modifying enzymes by CTIP2 promotes HIV-1 transcriptional silencing. EMBO J 2007; 26:412–423.

197. Szulakowski P, Crowther AJ, Jimenez LA, et al. The effect of smoking on the transcriptional regulation of lung inflammation in patients with chronic obstructive pulmonary disease. Am J Respir Crit Care Med 2006; 174:41–50.

198. Ito K, Lim S, Caramori G, et al. A molecular mechanism of action of theophylline: Induction of histone deacetylase activity to decrease inflammatory gene expression. Proc Natl Acad Sci U S A 2002; 99:8921–8926.

199. Ito K, Yamamura S, Essilfie-Quaye S, et al. Histone deacetylase 2-mediated deacetylation of the glucocorticoid receptor enables NF-kappaB suppression. J Exp Med 2006; 203:7–13.

200. Carmichael J, Paterson IC, Diaz P, et al. Corticosteroid resistance in chronic asthma. Br Med J (Clin Res Ed) 1981; 282:1419–1422.

201. Lane SJ, Arm JP, Staynov DZ, et al. Chemical mutational analysis of the human glucocorticoid receptor cDNA in glucocorticoid-resistant bronchial asthma. Am J Respir Cell Mol Biol 1994; 11:42–48.

202. Hakonarson H, Bjornsdottir US, Halapi E, et al. Profiling of genes expressed in peripheral blood mononuclear cells predicts glucocorticoid sensitivity in asthma patients. Proc Natl Acad Sci U S A 2005; 102:14789–14794.

203. Donn R, Berry A, Stevens A, et al. Use of gene expression profiling to identify a novel glucocorticoid sensitivity determining gene, BMPRII. FASEB J 2007; 21:402–414.

204. Irusen E, Matthews JG, Takahashi A, et al. p38 Mitogen-activated protein kinase-induced glucocorticoid receptor phosphorylation reduces its activity: role in steroid-insensitive asthma. J Allergy Clin Immunol 2002; 109:649–657.

205. Webster JC, Oakley RH, Jewell CM, et al. Proinflammatory cytokines regulate human glucocorticoid receptor gene expression and lead to the accumulation of the dominant negative beta isoform: a mechanism for the generation of glucocorticoid resistance. Proc Natl Acad Sci U S A 2001; 98:6865–6870.

206. Goleva E, Li LB, Eves PT, et al. Increased glucocorticoid receptor beta alters steroid response in glucocorticoid-insensitive asthma. Am J Respir Crit Care Med 2006; 173:607–616.

207. Lane SJ, Adcock IM, Richards D, et al. Corticosteroid-resistant bronchial asthma is associated with increased c-fos expression in monocytes and T lymphocytes. J Clin Invest 1998; 102:2156–2164.

208. Barnes PJ, Ito K, Adcock IM. Corticosteroid resistance in chronic obstructive pulmonary disease: inactivation of histone deacetylase. Lancet 2004; 363:731–733.

209. Rahman I, Adcock IM. Oxidative stress and redox regulation of lung inflammation in COPD. Eur Respir J 2006; 28:219–242.

210. Hawrylowicz CM. Regulatory T cells and IL-10 in allergic inflammation. J Exp Med 2005; 202:1459–1463.

211. Loke TK, Mallett KH, Ratoff J, et al. Systemic glucocorticoid reduces bronchial mucosal activation of activator protein 1 components in glucocorticoid-sensitive but not glucocorticoid-resistant asthmatic patients. J Allergy Clin Immunol 2006; 118:368–375.

212. Goleva E, Kisich KO, Leung DY. A role for STAT5 in the pathogenesis of IL-2-induced glucocorticoid resistance. J Immunol 2002; 169:5934–5940.

213. Cosio BG, Tsaprouni L, Ito K, et al. Theophylline restores histone deacetylase activity and steroid responses in COPD macrophages. J Exp Med 2004; 200:689–695.

214. Fox JC, Spicer D, Ito K, et al. Oral or inhaled corticosteroid combination therapy with low dose theophylline reverses corticosteroid insensitivity in a smoking mouse model. Proc Am Thorac Soc 2007; 2:A637.

215. Ahmad T, Barnes PJ, Adcock IM. Overcoming steroid insensitivity in smoking asthmatics. Curr Opin Investig Drugs 2008; 9:470–477.

216. Marone R, Cmiljanovic V, Giese B, et al. Targeting phosphoinositide 3-kinase: moving towards therapy. Biochim Biophys Acta 2008; 1784:159–185.

217. Barnes PJ. Emerging targets for COPD therapy. Curr Drug Targets Inflamm Allergy 2005; 4:675–683.

218. Adcock IM, Caramori G, Chung KF. New targets for drug development in asthma. Lancet 2008; 372:1073–1087.

219. Caramori G, Adcock I. Pharmacology of airway inflammation in asthma and COPD. Pulm Pharmacol Ther 2003; 16:247–277.

220. Paul-Clark MJ, Roviezzo F, Flower RJ, et al. Glucocorticoid receptor nitration leads to enhanced anti-inflammatory effects of novel steroid ligands. J Immunol 2003; 171:3245–3252.

221. Nevin BJ, Broadley KJ. Comparative effects of inhaled budesonide and the NO-donating budesonide derivative, NCX 1020, against leukocyte influx and airway hyperreactivity following lipopolysaccharide challenge. Pulm Pharmacol Ther 2004; 17:219–232.

222. Derendorf H. Pharmacokinetic and pharmacodynamic properties of inhaled ciclesonide. J Clin Pharmacol 2007; 47:782–789.

223. Schacke H, Schottelius A, Docke WD, et al. Dissociation of transactivation from transrepression by a selective glucocorticoid receptor agonist leads to separation of therapeutic effects from side effects. Proc Natl Acad Sci U S A 2004; 101:227–232.

224. Schacke H, Docke WD, Asadullah K. Mechanisms involved in the side effects of glucocorticoids. Pharmacol Ther 2002; 96:23–43.

225. Miner JN, Ardecky B, Benbatoul K, et al. Antiinflammatory glucocorticoid receptor ligand with reduced side effects exhibits an altered protein-protein interaction profile. Proc Natl Acad Sci U S A 2007; 104:19244–19249.

226. Ogawa S, Lozach J, Benner C, et al. Molecular determinants of crosstalk between nuclear receptors and toll-like receptors. Cell 2005; 122:707–721.

227. Farrow SN. Nuclear receptors: doubling up in the lung. Curr Opin Pharmacol 2008; 8:275–279.

228. Renda T, Baraldo S, Pelaia G, et al. Increased activation of p38 MAPK in COPD. Eur Respir J 2008; 31:62–69.

229. Ito K, Caramori G, Adcock IM. Therapeutic potential of phosphatidylinositol 3-kinase inhibitors in inflammatory respiratory disease. J Pharmacol Exp Ther 2007; 321:1–8.

230. Marwick JA, Caramori G, Stevenson CS, et al. Inhibition of PI3Kdelta restores glucocorticoid function in smoking-induced airway inflammation in mice. Am J Respir Crit Care Med 2009; 179:542–548.

231. Rothschild BM. Review: individual DMARDs have similar efficacy for RA, but combination therapy improves response. Evid Based Med 2008; 13:76.

7

Bronchodilator Therapy of Airway Diseases

JAMES F. DONOHUE
University of North Carolina at Chapel Hill, Chapel Hill, North Carolina, U.S.A.

JILL OHAR
Wake Forest University School of Medicine, Winston-Salem, North Carolina, U.S.A.

I. Introduction

Both short-acting and long-acting bronchodilators have been used for many years for the treatment of asthma and chronic obstructive pulmonary disease (COPD). Patient response to these agents is characterized by a large degree of heterogeneity due in part to genetic variability and differences in disease severity. Furthermore, initiation of guideline-based treatment is often poorly applied in developed countries because of lack of awareness and in developing countries because of cost or cultural preferences. Increasing emphasis is placed on "asthma control," that is, the extent to which the manifestations of asthma have been reduced or removed by treatment (1). Its assessment should incorporate the dual components of current clinical control (i.e., symptoms, reliever use, and lung function) and future risk (e.g., exacerbations and lung function decline). The most clinically useful concept of severity is based on the intensity of treatment required to achieve good control, that is, severity is assessed during treatment. For example, severe asthma requires high-intensity treatment. Severity may be influenced by underlying disease activity and patient phenotype (1).

There are many benefits of short-acting β-adrenergics (SABAs) as lifesaving medications, and their role as rescue agents in both conditions is unquestioned (Table 1). However, regular SABA use is not recommended in asthma because of safety concerns and the effectiveness of controller medications. In COPD, regular use is common especially via nebulizer in older and more severely ill patients, while in asthma, nebulizers are used in the very young and in the acute setting. Long-acting β-adrenergics (LABAs) are effective controller medications when used with ICS in asthma but safety issues also exist prompting multiple safety reviews at the FDA. Because of this, LABA use should be restricted to those who are not optimally controlled on first-line controllers such as inhaled corticosteroids (ICSs). In COPD use of LABA/long-acting muscarinic agents (LAMAs) alone or together, often with an ICS, is commonplace. The role of the β-receptor genotype in affecting β-agonist response is unclear but could hold promise in the future for optimal patient management. Long- and short-acting anticholinergics are more effective in COPD but can have a role in asthma. Oral methylxanthines also have a therapeutic role in both and are widely used in developing nations.

Table 1   Effects of β-Adrenergic Agonists on Airways

Relaxes airway smooth-muscle (proximal and distal airways)
Inhibitors mast-cell mediator release
Inhibitors plasma exudation and airway edema
Increases mucociliary clearance
Increase mucus secretion
Decreases cholinergic neurotransmission
Decrease cough
No effect on chronic inflammation

Source: Adapted from Ref. 2.

II.   β₂-Agonists and the Airway

The safety of β_2-agonists along with the heterogeneity of responses has become once again the focus of concern. Clearly, these agents are effective in both asthma and COPD. These sympathomimetic agents stimulate β_2-receptors in airway cells to produce a variety of effects (2). Chief among these are smooth muscle relaxation and broncho-dilation caused by activation of adenylyl cyclase to produce cyclic 3′,5′-adenosine monophosphate (AMP). β_2-agonists are differentiated as SABAs with 3- to 6-hour duration of action and LABAs with duration of action of or exceeding 12 hours. Figure 1 depicts the evolution of the most commonly used SABA, albuterol, from the less selective agents, epinephrine, norepinephrine, and isoproterenol. Figure 1 also depicts the structure of the two currently available LABAs, salmeterol and formoterol. In the future, new 24-hour ultra-long-acting β-agonists such as indacaterol, GSK 444, com-bined with novel anticholinergics such as aclidinium bromide, stereoisomeric for-mulations including arformoterol and levalbuterol, and new combination platforms such as M3 muscarinic antagonist and β_2-agonist (MABA) are likely to be introduced for both asthma and COPD.

III.   Short-Acting β-Agonists

A.   Efficacy

SABAs are highly effective rescue agents that can be given by oral, parenteral, or inhalation routes of administration. However, the inhalational route is generally pre-ferred as it has the highest therapeutic ratio (beneficial effects/side effects). SABAs use is widespread in a variety of conditions that have airway abnormalities and have con-sistently been shown to produce effective bronchodilation with improved lung function as well as bronchoprotection against a variety of stimuli. Because of their short duration of action, however, they are not considered maintenance medication in asthma and COPD and are generally reserved for "as-needed" use. Guidelines such as GINA and NAEPP recommend the SABAs be used as needed in all stages of asthma for adults and children. Furthermore, frequency of SABA use is one component of classifying severity and initiating treatment as well as an indicator of asthma control used to adjust treat-ment. As for classification, short-acting β_2-agonist use of <2 days a week is intermittent; >2 days a week but not daily or more than once on any day is mild persistent; daily use is moderate persistent and several times per day is severe persistent. As for impairment

CORRECT Albuterol

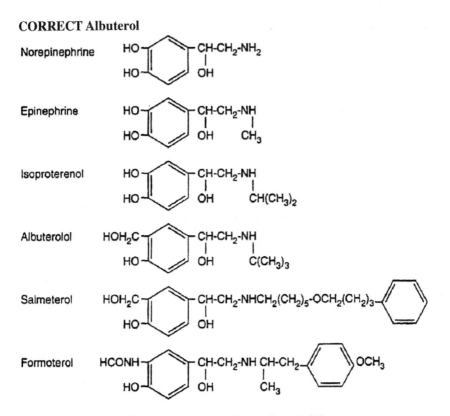

Figure 1   Structures of β-adrenergic agonists. *Source*: From Ref. 2.

and control, <2 days a week is well controlled, >2 days a week is not well controlled, and several times a day is very poorly controlled (3,4).

B. Mild Asthma

Treatment strategies in mild asthma are undergoing intense scrutiny. Mild asthma has been divided into mild intermittent and mild persistent for which regular use of low-dose ICS was recommended. Recent trials have questioned the assumption that that all patients at the mild end of the spectrum should be subjected to regular use of ICS (5). Options include as-needed inhaled beclomethasone plus albuterol, oral leukotriene receptor antagonist plus as-needed albuterol, or once-daily corticosteroid plus LABA in a single inhaler (6). The combined use of beclomethasone and albuterol in a single inhaler was effective as rescue in mild asthma (7). In a study of 455 patients with mild asthma with a forced expiratory volume in one second (FEV$_1$) of 88% of predicted, the combination of BDP and albuterol when used as needed had a higher AM peak flow rate in the last two weeks of the study and lower numbers of exacerbations over six months than as-needed albuterol alone. No significant differences from those on regular beclomethasone or regular combination therapy were noted. Therefore, symptom-driven use of a single inhaler with low-dose BDP and SABA might be an attractive step-down steroid-sparing therapy for mild persistent asthma (7).

C. Safety of SABAs

In asthma the safety profile of SABAs has been adequate for most patients although there have been concerns for decades that some patients may experience serious adverse effects (8). β-Adrenergic bronchodilators, even when inhaled, can have systemic as well as local effects. Older asthmatics may experience more adverse effects due to pharmacodynamic as well as pharmacokinetic changes with drug-drug and drug-disease interactions. β-Adrenergic agonists have inotropic and chronotropic effects that can increase arrhythmias and aggravate cardiomyopathy in some patients with cardiovascular disease (9). Tremor can be bothersome to some while some older patients can have anxiety with regular use. The effects of long-term use on tolerance, deteriorating disease control, and deaths are controversial. For example, SABAs were implicated in two epidemics of deaths due to asthma in the 1960s and 1970s in the United Kingdom and New Zealand (10,11). The mechanism(s) of death, however, were not clear but could include excessive β-agonist use in very sick asthmatics, rebound hyperresponsiveness due to short duration of action, tachyphylaxis, lack of anti-inflammatory corticosteroid use, or some other ill-defined process (12,13). The effect may have also been more common with specific β-agonists such as isoproterenol and fenoterol, so-called complete β_2-agonist. In one epidemic, there was a correlation between fenoterol prescriptions and market share and asthma mortality. When high-dose fenoterol was withdrawn from the market, the asthma mortality returned back to baseline (14).

More focused studies in the early 1990s also suggested that regular use of SABAs may produce serious adverse effects. Taylor et al. in a study of 64 patients, 50 of whom were on ICSs, analyzed the number of subjects without exacerbations versus the number of days of treatment (15). When β-agonists were used as needed as opposed to "regular use," a corresponding marked reduction in the frequency of exacerbations was noted. The possibility was raised that there were more exacerbations, occurring earlier and with greater severity, with a greater decline in FEV_1, more diurnal variation in peak expiratory flow (PEF), and greater sensitivity to methacholine with regular use of β-agonists in asthma.

In the United States, the NIH Asthma Clinical Research Network (ACRN) also noted some conflicting signals with regular use of SABAs. The β-agonists in mild asthma (BAGS) trial was designed to compare regular albuterol versus as-needed in 255 patients with mild asthma (16). After a 6-week run-in period patients were randomized to the therapy for 16 weeks followed by an additional 4-week run-out period. In this study, PEF was higher with as-needed albuterol versus regular treatment with albuterol. However, there were no differences in the primary outcome of PEF variability, FEV_1, number of puffs of albuterol, or symptoms. The conclusion was that as-needed SABA therapy was preferable to regular SABA use.

D. Genetic Variation in the β_2-Receptor and SABA Responses

Over the last decade, there has been a growing interest in genetic variations (polymorphisms) at several locations in the β_2-receptor ADRB2 (Fig. 2) and whether these variations might explain different β-agonist responses (17). The ADRB2 is a small

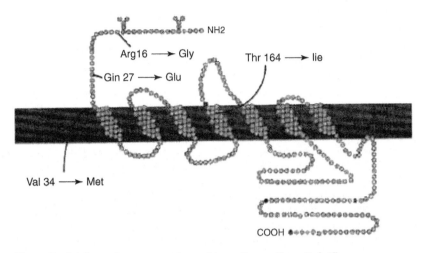

NH2

Arg16 ——▶ Gly   Thr 164 ——▶ Iie

Gin 27 ——▶ Glu

Val 34 ——▶ Met

COOH

Figure 2 β-Adrenergic receptor polymorphisms. *Source*: From Ref. 17.

intronless gene having many polymorphisms, two of which at amino acid 16 (GLY16ARG) and 27 (GLN27GLU) have functional relevance. Taylor noted that differences at position B16 between Arg/Arg and Gly/Gly may be important in the response to β-agonists (18). This led to a retrospective genetic analysis of the BAGS data (19). There was no effect seen with variations at the B27 locus, and no effect seen with B16 heterozygotes (Arg/Gly). However, when B16 Arg/Arg patients (1/6 of the population) were compared to B16 Gly/Gly patients, a difference was found in the primary outcome variable, a lower PEF, particularly noticeable during the four-week run-out period. Taylor et al. studied the influence of β-adrenergic receptor polymorphisms on asthma exacerbations (20). Those with the Arg/Arg at position B16 who received regular albuterol had more exacerbations than those with placebo and those on salmeterol. Individuals with Gly/Arg or Gly/Gly showed no such differences.

The β-Adrenergic Response by Genotype (BARGE) prospective analysis studied regular scheduled albuterol versus as-needed albuterol (21). Patients were screened and genotyped. They had six-week run-in period while on placebo. Then they received 16 weeks of treatment on active drug or placebo and an 8-week run-out. Then there was a crossover to 16 weeks receiving placebo or active treatment and a second 8-week run-out. Those on regular albuterol with B16 Arg/Arg had a much lower PEF than those on placebo or those with regular albuterol and B16 Gly/Gly. The conclusions of the BARGE study were as follows: the PEF, FEV_1, symptoms, and rescue inhaler use improved significantly in B16 Arg/Arg patients with asthma when regular β-agonists were withdrawn and ipratropium was substituted. The pattern was reversed in B16 Gly/Gly patients with asthma. These findings suggested that B-16 Arg/Arg patients (1/6 of asthmatics) may benefit from minimizing (SABA) use. More recent studies including genome-wide association studies implicate variants in other genes that contribute to bronchodilator response heterogeneity and have not replicated the worsening of asthma with continuous β-agonist use seen in earlier trials.

E. Stereoisomers

The SABA albuterol exists as a racemic mixture containing 2 enantiomers (R)-albuterol or levalbuterol and (S)-albuterol. Some have found the S-isomer to be proinflammatory while others question the relative clinical value compared with racemic albuterol (22). The lower doses (1.25, 0.63) available with levalbuterol have lead to widespread use in pediatrics; the (R)-albuterol form is available in some countries as a PMDI and solution. This isomer when compared in clinical trials with the racemic mixture is a little longer acting (6–8 vs. 4–6 hours duration) but is more expensive (23). Some studies suggest a benefit when used in the emergency room and in inpatient services (24). Adverse event profiles are similar with little safety advantage over the racemic mixture. Stereoisomeric forms of LABAs such as arformoterol and carmoterol are presently being evaluated in both asthma and COPD (25).

F. Conclusions on SABAs

SABAs bronchodilators are essential as rescue medications to relieve symptoms, prevent exercise-induced bronchospasm, and treat acute exacerbations. Usually in these acute settings, high doses can be given at short intervals. In contrast, there appears to be no benefit of regular use of SABAs in the maintenance therapy of asthma. Additional research should clarify the role of β receptor polymorphisms but it does appear that regular use can be associated with loss of control with some polymorphisms. There appears to be limited loss of efficacy in COPD with regular use and only modest effect of polymorphism although less well studied. The frequency of use of SABA can be used to classify asthma severity and assess control. Recent studies suggest a possible role of the combination of SABA/ICS in mild persistent and intermittent asthma.

IV. Long-Acting β-Agonists

A. Efficacy

The LABAs have been developed as maintenance therapy for obstructive airway disease. As with SABAs, the inhalational route provides the highest therapeutic ratio. These agents act by effecting prolonged stimulation of the β_2-adrenergic receptor. In clinical trials these agents have diminished symptoms, improved lung function, and reduced exacerbations when combined with ICS in asthmatics. A recent Cochrane review of 67 studies involving over 42,000 patients concluded that LABAs indeed were effective in the control of chronic asthma, and their use (both with and without ICSs) was associated with better pulmonary function, fewer symptoms, less rescue medications, and higher quality of life scores (26). Similarly, a Cochrane review in COPD also affirms modest efficacy and safety (27) although not all share this conclusion (28). The additive effect of LABAs in combination with ICS in asthma was first noted by Greening (29). Systematic reviews of LABA/ICS combinations in asthma show superiority over placebo and over doubling the dose of ICS in adults (30). In fact, the Formoterol and Corticosteroid Establishing Therapy (FACET) trial compared asthma control with up to a fourfold increase in the budesonide dose with low-dose budesonide and formoterol. Time with well-controlled asthma was increased by 19% while time with poorly controlled was significantly reduced by 43% (31).

This combination also leads to more patients with "well-controlled" asthma. These observations have been incorporated into asthma Guidelines where LABAs may be added to ICS or other controllers for those not controlled on ICS alone or those whose severity warrants a combination. In youths aged 12 years and adults, step 3 preferred therapy is either low-dose ICs and LABA or medium-dose ICS. For steps 4 to 6, LABAs plus increasing dose of ICS is preferred. In children, the benefits of combinations of ICS/LABA is less robust and the guideline recommendation for children aged 5 to 11 for step 3 is either low-dose ICS plus LABA or LTRA or theophylline or medium-dose ICS. The combination of salmeterol/fluticasone (SFC) 50/100 μg b.i.d. compared favorably with twice the steroid dose [fluticasone propionate (FP) 200 μg b.i.d.] in clinical outcomes (MEF 50%, vital capacity, rescue free days) and overall control in 321 children aged 4 to 11 (32).

For many patients, asthma may not be controlled as defined by guidelines; the Gaining Optimal Asthma Control (GOAL) study attempted to look at control prospectively (33). In this one-year stratified double blind, parallel-group study of 3421 patients with uncontrolled asthma SFC was compared with FP in achieving two rigorous, composite, guideline based measures of control: totally and well-controlled asthma. Significantly, more patients in each stratum (previously steroid-free, and low- and moderate-dose corticosteroid users) achieved control with SFC than FP alone. Total control at one year was 41% versus 28% and well-controlled was 71% versus 59% for SFC and FP, respectively. Exacerbation rates and improvements in health status were significantly better with SFC. In a post hoc analysis, patients achieving well-controlled or totally controlled asthma, at least well-controlled asthma was maintained for months with regular stable dosing (34) and this study illustrates the effectiveness of LABA when added to ICS.

B. Novel Uses

A potential novel use of LABA is combined with ICS and given once daily in mild asthma. In a study by the American Lung Association Asthma Clinical Research Centers, once-daily use of a combination inhaler of low-dose ICS and LABA SFC provided better asthma control than once-daily montelukast and greater convenience than twice daily ICS (6). Theoretically lower doses of ICS could be used while affording comparable control with this approach. Although once-daily dosing of ICS/LABA is not presently approved by FDA, longer-acting once-daily agents are in clinical trials such as GSK's Horizon and indacaterol (QAB)/mometasone (QMF). Another potential use of ICS/LABA is in flexible dosing, a maintenance and rescue (M&R) use of the same combination inhaler. In a double-blind, randomized, parallel group study, 2760 patients with asthma aged 4 to 80 years, with FEV_1 ranging from 60% to 100%, received budesonide 320 μg b.i.d. with SABA, BUD/FORM 80/4.5 μg b.i.d. with terbutaline as SABA, or BUD/FORM 80/4.5 μg b.i.d. and as needed (BUD/FORM maintenance and relief). BUD/FORM M&R prolonged time to first severe exacerbation ($p < 0.0010$), resulting in a 45% to 47% lower exacerbation risk versus BUD/FORM + SABA [hazard ratio (HR), 0.55; 95% confidence interval (CI), 0.44, 0.67] or BUD + SABA (HR, 0.53; 95% CI, 0.43, 0.65). BUD/FORM M&R also prolonged the time to first, second, and third exacerbation requiring medical intervention, reduced severe exacerbation rate, and improved symptoms, awakenings, and lung function compared with both fixed dose regimens (35).

C. Safety of LABAs

As with SABAs, safety concerns exist for LABAs in asthma. For example, the use of LABA alone might offer false reassurance by improving symptom scores, morning PEF, and even composite control scores but, because they do not treat the underlying disease process, they may expose the patient to a greater risk of exacerbation. Thus, there is widespread agreement that LABA should never be used as monotherapy for patients with asthma. The first pertinent large safety study was the Serevent surveillance study or the SNS study by Castle et al. (36). In the SNS, there was no run-in and there was a requirement for regular use of bronchodilators. Of those participating, 69% were on concurrent inhaled steroids. In the SNS 16,787 patients received salmeterol and 8393 received albuterol. There were no significant differences in overall serious events, withdrawals, or asthma-related hospitalizations, but there was a slight increase in asthma-related deaths with 12 in the salmeterol group and 2 in the albuterol group. The relative risk (RR) was 3.0 but it was not statistically significant ($p = 0.105$). Asthma-related withdrawals were much greater in the albuterol group and this was statistically significant ($p = 0.0002$).

The Salmeterol Multicenter Asthma Research Trial (SMART) study was performed in the United States following the approval of salmeterol for asthma maintenance (37). This large study included 13,176 patients who were randomized to salmeterol and a similar number who received placebo plus usual care for a 28-week period. Patients were followed with phone contacts every four weeks and case reports of serious adverse events were collected. The primary outcomes were respiratory deaths or life-threatening experiences (intubations). Secondary endpoints were: (*i*) respiratory deaths, (*ii*) asthma death or life-threatening experience, or (*iii*) asthma death. A morbidity and mortality review committee (MMRC) reviewed all the events and determined if respiratory and/or asthma-related using a scale of (*i*) unrelated, (*ii*) unlikely related, (*iii*) possibly related, and (*iv*) almost certainly related. The Data Safety Monitoring Board (DSMB) performed a study oversight interim analysis. While the SMART did not reach predetermined stopping criterion at the interim analysis, the study was discontinued due to difficulties in enrollment and safety concerns especially in African-American patients.

The results of SMART have been controversial. There were differences in baseline asthma characteristics between Caucasians and African-American with the latter group having a lower PEF at baseline, more nocturnal symptoms, more emergency department (ED) visits, and hospitalizations in their lifetime. Also in the previous 12 months, African-Americans had more hospitalizations, and more ED visits and over lifetime more intubations. There were differences in baseline in ICS use (Caucasians, 49%; African-Americans, 38%). In SMART, 13 died in the Salmeterol arm versus 3 in the placebo arm (RR 4.37; 95% CI, 1.25–15.34). On the primary end point of respiratory death or life-threatening experiences, there was no significant difference overall (RR 1.40, 0.91–2.14) but in the African-American patients, there were important changes between salmeterol and placebo: RR 4.1(1.54–10.90). SMART was not designed to assess the effects of ICSs when added to LABAs, but they did appear to provide a protective effect that has been supported by a subsequent meta-analysis (38). Data from 62 studies of over 29,000 participants of which 15,710 were on LABAs, revealed only 3 asthma-related deaths, 2 intubations with no significant difference in asthma-related serious asthma events such as hospitalization. The odds ratio (OR) for total mortality was 1.26 (95% CI, 0.58–2.74).

A meta-analysis of 19 studies involving LABA use in over 33,000 patients concluded that LABA use was associated with increased exacerbations and asthma deaths (39). Of note is that these conclusions were driven heavily by the SMART results and the authors noted that asthma deaths were a very rare event in all studies. Other meta-analyses do not find a mortality effect resulting from LABA use (40,41). Within this backdrop, the U.S. Food and Drug Administration (FDA) issued a "black box" warning for all LABAs (42).

Importantly, the finding of excessive deaths with salmeterol in SMART contrasts with national statistical data comparing U.S. prescriptions for salmeterol and salmeterol/ICS combination products and asthma deaths. Whereas the number of asthma deaths peaked above 5000 in the middle 1990s in the United States, the death rates have declined below 4000 in the 2000s as the prescriptions for salmeterol and ICS/salmeterol have increased. Extrapolation of the mortality data from SMART suggests that in 2004 there would have been two- to threefold more asthma deaths than were actually reported in the national statistics. It is reassuring to note that this did not occur.

Safety concerns for the other available LABA, formoterol, focus less on excess deaths and more on serious asthma exacerbations (43). In the three pivotal studies plus the postmarketing 16-week phase IV study, there seemed to be a signal that with formoterol serious asthma exacerbations were more common, especially with higher doses in the pediatric study (44,45). However, in the large postmarketing study, serious asthma-related adverse events requiring hospitalizations were rarely seen in any group (46). In phase III studies, serious asthma exacerbations occurred more frequently with formoterol 24 µg b.i.d. than formoterol 12 µg b.i.d. The 24 µg b.i.d. dose is not approved in the United States nor is the M&R approach.

A review of formoterol safety data from all AstraZeneca clinical trials of 3 to 12 months in duration found no increase in asthma-related deaths in 49,906 patients exposed to formoterol versus 18,098 not exposed. Asthma-related severe adverse events (SAEs) such as hospitalization were significantly fewer among formoterol exposed (0.75% vs. 1.10%). All-cause mortality was similar. There was neither increasing dose response for asthma SAEs nor significant cardiac-related SAEs. However, despite data on >68,000 patients the power was insufficient to conclude that there was no increased mortality with formoterol (47).

As with salmeterol, when ICSs are added to formoterol, risks of asthma deaths and serious adverse events such as hospitalization and intubation seen with LABA mono-therapy seem to be diminished (38). A systematic review and meta-analysis of LABA (both salmeterol and formoterol) concluded that in 15,710 patients using ICS, LABA did not increase the risk of asthma-related hospitalization (OR, 0.74; 95%; CI, 0.53 to 1.03). There were few asthma-related deaths and intubations but events were too infrequent to establish LABA's relative effect on these outcomes.

The recent FDA joint meeting of the Pediatric Advisory Committee, Drug Safety and Risk Management Committee, and the Pulmonary-Allergy Drug Advisory Committee was conducted to review benefits and the risks of LABA including asthma deaths, intubations, and hospitalizations in adults as well as children. The FDA conducted a meta-analysis of 110 randomized parallel controlled trials involving 60,954 patients and noted a composite risk of 2.80 more events per 1000 patients with LABA (48) (Fig. 3). In trials comparing those with LABA to non-LABA therapy, the difference in rates was 3.63 per 1000 subjects. In trials of LABA plus ICS versus ICS alone, the difference was only 0.25 per 1000 subjects. For single agent LABA, the benefits do not appear to outweigh the risk particularly in children. While fixed drug combinations appeared to be beneficial and safe in adults and adolescents, the efficacy/safety data are less robust in

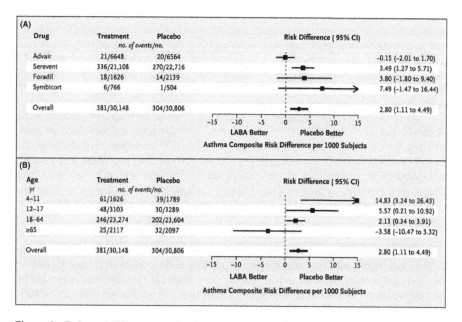

Figure 3 Estimated differences in the risk of asthma-related death, intubation, or hospitalization according to medication used (panel A) and age group (panel B).

children. Despite 20 years of debate, several hearings, black box warnings, and meta-analysis, controversy over LABA safety continues provoking yet another call for a large and definitive study (49,50), which may not be practical.

D. Pharmacogenetics of LABAs

As with SABAs, the effect of LABA therapy on asthmatic control by ADRB2genotype is under intense scrutiny. Taylor et al. compared the PEF response in patients with differing genotypes at B-16 receiving albuterol or salmeterol (18). The patients, who received regular albuterol for 26 weeks, who had the B-16 Arg/Arg genotypes had lower PEF than those who had Arg/Gly or Gly/Gly genotypes. In contrast no such reduction in PEF was noted when salmeterol was given regularly. There was no unusual drop off in PEF during the run-out period. These contrasts with the NIH ACRN's two studies (SOCS and SLIC) of salmeterol: one of salmeterol monotherapy after discontinuing ICS and the second combined with ICS. Compared with Gly/Gly individuals, Arg/Arg homozygous patients retrospectively studied did not benefit from salmeterol and had decreased PEF flow, increased PEF variability, and increased exhaled nitric oxide. The difference in PEF and PEF variability was accentuated in the run-out period (51).

Retrospective pharmacogenetic analysis in all racial groups and in both adults and children have not found an association between ADBR2 Gly16Arg genotype and poor asthma control with salmeterol and formoterol but a prospective trial by the NIH ACRN has been initiated. Recent large pharmaceutical studies have revealed no effect of β-receptor genotype on the response to LABAs when combined with ICS (52,53). In one study, 2250 asthmatics were randomized to fixed combination of budesonide/formoterol, fixed-dose fluticasone/salmeterol, budesonide plus formoterol maintenance and as rescue. In this study, B16 polymorphisms had no effects on exacerbations, lung function, or the use of rescue medications. In a second trial of 405 asthmatics, an open label extension for seven months also did not show any pharmacogenetic effects of variation at site B16.

A number of new so-called ultra-LABAs are in phase III trials and are soon to be available. Because of safety concerns, most new LABA agents are submitted as monotherapy for COPD alone and in combination with an ICS for asthma. For example, the LABA GW642444 is being combined with the ICS GW685698 in a fixed drug product in the horizon development program. Indacaterol is combined with mometasone (QMF) in another fixed drug asthma program. Agents such as arformoterol are also available with similar safety and efficacy profiles as formoterol but are licensed for COPD only at this time.

E. Conclusions on LABAs

LABAs are highly effective maintenance agents in asthma. However, they should be used only in combination with an ICS and not as monotherapy in asthma as suggested by the National Asthma Guidelines for patients with step 3 or greater severity (3). Several large ongoing studies of LABA use and B16 polymorphisms are underway, which should clarify some of these issues. At the present time, ADRB2 variants do not appear to be associated with poor asthma control with LABAs.

V. Theophylline

Theophylline continues to be widely used in standard doses in asthma as a bronchodilator but it can also modulate the immune response. This agent is available worldwide and is inexpensive. However, the frequency of side effects with oral delivery limits its use. Effects due to adenosine receptor antagonism and phosphodiesterase inhibition are not clarified. Low-dose theophylline can control asthma through increasing activation of the histone deacetylase, which is subsequently recruited by corticosteroids to suppress inflammatory genes. Theophylline may have a role in special populations. Cigarette smoke reduces histone deacetylase (HDAC) activity; smokers with asthma are often poorly controlled with increased symptoms, frequent emergency room visits, and an impaired response to oral and ICSs. When low-dose (400 mg/day) theophylline was added to beclomethasone in a pilot study, improvements in PEF (39.9 L/min, 95% CI, 10.9 to 68.8) and ACQ scores (−0.47, 95% CL, −0.91 to −0.04) while increasing prebronchodilator FEV_1 (165 mL, 95% CL, −13 to 342) relative to ICS alone (54).

Novel approaches including using the inhalation route to reduce side effects and combining with ICS are undergoing study (55). Recently the combination of ICS and LABA was shown to be more effective than ICS and theophylline in moderate asthma patients (56).

VI. Bronchodilators in Asthma—Conclusions

The two combinations presently available of fluticasone and salmeterol and budesonide and formoterol appear to have similar effectiveness (57). As noted by O'Byrne in an editorial, "Asthma continues to be poorly controlled as reflected in surveys and in the baseline characteristics of most patient populations in insurance databases or clinical trials" (58). Less than half of the patients in most trials report ICS use at baseline. Compliance with ICS therapy during most studies has not been well-documented but it appears from pharmacy databases that refill rates are less than 50% of prescribed medications. The SMART study did not assess whether combination therapy of an ICS plus LABA carries the same risk as using LABA as monotherapy. At baseline, African-Americans had more severe asthma compared with the overall population. It is unclear whether this or other factors attributed to the increased risk of deaths in the subgroup. It is also unclear whether the results of SMART apply to all LABAs. The best guidance for practitioners is to follow the new Asthma Guidelines (3). LABAs and fixed drug combinations with ICS/LABAS are not indicated in patients with step 1 and 2 asthma, which is controlled by ICS alone or with other recommended agents. For those with step 3 and higher severity, ICS /LABA combinations appear safe and effective. These combinations can successfully control asthma symptoms.

VII. Acute Bronchodilator Testing

Guidelines emphasize the comprehensive and stepwise approach to the management of COPD and stipulate that all patients who are symptomatic merit a trial of pharmacologic intervention (Table 2). Choice of bronchodilator therapy is based on severity of disease quantified by postbronchodilator FEV_1. Bronchodilators work through their direct relaxation effect on airway smooth muscle cells (Table 3) but the lack of an acute bronchodilator response does not necessarily imply nonresponsiveness to bronchodilator therapy. Donohue and colleagues (60) reported that 73% of 813 COPD patients demonstrated a significant acute bronchodilator response (increased their FEV_1 by $\geq$12% or 200 mL); 11% of patients showed a response to ipratropium, 27% to albuterol, and 35% to both drugs combined. Calverley et al. (61) have shown that a patient's FEV_1 response to acute bronchodilator therapy does not predict long-term response to bronchodilator

Table 2 Stepwise Approach to the Pharmacologic Management of COPD and the Position of Bronchodilators

Severity	Spirometric findings	Pharmacologic intervention
Stage I: Mild	$FEV_1/FVC < 70\%$ $FEV_1 \geq 80\%$	Add a *short-acting bronchodilator* to be used when needed; anticholinergic or β_2-adrenoceptor agonist
Stage II: Moderate	$FEV_1/FVC < 70\%$ $50\% \leq FEV_1 < 80\%$	Add *one or more long-acting bronchodilators* on a scheduled basis Consider pulmonary rehabilitation
Stage III: Severe	$FEV_1/FVC < 70\%$ $30\% \leq FEV_1 < 50\%$	Add inhaled steroids if repeated exacerbations
Stage IV: Very severe	$FEV_1/FVC < 70\%$ $FEV_1 < 30\%$	Evaluate for adding oxygen Consider surgical options

Abbreviation: FEV_1, forced expiratory volume in one second.
Source: Adapted from Ref. 59.

Table 3 Rationale for the Use of Bronchodilators in COPD

1. Physiologic effects
    a. Airway smooth muscle relaxation
        • Bronchodilation: improve FEV_1, lung volumes
        • Decreased air trapping and dynamic hyperinflation
    b. Nonbronchodilator effects
2. Clinical effects
        • ↓ Breathlessness (↓ airway resistance, ↓ hyperinflation)
        • ↑ Exercise tolerance (↓ dynamic hyperinflation)
        • ↑ Sleep quality (↓ nocturnal bronchospasm)
        • ↑ Health-related quality of life
        • ↓ Frequency of acute exacerbations

Abbreviations: FEV_1, forced expiratory volume in one second; COPD, chronic obstructive pulmonary disease.

therapy and may vary from day to day. Acute bronchodilator testing using albuterol, ipratropium bromide, or a combination of the two was performed on 660 COPD patients who had been classified according to both European Respiratory Society (ERS) and American Thoracic Society (ATS) spirometric criteria. Over the two-month study period, 55% of patients classified as irreversible under ATS criteria changed to reversible status on at least one of the visits. In summary, the acute response to short-acting bronchodilators is of limited value in deciding future response to long-acting agents.

VIII. Bronchodilators in COPD

Three classes of bronchodilators—β_2-adrenoceptoragonists, anticholinergics, and methylxanthines—are currently available and can be used individually or in combination (Tables 4 and 5). Several novel bronchodilators are under development (63).

Table 4 Summary of the Effects of Commonly Used Bronchodilators on Clinical Outcomes in COPD

Bronchodilator	FEV_1	Lung volume	Dyspnea	HRQoL	Exercise endurance
Short-acting β_2AR agonist	Yes[a]	Yes[b]	Yes[a]	–	Yes[b]
Ipratropium bromide	Yes[a]	Yes[b]	Yes[a]	No[b]	Yes[b]
Long-acting β_2AR agonist	Yes[a]	Yes[a]	Yes[a]	Yes[a]	Yes[b]
Tiotropium	Yes[a]	Yes[a]	Yes[a]	Yes[a]	Yes[b]
Theophylline	Yes[a]	Yes[b]	Yes[a]	Yes[b]	Yes[b]

[a]Randomized clinical trial, substantial numbers of studies with large study populations.
[b]Randomized clinical trial, few studies, or studies with small study populations.
Abbreviations: FEV_1, forced expiratory volume in one second; COPD, chronic obstructive pulmonary disease.
Source: Adapted from Ref. 62.

Table 5 Commonly Used Bronchodilators in COPD

Short-acting agents	Long-acting agents
$\beta_2 AR$ agonists	$\beta_2 AR$ agonists
Albuterol (MDI, NS)	Salmeterol (DPI)
Terbutaline (MDI, DPI)	Formoterol (DPI)
Levalbuterol (MDI, NS)	Arformoterol (NS)
Pirbuterol (MDI)	
Anticholinergic	Anticholinergic
Ipratropium bromide (MDI, NS)	Tiotropium bromide (DPI)
Fixed combination	Fixed combination
Albuterol/ipratropium (MDI, NS)	Salmeterol/fluticasone[a] (DPI, MDI)
	Formoterol/budesonide[b] (DPI, MDI)
	Methylxanthines
	Theophylline (PO)

[a]Only one dose formulation (250/50) approved for COPD in the Unites States.
[b]Not currently approved for COPD in the Unites States.
Abbreviations: MDI, metered dose inhaler; DPI, dry powder inhaler; NS, nebulized solution; PO, oral preparation; COPD, chronic obstructive pulmonary disease.

A. β₂-Adrenoceptor Agonists
Pharmacology

β_2-adrenergic receptor ($\beta_2 AR$) agonists act through binding to the $\beta_2 AR$ that is a member of the seven transmembrane domains, G protein–coupled family of receptors. Adenylyl cyclase is activated via the signal transducing G_s protein, which results in a rise in cellular cyclic AMP levels and activation of protein kinase A (PKA) when ligand binds to the $\beta_2 AR$. The precise PKA phosphorylation targets mediating bronchial smooth muscle relaxation are not fully understood but are likely to include myosin light chain kinase and Ca^{2+}-dependent K^+ (K_{ca}) channels (64). Although $\beta_2 AR$s are present in high density in airway smooth muscle cells, they are also present in submucosal glands, vascular endothelium, ciliated epithelium, mast cells, circulating inflammatory cells such as eosinophils and lymphocytes, Clara cells, type II pneumocytes, and cholinergic ganglia. $\beta_2 AR$ agonists are delivered through the inhaled or oral route; although use of the latter is limited because of the increased risk of adverse effects.

There are several important pharmacologic differences among the existing agents (64,65). The onset of action is short (1–5 minutes) with albuterol and formoterol while it is more prolonged with salmeterol (30–45 minutes). The difference in onset of action is related to the lipophilicity of each of these agents and their ability to activate the $\beta_2 AR$ in the aqueous phase (albuterol and formoterol). Albuterol has a short duration of action lasting less than 6 hours while the duration of action of salmeterol and formoterol is approximately 12 hours. These agents also differ significantly in their ability to active the $\beta_2 AR$ (intrinsic efficacy), which is dependent on their affinity and potency (64). While formoterol has a high intrinsic efficacy (strong agonist), albuterol and salmeterol have a very low intrinsic efficacy (weak agonists). The clinical relevance of this difference needs to be further explored in future trials.

Clinical Benefits

Because of their rapid onset of action, short-acting β_2-adrenoceptor agonists are very effective for rescue from symptoms of COPD. Albuterol is the most commonly used agent. In addition to their bronchodilatory properties, these agents are effective in increasing mucociliary clearance. A systematic review showed that regular use of short-acting β_2AR agonists in COPD was associated with improvement in lung function and dyspnea (66). The two currently available LABAs—salmeterol and formoterol—have been shown in some studies to significantly improve lung function, health status, and symptom reduction, compared with both placebo (67–70) and ipratropium (71,72). However, a recent Cochrane meta-analysis concluded that while salmeterol is more effective in improving lung function variables than ipratropium, there was no significant difference in these agents' effect on quality of life, exacerbation frequency, or symptoms (73). Because of formoterol's fast onset of action, it has a potential role as monotherapy or in combination with another bronchodilator in the management of acute COPD exacerbations (74–76) and for use as both a rescue and maintenance medication (77). A recent study demonstrated a superior effect of formoterol compared with tiotropium bromide in improving FEV_1 in the first two hours after administration; however the area under the curve (AUC) FEV_1 over 12 hours was similar between these two agents (78). Several systematic reviews of LABAs reveal that these agents can reduce the rate of COPD exacerbations (27,79). This has been confirmed by a recent Cochrane systematic review and meta-analysis of 27 trials (80). This study went on to show that LABAs had significant benefits on airflow limitation measures, quality of life, and use of rescue medication (80). In a study of 634 patients with COPD, the administration of salmeterol for 12 months improved health outcomes including exacerbations especially in patients who complied with therapy (81).

Role of Stereoisomers

The majority of currently used β_2AR agonists are racemic compounds, which contain a 50-50 mixture of the R- and S-enantiomers of the agonist. Recently, the R-enantiomer of albuterol (levalbuterol) (82,83) and the R,R-enantiomer of formoterol (arformoterol) were approved for clinical use in the management of COPD (84). Much of the pharmacologic activity of the agonist usually resides in the effects of the R-enantiomer; the S-enantiomer is believed to have no bronchodilator effects but in fact may induce deleterious effects. An in vitro study suggests that S,S-formoterol is not biologically inert, such that in racemic mixtures, it inhibited the beneficial effects of R,R,-formoterol on proliferation, anti-inflammatory cellular surface marker expression, and cytokine secretion (85). A recent study by Donohue and coworkers showed that patients hospitalized for COPD or asthma exacerbations could receive less frequent levalbuterol nebulized treatments than those treated with racemic albuterol (24). However, there was no significant difference between the groups for length of stay and hospital costs. The effectiveness and cost-effectiveness of isomeric versus racemic β_2AR agonists in the management of airway diseases such as COPD remain controversial and need to be further explored (22,86). A recent trial investigating the efficacy and safety of different dose formulations of arformoterol nebulization solution administered over 12 weeks to patients with moderate to severe COPD demonstrated a significant sustained improvement in FEV_1 compared with placebo but comparable to salmeterol (87).

Nonbronchodilator Effects of β_2AR Agonists

Although the major action of β_2AR agonists on airways is relaxation of airway smooth muscles, they also exert several effects mediated through the activation of β_2ARs expressed on resident airway cells such as epithelial cells and mast cells and circulating inflammatory cells such as eosinophils and neutrophils (88,89). These effects include inhibition of airway smooth muscle cell proliferation and inflammatory mediator release, as well as nonsmooth muscle effects, such as stimulation of mucociliary transport (90) cytoprotection of the respiratory mucosa, and attenuation of neutrophil recruitment and activation (89). However, many of these effects have been described in vitro studies and in vivo studies are still needed to fully explore these effects.

Novel β_2-Adrenoceptor Agonists

A variety of β_2AR agonists with longer half lives are currently under development with the hopes of achieving once-daily dosing (63). These include carmoterol, indacaterol, GSK-159797, GSK-597901, GSK-159802, GSK-642444, and GSK-678007. These compounds are mainly (R,R)-enantiomers, have high intrinsic efficacy, and quick onset of action. While a quick onset of action and a prolonged 24-hour effect are desirable in the management of COPD, the use of agonists with high intrinsic efficacy may theoretically be associated with a rapid onset of tolerance, the fact that may limit their clinical use (64). This needs to be taken in consideration in the evaluation of new agents under development. However, it is likely that once-daily dosing of a LABA will lead to enhancement of compliance with therapy and may have advantages leading to improved overall clinical outcomes in patients with COPD.

B. Anticholinergics

Pharmacology

Parasympathetic activity in the large- and medium-size airways is mediated through the muscarinic receptors (M_1 and M_3) and results in airway smooth-muscle contraction, mucus secretion, and possibly increased ciliary activity. M_2 receptors inhibit acetylcholine release from nerve terminals. Increased cholinergic tone is important in the pathogenesis of COPD, contributing both to increased bronchial smooth muscle tone and to mucus hypersecretion (91,92). Thus, anticholinergics reduce airway tone and improve expiratory flow limitation, hyperinflation, and exercise capacity in patients with COPD.

Two anticholinergic bronchodilators are currently available in the United States for clinical use. These are ipratropium bromide and tiotropium. The short-acting anticholinergic agent, ipratropium bromide, acts on all three muscarinic receptors. Its short duration of action requires dosing every six hours and its delayed onset of action (peak at 45 minutes) precludes its use as rescue therapy. Tiotropium also binds to all three receptor subtypes; however it dissociates rapidly from M_2 receptors. In contrast, its dissociation half-life from M_3 receptors is close to 35 hours that results in a prolonged bronchodilatory effect. Its peak bronchodilatory effect is in 1 to 3 hours, and continues for up to 32 hours with a dip between 16 to 24 hours related to circadian change. However, its bronchoprotective effect against a bronchospastic agent continues up to 48 hours (93).

Clinical Benefits

The short-acting ipratropium has for a long time been used as monotherapy or in combination with albuterol in the maintenance therapy of COPD (73,94,95). Like ipratropium monotherapy, the fixed combination is available in both metered dose inhaler and nebulizer solution. Unlike ipratropium monotherapy, the fixed combination can be used as rescue therapy because of the rapid onset of action of the albuterol component. Several studies have now shown that the use of long-acting bronchodilators is superior in improving health outcomes. The use of tiotropium in patients with COPD results in improved health status, dyspnea, and exercise capacity, and reduced hyperinflation and COPD exacerbation rate in patients with moderate to severe COPD relative to placebo (96–98) and ipratropium (99). Data from large long-term trials showed that trough FEV_1 increased by 100 to 150 mL, and the peak FEV_1 increased by 150 to 200 mL above trough level after inhalation of 18 micrograms of tiotropium. No loss of efficacy was seen over the course of one year of regular treatment with tiotropium. Furthermore, in a multicenter Veterans Administration trial involving 1829 patients with severe COPD, the addition of tiotropium to other COPD therapies significantly reduced acute COPD exacerbations and reduced COPD hospitalizations when compared with placebo (100). Data from three more recent studies, specifically designed to explore the potential differences between tiotropium and salmeterol, seem to indicate a greater efficacy of tiotropium (101–103). A meta-analysis that contained these studies and others concluded that tiotropium reduced the odds of a COPD exacerbation, related hospitalizations but not pulmonary, or all-cause mortality compared with ipratropium and placebo (104). It yielded greater increases in FEV_1 and FVC than ipratropium, placebo, and LABAs. The effect of tiotropium on odds of a COPD exacerbation and related hospitalizations in this meta-analysis were not different from LABAs (104). In a conflicting analysis, Rodrigo and colleagues concluded that tiotropium did decrease the incidence of severe COPD exacerbations compared with LABAs (80). A recent large clinical trial designed to evaluate the effect of tiotropium on the decline of lung function over a four-year period failed to meet its primary endpoint; however, this study did show a significant mortality benefit at the end of treatment that was lost at the end of the study (105). Consistent with these findings are the results of the longitudinal, population cohort study in Ontario, Canada. This study showed that patients who received tiotropium were 20% less likely to die than those receiving a LABA (106).

Nonbronchodilator Effects of Anticholinergics

Some nonbronchodilator effects for the existing anticholinergics have been reported (107). Furthermore, results from a recent study performed on sputum cells obtained from COPD patients demonstrate that muscarinic receptors may be involved in airway inflammation in subjects with COPD through acetylcholine-induced ERK1/2-dependent leukotriene B4 release (108). These results suggest that anticholinergic therapy may contribute to reduced neutrophilic inflammation in COPD; however these findings need to be further evaluated.

Novel Anticholinergics

Several new long-acting anticholinergic agents are under development and these include LAS-34273, LAS-35201, GSK656398, GSK233705, and NVA-237 (glycopyrrolate). Although clinical details are still not available, potential advantages of such agents over tiotropium may include a quicker onset of action and a better safety profile.

Pharmacology
Theophylline is a nonselective phosphodiesterase inhibitor that acts both as a weak bronchodilator and a respiratory stimulant. It has been shown to improve diaphragmatic contractility and has some anti-inflammatory properties (109). Because of its potential ability to activate the HDAC system, theophylline may have the ability of enhancing the effects of ICSs in patients with COPD. However, because of its potential adverse effects and narrow therapeutic index, it should only be used when symptoms persist despite optimal bronchodilator therapy.

Clinical Benefits
Relative to other available agents such as LABAs and tiotropium, the bronchodilatory effect of theophylline is weak. Several studies have demonstrated the additive effect for theophylline when used in combination with other treatments in patients with COPD (110,111). Analysis of a large ($n = 36,492$) health administration database revealed that users of theophylline were less likely than the users of LABAs but more likely than users of inhaled glucocorticoids to suffer an exacerbation (112).

Nonbronchodilator Effects of Methylxanthines
The salutary effects of theophylline may be due as much to its nonbronchodilator as to its bronchodilator activity (109,113–116). In addition to its steroid-sparing effects on histone deacetylase, theophylline has both ionotropic and chronotropic cardiac effects. It enhances mucociliary sweep, diaphragmatic contractility, and central respiratory drive.

C. Combination Therapies
Current guidelines highlight the fact that for COPD patients uncontrolled by broncho-dilator monotherapy, the use of a combination therapy is recommended. The combination of LABA and ICS is the most common in use for both COPD and asthma. The physiologic and clinical benefits of LABAs have been shown to be enhanced when administered in conjunction with ICS (117–120), which translates into clinical benefits. ICS and LABA combination products have been shown to improve lung function, symptoms health status, and reduce exacerbations in patients with moderate to severe COPD (121–124). This is discussed in depth in chapter 6. Combination of more than one class of bronchodilators such as an inhaled anticholinergic with a β_2AR agonist may be more effective than the use of single agents with respect to improvements in lung function, symptoms, and reducing the risk of adverse events (59,125,126). Large studies have demonstrated that the combination of the short-acting β_2AR agonist albuterol with the short-acting anticholinergic ipratropium is superior to either single agent alone (127). Some trials have highlighted that the addition of LABAs to ipratropium is more effective than either agent used alone (128,129). In a 12-week trial, ZuWallack and colleagues showed that salmeterol plus theophylline caused significantly greater improvements in pulmonary function and symptoms, compared with either single agent (130).

The onset of action for formoterol is quicker (in 5 minutes) than tiotropium but it has comparable bronchodilation over 12 hours (78). Cazzola and coworkers therefore examined the bronchodilator effect of single doses of formoterol 12 µg and tiotropium 18 µg, and formoterol 12 µg + tiotropium 18 µg given together in stable COPD (131). Formoterol and tiotropium appeared complementary with regard to lung function indices. van Noord et al. (132) explored these effects elicited by six weeks of treatment with tiotropium 18 μg once daily in the morning, formoterol 12 μg twice a day, and tiotropium 18 μg + formoterol 12 μg once daily in the morning in patients suffering from moderate-to-severe COPD. Patients receiving combination treatment had a greater improvement in FEV_1 and FVC compared with those receiving the individual agents over 24 hours. Tiotropium was superior to formoterol for FEV_1 response over 0 to 12 hours (owing to significant differences from 8 to 12 hours), but the two treatments were not significantly different for FEV_1 over 12 to 24 hours or 0 to 24 hours. A similar observation was documented from a recently published two-week study with tiotropium alone or tiotropium plus formoterol once- or twice-daily following a two-week pretreatment period with tiotropium. In this study, the use of an additional evening dose of formoterol had clear added benefit compared with once a day formoterol (133). Nebulized formoterol (20 μg) was combined with tiotropium compared with tiotropium with placebo for six weeks (134). This combination yielded a better FEV_1 AUC, mean TDI score, and lower SGRQ symptom score compared with tiotropium plus nebulized placebo. Results were similar in a 12-week study where tiotropium was added to formoterol (12 μg) compared with tiotropium alone (135). A recent study by Rabe and coworkers highlights the superiority of combining two agents from differing bronchodilator classes to a bronchodilator plus an ICS (136). Tiotropium plus formoterol was compared with SFC. After six weeks, the 12-hour FEV_1 AUC, FVC AUC, and peak FEV_1 and FVC were all significantly greater in the group receiving tiotropium plus formoterol.

Emerging evidence from in vitro studies suggests an interaction between corticosteroid and muscarinic receptors that may provide a rationale for use of anticholinergic/corticosteroid combination therapies (119). This is illustrated by three studies evaluating the benefits of "triple therapy" (tiotropium, salmeterol, and fluticasone) compared with the three component parts (137–139) FEV_1, inspiratory capacity (IC), and airway conductances were all significantly greater in the triple combination compared with tiotropium monotherapy and SCF (138). Perng showed that adding tiotropium in patients with severe COPD already treated with a LABA/ICS combination yielded improvements in FVC, FEV_1, IC, and SGRQ (137). The Canadian Respiratory Clinical Research Consortium in collaboration with the Canadian Thoracic Society evaluated tiotropium monotherapy, tiotropium plus salmeterol, and tiotropium plus SFC (139). There was no significant difference in the proportion of participants suffering an exacerbation (the primary endpoint in the study) among the three groups. However, tiotropium + SFC improved lung function and disease-specific quality of life, and reduced hospitalization for COPD exacerbations and all-cause hospitalizations compared with tiotropium monotherapy. The clinical effects of such interaction need to be investigated in future clinical trials.

IX. Safety of Bronchodilator Therapy in COPD

It has been reported that the continued use of β_2AR agonists may be associated with an increase in cardiovascular risk compared with placebo (140). In general, the short-acting β_2AR agonists are well tolerated, except for occasional episodes of tachycardia and tremor. One out of a series of meta-analyses (141) that included randomized controlled trials of at least three-month duration that evaluated anticholinergic or β_2-agonist use compared with placebo or each other in patients with COPD, documented that while inhaled anticholinergics significantly reduced severe exacerbations and respiratory deaths in patients with COPD, β_2AR agonists were associated with an increased risk for respiratory deaths. However, as highlighted by the authors themselves, meta-analyses have several problems that limit their validity. Clearly, the use of LABAs as monotherapy in asthma can be considered unsafe (37); however, the use of these medications in COPD has generally been described as safe. Data from the TORCH study suggests that chronic use of salmeterol as monotherapy in patients with COPD for three years produced no increase in mortality (142). This is in conflict with a reported corresponding increase in asthma that shows an increase in deaths in the salmeterol monotherapy group (37). Further, a meta-analysis ($N = 2853$) of data from seven clinical trials examining the effects of salmeterol in patients with COPD showed no clinically significant difference in the incidence of cardiovascular events between salmeterol and placebo (143). This was confirmed by a more recent meta-analysis of 27 COPD studies listed in the Cochrane Controlled Trials Register (78). This meta-analysis showed no difference in respiratory deaths between LABA and placebo groups. Additionally, the use of LABAs with ICS reduced the risk of respiratory death compared with LABAs alone (80). The safety of nebulized formoterol has also been studied and found to be similar to that of the dry powdered formulation (144). Nevertheless, β-agonists should be used with caution in patients with underlying cardiac disorders including ischemic heart disease (140,145). It has also been suggested that tolerance to the bronchodilator effects of LABAs may occur with their prolonged use in COPD (101,146). However, a recent study examining the bronchodilator effect of long-term use of salmeterol demonstrated a sustained bronchodilator effect for salmeterol administered for six months (70).

Class effects of anticholinergics are dry mouth, an increased risk of glaucoma, and urinary retention; however, the quaternary nitrogen atom prevents them from being systemically absorbed. Therefore, currently available agents when used in recommended doses are generally safe. These agents should also be used with caution in patients with bladder neck obstruction due to prostatism, and patients with glaucoma. The safety of these agents (both long- and short-acting anticholinergics) was questioned by a recent meta-analysis (147). This study analyzed 13,645 subjects enrolled into 17 trials and found that inhaled anticholinergics significantly increased the risk of myocardial infarction (RR, 1.52; CI 1.04–2.22) and cardiovascular death (RR, 1.92; CI 1.23–3.0). In direct conflict with the results of this meta-analysis is the "UPLIFT" study, a four-year, prospective, head-to-head comparison study of tiotropium and placebo (105). Mortality at the end of the treatment phase was significantly *lower* in this study in subjects receiving tiotropium compared with placebo. The mortality benefit was lost at the end of the trial of 30 days after cessation of therapy.

Theophylline is associated with tremors and nausea, and less frequently with cardiac arrhythmias and seizures (148). The fact that serum toxicity levels overlap therapeutic levels explains the high incidence of toxic side effects. The risk of such adverse events can be reduced by monitoring the drug's plasma levels and reducing the dose accordingly; however, the high frequency of drug interactions and clinical conditions that interfere with hepatic metabolism of theophylline limit its extensive use in clinical practice (149).

X. Bronchodilators in COPD: Conclusions

The use of bronchodilators is central in the symptomatic management of COPD and currently available agents have been shown to have significant effects on the long-term outcome and management of COPD. The use of the inhaled route is currently preferred to minimize systemic effects. Quick-acting and short-acting agents are best used for rescue of symptoms while long-acting agents are best used for maintenance therapy. The choice of agents may be based primarily on individual response, cost, side effect profile, and availability.

Several new bronchodilators are currently being studied in ongoing clinical trials that may improve the future treatment of COPD. The current opinion is that it will be advantageous to develop inhalers containing combination of several classes of long-acting bronchodilator drugs in an attempt to simplify treatment regimes as much as possible. Specific future research should examine the long-term efficacy and long-term safety of the different combination of bronchodilators ± ICSs, as well as their effects on the natural history of COPD when used early in the disease progression. Furthermore, future studies should also identify more sensitive methods to assess response to bronchodilators and identify through responder analyses specific groups based on gender, age, race, or pharmacogenetic makeup.

References

1. Taylor DR, Bateman E, Boulet LP, et al. A new perspective on concepts of asthma severity and control. Eur Respir J 2008; 32:545–554.
2. Barnes PJ. Airway Pharmacology. 4th ed. Philadelphia: Saunders, 2005.
3. Guidelines for the diagnosis and management of asthma 2007. Available at: http://nhlbi.nih.gov/guidelines/asthma/asthgdln.pdf. Accessed March 12, 2008, 2008.
4. Bateman ED, Hurd SS, Barnes PJ, et al. Global strategy for asthma management and prevention: GINA executive summary. Eur Respir J 2008; 31:143–178.
5. Papi A. Treatment strategies in mild asthma. Curr Opin Pulm Med 2009; 15:290–234.
6. American Lung Association Asthma Clinical Research Centers, Peters SP, Anthonisen N, et al. Randomized comparison of strategies for reducing treatment in mild persistent asthma. N Engl J Med 2007; 356:2027–2039.
7. Papi A, Canonica GW, Maestrelli P, et al. Rescue use of beclomethasone and albuterol in a single inhaler for mild asthma. N Engl J Med 2007; 356:2040–2052.
8. Taylor DR, Sears MR, Cockcroft DW. The beta-agonist controversy. Med Clin North Am 1996; 80:719–748.
9. Gupta P, O'Mahony MS. Potential adverse effects of bronchodilators in the treatment of airways obstruction in older people: recommendations for prescribing. Drugs Aging 2008; 25:415–443.
10. Stolley PD, Schinnar R. Association between asthma mortality and isoproterenol aerosols: a review. Prev Med 1978; 7:519–538.
11. Keating G, Mitchell EA, Jackson R, et al. Trends in sales of drugs for asthma in new zealand, australia and the united kingdom. Br Med J (Clin Res Ed) 1984; 289:348–351.
12. Hancox RJ. Concluding remarks: can we explain the association of beta-agonists with asthma mortality? A hypothesis. Clin Rev Allergy Immunol 2006; 31:279–288.
13. Stolley PD. Asthma mortality. Why the United States was spared an epidemic of deaths due to asthma. Am Rev Respir Dis 1972; 105:883–890.
14. Pearce N, Beasley R, Crane J, et al. End of the New Zealand asthma mortality epidemic. Lancet 1995; 345:41–44.
15. Taylor DR, Sears MR, Herbison GP, et al. Regular inhaled beta agonist in asthma: effects on exacerbations and lung function. Thorax 1993; 48:134–138.
16. Drazen JM, Israel E, Boushey HA, et al. Comparison of regularly scheduled with as-needed use of albuterol in mild asthma. Asthma Clinical Research Network. N Engl J Med 1996; 335:841–847.

17. Larj MJ, Bleecker ER. Pharmacogenetics of asthma: where are we now? Clin Chest Med 2006; 27:109–117, vii.
18. Taylor DR. Pharmacogenetics of beta2-agonist drugs in asthma. Clin Rev Allergy Immunol 2006; 31:247–258.
19. Israel E, Drazen JM, Liggett SB, et al. The effect of polymorphisms of the beta(2)-adrenergic receptor on the response to regular use of albuterol in asthma. Am J Respir Crit Care Med 2000; 162:75–80.
20. Taylor DR, Drazen JM, Herbison GP, et al. Asthma exacerbations during long term beta agonist use: influence of beta(2) adrenoceptor polymorphism. Thorax 2000; 55:762–767.
21. Israel E, Chinchilli VM, Ford JG, et al. Use of regularly scheduled albuterol treatment in asthma: genotype-stratified, randomised, placebo-controlled cross-over trial. Lancet 2004; 364:1505–1512.
22. Barnes PJ. Treatment with (R)-albuterol has no advantage over racemic albuterol. Am J Respir Crit Care Med 2006; 174:969–972; discussion 72–74.
23. Nelson HS, Bensch G, Pleskow WW, et al. Improved bronchodilation with levalbuterol compared with racemic albuterol in patients with asthma. J Allergy Clin Immunol 1998; 102:943–952.
24. Donohue JF, Hanania NA, Ciubotaru RL, et al. Comparison of levalbuterol and racemic albuterol in hospitalized patients with acute asthma or COPD: a 2-week, multicenter, randomized, open-label study. Clin Ther 2008; 30 Spec No:989–1002.
25. Cazzola M, Matera MG. Novel long-acting bronchodilators for COPD and asthma. Br J Pharmacol 2008; 155:291–299.
26. Walters EH, Gibson PG, Lasserson TJ, et al. Long-acting beta2-agonists for chronic asthma in adults and children where background therapy contains varied or no inhaled cortico-steroid. Cochrane Database Syst Rev 2007:CD001385.
27. Stockley RA, Whitehead PJ, Williams MK. Improved outcomes in patients with chronic obstructive pulmonary disease treated with salmeterol compared with placebo/usual ther-apy: results of a meta-analysis. Respir Res 2006; 7:147.
28. Salpeter SR. Bronchodilators in COPD: impact of beta-agonists and anticholinergics on severe exacerbations and mortality. Int J Chron Obstruct Pulmon Dis 2007; 2:11–18.
29. Greening AP, Ind PW, Northfield M, et al. Added salmeterol versus higher-dose cortico-steroid in asthma patients with symptoms on existing inhaled corticosteroid. Allen & Hanburys Limited UK Study Group. Lancet 1994; 344:219–224.
30. Ni CM, Greenstone IR, Ducharme FM. Addition of inhaled long-acting beta2-agonists to inhaled steroids as first line therapy for persistent asthma in steroid-naive adults. Cochrane Database Syst Rev 2005:CD005307.
31. O'Byrne PM, Naya IP, Kallen A, et al. Increasing doses of inhaled corticosteroids compared to adding long-acting inhaled beta2-agonists in achieving asthma control. Chest 2008; 134:1192–1199.
32. de Blic J, Ogorodova L, Klink R, et al. Salmeterol/fluticasone propionate vs. double dose fluticasone propionate on lung function and asthma control in children. Pediatr Allergy Immunol 2009.
33. Bateman ED, Boushey HA, Bousquet J, et al. Can guideline-defined asthma control be achieved? The Gaining Optimal Asthma ControL study. Am J Respir Crit Care Med 2004; 170:836–844.
34. Bateman ED, Bousquet J, Busse WW, et al. Stability of asthma control with regular treatment: an analysis of the Gaining Optimal Asthma controL (GOAL) study. Allergy 2008; 63:932–938.
35. O'Byrne PM, Bisgaard H, Godard PP, et al. Budesonide/formoterol combination therapy as both maintenance and reliever medication in asthma. Am J Respir Crit Care Med 2005; 171:129–136.

36. Castle W, Fuller R, Hall J, et al. Serevent nationwide surveillance study: comparison of salmeterol with salbutamol in asthmatic patients who require regular bronchodilator treatment. BMJ 1993; 306:1034–1037.
37. Nelson HS, Weiss ST, Bleecker ER, et al. The Salmeterol Multicenter Asthma Research Trial: a comparison of usual pharmacotherapy for asthma or usual pharmacotherapy plus salmeterol. Chest 2006; 129:15–26.
38. Jaeschke R, O'Byrne PM, Mejza F, et al. The safety of long-acting beta-agonists among patients with asthma using inhaled corticosteroids: systematic review and metaanalysis. Am J Respir Crit Care Med 2008; 178:1009–1016.
39. Salpeter SR, Buckley NS, Ormiston TM, et al. Meta-analysis: effect of long-acting beta-agonists on severe asthma exacerbations and asthma-related deaths. Ann Intern Med 2006; 144:904–912.
40. Ernst P, McIvor A, Ducharme FM, et al. Safety and effectiveness of long-acting inhaled beta-agonist bronchodilators when taken with inhaled corticosteroids. Ann Intern Med 2006; 145:692–694.
41. Bateman E, Nelson H, Bousquet J, et al. Meta-analysis: effects of adding salmeterol to inhaled corticosteroids on serious asthma-related events. Ann Intern Med 2008; 149:33–42.
42. FDA public health advisory.Severvent diskus (salmeterol xinafoate inhalation powder), Advair diskus (fluticasone propionate and salmeterol inhalation powder), Foradil aerolizer (formoterol fumarste inhalation powder). 2006. Available at: http://www.fda.gov/cder/drug/advisory/laba.htm. Accessed March 14, 2008, 2006.
43. Mann M, Chowdhury B, Sullivan E, et al. Serious asthma exacerbations in asthmatics treated with high-dose formoterol. Chest 2003; 124:70–74.
44. Bensch G, Lapidus RJ, Levine BE, et al. A randomized, 12-week, double-blind, placebo-controlled study comparing formoterol dry powder inhaler with albuterol metered-dose inhaler. Ann Allergy Asthma Immunol 2001; 86:19–27.
45. Bensch G, Berger WE, Blokhin BM, et al. One-year efficacy and safety of inhaled formoterol dry powder in children with persistent asthma. Ann Allergy Asthma Immunol 2002; 89:180–190.
46. Wolfe J, Laforce C, Friedman B, et al. Formoterol, 24 microg bid, and serious asthma exacerbations: similar rates compared with formoterol, 12 microg bid, with and without extra doses taken on demand, and placebo. Chest 2006; 129:27–38.
47. Sears MR, Ottosson A, Radner F, et al. Long-acting beta-agonists: a review of formoterol safety data from asthma clinical trials. Eur Respir J 2009; 33:21–32.
48. Kramer JM. Balancing the benefits and risks of inhaled long-acting beta-agonists–the influence of values. N Engl J Med 2009; 360:1592–1595.
49. Drazen JM, O'Byrne PM. Risks of long-acting beta-agonists in achieving asthma control. N Engl J Med 2009; 360:1671–1672.
50. Sears MR. Safety of Long-Acting Beta-Agonists: Are New Data Really Required? Chest 2009; 136 (2):604–607.
51. Wechsler ME, Lehman E, Lazarus SC, et al. beta-Adrenergic receptor polymorphisms and response to salmeterol. Am J Respir Crit Care Med 2006; 173:519–526.
52. Bleecker ER, Postma DS, Lawrance RM, et al. Effect of ADRB2 polymorphisms on response to longacting beta2-agonist therapy: a pharmacogenetic analysis of two randomised studies. Lancet 2007; 370:2118–2125.
53. Bleecker ER, Yancey SW, Baitinger LA, et al. Salmeterol response is not affected by beta2-adrenergic receptor genotype in subjects with persistent asthma. J Allergy Clin Immunol 2006; 118:809–816.
54. Spears M, Donnelly I, Jolly L, et al. Effect of low-dose theophylline plus beclometasone on lung function in smokers with asthma: a pilot study. Eur Respir J 2009; 33:1010–1017.

55. Momeni A, Mohammadi MH. Respiratory delivery of theophylline by size-targeted starch microspheres for treatment of asthma. J Microencapsul 2009:1–10.

56. Adachi M, Aizawa H, Ishihara K, et al. Comparison of salmeterol/fluticasone propionate (FP) combination with FP+sustained release theophylline in moderate asthma patients. Respir Med 2008; 102:1055–1064.

57. Suissa S, Dell'Aniello S, Ernst P. Effectiveness of combination therapies in asthma: an observational study. Pulm Pharmacol Ther 2009; 22:194–198.

58. O'Byrne PM, Adelroth E. Beta2 deja vu. Chest 2006; 129:3–5.

59. Fabbri L, Pauwels RA, Hurd SS, et al. Global Strategy for the Diagnosis, Management, and Prevention of Chronic Obstructive Pulmonary Disease: GOLD Executive Summary updated 2003. COPD 2004; 1:105–141; discussion 3–4.

60. Donohue JF. Therapeutic responses in asthma and COPD. Bronchodilators Chest 2004; 126: (2 suppl):125S–137S.

61. Calverley PM, Burge PS, Spencer S, et al. Bronchodilator reversibility testing in chronic obstructive pulmonary disease. Thorax 2003; 58:659–664.

62. Celli BR, MacNee W, Force AET. Standards for the diagnosis and treatment of patients with COPD: a summary of the ATS/ERS position paper. Eur Respir J 2004; 23:932–946.

63. Cazzola M, Matera MG, Lotvall J. Ultra long-acting beta 2-agonists in development for asthma and chronic obstructive pulmonary disease. Expert Opin Investig Drugs 2005; 14:775–783.

64. Hanania NA, Sharafkhaneh A, Barber R, et al. Beta-agonist intrinsic efficacy: measurement and clinical significance. Am J Respir Crit Care Med 2002; 165:1353–1358.

65. Lotvall J. Pharmacology of bronchodilators used in the treatment of COPD. Respir Med 2000; 94(suppl E):S6–S10.

66. Sestini P, Renzoni E, Robinson S, et al. Short-acting beta 2 agonists for stable chronic obstructive pulmonary disease. Cochrane Database Syst Rev 2002:CD001495.

67. Ramirez-Venegas A, Ward J, Lentine T, et al. Salmeterol reduces dyspnea and improves lung function in patients with COPD. Chest 1997; 112:336–340.

68. Boyd G, Morice AH, Pounsford JC, et al. An evaluation of salmeterol in the treatment of chronic obstructive pulmonary disease (COPD). Eur Respir J 1997; 10:815–821.

69. Cazzola M, Matera MG, Santangelo G, et al. Salmeterol and formoterol in partially reversible severe chronic obstructive pulmonary disease: a dose-response study. Respir Med 1995; 89:357–362.

70. Hanania NA, Kalberg C, Yates J, et al. The bronchodilator response to salmeterol is maintained with regular, long-term use in patients with COPD. Pulm Pharmacol Ther 2005; 18:19–22.

71. Mahler DA, Donohue JF, Barbee RA, et al. Efficacy of salmeterol xinafoate in the treatment of COPD. Chest 1999; 115:957–965.

72. Dahl R, Greefhorst LA, Nowak D, et al. Inhaled formoterol dry powder versus ipratropium bromide in chronic obstructive pulmonary disease. Am J Respir Crit Care Med 2001; 164:778–784.

73. Appleton S, Jones T, Poole P, et al. Ipratropium bromide versus long-acting beta-2 agonists for stable chronic obstructive pulmonary disease. Cochrane Database Syst Rev 2006; 3:CD006101.

74. Cazzola M, Santus P, Matera MG, et al. A single high dose of formoterol is as effective as the same dose administered in a cumulative manner in patients with acute exacerbation of COPD. Respir Med 2003; 97:458–462.

75. Di Marco F, Verga M, Santus P, et al. Effect of formoterol, tiotropium, and their combination in patients with acute exacerbation of chronic obstructive pulmonary disease: a pilot study. Respir Med 2006; 100:1925–1932.

76. Berger WE, Nadel JA. Efficacy and safety of formoterol for the treatment of chronic obstructive pulmonary disease. Respir Med 2008; 102:173–188.

77. Campbell M, Eliraz A, Johansson G, et al. Formoterol for maintenance and as-needed treatment of chronic obstructive pulmonary disease. Respir Med 2005; 99:1511–1520.

78. Richter K, Stenglein S, Mucke M, et al. Onset and duration of action of formoterol and tiotropium in patients with moderate to severe COPD. Respiration 2006; 73:414–419.

79. Sin DD, McAlister FA, Man SF, et al. Contemporary management of chronic obstructive pulmonary disease: scientific review. JAMA 2003; 290:2301–2312.

80. Rodrigo GJ, Nannini LJ, Rodriguez-Roisin R. Safety of long-acting beta-agonists in stable COPD: a systematic review. Chest 2008; 133:1079–1087.

81. Stockley RA, Chopra N, Rice L. Addition of salmeterol to existing treatment in patients with COPD: a 12 month study. Thorax 2006; 61:122–128.

82. Costello J. Prospects for improved therapy in chronic obstructive pulmonary disease by the use of levalbuterol. J Allergy Clin Immunol 1999; 104:S61–S68.

83. Truitt T, Witko J, Halpern M. Levalbuterol compared to racemic albuterol: efficacy and outcomes in patients hospitalized with COPD or asthma. Chest 2003; 123:128–135.

84. Arformoterol: (R,R)-eformoterol, (R,R)-formoterol, arformoterol tartrate, eformoterol-sepracor, formoterol-sepracor, R,R-eformoterol, R,R-formoterol. Drugs R D 2004; 5:25–27.

85. Steinke JW, Baramki D, Borish L. Opposing actions of (R,R)-isomers and (S,S)-isomers of formoterol on T-cell function. J Allergy Clin Immunol 2006; 118:963–965.

86. Ameredes BT, Calhoun WJ. (R)-albuterol for asthma: pro [a.k.a. (S)-albuterol for asthma: con]. Am J Respir Crit Care Med 2006; 174:965–969; discussion 72–74.

87. Baumgartner RA, Hanania NA, Calhoun WJ, et al. Nebulized arformoterol in patients with COPD: a 12-week, multicenter, randomized, double-blind, double-dummy, placebo- and active-controlled trial. Clin Ther 2007; 29:261–278.

88. Johnson M, Rennard S. Alternative mechanisms for long acting beta (2)-adrenergics agonists in COPD. Chest 2001; 120:258–270.

89. Hanania NA, Moore RH. Anti-inflammatory activities of beta2-agonists. Curr Drug Targets Inflamm Allergy 2004; 3:271–277.

90. Bennett WD, Almond MA, Zeman KL, et al. Effect of salmeterol on mucociliary and cough clearance in chronic bronchitis. Pulm Pharmacol Ther 2006; 19:96–100.

91. Gross NJ, Co E, Skorodin MS. Cholinergic bronchomotor tone in COPD. Estimates of its amount in comparison with that in normal subjects. Chest 1989; 96:984–987.

92. Gross NJ, Skorodin MS. Role of the parasympathetic system in airway obstruction due to emphysema. N Engl J Med 1984; 311:421–425.

93. O'Connor BJ, Towse LJ, Barnes PJ. Prolonged effect of tiotropium bromide on methacholine-induced bronchoconstriction in asthma. Am J Respir Crit Care Med 1996; 154:876–880.

94. O'Donnell DE, Lam M, Webb KA. Spirometric correlates of improvement in exercise performance after anticholinergic therapy in chronic obstructive pulmonary disease. Am J Respir Crit Care Med 1999; 160:542–549.

95. Ayers ML, Mejia R, Ward J, et al. Effectiveness of salmeterol versus ipratropium bromide on exertional dyspnoea in COPD. Eur Respir J 2001; 17:1132–1137.

96. Casaburi R, Mahler DA, Jones PW, et al. A long-term evaluation of once-daily inhaled tiotropium in chronic obstructive pulmonary disease. Eur Respir J 2002; 19:217–224.

97. O'Donnell DE, Voduc N, Fitzpatrick M, et al. Effect of salmeterol on the ventilatory response to exercise in chronic obstructive pulmonary disease. Eur Respir J 2004; 24:86–94.

98. Anzueto A, Tashkin D, Menjoge S, et al. One-year analysis of longitudinal changes in spirometry in patients with COPD receiving tiotropium. Pulm Pharmacol Ther 2005; 18:75–81.

99. Vincken W, van Noord JA, Greefhorst AP, et al. Improved health outcomes in patients with COPD during 1 yr's treatment with tiotropium. Eur Respir J 2002; 19:209–216.

100. Niewoehner DE, Rice K, Cote C, et al. Prevention of exacerbations of chronic obstructive pulmonary disease with tiotropium, a once-daily inhaled anticholinergic bronchodilator: a randomized trial. Ann Intern Med 2005; 143:317–326.
101. Donohue JF, van Noord JA, Bateman ED, et al. A 6-month, placebo-controlled study comparing lung function and health status changes in COPD patients treated with tiotropium or salmeterol. Chest 2002; 122:47–55.
102. Brusasco V, Hodder R, Miravitlles M, et al. Health outcomes following treatment for six months with once-daily tiotropium compared with twice daily salmeterol in patients with COPD. Thorax 2003; 58:399–404.
103. Briggs DD Jr., Covelli H, Lapidus R, et al. Improved daytime spirometric efficacy of tiotropium compared with salmeterol in patients with COPD. Pulm Pharmacol Ther 2005; 18:397–404.
104. Barr RG, Bourbeau J, Camargo CA, et al. Tiotropium for stable chronic obstructive pulmonary disease: a meta-analysis. Thorax 2006; 61:854–862.
105. Tashkin DP, Celli B, Senn S. A 4 year trial of tiotropium in chronic obstructive pulmonary disease. N Engl J Med 2008; 359:1543–1554.
106. Gershon AS, Wang L, To T, et al. Survival with tiotropium compared to long-acting Beta-2-agonists in Chronic Obstructive Pulmonary Disease. COPD 2008; 5:229–234.
107. Belmonte KE. Cholinergic pathways in the lungs and anticholinergic therapy for chronic obstructive pulmonary disease. Proc Am Thorac Soc 2005; 2:297–304; discussion 11–12.
108. Profita M, Giorgi RD, Sala A, et al. Muscarinic receptors, leukotriene B4 production and neutrophilic inflammation in COPD patients. Allergy 2005; 60:1361–1369.
109. Barnes PJ. Theophylline for COPD. Thorax 2006; 61:742–744.
110. Cazzola M, Gabriella Matera M. The additive effect of theophylline on a combination of formoterol and tiotropium in stable COPD: a pilot study. Respir Med 2007; 101:957–962.
111. Man GC, Champman KR, Ali SH, et al. Sleep quality and nocturnal respiratory function with once-daily theophylline (Uniphyl) and inhaled salbutamol in patients with COPD. Chest 1996; 110:648–653.
112. Cyr MC, Beauchesne MF, Lemiere C, et al. Effect of theophylline on the rate of moderate to severe exacerbations among patients with chronic obstructive pulmonary disease. Br J Clin Pharmacol 2008; 65:40–50.
113. Hanania NA, Ambrosino N, Calverley P, et al. Treatments for COPD. Respir Med 2005; 99(suppl B):S28–S40.
114. Barnes PJ. Targeting histone deacetylase 2 in chronic obstructive pulmonary disease treatment. Expert Opin Ther Targets 2005; 9:1111–1121.
115. Barnes PJ. Theophylline in chronic obstructive pulmonary disease: new horizons. Proc Am Thorac Soc 2005; 2:334–339; discussion 40–41.
116. Barnes PJ. Theophylline: new perspectives for an old drug. Am J Respir Crit Care Med 2003; 167:813–818.
117. Barnes NC, Qiu YS, Pavord ID, et al. Antiinflammatory effects of salmeterol/fluticasone propionate in chronic obstructive lung disease. Am J Respir Crit Care Med 2006; 173:736–743.
118. Johnson M. Interactions between corticosteroids and beta2-agonists in asthma and chronic obstructive pulmonary disease. Proc Am Thorac Soc 2004; 1:200–206.
119. Johnson M. Corticosteroids: potential beta2-agonist and anticholinergic interactions in chronic obstructive pulmonary disease. Proc Am Thorac Soc 2005; 2:320–325; discussion 40–41.
120. Sin DD, Johnson M, Gan WQ, et al. Combination therapy of inhaled corticosteroids and long-acting beta2-adrenergics in management of patients with chronic obstructive pulmonary disease. Curr Pharm Des 2004; 10:3547–3560.
121. Hanania NA, Darken P, Horstman D, et al. The efficacy and safety of fluticasone propionate (250 microg)/salmeterol (50 microg) combined in the Diskus inhaler for the treatment of COPD. Chest 2003; 124:834–843.

122. Mahler DA, Wire P, Horstman D, et al. Effectiveness of fluticasone propionate and salmeterol combination delivered via the Diskus device in the treatment of chronic obstructive pulmonary disease. Am J Respir Crit Care Med 2002; 166:1084–1091.

123. Calverley P, Pauwels R, Vestbo J, et al. Combined salmeterol and fluticasone in the treatment of chronic obstructive pulmonary disease: a randomised controlled trial. Lancet 2003; 361:449–456.

124. Calverley PM, Boonsawat W, Cseke Z, et al. Maintenance therapy with budesonide and formoterol in chronic obstructive pulmonary disease. Eur Respir J 2003; 22:912–919.

125. Global Initiative for Chronic Obstructive Lung Disease. Global strategy for the diagnisis, management and prevention of chronic obstrictive pulmonary disease. 2004. Available at: http://www.goldcopd.org. Accessed 4-24-2005, 2005.

126. Donohue JF. Combination therapy for chronic obstructive pulmonary disease: clinical aspects. Proc Am Thorac Soc 2005; 2:272–281; discussion 90–91.

127. In chronic obstructive pulmonary disease, a combination of ipratropium and albuterol is more effective than either agent alone. An 85-day multicenter trial. COMBIVENT Inhalation Aerosol Study Group. Chest 1994; 105:1411–1419.

128. D'Urzo AD, De Salvo MC, Ramirez-Rivera A, et al. In patients with COPD, treatment with a combination of formoterol and ipratropium is more effective than a combination of salbutamol and ipratropium : a 3-week, randomized, double-blind, within-patient, multicenter study. Chest 2001; 119:1347–1356.

129. van Noord JA, de Munck DR, Bantje TA, et al. Long-term treatment of chronic obstructive pulmonary disease with salmeterol and the additive effect of ipratropium. Eur Respir J 2000; 15:878–885.

130. ZuWallack RL, Mahler DA, Reilly D, et al. Salmeterol plus theophylline combination therapy in the treatment of COPD. Chest 2001; 119:1661–1670.

131. Cazzola M, Di Marco F, Santus P, et al. The pharmacodynamic effects of single inhaled doses of formoterol, tiotropium and their combination in patients with COPD. Pulm Pharmacol Ther 2004; 17:35–39.

132. van Noord JA, Aumann JL, Janssens E, et al. Comparison of tiotropium once daily, formoterol twice daily and both combined once daily in patients with COPD. Eur Respir J 2005; 26:214–222.

133. van Noord JA, Aumann JL, Janssens E, et al. Effects of tiotropium with and without formoterol on airflow obstruction and resting hyperinflation in patients with COPD. Chest 2006; 129:509–517.

134. Tashkin DP, Littner M, Andrews CP, et al. Concomitant treatment with nebulized formoterol and tiotropium in subjects with COPD: a placebo-controlled trial. Respir Med 2008; 102:479–487.

135. Tashkin DP, Pearle J, Iezzoni D, et al. Formoterol and tiotropium compared with tiotropium alone for treatment of COPD. COPD 2009; 6:17–25.

136. Rabe KF, Timmer W, Sagkriotis A, et al. Comparison of a combination of tiotropium plus formoterol to salmeterol plus fluticasone in moderate COPD. Chest 2008; 134:255–262.

137. Perng DW, Wu CC, Su KC, et al. Additive benefits of tiotropium in COPD patients treated with long-acting beta agonists and corticosteroids. Respirology 2006; 11:598–602.

138. Singh D, Brooks J, Hagan G, et al. Superiority of "triple" therapy with salmeterol/fluticasone propionate and tiotropium bromide versus individual components in moderate to severe COPD. Thorax 2008; 63:592–598.

139. Aaron SD, Vandemheen KL, Fergusson D, et al. Tiotropium in combination with placebo, salmeterol, or fluticasone-salmeterol for treatment of chronic obstructive pulmonary disease: a randomized trial. Ann Intern Med 2007; 146:545–555.

140. Salpeter SR. Cardiovascular safety of beta(2)-adrenoceptor agonist use in patients with obstructive airway disease: a systematic review. Drugs Aging 2004; 21:405–414.

141. Salpeter SR, Buckley NS, Salpeter EE. Meta-analysis: anticholinergics, but not beta-agonists, reduce severe exacerbations and respiratory mortality in COPD. J Gen Intern Med 2006; 21:1011–1019.
142. Calverley PM, Anderson JA, Celli B, et al. Salmeterol and fluticasone propionate and survival in chronic obstructive pulmonary disease. N Engl J Med 2007; 356:775–789.
143. Ferguson GT, Funck-Brentano C, Fischer T, et al. Cardiovascular safety of salmeterol in COPD. Chest 2003; 123:1817–1824.
144. Donohue JF, Hanania NA, Fogarty C, et al. Long-term safety of nebulized formoterol: results of a twelve-month open-label clinical trial. Ther Adv Respir Dis 2008; 2:199–208.
145. Cazzola M, Matera MG, Donner CF. Inhaled beta2-adrenoceptor agonists: cardiovascular safety in patients with obstructive lung disease. Drugs 2005; 65:1595–1610.
146. Donohue JF, Menjoge S, Kesten S. Tolerance to bronchodilating effects of salmeterol in COPD. Respir Med 2003; 97:1014–1020.
147. Singh S, Loke YK, Furberg CD. Inhaled anticholinergics and risk of major adverse cardiovascular events in patients with chronic obstructive pulmonary disease: a systematic review and meta-analysis. JAMA 2008; 300:1439–1450.
148. Barnes PJ. Current therapies for asthma. Promise and limitations. Chest 1997; 111:17S–26S.
149. Charytan D, Jansen K. Severe metabolic complications from theophylline intoxication. Nephrology (Carlton) 2003; 8:239–242.

8

Anti-Mediator Therapy

NEIL C. THOMSON
University of Glasgow, Glasgow, U.K.

I. Introduction

Many inflammatory mediators have been implicated as having an important role in the pathogenesis of asthma, and this has led the pharmaceutical industry to develop specific mediator antagonists as potential therapeutic agents for asthma. Of particular importance is whether these agents can be used as alternative therapies to inhaled corticosteroids and/or as add-on treatments for patients in whom asthma control remains inadequate despite inhaled corticosteroid therapy. The role of these drugs in the treatment of chronic obstructive pulmonary disease (COPD) is largely untested. This chapter will concentrate on the therapeutic effects of currently licensed mediator antagonists and modulators in the treatment of asthma.

II. Leukotriene-Receptor Antagonists and Leukotriene Synthesis Inhibitors

A. Leukotrienes and Asthma

Leukotrienes are inflammatory mediators that play a role in the pathogenesis of asthma (1–4). The cysteinyl leukotrienes (Cys-LTs), leukotriene C_4, leukotriene D_4, and leukotriene E_4 are synthesized from arachidonic acid by 5-lipoxygenase and 5-lipoxygenase-activating protein (FLAP) in inflammatory cells such as eosinophils, alveolar macrophages, and mast cells (Fig. 1). The Cys-LTs act on target cells, including smooth muscle cells, leukocytes, epithelial cells, or endothelial cells and contribute to the pathogenesis of asthma by causing bronchial smooth muscle contraction, mucus hypersecretion, and edema formation. In addition, the leukotrienes can cause eosinophil recruitment, smooth muscle proliferation, and airway remodeling. Leukotriene A_4, which is an unstable compound, is converted by leukotriene C_4 synthase to leukotriene C_4 or by leukotriene A_4 hydrolase to leukotriene B_4. Leukotriene B_4 is a potent chemotactic factor for neutrophils as well as also being implicated in causing eosinophil chemotaxis, mucus secretion, and airway hyperreactivity (2,4).

Leukotriene levels are increased in biological fluids from individuals with asthma including elevated urinary leukotriene E_4 after allergen challenge and in aspirin-sensitive asthma, nocturnal asthma, and severe asthma (2,4). Furthermore, increased leukotriene concentrations are found in bronchoalveolar lavage, sputum, and exhaled breath condensate samples from subjects with asthma (2,4). In view of the potential involvement of

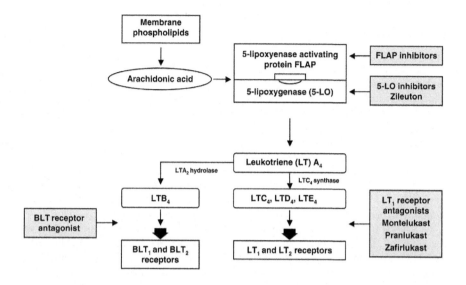

Figure 1 Site of action of leukotriene synthesis inhibitors and leukotriene-receptor antagonists.

leukotrienes in asthma, a number of drugs have been developed to block their effects or inhibit their synthesis, in the hope that these agents will be beneficial for the treatment of asthma.

B. Drugs Acting on the 5-Lipoxygenase Pathway

The effects of the leukotrienes on the lungs can be inhibited in two ways (Fig. 1).

Leukotriene-Receptor Antagonists

There are two subtypes of Cys-LT receptors termed the Cys-LT$_1$ receptor and the Cys-LT$_2$ receptor. Leukotriene C$_4$, leukotriene D$_4$, and leukotriene E$_4$ act on the Cys-LT$_1$ receptor to cause bronchoconstriction, mucus secretion, and edema (3). Montelukast, pranlukast, and zafirlukast are orally active leukotriene-receptor antagonists that act at the Cys-LT$_1$ receptor (Fig. 1). The chemical structures of these drugs are different although they have similar receptor binding affinities. They are metabolized by cytochrome P450 enzymes in the liver and metabolites are excreted largely in bile. Pranlukast and zafirlukast are administered twice daily whereas montelukast is administered once daily at bedtime. Montelukast and zafirlukast are licensed worldwide for the treatment of asthma. Pranlukast is approved only in Japan. Activation of Cys-LT$_2$ receptors, which are expressed in eosinophils, mast cells, and endothelial cells, increases vascular permeability and contributes to inflammation and tissue fibrosis (3). There are no specific Cys-LT$_2$ receptor antagonists. The high-affinity B leukotriene-receptors 1 (BLT$_1$) are expressed in neutrophils, macrophages, mast cells, and T lymphocytes, and when activated by leukotriene B$_4$ mediates the recruitment of eosinophils, neutrophils, mast cells, or macrophages (3,5). The actions of the low-affinity B leukotriene-receptor 2 (BLT$_2$) are not known. Several

LTB$_4$ receptor antagonists have been synthesized including LY293111 (6) and SB225002, but none are so far licensed for the treatment of asthma or COPD.

Leukotriene Synthesis Inhibitors

Leukotriene synthesis is blocked by inhibition of either 5-lipoxygenase or FLAP. The 5-lipoxygenase inhibitors block the enzyme directly whereas the FLAP inhibitors prevent 5-lipoxygenase binding with FLAP on the nuclear membrane (Fig. 1). The orally active 5-lipoxygenase inhibitor zileuton, which can be administered twice or four times daily, is licensed in the United States for use in adults and children 12 years of age and older. In addition to inhibiting the production of the Cys-LTs, the 5-lipoxygenase inhibitors also prevent the formation of leukotriene B$_4$ and other 5-lipoxygenase products. It has been proposed that the additional pharmacological properties of 5-lipoxygenase inhibitors compared with leukotriene-receptor antagonists may of relevance in the treatment of airway hyperresponsiveness and nasal symptoms in aspirin-induced asthma (7).

Several FLAP inhibitors have been developed, but none has been licensed for the treatment of airway disease. A selective leukotriene A$_4$ hydrolase inhibitor JNJ-26993135, targeted at reducing LTB$_4$ levels in inflammatory diseases, is undergoing preclinical evaluation (8). The clinical importance of the different pharmacological effects of 5-lipoxygenase inhibitors, FLAP inhibitors, or selective leukotriene A$_4$ hydrolase inhibitors compared to leukotriene-receptor antagonists for the treatment of chronic airway diseases is uncertain.

C. Anti-leukotriene Drugs on Airway Inflammation and Remodeling

A number of studies have investigated the effects of drugs modifying the 5-lipoxygenase pathway on inflammatory responses in allergen-induced asthma and chronic asthma (9). Montelukast has no effect on allergen-induced increases in sputum eosinophil counts when administered for 36 hours before allergen exposure (10), whereas more prolonged treatment for up to 10 days decreases sputum eosinophil counts induced by allergen challenge (11,12). Zafirlukast administered at a dose of 20 mg twice daily for one week reduces bronchoalveolar lavage lymphocyte and basophil counts, but not eosinophil influx after segmental allergen challenge (13). Zileuton decreases the influx of eosinophils following segmental allergen challenge (14), particularly in subjects with asthma in whom leukotriene levels are elevated within the airways by allergen (15). Chronic treatment with leukotriene-receptor antagonists or zileuton reduces circulating blood eosinophil counts (16–19), induced sputum eosinophil counts (16,20), exhaled nitric oxide concentrations (21–23), nocturnal bronchoalveolar lavage eosinophil counts (24), and urinary leukotriene E$_4$ excretion (25–27). Taken together, these findings indicate that drugs modifying the 5-lipoxygenase pathway have anti-inflammatory activity in asthma.

The anti-inflammatory effect of 5-lipoxygenase blockers on airway inflammation in asthma is generally less marked than that produced by inhaled corticosteroids. Daily budesonide reduces markers of airway inflammation including sputum eosinophil counts and exhaled nitric oxide, which was not found with daily zafirlukast (28). Similarly, montelukast is not as effective as low-dose fluticasone in reducing or maintaining an anti-inflammatory effect on induced sputum eosinophil counts and exhaled nitric oxide levels in patients with steroid naïve asthma (29,30). The reduction of inflammatory cell numbers in the bronchial mucosa achieved with fluticasone plus montelukast is not significantly different from that observed with fluticasone alone in adults with mild asthma (31). The addition of montelukast to existing moderate-dose corticosteroid therapy or to high-dose corticosteroid therapy in adults with asthma with normal or elevated sputum eosinophils is not effective in providing an additional reduction in airway eosinophil counts (32,33). Salmeterol plus fluticasone propionate versus fluticasone propionate plus montelukast administered for three months to adults with asthma poorly controlled on low-dose inhaled corticosteroids led to similar minor effects on eosinophilic airway inflammation (34). However, in children with asthma there may be an anti-inflammatory effect of montelukast, additive to that of moderate doses of inhaled corticosteroids (35).

In a mouse model of allergen-induced chronic inflammation and fibrosis, montelukast reverses established airway smooth muscle cell layer thickening and subepithelial fibrosis, which in this model was not affected by corticosteroids (36). These findings suggest that anti-leukotriene drugs could prevent or reverse airway remodeling in asthma. In support of this hypothesis, a bronchial biopsy study in patients with mild asthma reported a reduction in low-dose allergen-induced myofibroblast numbers following treatment with montelukast (37). However, recent in vitro studies on human bronchial fibroblasts suggest that current leukotriene-receptor antagonists might not block all the effects of leukotrienes on airway remodeling (38). Further evidence from larger clinical trials is required to establish whether leukotriene-receptor antagonists have a role in treating airway remodeling in asthma.

D. Anti-leukotriene Drugs on Triggers of Asthma and Associated Comorbidities

Leukotriene-receptor antagonists and 5-lipoxygenase inhibitors attenuate the bronchoconstrictor response to a number of trigger factors including allergen, exercise, cold air, aspirin, ultrasonically nebulized distilled water, or adenosine (2,9,39–42).

Allergen-Induced Asthma

A single oral dose of zafirlukast administered two hours before allergen challenge inhibits both early and late responses (43). Chronic dosing with zafirlukast for one week protects against symptoms of asthma and alterations in pulmonary function induced by natural exposure to cat allergen (44). Similar results to those obtained with zafirlukast on acute allergen challenge have been reported with montelukast in both adults and children (10,12,45). A single dose of montelukast given orally, immediately after the early allergic response, can significantly inhibit the late allergic response after bronchial allergen challenge (46). However, a single 800 mg dose of zileuton has no effect on either the early or the late airway response to allergen (47).

Montelukast and budesonide 400 µg daily for 10 days attenuate allergen-induced asthmatic responses, airway hyperresponsiveness, and sputum eosinophilia, although combination treatment did not provide greater anti-inflammatory effects than either drug alone (11). High-dose inhaled corticosteroid therapy in the form of inhaled fluticasone 250 µg twice daily administered for eight days had overall greater efficacy in attenuating allergen-induced airway responses compared to montelukast 10 mg daily in subjects with mild asthma (12).

The effect of the LTB_4 receptor antagonist, LY293111, on allergen challenge demonstrated a reduction in the number and degree of activation of neutrophils, but there was no measured physiological benefit (48).

Exercise-Induced Asthma

Montelukast and zafirlukast attenuate exercise-induced asthma in both children and adults (49–53). The mean maximal percentage fall in FEV_1 (forced expiratory volume in one second) after exercise following a single dose of zafirlukast was 22% compared with 36% after placebo, although the degree of protection against exercise-induced asthma varies between individuals (49). Following three months treatment with montelukast, the maximal fall in FEV_1 after exercise was 22% compared with 32% after placebo (51). The results remained consistent throughout the study and tolerance did not develop. In patients with mild asthma who were not receiving inhaled corticosteroid therapy, the inhaled long-acting β_2-agonist salmeterol, but not montelukast, showed attenuation of bronchoprotection after four and eight weeks of treatment (52). Acute and long-term treatment with zileuton has been shown to decrease the response to isocapnic hyperventilation (54). Single doses of zileuton and montelukast are equally effective in attenuating exercise-induced asthma, but zileuton has a shorter duration of action (55).

Aspirin-Induced Asthma

Aspirin-induced asthma is associated with elevated formation of the Cys-LTs and this may be related to upregulation of leukotriene C_4 synthase (56). Both 5-lipoxygenase inhibitors and leukotriene-receptor antagonists can inhibit acute aspirin-induced bronchoconstriction, but the degree of protection varies between individuals (57). The addition of montelukast treatment for four weeks improves lung function and asthma symptoms in aspirin-intolerant patients over and above that achieved by corticosteroids (58). In one study, pretreatment with zileuton not only prevented the fall in FEV_1 after aspirin challenge but also reduced urinary leukotriene E_4 levels at baseline and after aspirin challenge (27).

Allergic Rhinitis

Leukotriene-receptor antagonists are effective therapies for allergic rhinitis (59). In patients with coexistent asthma, montelukast improves symptoms of seasonal allergic rhinitis and chronic asthma (60), and the combination of montelukast and budesonide provided slightly greater improvement in lung function compared with doubling the dose of budesonide (61). However, in another study of patients with persistent asthma treated with fluticasone propionate/salmeterol, the addition of montelukast or fluticasone propionate aqueous nasal spray for the treatment of seasonal allergic rhinitis resulted in no additional improvements in overall asthma control compared with fluticasone propionate/salmeterol alone (62).

E. Anti-leukotriene Drugs on Baseline Lung Function

The finding that drugs that modify the 5-lipoxygenase pathway can cause mild bronchodilation suggests that leukotriene release within the airways contributes to bronchoconstriction in asthma (25,26,63,64). A single 40-mg oral dose of zafirlukast produces a small bronchodilator effect, increasing the mean FEV_1 value by 8% (25). In

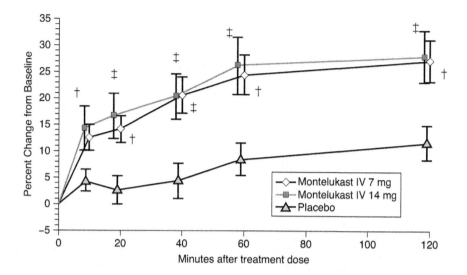

Figure 2 Effect of intravenous montelukast (7- and 14-mg doses) and placebo in addition to standard therapy on percentage change in FEV_1 in patients with acute asthma. $^\dagger p < 0.05$ for montelukast versus placebo; $^\ddagger p < 0.01$ for montelukast versus placebo. No differences between the montelukast treatment groups. *Source*: From Ref. 65.

this study, the increase in FEV_1 after nebulized albuterol and zafirlukast was 26% compared with 18% after nebulized albuterol and placebo. This finding suggests that the bronchodilator effect of β_2-agonists and leukotriene-receptor antagonists might be additive. Single oral doses of montelukast cause bronchodilation irrespective of the concurrent use of inhaled corticosteroids in asthmatic subjects with airflow limitation (63). In a group of 139 asthmatic patients whose baseline FEV_1 values were approximately 60% of predicted, a single 600-mg dose of zileuton increased mean FEV_1 values by 14.6% in one hour, which was significantly greater than the change with placebo (26). Further improvements in FEV_1 values occurred during the following four weeks of chronic dosing with zileuton.

The finding that intravenous montelukast produces a rapid onset of bronchodilation in patients with chronic asthma raised the possibility that leukotriene-receptor antagonists might have a role as a treatment for acute asthma (64). In support of this suggestion, intravenous montelukast, in addition to standard therapy, causes rapid improvement in lung function and is well tolerated in adults with acute asthma (Fig. 2) (65).

F. Therapeutic Effects of Anti-leukotriene Drugs in Chronic Asthma

The leukotriene-receptor antagonists, montelukast, and zafirlukast are effective anti-asthma agents in both children and adults (18,66–71). In a group of 681 adult patients with chronic stable asthma, 23% of whom were receiving inhaled corticosteroids, montelukast, compared with placebo, significantly improved asthma control [FEV_1, morning and evening peak expiratory flow (PEF), asthma symptoms, and exacerbation rates] during a three-month treatment period (18). Montelukast produces dose-related improvements in asthma control in patients with mild persistent asthma (68,71). In a six-week trial of zafirlukast, significant improvements in symptoms and lung function were seen in the highest dose group (40 mg daily) (66). Treatment with zafirlukast in a dose of 40 mg daily for three months was also found to reduce the rate of exacerbations of asthma (67). Montelukast has improved asthma control in 6- to 14-year-old children with chronic asthma (69) as well as in younger asthmatic children aged 2 to 5 years (70). A short course of montelukast, introduced at the first signs of an asthma symptoms or upper respiratory tract infection, results in a modest reduction in symptoms, time off from school, and acute health care resource utilization in children with intermittent asthma (72).

Three large multicenter trials using zileuton in mild-to-moderate chronic asthma have shown evidence of efficacy (17,26,73). The durations of the trials were 4, 13, and 26 weeks, respectively, and each employed a double blind, parallel group, and placebo-controlled study design. Zileuton was shown to improve daily symptoms of asthma, night waking, and PEF measurements, and to reduce the use of rescue inhaled β_2-agonists and the number of exacerbations of asthma requiring corticosteroids. In general, the 5-lipoxygenase inhibitors and leukotriene-receptor antagonists appear to produce similar clinical effects, although to date there have been no comparative studies.

Comparison with Inhaled Corticosteroids

The clinical efficacy of montelukast and zafirlukast is less than that seen with low doses of inhaled corticosteroids (equivalent to 400 µg daily of inhaled beclometasone) (74–79). For example, in a group of 895 adult patients with chronic stable asthma, montelukast 10 mg once daily, compared with inhaled beclometasone 200 µg twice daily, increased mean FEV_1 values by 7.5% compared with the larger increase of 13.3% after the inhaled corticosteroid following three months of treatment (75). Multicenter randomized controlled trial of zafirlukast (20 mg twice daily) or montelukast (10 mg once daily) for three and six months, respectively, when compared with inhaled fluticasone (100 µg twice daily) found that the improvement in asthma control was greater in the inhaled corticosteroid groups (76–78).

A systematic review of 27 randomized controlled trials that compared anti-leukotrienes with inhaled corticosteroids during a minimal 30-day intervention period in asthmatic patients aged two years and older concluded that inhaled corticosteroids at a dose of 400 µg daily of beclometasone or equivalent are more effective than anti-leukotriene agents given in the usual licensed doses (79). Inhaled corticosteroids resulted in greater improvements in lung function, symptoms, nocturnal awakenings, rescue medication use, symptom-free days, and quality of life compared with anti-leukotriene agents. Patients treated with anti-leukotrienes were 65% more likely to suffer an exacerbation requiring systemic steroids. Anti-leukotriene therapy was associated with 160% increased risk of withdrawals due to poor asthma control. A recent clinical trial in children confirmed the conclusion that inhaled corticosteroid therapy is superior to montelukast in treating children with mild-to-moderate persistent asthma with $FEV_1 \geq$ 80% predicted (80). In patients with mild persistent asthma, short intermittent therapy with inhaled budesonide and daily zafirlukast over a period of one year produced equivalent effects on asthma control and markers of inflammation (28).

Anti-leukotrienes: An Add-on Therapy

The efficacy of leukotriene-receptor antagonists as add-on treatment to inhaled corticosteroids has been assessed using a number of different protocols.

Add-on to Low-Dose Inhaled Corticosteroids

In a randomized, placebo-controlled trial lasting 16 weeks, of 642 adult asthmatic patients not adequately controlled on inhaled beclometasone 400 µg daily, the addition of montelukast 10 mg daily resulted in an improvement in mean FEV_1 of 5% compared with 1% for inhaled corticosteroids alone and also caused modest improvements in PEF and reductions in β_2-agonist use (74). In children with persistent asthma, the addition of montelukast 5 mg daily to inhaled budesonide 400 µg daily produced modest improvements in PEF and reductions in β_2-agonist use over a four-week treatment period (19). The results of these published studies suggest a modest additional effect of licensed doses of montelukast in symptomatic children and adults. A Cochrane systematic review of randomized controlled trials identified up until 2003 of leukotriene-receptor antagonists as add-on therapy in children and adults with chronic asthma found that the addition of licensed doses of anti-leukotrienes to inhaled corticosteroids resulted in a nonsignificant reduction in the risk of exacerbations requiring systemic corticosteroids and modest improvement in lung function (81). The meta-analysis concluded that the addition of licensed doses of anti-leukotrienes to add-on therapy to inhaled corticosteroids brings modest improvement in lung function.

Compared with a Long-Acting β_2-Agonist as an Add-on to Low-Dose Inhaled Corticosteroids

A study of a small group of 20 patients with persistent asthma found that the addition of montelukast or inhaled salmeterol over a two-week treatment period produced similar improvements in the asthma control of patients not controlled with inhaled corticosteroids, but only montelukast therapy reduced blood eosinophil counts (82). The effect of montelukast versus salmeterol added to inhaled fluticasone propionate on asthma exacerbation in patients whose symptoms are inadequately controlled with fluticasone 100 µg daily alone was equivalent over a period of one year. However, improvements in lung function were greater with the addition of salmeterol and the reduction in peripheral blood eosinophil counts was greater with the addition of montelukast (83).

A systematic review and meta-analysis of 15 randomized controlled trials in adults and children with asthma, inadequately controlled on low doses of inhaled corticosteroids, the addition of long-acting β_2-agonist was superior to a leukotriene-receptor antagonist for preventing exacerbations requiring systemic corticosteroids, and for improving lung function, symptoms, and the use of rescue β_2-agonists (84). The risk of exacerbations requiring systemic corticosteroids was significantly lower with the inhaled corticosteroids and long-acting β_2-agonist combination when compared to the leukotriene-receptor antagonist and inhaled corticosteroid combination (84).

As an Add-on to Low-Dose Inhaled Corticosteroids Vs. Double Dose of Inhaled Corticosteroid

A Cochrane systematic review of randomized controlled trials identified up until 2003 found that only three trials compared the use of licensed doses of anti-leukotrienes with increased doses of inhaled corticosteroids, and no firm conclusion could be drawn about the equivalence of both treatment options. The review concluded that although the addition of anti-leukotrienes to inhaled corticosteroids appears comparable to increasing the dose of inhaled corticosteroids, the power of the review was insufficient to confirm the equivalence of both treatment options (81).

Over a three-month period the addition of montelukast to inhaled budesonide 800 µg daily was as effective as doubling the dose of inhaled budesonide 800 µg daily in adult asthma patients experiencing symptoms and inadequate control on budesonide alone (85). However, the duration of the trial may have been too short to detect differences in exacerbation rates (86). The addition of zileuton to low-dose beclometasone 400 µg daily compared with higher doses of inhaled beclometasone 800 µg daily in patients unable to achieve asthma control on low-dose inhaled corticosteroid therapy produced a similar level of asthma control (87).

As an Add-on to Low-Dose Inhaled Corticosteroids Vs. Other Add-on Therapies

A clinical trial of the efficacy of once-daily oral controller therapy with either montelukast or low-dose theophylline added to existing medications in patients with poorly controlled found that neither drug improved asthma control. Both montelukast and theophylline caused small improvements in lung function (88). In a three-month trial, zileuton and theophylline were found to be equally effective in the control of chronic asthma (89).

As an Add-on to High-Dose Inhaled Corticosteroids Plus Other Add-on Therapies

In a group of 72 patients with symptomatic chronic persistent asthma already taking high-dose inhaled corticosteroids and other add-on therapies such as inhaled long-acting β_2-agonists, the addition of montelukast for two weeks did not improve symptoms or PEF recordings (90). This result suggests that leukotriene-receptor antagonists might be less effective or ineffective in patients with moderate or severe asthma. Another randomized controlled study in patients with mild-to-moderate persistent asthma found that the addition of montelukast to daily fluticasone propionate, 500 µg, plus salmeterol produced no additional effects on lung function although did find improvements in inflammatory biomarkers and airway hyperresponsiveness (91). However, zafirlukast administered for two weeks, at an unlicensed dose of 80 mg twice daily, was found to improve asthma control as assessed by reduced exacerbations, improvements in PEF readings, and reduction in both β_2-agonist usage and symptoms in patients with severe persistent asthma receiving high-dose inhaled corticosteroids ($\geq$1200 µg daily) (92). Possibly patients with chronic severe asthma may require higher than currently licensed doses of leukotriene-receptor antagonists.

Add-on to a Long-Acting β_2-Agonist Vs. Inhaled Corticosteroids Plus a Long-Acting β_2-Agonist

In a randomized controlled crossover trial of 192 patients with moderate asthma, the combination of montelukast and salmeterol compared to combination of an inhaled beclometasone 160 µg daily and salmeterol was less effect in preventing treatment failure and in improving lung function, airway hyperresponsiveness, and markers of inflammation (93).

To Allow Tapering of Inhaled Corticosteroids

Several short-term studies have reported modest inhaled corticosteroid sparing effects with the addition of montelukast daily for 12 weeks (94) or pranlukast administered daily for 6 weeks (95). However, a Cochrane systematic review of inhaled corticosteroid sparing studies of patients who were well controlled at baseline found that the addition of anti-leukotrienes produced no overall difference in dose of inhaled corticosteroids, but it was associated with fewer withdrawals due to poor asthma control (81). The review concluded that a corticosteroid-sparing effect cannot be quantified at present (81).

Factors Predicting a Therapeutic Response to Anti-leukotrienes

Recent studies in asthma have noted a highly variable therapeutic response to leukotriene-receptor antagonists and to inhaled corticosteroids in individuals with both adult and childhood asthma (96–98). A higher proportion of subjects obtain a better response to inhaled corticosteroid therapy, as assessed by improvement in lung function or asthma control days, but some individuals respond better to montelukast (Fig. 3) (97). Several factors have been implicated in predicting a beneficial therapeutic response to anti-leukotrienes (Table 1):

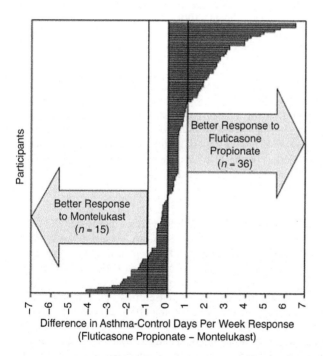

Figure 3 Difference in asthma control days between inhaled fluticasone and montelukast (fluticasone minus montelukast) for individual participants with mild-to-moderate persistent childhood asthma. Each *line* designates a single participant. *Source*: From Ref. 97.

Table 1 Factors Reported to Predict a Favorable Therapeutic Response to Anti-leukotriene Drugs

- Increased urinary leukotriene E_4 concentrations or exhaled breath condensate leukotriene E_4 levels
- Corticosteroid insensitivity
- Cigarette smokers
- Genetic polymorphisms
- Children
- Obesity
- Severity of disease

Leukotriene Production

A raised urinary leukotriene E_4 concentrations predict the response to leukotriene-receptor antagonist in same studies in adults with asthma, but not on others (58,99). In children with asthma, a favorable clinical response to montelukast was associated with high urinary leukotriene E_4 levels (98). In an open label study, montelukast decreased exhaled breath condensate leukotriene E_4 levels in atopic children with asthma who had raised baseline exhaled leukotriene E_4 levels (100). The reduction by zileuton in bronchoalveolar lavage eosinophil count after segmental allergen challenge occurs in those in whom airway leukotriene levels were elevated by allergen (15).

Corticosteroid Insensitivity

In aspirin-sensitive asthma, chronic dosing with montelukast for four weeks (58) or with zileuton for six weeks (101) has been shown to improve asthma control over that achieved with medium-to-high doses of inhaled corticosteroids. These findings are of interest in view of the observation that corticosteroids do not inhibit leukotriene formation and airway responsiveness in vivo (102,103), and aspirin-intolerant asthma is associated with increased formation of the Cys-LTs. These findings suggest that the biosynthesis and actions of leukotrienes are less sensitive to corticosteroids.

Genetic Factors

Naturally occurring mutations in the promoter of 5-lipoxygenase gene (ALOX5) may influence the clinical response to drugs modifying the 5-lipoxygenase pathway (104–106). Polymorphisms of 5-lipoxygenase and also cys-LT_2 receptor, however, predispose to only a small subset of <15% of asthma patients to respond better to montelukast (106). Genetic variability in leukotriene C4 synthetase has been reported to be more commonly associated with a good therapeutic response to a leukotriene-receptor antagonist in a small group of patients with severe asthma (107), although this association has not been found by others (106,108). Variation in the genes that encode membrane efflux and uptake transport proteins could influence the absorption of oral leukotriene-receptor antagonists and might contribute to heterogeneity in therapeutic response (105,109). In patients taking montelukast polymorphisms of leukotriene A_4 hydrolase, the enzyme that catalyzes the formation of leukotriene B_4, are associated with an increased risk of an exacerbation of asthma (105). It has been suggested that racial and geographic origin of study populations may account for the variable results from different pharmacogenetic association studies (3). Certain thromboxane (Tx) A_2 receptor gene polymorphisms may predict an impaired response to montelukast in attenuating exercise-induced asthma among Korean children (110).

Children

Montelukast may be of particular benefit in 2- to 5-year-old children where it has been shown to reduce the number of viral-induced exacerbations by 31.9% compared with placebo (111). Children aged 6 to 17 year of age with low pulmonary function or high levels of exhaled nitric oxide or other biomarkers of airway inflammation responded better to inhaled corticosteroid therapy compared to a leukotriene-receptor antagonist, whereas other children respond to either drug (97,98).

Cigarette Smokers

Lazarus and colleagues (112) report for the first time that the leukotriene-receptor agonist montelukast shows efficacy in smokers with mild asthma, which is important in view of the data showing corticosteroid insensitivity in this group (113,114). However, the beneficial effect on morning PEF of montelukast in the smokers with asthma was not large nor did the study include supportive data on urinary or sputum leukotrienes in smokers versus nonsmokers. The generalizability of their findings is uncertain, in particular whether a similar beneficial effect would be found in smokers with more severe asthma (114).

Obesity

The response to leukotriene-receptor antagonists remained unaltered with increasing body mass index, whereas the response to inhaled corticosteroids is reduced (115).

Severity of Disease

A post hoc analysis of two phase III studies of zileuton in asthma suggested that patients with more severe disease ($FEV_1 \leq 50\%$) had a better response compared to subjects with milder asthma (116). A neutrophilic airway phenotype associated with increased LTB_4 levels is a possible mechanism to explain improved efficacy of zileuton in severe asthma.

G. Adverse Effects

In clinical trials zafirlukast, montelukast, and zileuton have been well tolerated. The main side effects with the use of zafirlukast are headache and gastrointestinal disturbance. Zafirlukast can interact with other drugs including warfarin (increases the prothrombin time by approximately 35%), aspirin (increases the plasma levels of zafirlukast by approximately 45%), theophylline (decreases the plasma levels of zafirlukast by approximately 30%), and erythromycin (decreases the plasma levels of zafirlukast by approximately 40%). Cigarette smokers exhibit increased clearance of zafirlukast. In clinical trials with montelukast, abdominal pain and headache are reported in a small proportion of patients, and the incidence is only slightly higher from those receiving placebo. In small study sample of 96 women who took leukotriene-receptor antagonists during pregnancy, there were no associated increased structural anomalies or other adverse perinatal outcomes in comparison to women who only took short-acting β_2-agonists (117).

Zileuton has been associated with rises in liver enzymes that return to normal on stopping the drug (26,73). The incidence of zileuton-induced hepatitis is approximately 3%. In the United States, the Food and Drug Administration recommend that liver function tests be monitored regularly during the first year of treatment. Zileuton increases theophylline and warfarin levels.

The administration of leukotriene-receptor antagonists has been associated with the development of the Churg–Strauss syndrome (118–121). In each case, the patient was reducing their dose of oral corticosteroids for asthma and it is likely that the reduction in oral corticosteroid dose resulted in unmasking the syndrome.

H. Leukotrienes and COPD

There is very limited data on the efficacy of anti-leukotrienes in COPD. Urinary and breath condensate concentrations of leukotriene E_4 are not elevated in patients with COPD compared with healthy controls (122,123). However, a randomized controlled single blind study of montelukast added to treatment with ipratropium bromide and formoterol to patients with moderate to severe COPD produced increases in FEV_1 and vital capacity values and symptoms of dyspnea (124). In patients with stable COPD, zafirlukast has a slight bronchodilator effect suggesting that Cys-LTs may contribute to bronchoconstriction in COPD (125).

Leukotriene B_4 levels are increased in sputum and exhaled breath of patients with COPD (123,126). In a small pilot clinical trial, an oral leukotriene synthesis inhibitor BAYx1005 administered for 14 days produced modest reductions in sputum leukotriene B_4 levels in patients with COPD (127). LTB_4 receptor antagonists, BLT_1 antagonists, such as LY29311 (6) and SB 201146, inhibit the neutrophil chemotactic activity of sputum from COPD patients (128,129), and these agents may have a role in the treatment of COPD.

I. Conclusions

In the treatment of asthma, leukotriene-receptor antagonists and 5-lipoxygenase inhibitors produce mild bronchodilation in patients with airflow obstruction and attenuate bronchoconstriction induced by exercise, allergen, and aspirin. Systemic administration of drugs acting on the 5-lipoxygenase pathway may also improve coexisting disease such as allergic rhinitis. There is also some evidence to indicate that they have anti-inflammatory actions. Several therapeutic studies in mild-to-moderate asthma have shown evidence of efficacy. A theoretical advantage of the oral formulation of these drugs, and for some agents, the infrequent dose scheduling, is improved concordance with therapy, but this potential beneficial on improved outcome has not been demonstrated (130). In clinical trials, the leukotriene-receptor antagonists, zafirlukast and montelukast, and the 5-lipoxygenase inhibitor, zileuton, are well tolerated. There is little data on the effects of anti-leukotrienes in COPD.

The clinical effectiveness of these drugs appears to be quite variable between individuals. There is some evidence that levels of leukotriene production, corticosteroid sensitivity, naturally occurring mutations in the 5-lipoxygenase gene, cigarette smoking, age, or severity of disease may influence the therapeutic response to anti-leukotrienes. Current guidelines suggest a role for anti-leukotrienes in adults and children older than five years as alternative, but less effective first line prophylactic agents to inhaled corticosteroids (131). Anti-leukotrienes are alternative add-on drugs for adults and children with persistent symptoms despite low-dose inhaled cortico-steroid therapy, but in adults are less effective than long-acting β_2 agonists. In children five years of age and under, anti-leukotrienes also reduce exacerbation due to viral infections. Zileuton may be a less desirable alternative to leukotriene-receptor antagonists because of the need to monitor liver function. The role of the leukotriene-receptor antagonists and the 5-lipoxygenase inhibitors in moderate to severe asthma is less well-established.

III. Prostaglandin and Thromboxane Antagonists

Arachidonic acid is metabolized by prostaglandin H synthase (PGHS) to form prosta-glandin (PG) endoperoxidases (132). There are two isoforms of PGHS, the constitutive isoform cyclooxygenase (COX)-1 and the largely inducible isoform COX-2. COX-1 is expressed in airway epithelial cells, whereas COX-2 expression is induced in epithelial and airway smooth muscle cells by inflammatory mediators such as IL-1β and TNFα (133). PG endoperoxidases are metabolized by tissue-specific isomerize and synthases to generate distinct prostanoids such as prostacyclin, Tx A$_2$, PGD$_2$, PGE$_2$, and PDF$_{2\alpha}$ (132). Each prostanoid acts on distinct G protein coupled receptors. For examples, PGD$_2$ activates DP$_1$ or DP$_2$ receptors, PGE$_2$ activates EP$_1$, EP$_2$, EP$_3$, or EP$_4$ receptors, PDF$_{2\alpha}$ activates FP$_\alpha$ or FP$_\beta$ receptors, and TxA$_2$ activates TP$_\alpha$ or TP$_\beta$ receptor.

PGE$_2$ causes airway smooth muscle relaxation by activating EP$_2$ receptors and in vivo in asthma inhaled PGE$_2$ can attenuate bronchoconstriction induced by allergen and exercise. In addition, PGE$_2$ induces airway smooth muscle proliferation, vasodilatation, inhibits cholinergic nerve contraction of human airways, and inhibits the release of mediators from eosinophils, mast cells, and neutrophils. In contrast PGD$_2$, PDF$_{2\alpha}$, and TxA$_2$ cause bronchoconstriction that is inhibited by TP receptor antagonists.

Prostanoid levels are increased in biological fluids from individuals with asthma including elevated bronchoalveolar lavage concentrations PGD$_2$, PDF$_{2\alpha}$, and TXB$_2$ in basal conditions and after allergen challenge (134). Urinary metabolites of TxA$_2$ are increased in COPD (135). Several TP-receptor antagonists and TX synthase inhibitors have been synthesized, but none are so far licensed out with Japan for the treatment of asthma or COPD (134). Ozagrel is a TX synthase inhibitor, but with additional effects in inhibiting other mediators such as the leukotrienes can attenuate bronchial hyper-responsiveness to methacholine (136). The TP-receptor antagonist seratrodast can improve asthma control and reduce the infiltration of activated eosinophil in the airways (137), although the beneficial effects on lung function are small (138). Ramatroban, a TP-receptor antagonist and PGD2 receptor, chemoattractant receptor-homologous molecule expressed on Th2 cells (CRTh2) antagonist, has also been shown to be effective in attenuating induced bronchoconstriction to allergen and exercise and is marketed in Japan for the treatment of allergic rhinitis (134). Possibly the combination of a Tx modulator with a leukotriene D$_4$ receptor antagonist may have greater thera-peutic effects in the treatment of asthma (134,139,140).

IV. Histamine Receptor Antagonists

Histamine is an inflammatory mediator that plays a role in allergic inflammation (133,141). The majority of histamine is stored preformed in cytoplasmic granules of mast cells and basophils. Many stimuli, including antigen, cause mast cell degranulation and histamine release. Histamine has several properties that might contribute to the pathogenesis of asthma including bronchial smooth muscle contraction, increased vascular permeability leading to mucosal oedema, and mucus hypersecretion. Four subtypes of histamine receptor (H_1, H_2, H_3, H_4) have been identified (142). Clinical studies evaluating the efficacy of histamine-receptor antagonists in asthma have concentrated predominately on drugs acting at the H_1 receptor, which mediates bronchoconstriction and microvascular leakage. Non-sedating antihistamines, such as astemizole, azelastine, cetirizine, loratadine, and terfenadine, act as histamine H_1-receptor antagonists. A number of these compounds possess additional pharmacological properties (143). For example, cetirizine has been reported to inhibit eosinophil chemotaxis in vitro and adhesion molecule expression by epithelial cells in vivo (144), and loratadine inhibits leukotriene release (145). H_1-receptor antagonists have also been shown to downregulate nuclear factor kappa B (NF-κB) expression (143). The exact mode of action of ketotifen in vivo is uncertain, although the main pharmacological effects are likely to be due to H_1-receptor antagonism (146).

Antihistamines have been shown to attenuate early and late responses to allergen, although the combination of H_1-receptor antagonists, loratadine, and the leukotriene-receptor antagonist, zafirlukast, was found to be more effective than either drug alone (147). H_1-receptor antagonists also inhibit exercise-induced asthma (148) and broncho-constriction mediated by cold-air challenge (149). Pretreatment with oral terfenadine attenuates adenosine-induced bronchoconstriction in smokers with COPD (150). H_1-receptor antagonists administered both orally or by inhalation cause modest bronchodilation in patients with asthma (151). A meta-analysis of 19 randomized controlled trials found that antihistamines had little effect on lung function or on the use of inhaled β_2-agonists and that sedation occurred more often than with placebo (152). A systematic review of 26 randomized controlled trial indicates that ketotifen alone or in combination with other therapies improves control of asthma and wheezing in children with mild and moderate asthma, but the studies were of low methodological quality (153). Taken together, current evidence indicates that H_1-receptor antagonists do not have a place in the treatment of chronic persistent asthma. The role of combination therapy with H_1-receptor antagonist and leukotriene-receptor antagonist in chronic asthma therapy remains to be established. The finding that H_4-receptor activation induces recruitment of regulatory T cells and inhibits allergic asthma in a murine model (154) suggests that H_4-receptor antagonists might have a potential role in the treatment of asthmatic inflammation (141).

V. New Prospects

A number of new mediator receptor antagonists and synthesis inhibitors are under development for the treatment of airway disease.

A. Adenosine Receptor Antagonists

Adenosine has been implicated in having a pathogenic role in asthma and COPD (155). Adenosine exerts its proinflammatory and anti-inflammatory biological activities by interacting with G protein–coupled receptors of which there are four subtypes: termed

A_1, A_{2A}, A_{2B}, and A_3. Adenosine A_1 receptor expression is increased in the bronchial epithelium and smooth muscle in patients with mild asthma compared to healthy controls (156). Adenosine induces the release of inflammatory mediators from mast cells via stimulation of adenosine A_2 receptors, particularly the A_{2B} subtype. A specific adenosine A_{2B} receptor antagonists CVT-6883 attenuate allergen-induced airway inflammation in a mouse model (157) and other selective adenosine A_{2B} receptor antagonists have been developed (155). The clinical effects of adenosine A_{2B} receptor antagonists in asthma and COPD are under investigation. The inhaled A_{2A} receptor agonist, GW328267X, does not affect the allergen-induced late asthmatic response or the associated inflammatory response in asthma (158).

B. Endothelin Receptor Antagonists

Endothelin-1 (ET) mimics several of the features of asthma including bronchoconstriction (159,160). The biological effects of ET are mediated by the two receptor subtypes: ET_A and ET_B, which are found in human lung. Increased levels and expression of ET are found in patients with asthma, particularly in subjects with refractory disease (161). The expression of ET in bronchial epithelium correlates with indices of airway remodeling, suggesting that ET receptor antagonists might be of value in the treatment of severe asthma (161). ET receptor antagonists, although effective in animal models of eosinophilic inflammation (160,162), have not been evaluated in patients with asthma.

C. Neurokinin Receptor Antagonists

The neuropeptides substance P and neurokinin A (NKA) are implicated in the pathophysiology of asthma. Neurokinin NK_1 and NK_2 receptor antagonists have been developed for the treatment of asthma and COPD. NK_1 or NK_2 receptor antagonists can attenuate the bronchoconstrictor response to NKA. In patients with allergic asthma, a tachykinin NK(1)/NK(2) receptor antagonist AVE5883 paradoxically increased allergen-induced early and late airway responses without affecting markers of airway hyperresponsiveness and airway inflammation (163). These results do not support a role for dual tachykinin antagonists in the treatment of asthma.

D. Bradykinin Receptor Antagonists

Kinins are proinflammatory peptides that mediate a variety of pathophysiological responses in airway disease. Kinins act through stimulation of two distinct receptor subtypes B1 and B2. A large number of peptide and nonpeptide bradykinin B2 receptor antagonists have been developed including HOE140, FK3657, and B-9430 (dual B1/B2) (164). The selective bradykinin B2 receptor antagonist HOE140 (Icatibant) administered by inhalation attenuates the bradykinin-induce bronchoconstriction and allergen challenge in the nose (165). None of these agents have been licensed for use in asthma or COPD.

E. Vanilloid Receptor Antagonists

Transient receptor potential vanilloid type channels (TRPVs) are expressed in several cell types in the lungs and they may be involved in the pathogenesis of asthma and chronic cough (166). Activation of these channels, particularly TRPV1 and TRPV4, by changes in temperature and osmolarity as well as by inflammatory mediators induces cough, reflex bronchoconstriction, and neurogenic inflammation. Several TRPV antagonists have been discovered and could have a role in the treatment of airway disease (166).

Summary

The potential involvement of many inflammatory mediators in the pathogenesis of asthma has led the pharmaceutical industry to develop specific mediator antagonists and synthesis inhibitors as possible new therapeutic agents for asthma. The role of specific mediator antagonists in the treatment of chronic obstructive pulmonary disease (COPD) is largely untested. In patients with asthma, the leukotriene-receptor antagonists, zafirlukast and montelukast, and the 5-lipoxygenase inhibitors, zileuton, attenuate bronchoconstriction induced by exercise, allergen, and aspirin and decrease some indices of airway inflammation. Anti-leukotrienes are effective and well-tolerated in patients with mild-to-moderate asthma. International guidelines for asthma recommend anti-leukotrienes as alternative, but less effective first-line prophylactic agents to inhaled corticosteroids and as an alternative second-line add-on drug to long-acting β_2 agonists for patients with persistent symptoms despite low-dose inhaled corticosteroid therapy. The clinical effectiveness of these drugs appears variable between individuals, possibly because of multiple factors including levels of leukotriene production, corticosteroid sensitivity, naturally occurring mutations in the 5-lipoxygenase gene, cigarette smoking, age, or severity of disease. Current evidence indicates that H_1-receptor antagonists do not have a place in the treatment of chronic persistent asthma. A number of new mediator receptor antagonists and synthesis inhibitors are under development for the treatment of airway diseases including thromboxane-receptor antagonists, chemoattractant receptor–homologous molecule expressed on Th2 cells (CRTh2) antagonists, adenosine A_{2B} receptor antagonists, and endothelin-1 receptor antagonists. If new drugs are found to have a place in the treatment of airway diseases, it is likely that they will be used in combination with other therapies such as inhaled corticosteroids or other mediator antagonists rather than as monotherapy. New mediator antagonists may have a role in the treatment of specific phenotypes of asthma and COPD and on the systemic components of airway disease.

References

1. Hay DWP, Torphy TJ, Undem BJ. Cysteinyl leukotrienes in asthma: old mediators up to new tricks. Trends Pharmacol Sci 1995; 16(9):304–309.
2. Ogawa Y, Calhoun WJ. The role of leukotrienes in airway inflammation. J Allergy Clin Immunol 2006; 118(4):789–798.
3. Peters-Golden M, Henderson WR Jr. Leukotrienes. N Engl J Med 2007; 357(18):1841–1854.
4. Montuschi P, Sala A, Dahlen S-E, et al. Pharmacological modulation of the leukotriene pathway in allergic airway disease. Drug Discov Today 2007; 12(9–10):404–412.
5. Miyahara N, Miyahara S, Takeda K, et al. Role of the LTB4/BLT$_1$ pathway in allergen-induced airway hyperresponsiveness and inflammation. Allergol Int 2006; 55(2):91–97.
6. Silbaugh S, Stengel P, Cockerham S, et al. Pharmacologic actions of the second generation leukotriene B4 receptor antagonist LY29311: in vivo pulmonary studies. Naunyn Schmiedebergs Arch Pharmacol 2000; 361(4):397–404.
7. Dahlen S-E. Treatment of asthma with antileukotrienes: first line or last resort therapy? Eur J Pharmacol 2006; 533(1-3):40–56.
8. Rao NL, Dunford PJ, Xue X, et al. Anti-inflammatory activity of a potent, selective leukotriene A4 hydrolase inhibitor in comparison with the 5-lipoxygenase inhibitor zileuton. J Pharmacol Exp Ther 2007; 321(3):1154–1160.
9. Busse W, Kraft M. Cysteinyl leukotrienes in allergic inflammation: strategic target for therapy. Chest 2005; 127(4):1312–1326.

10. Diamant, Grootendorst, Veselic C, et al. The effect of montelukast (MK-0476), a cysteinyl leukotriene receptor antagonist, on allergen-induced airway responses and sputum cell counts in asthma. Clin Exp Allergy 1999; 29(1):42–51.

11. Leigh R, Vethanayagam D, Yoshida M, et al. Effects of montelukast and budesonide on airway responses and airway inflammation in asthma. Am J Repir Crit Care Med 2002; 166(9):1212–1217.

12. Palmqvist M, Bruce C, Sjostrand M, et al. Differential effects of fluticasone and montelukast on allergen-induced asthma. Allergy 2005; 60(1):65–70.

13. Calhoun William J, Lavins Bernard J, Minkwitz Margaret C, et al. Effect of zafirlukast (accolate) on cellular mediators of inflammation. bronchoalveolar lavage fluid findings after segmental antigen challenge. Am J Repir Crit Care Med 1998; 157(5):1381–1389.

14. Kane GC, Pollice M, Kim C-J, et al. A controlled trial of the effect of the 5-lipoxygenase inhibitor, zileuton, on lung inflammation produced by segmental antigen challenge in human beings. J Allergy Clin Immunol 1996; 97(2):646–654.

15. Hasday JD, Meltzer SS, Moore WC, et al. Anti-inflammatory effects of zileuton in a subpopulation of allergic asthmatics. Am J Respir Crit Care Med 2000; 161(4):1229–1236.

16. Pizzichini E, Leff JA, Reiss TF, et al. Montelukast reduces airway eosinophilic inflammation in asthma: a randomized, controlled trial. Eur Respir J 1999; 14(1):12–18.

17. Liu M, Dubé L, Lancaster J. Acute and chronic effects of a 5-lipoxygenase inhibitor in asthma: a 6-month randomized multicenter trial. Zileuton Study Group. J Allergy Clin Immunol 1996; 98(5):859–871.

18. Reiss TF, Chervinsky P, Dockhorn RJ, et al. Montelukast, a once-daily leukotriene receptor antagonist, in the treatment of chronic asthma: a multicenter, randomized, double-blind trial. Arch Intern Med 1998; 158(11):1213–1220.

19. Simons FER, Villa JR, Lee BW, et al. Montelukast added to budesonide in children with persistent asthma: a randomized, double-blind, crossover study. J Pediatr 2001; 138(5):694–698.

20. Minoguchi K, Kohno Y, Minoguchi H, et al. Reduction of eosinophilic inflammation in the airways of patients with asthma using montelukast. Chest 2002; 121(3):732–738.

21. Bisgaard H, Loland L, Oj JA. NO in exhaled air of asthmatic children is reduced by the leukotriene receptor antagonist montelukast. Am J Repir Crit Care Med 1999; 160(4):1227–1231.

22. Sandrini A, Ferreira IM, Gutierrez C, et al. Effect of montelukast on exhaled nitric oxide and nonvolatile markers of inflammation in mild asthma. Chest 2003; 124(4):1334–1340.

23. Straub DA, Moeller A, Minocchieri S, et al. The effect of montelukast on lung function and exhaled nitric oxide in infants with early childhood asthma. Eur Repir J 2005; 25(2):289–294.

24. Wenzel S, Trudeau J, Kaminsky D, et al. Effect of 5-lipoxygenase inhibition on bronchoconstriction and airway inflammation in nocturnal asthma. Am J Respir Crit Care Med 1995; 152(3):897–905.

25. Hui K, Barnes N. Lung function improvement in asthma with a cysteinyl-leukotriene receptor antagonist. Lancet 1991; 337:1062–1063.

26. Israel E, Rubin P, Kemp JP, et al. The effect of inhibition of 5-lipoxygenase by zileuton in mild-to-moderate asthma. Ann Intern Med 1993; 119(11):1059–1066.

27. Israel E, Fischer A, Rosenberg M, et al. The pivotal role of 5-lipoxygenase products in the reaction of aspirin-sensitive asthmatics to aspirin. Am Rev Respir Dis 1993; 148(6):1447–1451.

28. Boushey HA, Sorkness CA, King TS, et al. Daily versus as-needed corticosteroids for mild persistent asthma. N Engl J Med 2005; 352(15):1519–1528.

29. Jayaram L, Pizzichini E, Lemiere C, et al. Steroid naive eosinophilic asthma: anti-inflammatory effects of fluticasone and montelukast. Thorax 2005; 60(2):100–105.

30. Kanniess F, Richter K, Bohme S, et al. Montelukast versus fluticasone: effects on lung function, airway responsiveness and inflammation in moderate asthma. Eur Respir J 2002; 20(4):853–858.

31. O'Sullivan S, Akveld M, Burke CM, et al. Effect of the addition of montelukast to inhaled fluticasone propionate on airway inflammation. Am J Repir Crit Care Med 2003; 167(5): 745–750.

32. Jayaram L, Duong M, Pizzichini MMM, et al. Failure of montelukast to reduce sputum eosinophilia in high-dose corticosteroid-dependent asthma. Eur Respir J 2005; 25(1):41–46.

33. Barnes N, Laviolette M, Allen D, et al. Effects of montelukast compared to double dose budesonide on airway inflammation and asthma control. Respir Med 2007; 101(8):1652–1658.

34. Pavord I, Woodcock A, Parker D, et al. Salmeterol plus fluticasone propionate versus fluticasone propionate plus montelukast: a randomised controlled trial investigating the effects on airway inflammation in asthma. Respir Res 2007; 8(1):67.

35. Ghiro L, Zanconato S, Rampon O, et al. Effect of montelukast added to inhaled corticosteroids on fractional exhaled nitric oxide in asthmatic children. Eur Repir J 2002; 20(3): 630–634.

36. Henderson WR Jr., Chiang GKS, Tien Y-t, et al. Reversal of allergen-induced airway remodeling by CysLT1 receptor blockade. Am J Repir Crit Care Med 2006; 173(7):718–728.

37. Kelly MM, Chakir J, Vethanayagam D, et al. Montelukast treatment attenuates the increase in myofibroblasts following low-dose allergen challenge. Chest 2006; 130(3):741–753.

38. Yoshisue H, Kirkham-Brown J, Healy E, et al. Cysteinyl leukotrienes synergize with growth factors to induce proliferation of human bronchial fibroblasts. J Allergy Clin Immunol 2007; 119(1):132–140.

39. McGill KA, Busse WW. Zileuton. Lancet 1996; 348(9026):519–524.

40. Drazen JM, Israel E, O'Byrne PM. Treatment of asthma with drugs modifying the leukotriene pathway. N Engl J Med 1999; 340(3):197–206.

41. Dekhuijzen PN, Bootsma GP, Wielders PL, et al. Effects of single-dose zileuton on bronchial hyperresponsiveness in asthmatic patients treated with inhaled corticosteroids. Eur Respir J 1997; 10(12):2749–2753.

42. Rorke S, Jennison S, Jeffs JA, et al. Role of cysteinyl leukotrienes in adenosine 5′-monophosphate induced bronchoconstriction in asthma. Thorax 2002; 57(4):323–327.

43. Taylor I, O'Shaughnessy K, Fuller R, et al. Effect of cysteinyl-leukotriene receptor antagonist ICI 204.219 on allergen-induced bronchoconstriction and airway hyperreactivity in atopic subjects. Lancet 1991; 337:690–694.

44. Corren J, Spector S, Fuller L, et al. Effects of zafirlukast upon clinical, physiologic, and inflammatory responses to natural cat allergen exposure. Ann Allergy Asthma Immunol 2001; 87(3):211–217.

45. Phipatanakul W, Nowak-Wegrzyn A, Eggleston PA, et al. The efficacy of montelukast in the treatment of cat allergen-induced asthma in children. J Allergy Clin Immunol 2002; 109(5):794–799.

46. Rosewich M, Rose MA, Eickmeier O, et al. Montelukast as add-on therapy to {beta}-agonists and late airway response. Eur Respir J 2007; 30(1):56–61.

47. Hui K, Taylor I, Taylor G, et al. Effect of a 5-lipoxygenase inhibitor on leukotriene generation and airway responses after allergen challenge in asthmatic patients. Thorax 1991; 46(3):184–189.

48. Evans D, Barnes P, Spaethe S, et al. Effect of a leukotriene B4 receptor antagonist, LY293111, on allergen induced responses in asthma. Thorax 1996; 51(12):1178–1184.

49. Finnerty J, Wood-Baker R, Thomson H, et al. Role of leukotrienes in exercise-induced asthma. Inhibitory effect of ICI 204219, a potent leukotriene D4 receptor antagonist. Am Rev Respir Dis 1992; 145(4):746–749.

50. Kemp J, Dockhorn R, Shapiro G, et al. Montelukast once daily inhibits exercise-induced bronchoconstriction in 6- to 14-year-old children with asthma. J Pediatr 1998; 133(3): 424–428.

51. Leff JA, Busse WW, Pearlman D, et al. Montelukast, a leukotriene-receptor antagonist, for the treatment of mild asthma and exercise-induced bronchoconstriction. N Engl J Med 1998; 339(3):147–152.
52. Edelman JM, Turpin JA, Bronsky EA, et al. Oral montelukast compared with inhaled salmeterol to prevent exercise-induced bronchoconstriction: a randomized, double-blind trial. Ann Intern Med 2000; 132(2):97–104.
53. Melo RE, Sole D, Naspitz CK. Exercise-induced bronchoconstriction in children: montelukast attenuates the immediate-phase and late-phase responses. J Allergy Clin Immunol 2003; 111(2):301–307.
54. Fischer A, McFadden C, Frantz R, et al. Effect of chronic 5-lipoxygenase inhibition on airway hyperresponsiveness in asthmatic subjects. Am J Respir Crit Care Med 1995; 152(4): 1203–1207.
55. Coreno A, Skowronski M, Kotaru C, et al. Comparative effects of long-acting [beta]2-agonists, leukotriene receptor antagonists, and a 5-lipoxygenase inhibitor on exercise-induced asthma. J Allergy Clin Immunol 2000; 106(3):500–506.
56. Cowburn AS, Sladek K, Soja J, et al. Overexpression of leukotriene C4 synthase in bronchial biopsies from patients with aspirin-intolerant asthma. J Clin Invest 1998; 101(4):834–846.
57. Volkman JA, Pontikes PJ. Leukotriene modifiers to prevent aspirin-provoked respiratory reactions in asthmatics. Ann Pharmacother 2002; 36(9):1457–1461.
58. Dahlen S-E, Malmstrom K, Nizankowska EWA, et al. Improvement of aspirin-intolerant asthma by montelukast, a leukotriene antagonist. A randomized, double-blind, placebo-controlled trial. Am J Repir Crit Care Med 2002; 165(1):9–14.
59. Wilson AM, O'Byrne PM, Parameswaran K. Leukotriene receptor antagonists for allergic rhinitis: a systematic review and meta-analysis. Am J Med 2004; 116(5):338–344.
60. Busse W, Casale T, Dykewicz M, et al. Efficacy of montelukast during the allergy season in patients with chronic asthma and seasonal aeroallergen sensitivity. Ann Allergy Asthma Immunol 2006; 96(1):60–68.
61. Price DB, Swern A, Tozzi CA, et al. Effect of montelukast on lung function in asthma patients with allergic rhinitis: analysis from the COMPACT trial. Allergy 2006; 61(6):737–742.
62. Nathan RA, Yancey SW, Waitkus-Edwards K, et al. Fluticasone propionate nasal spray is superior to montelukast for allergic rhinitis while neither affects overall asthma control. Chest 2005; 128(4):1910–1920.
63. Reiss T, Sorkness C, Stricker W, et al. Effects of montelukast (MK-0476); a potent cysteinyl leukotriene receptor antagonist, on bronchodilation in asthmatic subjects treated with and without inhaled corticosteroids. Thorax 1997; 52(1):45–48.
64. Dockhorn RJ, Baumgartner RA, Leff JA, et al. Comparison of the effects of intravenous and oral montelukast on airway function: a double blind, placebo controlled, three period, crossover study in asthmatic patients. Thorax 2000; 55(4):260–265.
65. Camargo CA Jr., Smithline HA, Malice M-P, et al. A randomized controlled trial of intravenous montelukast in acute asthma. Am J Respir Crit Care Med 2003; 167(4):528–533.
66. Spector S, Smith L, Glass M. Effects of 6 weeks of therapy with oral doses of ICI 204,219, a leukotriene D4 receptor antagonist, in subjects with bronchial asthma. ACCOLATE Asthma Trialists Group. Am J Respir Crit Care Med 1994; 150(3):618–623.
67. Suissa S, Dennis R, Ernst P, et al. Effectiveness of the leukotriene receptor antagonist zafirlukast for mild-to-moderate asthma: a randomized, double-blind, placebo-controlled trial. Ann Intern Med 1997; 126(3):177–183.
68. Noonan MJ, Chervinsky P, Brandon M, et al. Montelukast, a potent leukotriene receptor antagonist, causes dose-related improvements in chronic asthma. Montelukast Asthma Study Group. Eur Respir J 1998; 11(6):1232–1239.
69. Knorr B, Matz J, Bernstein JA, et al. Montelukast for chronic asthma in 6- to 14-year-old children: a randomized, double-blind trial. JAMA 1998; 279(15):1181–1186.

70. Knorr B, Franchi LM, Bisgaard H, et al. Montelukast, a leukotriene receptor antagonist, for the treatment of persistent asthma in children aged 2 to 5 years. Pediatrics 2001; 108(3):e48.

71. Barnes N, Wei LX, Reiss TF, et al. Analysis of montelukast in mild persistent asthmatic patients with near-normal lung function. Respir Med 2001; 95(5):379–386.

72. Robertson CF, Price D, Henry R, et al. Short-course montelukast for intermittent asthma in children: a randomized controlled trial. Am J Respir Crit Care Med 2007; 175(4):323–329.

73. Israel E, Cohn J, Dubé L, et al. Effect of treatment with zileuton, a 5-lipoxygenase inhibitor, in patients with asthma. A randomized controlled trial. Zileuton Clinical Trial Group. JAMA 1996; 275(12):931–936.

74. Laviolette M, Malmstrom K, Lu S, et al. Montelukast added to inhaled beclomethasone in treatment of asthma. Am J Repir Crit Care Med 1999; 160(6):1862–1868.

75. Malmstrom K, Rodriguez-Gomez G, Guerra J, et al. Oral montelukast, inhaled beclomethasone, and placebo for chronic asthma: a randomized, controlled trial. Ann Intern Med 1999; 130(6):487–495.

76. Bleecker E, Welch M, Weinstein S, et al. Low-dose inhaled fluticasone propionate versus oral zafirlukast in the treatment of persistent asthma. J Allergy Clin Immunol 2000; 105(6): 1123–1129.

77. Busse W, Wolfe J, Storms W, et al. Fluticasone propionate compared with zafirlukast in controlling persistent asthma: a randomized double-blind, placebo-controlled trial. J Fam Pract 2001; 50(7):595–602.

78. Busse W, Raphael GD, Galant S, et al. Low-dose fluticasone propionate compared with montelukast for first-line treatment of persistent asthma: a randomized clinical trial. J Allergy Clin Immunol 2001; 107(3):461–468.

79. Ducharme F, Di Salvio F. Anti-leukotriene agents compared to inhaled corticosteroids in the management of recurrent and/or chronic asthma in adults and children. Cochrane Database Syst Rev 2004(1):Art. No.: CD002314. DOI: 10.1002/14651858.CD002314.pub2.

80. Sorkness CA, Lemanske RF Jr., Mauger DT, et al. Long-term comparison of 3 controller regimens for mild-moderate persistent childhood asthma: the pediatric asthma controller trial. J Allergy Clin Immunol 2007; 119(1):64–72.

81. Ducharme F, Schwartz Z, Hicks G, et al. Addition of anti-leukotriene agents to inhaled corticosteroids for chronic asthma. Cochrane Database Syst Rev 2004(1):Art. No.: CD003133. DOI: 10.1002/14651858.CD003133.pub2.

82. Wilson AM, Dempsey OJ, Sims EJ, et al. Evaluation of salmeterol or montelukast as second-line therapy for asthma not controlled with inhaled corticosteroids. Chest 2001; 119(4): 1021–1026.

83. Bjermer L, Bisgaard H, Bousquet J, et al. Montelukast and fluticasone compared with salmeterol and fluticasone in protecting against asthma exacerbation in adults: one year, double blind, randomised, comparative trial. BMJ 2003; 327(7420):891.

84. Ducharme F, Lasserson T, Cates C. Long-acting beta2-agonists versus anti-leukotrienes as add-on therapy to inhaled corticosteroids for chronic asthma. Cochrane Database Syst Rev 2006; (4):CD003137.

85. Price DB, Hernandez D, Magyar P, et al. Randomised controlled trial of montelukast plus inhaled budesonide versus double dose inhaled budesonide in adult patients with asthma. Thorax 2003; 58(3):211–216.

86. Thomson NC, Shepherd M. Leukotriene receptor antagonists as add-on therapy for adults with asthma. Thorax 2003; 58(3):190–192.

87. O'Connor BJ, Lofdahl C-G, Balter M, et al. Zileuton added to low-dose inhaled beclomethasone for the treatment of moderate to severe persistent asthma. Respir Med 2007; 101(6): 1088–1096.

88. The American Lung Association Asthma Clinical Research C. Clinical Trial of Low-Dose Theophylline and Montelukast in Patients with Poorly Controlled Asthma. Am J Respir Crit Care Med 2007; 175(3):235–242.

89. Schwartz HJ, Petty T, Dube LM, et al. for the Zileuton Study G. A randomized controlled trial comparing zileuton with theophylline in moderate asthma. Arch Intern Med 1998; 158(2): 141–148.

90. Robinson DS, Campbell D, Barnes PJ. Addition of leukotriene antagonists to therapy in chronic persistent asthma: a randomised double-blind placebo-controlled trial. Lancet 2001; 357(9273):2007–2011.

91. Currie GP, Lee DKC, Haggart K, et al. Effects of montelukast on surrogate inflammatory markers in corticosteroid-treated patients with asthma. Am J Respir Crit Care Med 2003; 167(9):1232–1238.

92. Christian Virchow J Jr., Prasse A, Naya IAN, et al. The Zafirlukast Study G. zafirlukast improves asthma control in patients receiving high-dose inhaled corticosteroids. Am J Respir Crit Care Med 2000; 162(2):578–585.

93. Deykin A, Wechsler ME, Boushey HA, et al. Combination therapy with a long-acting beta-agonist and a leukotriene antagonist in moderate asthma. Am J Respir Crit Care Med 2007; 175(3):228–234.

94. Lofdahl C-G, Reiss TF, Leff JA, et al. Randomised, placebo controlled trial of effect of a leukotriene receptor antagonist, montelukast, on tapering inhaled corticosteroids in asthmatic patients. BMJ 1999; 319(7202):87–90.

95. Tamaok IJ, Kondo M, Sakai N, et al. Leukotriene antagonist prevents exacerbation of asthma during reduction of high-dose inhaled corticosteroid. The Tokyo Joshi-Idai Asthma Research Group. Am J Respir Crit Care Med 1997; 155(4):1235–1240.

96. Malmstrom K, Rodriguez-Gomez G, Guerra J, et al. Oral montelukast, inhaled beclomethasone, and placebo for chronic asthma: a randomized, controlled trial. Ann Intern Med 1999; 130(6):487–495.

97. Zeiger RS, Szefler SJ, Phillips BR, et al. Response profiles to fluticasone and montelukast in mild-to-moderate persistent childhood asthma. J Allergy Clin Immunol 2006; 117(1):45–52.

98. Szefler SJ, Phillips BR, Martinez FD, et al. Characterization of within-subject responses to fluticasone and montelukast in childhood asthma. J Allergy Clin Immunol 2005; 115(2): 233–242.

99. Cai C, Yang J, Hu S, et al. Relationship between urinary cysteinyl leukotriene E4 levels and clinical response to antileukotriene treatment in patients with asthma. Lung 2007; 185(2): 105–112.

100. Montuschi P, Mondino C, Koch P, et al. Effects of a leukotriene receptor antagonist on exhaled leukotriene E4 and prostanoids in children with asthma. J Allergy Clin Immunol 2006; 118(2):347–353.

101. Dahlen B, Nizankowska EWA, Szczeklik A, et al. Benefits from adding the 5-lipoxygenase inhibitor zileuton to conventional therapy in aspirin-intolerant asthmatics. Am J Respir Crit Care Med 1998; 157(4):1187–1194.

102. O'Shaughnessy K, Wellings R, Gillies B, et al. Differential effects of fluticasone propionate on allergen-evoked bronchoconstriction and increased urinary leukotriene E4 excretion. Am Rev Respir Dis 1993; 147(6):1472–1476.

103. Gyllfors P, Dahlén S, Kumlin M, et al. Bronchial responsiveness to leukotriene D4 is resistant to inhaled fluticasone propionate. J Allergy Clin Immunol 2006; 118(1):78–83.

104. Drazen JM, Yandava CN, Dube L, et al. Pharmacogenetic association between ALOX5 promoter genotype and the response to anti-asthma treatment. Nat Genet 1999; 22(2): 168–170.

105. Lima JJ, Zhang S, Grant A, et al. Influence of leukotriene pathway polymorphisms on response to montelukast in asthma. Am J Repir Crit Care Med 2006; 173(4):379–385.

106. Klotsman M, York T, Pillai S, et al. Pharmacogenetics of the 5-lipoxygenase biosynthetic pathway and variable clinical response to montelukast. Pharmacogenet Genomics 2007; 17(3):189–196.

107. Sampson AP, Siddiqui S, Buchanan D, et al. Variant LTC4 synthase allele modifies cysteinyl leukotriene synthesis in eosinophils and predicts clinical response to zafirlukast. Thorax 2000; 55(90002):S28–S31.
108. Currie GP, Lima JJ, Sylvester JE, et al. Leukotriene C4 synthase polymorphisms and responsiveness to leukotriene antagonists in asthma. Br J Clin Pharmacol 2003; 56(4):422–426.
109. Lima J. Treatment heterogeneity in asthma: genetics of response to leukotriene modifiers. Mol Diagn Ther 2007; 11(2):97–104.
110. Kim JH, Lee SY, Kim HB, et al. TBXA2R gene polymorphism and responsiveness to leukotriene receptor antagonist in children with asthma. Clin Exp Allergy 2008; 38(1):51–59.
111. Bisgaard H, Zielen S, Garcia-Garcia ML, et al. Montelukast reduces asthma exacerbations in 2- to 5-year-old children with intermittent asthma. Am J Respir Crit Care Med 2005; 171(4): 315–322.
112. Lazarus SC, Chinchilli V, Rollings N, et al. Smoking affects response to inhaled corticosteroids or leukotriene receptor antagonists in asthma. Am J Respir Crit Care Med 2007; 175(8):783–190.
113. Thomson NC, Spears M. The influence of smoking on the treatment response in patients with asthma. Curr Opin Allergy Clin Immunol 2005; 5(1):57–63.
114. Thomson NC. Smokers with asthma: what are the management options? Am J Respir Crit Care Med 2007; 175(8):749–750.
115. Peters-Golden M, Swern A, Bird SS, et al. Influence of body mass index on the response to asthma controller agents. Eur Respir J 2006; 27(3):495–503.
116. Berger W, De Chandt MTM, Cairns CB. Zileuton: clinical implications of 5-Lipoxygenase inhibition in severe airway disease. Int J Clin Pract 2007; 61(4):663–676.
117. Bakhireva LN, Jones KL, Schatz M, et al. Safety of leukotriene receptor antagonists in pregnancy. J Allergy Clin Immunol 2007; 119(3):618–625.
118. Stirling RG, Chung KF. Leukotriene antagonists and Churg-Strauss syndrome: the smoking gun. Thorax 1999; 54(10):865–866.
119. Josefson D. Asthma drug linked with Churg-Strauss syndrome. BMJ 1997; 315:330.
120. Wechsler ME, Garpestad E, Flier SR, et al. Pulmonary infiltrates, eosinophilia, and cardiomyopathy following corticosteroid withdrawal in patients with asthma receiving Zafirlukast. JAMA 1998; 279(6):455–457.
121. Tuggey JM, Hosker HSR. Churg-Strauss syndrome associated with montelukast therapy. Thorax 2000; 55(9):805–806.
122. Gaki E, Papatheodorou G, Ischaki E, et al. Leukotriene E4 in urine in patients with asthma and COPD—The effect of smoking habit. Respir Med 2007; 101(4):826–832.
123. Montuschi P, Kharitonov SA, Ciabattoni G, et al. Exhaled leukotrienes and prostaglandins in COPD. Thorax 2003; 58(7):585–588.
124. Celik P, Sakar A, Havlucu Y, et al. Short-term effects of montelukast in stable patients with moderate to severe COPD. Respir Med 2005; 99(4):444–450.
125. Cazzola M, Boveri B, Carlucci P, et al. Lung function improvement in smokers suffering from COPD with zafirlukast, a CysLT(1)-receptor antagonist. Pulm Pharmacol Ther 2000; 13(6):301–305.
126. Kostikas K, Gaga M, Papatheodorou G, et al. Leukotriene B4 in exhaled breath condensate and sputum supernatant in patients with COPD and asthma. Chest 2005; 127(5):1553–1559.
127. Gompertz S, Stockley RA. A randomized, placebo-controlled trial of a leukotriene synthesis inhibitor in patients with COPD*. Chest 2002; 122(1):289–294.
128. Crooks SW, Bayley DL, Hill SL, et al. Bronchial inflammation in acute bacterial exacerbations of chronic bronchitis: the role of leukotriene B4. Eur Respir J 2000; 15(2):274–280.
129. Beeh KM, Kornmann O, Buhl R, et al. Neutrophil chemotactic activity of sputum from patients with COPD: role of interleukin 8 and leukotriene B4. Chest 2003; 123(4):1240–1247.

130. Rand C, Bilderback A, Schiller K, et al. Adherence with montelukast or fluticasone in a long-term clinical trial: results from the mild asthma montelukast versus inhaled corticosteroid trial. J Allergy Clin Immunol 2007; 119(4):916–923.

131. GINA Report, Global Strategy for Asthma Management and Prevention. 2006. Available at: http://www.ginasthma.com/Guidelineitem.asp??l1=2&l2=1&intId=60. Accessed December 12, 2007.

132. FitzGerald GA. COX-2 and beyond: approaches to prostaglandin inhibition in human disease. Nat Rev Drug Discov 2003; 2(11):879–890.

133. Barnes PJ, Chung KF, Page CP. Inflammatory mediators of asthma: an update. Pharmacol Rev 1998; 50(4):515–596.

134. Rolin S, Masereel B, Dogne J-M. Prostanoids as pharmacological targets in COPD and asthma. Eur J Pharmacol 2006; 533(1-3):89–100.

135. Davi G, Basili S, Vieri M, et al. Enhanced thromboxane biosynthesis in patients with chronic obstructive pulmonary disease. Am J Respir Crit Care Med 1997; 156(6):1794–1799.

136. Fujimura M, Sakamoto S, Matsuda T. Attenuating effect of a thromboxane synthetase inhibitor (OKY-046) on bronchial responsiveness to methacholine is specific to bronchial asthma. Chest 1990; 98(3):656–660.

137. Hoshino M, Sim J, Shimizu K, et al. Effect of AA-2414, a thromboxane A2 receptor antagonist, on airway inflammation in subjects with asthma. J Allergy Clin Immunol 1999; 103(6):1054–1061.

138. Tamaoki J, Kondo M, Nakata J, et al. Effect of a thromboxane A2 antagonist on sputum production and its physicochemical properties in patients with mild to moderate asthma. Chest 2000; 118(1):73–79.

139. Arakida Y, Ohga K, Okada Y, et al. Effect of combined leukotriene D4 and thromboxane A2 receptor antagonist on mediator-controlled resistance in guinea pigs. Eur J Pharmacol 2000; 403(1-2):169–179.

140. Ishimura M, Kataoka S, Suda M, et al. Effects of KP-496, a novel dual antagonist for leukotriene D4 and thromboxane A2 receptors, on contractions induced by various agonists in the guinea pig trachea. Allergol Int 2006; 55(4):403–410.

141. Zhang M, Thurmond RL, Dunford PJ. The histamine H4 receptor: a novel modulator of inflammatory and immune disorders. Pharmacol Ther 2007; 113(3):594–606.

142. Akdis CA, Simons FER. Histamine receptors are hot in immunopharmacology. Eur J Pharmacol 2006; 533(1–3):69–76.

143. Leurs R, Church MK, Taglialatela M. H1-antihistamines: inverse agonism, anti-inflammatory actions and cardiac effects. Clin Exp Allergy 2002; 32(4):489–498.

144. Walsh G. The effects of cetirizine on the function of inflammatory cells involved in the allergic response. Clin Exp Allergy 1997; 27(suppl 2):47–53; discussion 54–56.

145. Temple D, McCluskey M. Loratadine, an antihistamine, blocks antigen-and ionophore-induced leukotriene release from human lung in vitro. Prostaglandins 1988; 35(4):549–554.

146. Grant S, Goa K, Fitton A, et al. Ketotifen. A review of its pharmacodynamic and pharmacokinetic properties, and therapeutic use in asthma and allergic disorders. Drugs 1990; 40(3):412–448.

147. Roquet A, Dahlén B, Kumlin M, et al. Combined antagonism of leukotrienes and histamine produces predominant inhibition of allergen-induced early and late phase airway obstruction in asthmatics. Am J Respir Crit Care Med 1997; 155(6):1856–1863.

148. Ghosh S, De Vos C, McIlroy I, et al. Effect of cetirizine on exercise induced asthma. Thorax 1991; 46(4):242–244.

149. O'Byrne P, Thomson N, Morris M, et al. The protective effect of inhaled chlorpheniramine and atropine on bronchoconstriction stimulated by airway cooling. Am Rev Respir Dis 1983; 128(4):611–617.

150. Rutgers SR, Koeter GH, Van Der M TW, et al. Protective effect of oral terfenadine and not inhaled ipratropium on adenosine 5'-monophosphate-induced bronchoconstriction in patients with COPD. Clin Exp Allergy 1999; 29(9):1287–1292.

151. Thomson N, Kerr J. Effect of inhaled H1 and H2 receptor antagonist in normal and asthmatic subjects. Thorax 1980; 35(6):428–434.

152. Van Ganse E, Kaufman L, Derde MP, et al. Effects of antihistamines in adult asthma: a meta-analysis of clinical trials. Eur Respir J 1997; 10(10):2216–2224.

153. Bassler D, Mitra A, Ducharme F, et al. Ketotifen alone or as additional medication for long-term control of asthma and wheeze in children. Cochrane Database Syst Rev 2004(1):Art. No.: CD001384. DOI: 10.1002/14651858.CD001384.pub2.

154. Morgan RK, McAllister B, Cross L, et al. Histamine 4 receptor activation induces recruitment of FoxP3+ T cells and inhibits allergic asthma in a murine model. J Immunol 2007; 178(12):8081–8089.

155. Spicuzza L, Di Maria G, Polosa R. Adenosine in the airways: implications and applications. Eur J Pharmacol 2006; 533(1-3):77–88.

156. Brown RA, Clarke GW, Ledbetter CL, et al. Elevated expression of adenosine A1 receptor in bronchial biopsy specimens from asthmatic subjects. Eur Respir J 2008; 31(2):311–319.

157. Mustafa SJ, Nadeem A, Fan M, et al. Effect of a specific and selective A2B adenosine receptor antagonist on adenosine agonist AMP and allergen-induced airway responsiveness and cellular influx in a mouse model of asthma. J Pharmacol Exp Ther 2007; 320(3):1246–1251.

158. Luijk B, van den Berge M, Kerstjens HAM, et al. Effect of an inhaled adenosine A2A agonist on the allergen-induced late asthmatic response. Allergy 2008; 63(1):75–80.

159. Chalmers George W, Little Stuart A, Patel Kantilal R, et al. Endothelin-1-induced bronchoconstriction in asthma. Am J Respir Crit Care Med 1997; 156(2):382–388.

160. Hay DWP. Putative mediator role of endothelin-1 in asthma and other lung diseases. Clin Exp Pharmacol Physiol 1999; 26(2):168–171.

161. Pegorier S, Arouche N, Dombret M-C, et al. Augmented epithelial endothelin-1 expression in refractory asthma. J Allergy Clin Immunol 2007; 120(6):1301–1307.

162. Finsnes F, Lyberg T, Christensen G, et al. Effect of endothelin antagonism on the production of cytokines in eosinophilic airway inflammation. Am J Physiol Lung Cell Mol Physiol 2001; 280(4):L659–L665.

163. Boot JD, de Haas S, Tarasevych S, et al. Effect of an NK1/NK2 receptor antagonist on airway responses and inflammation to allergen in asthma. Am J Respir Crit Care Med 2007; 175(5):450–457.

164. Abraham WM, Scuri M, Farmer SG. Peptide and non-peptide bradykinin receptor antagonists: role in allergic airway disease. Eur J Pharmacol 2006; 533(1-3):215–221.

165. Turner P, Dear J, Scadding G, et al. Role of kinins in seasonal allergic rhinitis: Icatibant, a bradykinin B2 receptor antagonist, abolishes the hyperresponsiveness and nasal eosinophilia induced by antigen. J Allergy Clin Immunol 2001; 107(1):105–113.

166. Jia Y, Lee L-Y. Role of TRPV receptors in respiratory diseases. Biochim Biophys Acta 2007; 1772(8):915–927.

9

Antiallergic Approaches in Airway Disease

CHRIS J. CORRIGAN
MRC and Asthma UK Centre for Allergic Mechanisms of Asthma, King's College London School of Medicine, London, U.K.

I. Introduction

It is proposed in this chapter to examine the proposition that IgE plays a role in the causation of asthma, and to attempt to define the nature of this role. The worth of allergen avoidance as a primary and secondary preventative measure for asthma will then be examined, as will the role of allergen immunotherapy. There will follow an account of studies of clinical efficacy and controversies surrounding the use of anti-IgE therapy for asthma. The chapter will conclude with an overview of the definition of anaphylaxis and its immediate and longer-term management.

II. What Is the Role of IgE in Asthma Pathogenesis?
A. Asthma and the Atopic Diathesis

The frequent association of atopy, defined conventionally as the propensity of some individuals to make IgE specific for certain antigens ("allergens") encountered at mucosal surfaces and detected by skin prick or in vitro tests to arrange of common local aeroallergens (1), with asthma invites the assumption of a causal mechanistic relationship that is widely assumed but not necessarily justifiable. A body of evidence (2) suggests that allergic sensitization (i.e., the production of allergen-specific IgE) is associated with asthma, and that allergen exposure is related to sensitization. It is therefore difficult to separate the effects of allergen sensitization and exposure on the initiation of asthma, and even if it were not, associations do not necessarily prove causality. This assumption has been extended to invoke allergens as the primary driving force to bronchial mucosal T-cell activation in asthma, which is again not necessarily the case: although allergen-specific T cells can be recovered from the bronchial mucosa and lumen of asthmatic and indeed nonasthmatic individuals, the full antigenic repertoire of T cells in this disease, let alone which antigens cause T-cell activation in different individuals, will never be known for certain until this can be investigated directly, for example, by peptide/tetramer binding studies. Doubts about the prominence of atopy and allergen exposure as exacerbating or causative factors for asthma have been voiced over the years (3,4) and increasingly ratified by modern epidemiological studies (5). Thus, while exposure to allergens in some IgE-sensitized individuals may be a mechanism for acute exacerbation of asthma, the role of allergen-specific IgE in asthma causation remains unclear. This is arguably of little practical importance from the point of view of clinical management of established asthma, but is of vital importance when considering what role allergen avoidance, allergen immunotherapy, and anti-IgE strategies have to play in the primary prevention of asthma as well as modification of its natural history.

B. Molecular Mechanisms of "Nonatopic" Asthma

The physician Rackeman (6) is accredited with first penning (publicly) the observation familiar to clinicians dealing with asthma, namely, that environmental influences alter disease severity in the short term in some patients more prominently than others. His distinction between "extrinsic" and "intrinsic" asthma has again become equated nowadays with the presence or absence of coexisting atopy, which is a pity because, numerically, viral infections are the commonest cause of asthma exacerbation, and modern epidemiological studies (7) have shown that both atopic and nonatopic asthma show seasonal variability (atopic asthma tends to be more severe in the summer months, when pollens abound, whereas nonatopic asthma tends to be worse in the winter, perhaps reflecting the influence of viral infections). In this sense, intrinsic asthma is a misnomer since like extrinsic disease it is clearly susceptible to environmental influences.

These clinical distinctions between atopic and nonatopic asthma led to speculation (8) about the possibility of fundamental differences in disease pathogenesis. Research conducted over the past 15 years, to which this author and his colleagues have made a significant contribution, has however suggested remarkable similarity in the cellular and molecular immunopathology of atopic and nonatopic asthma and the possibility of a role for IgE in both types of disease. Specifically, the bronchial mucosal inflammatory cellular infiltrate is identical save for an excess of tissue macrophages in nonatopic patients (9). Furthermore, there appears to be equivalent, elevated expression not only of the key eosinophil-active cytokine IL-5 but also of the two B-cell IgE-switching cytokines IL-4 and IL-13 in the bronchial mucosa of both atopic and nonatopic asthmatics as compared with atopy-matched controls (10–12). Submucosal expression of mRNA encoding the α-subunits of the IL-4 (13) and IL-5 receptors (14) is also elevated in both patient groups. Mucosal expression of the eosinophil chemotactic chemokines eotaxin, eotaxin-2, RANTES, MCP-3, and MCP-4, as well as expression of the chemokine receptor CCR3, a ligand for these chemokines expressed on eosinophils and Th2-type T cells, is also similarly elevated in both patient groups (15,16) and these molecules show a similar cellular distribution. Further to this, there is now abundant evidence that B cells in the human respiratory mucosa undergo class switching to IgE synthesis and secrete mature IgE in both atopic and nonatopic asthmatics. Cells in the bronchial mucosa of nonatopic as well as atopic asthmatics show elevated expression of the high-affinity IgE receptor FcɛRI (17). Since IgE upregulates expression of its own receptor, this is indirect evidence of IgE synthesis. More compelling evidence for local IgE synthesis has come from the demonstration of elevated expression of IgE ɛ-heavy-chain germ line gene transcripts and mature IgE mRNA in the bronchial mucosa of both nonatopic and atopic asthmatics compared with controls, in the absence of elevated numbers of B cells (18). This observation has been further ratified by our recent demonstration of IgE circle transcripts in the bronchial mucosa of atopic and nonatopic asthmatics but not controls (19), confirming that the mucosal environment in asthmatics appears to be conducive to IgE switching. B-cell IgE class switching, as shown by the production of circle switch transcripts, has also been detected in the nasal mucosa of patients with allergic rhinitis (20). This was increased in isolated nasal biopsies following culture with an allergen to which the patient was sensitized ex vivo, precluding the possibility that it could have occurred anywhere other than in the mucosa itself. Synthesis and secretion of mature, allergen-specific IgE have also been demonstrated in such biopsies cultured with allergen ex vivo (21). Interestingly, the fraction of IgE expressed as a proportion of the total immunoglobulin secreted by these biopsies far exceeded that observed in the circulation, consistent with the hypothesis that circulating IgE originates largely from the respiratory mucosa.

It has long been known from epidemiological studies (22,23) that although total serum IgE concentrations in populations diminish with age, higher concentrations remain a predictor of poorer lung function at all ages, regardless of the presence or absence of asthma. A more recent study (24) showed that in a large, unselected cohort of patients defined as nonatopic on the basis of skin prick testing, asthma was fivefold more prevalent and airways obstruction was more severe in subjects with serum IgE concentrations in excess of the "normal" upper limit of 150 IU/mL as compared with subjects with total serum IgE concentrations below this threshold. It is worth noting that these studies make no reference to the antigen specificity of the IgE, and indeed suggest that inappropriate IgE production is a risk factor for asthma independently of IgE-mediated responses to allergens.

C. Conclusion

The evidence implicating IgE a causative factor for asthma is compelling but so far only associative. More definite information will be gleaned from observing and understanding the effects of anti-IgE therapy (see sections below). All of the above observations have led us to hypothesize (25) that most IgE is synthesized and sequestered in mucosal tissues bound to high- and low-affinity IgE receptors, and that IgE in the serum represents no more than the "spillover" from this process. Further considerations of the possible role of IgE in asthma might be better considered in this light, specifically the following:

1. IgE elaborated in the respiratory mucosa might not always escape into the periphery in sufficient quantities to be detectable by skin prick or in vitro tests. Thus, conventional distinctions between atopic and nonatopic patients may be worthless in terms of mechanisms of asthma.

2. There is no reason to suppose that all IgE responses relevant to asthma pathogenesis are directed against allergens: for example, there is evidence that IgE against respiratory tract viruses (26), staphylococcal superantigens [which we have shown cause local oligoclonal activation of mucosal IgE+ B cells (27,28)], and even autoantigens (29) may play a role in asthma pathogenesis. Finally, certain species of so-called "highly cytokinergic" IgE can affect the function of mast cells by mechanisms other than surface cross-linking (30).

Setting healthy skepticism aside, on the other side of the coin, these data also suggest the possibility that IgE plays an important mechanistic role in asthma regardless of conventional atopic status. A corollary of this hypothesis is that anti-IgE strategies will be effective in treating patients with nonatopic, as well as atopic asthma.

III. Allergen Avoidance and Asthma Prevention

There are numerous problems of interpretation when assessing the possible worth of allergen avoidance as a therapeutic or preventative strategy for asthma. Studies have addressed the relationship between allergen exposure and the likelihood of allergic sensitization (i.e., the production of allergen-specific IgE antibody), the relationship between allergic sensitization and the risk of asthma, and the impact of allergen avoidance on asthma.

A. Allergen Exposure and the Risk of Sensitization

Intuitively, one might expect that the likelihood of sensitization to a particular allergen (defined as allergen-specific IgE production detectable by a positive skin prick test) will depend on the degree of exposure to that allergen. In practice, the problem is more complex. An exposure/risk relationship has been reported in the case of some allergens such as house-dust mite (31) but not others such as cat (32), with which there are suggestions that high exposure is protective (33). High exposure to an allergen, perhaps at a critical period of immune development, could conceivably induce "tolerance" to the clinical effects of subsequent exposure, a process that may be recapitulated in allergen immunotherapy (see below). Confusion also arises from methodological problems with epidemiological studies that compare spot prevalences of sensitization with environmental allergen concentrations. The total amount of exposure to allergen, reflecting mean ambient concentrations over time, the precise timing of exposure, and heritable predisposing factors may also influence whether or not an IgE response is seen. Assessment of personal exposure to allergens is inevitably imprecise and there are few data on the relative "potency" of different allergens in terms of their liability to induce an IgE response. Furthermore, there are many confounding factors such as urbanization, which is popularly believed to be associated with high allergen exposure and risk of allergic disease, although several studies refute this (34,35), suggesting that in fact allergen exposure may be greater in some rural environments where the prevalence of allergic diseases is generally lower. Another area of uncertainty is whether there is a critical time period during which exposure to allergens causes sensitization. Numerous studies (36,37) suggest that allergen-specific T-cell responses can be detected in umbilical cord blood of neonates, implying that sensitization, at least at the T-cell level, to some allergens may occur in utero. On the other hand, T-cell responses to antigens to which infants cannot have been exposed in utero, such as tetanus toxoid or diphtheria toxin, have also been reported in cord blood (38,39). Furthermore, infants born to mothers exposed to tree and grass pollens during the hay fever season are no more likely to be sensitized to tree and grass pollen allergens than those whose mothers were not so exposed (40). Overall, then, these data question whether T-cell responses detected in cord blood reflect allergen exposure or the normal development of the T-cell repertoire. A review of the subject (41) concluded that there was no convincing evidence that cord blood T-cell responses to allergens (at least aeroallergens) reflect maternal exposure or the likelihood of sensitization or subsequent allergic disease. Since many allergic diseases develop early in infancy and childhood, there is a popular belief that this may be a critical period in which allergen exposure exerts an effect on the risk of subsequent allergic disease and in which intervention in this regard may be effective.

An additional large gap in knowledge concerns the relationship between sensitization to allergens, as defined by the ability to detect allergen-specific IgE in the periphery, and "clinical" sensitization, that is, whether exposure to particular allergens actually causes clinical symptoms in sensitized individuals. Many subjects with positive skin prick tests to ingested or inhaled allergens evince no symptoms on allergen exposure, which is why the positive predictive value of skin prick or in vitro tests for these symptoms is so poor. The reason for this anomaly is entirely unknown but it does clearly demonstrate that clinical allergy does not simply depend on the presence or absence of allergen-specific IgE. An extension of this problem is that the severity of clinical reactions to allergen exposure varies greatly between individuals, and this is only very loosely related to total allergen-specific IgE concentrations detected in the periphery. As speculated above, because of possible sequestration of IgE at sites of synthesis such as the respiratory mucosa, its concentration in target organs may differ very greatly from that detected in the periphery. Alternatively or in addition, there may be variability in some aspect of the environment of the target organ itself, which governs the severity of clinical reactions to allergen exposure.

In summary, experimental evidence does not clearly support the hypothesis that allergen avoidance is necessarily the best approach to prevention of allergic disease. Clinical tolerance, however caused, to allergens may also result from high allergen exposure, and at the time of writing of this chapter trials are under way to investigate the effects of administration of high dosages of aeroallergens and food allergens to infants (*per orem*) on the subsequent development of allergic diseases.

B. Allergen Sensitization and the Risk of Asthma

Many studies (42,43) have shown that allergic sensitization (defined as the production of allergen-specific IgE) particularly to perennial allergens such as cat or house-dust mite, although not so much to seasonal allergens, is associated with increased risk of expression of clinical asthma, at least in children. Such observations do not, however, imply causality, as emphasized above. A safer conclusion is that allergic sensitization and asthma commonly coexist. This means that allergen sensitization may be an important exacerbating factor for asthma in certain allergic individuals, and that in these individuals allergen avoidance may play a legitimate role in asthma control. Unfortunately, these are no universal guidelines based on a firm body of evidence to mandate what is both effective and practicable with allergen avoidance in asthma, but most clinicians would agree that all asthmatics should try and avoid exposure to allergens that clearly exacerbate their symptoms. This is particularly relevant in the case of occupational allergens and other sensitizing agents. Food allergies may be an important cause of exacerbation of asthma (as well as rhinitis and eczema) in infants and young children. These measures relate to avoidance of provoking agents in established asthma. The key question to be considered here, however, is whether or not allergen avoidance has any role to play in the primary prevention of asthma.

C. Allergen Avoidance and Primary Prevention of Asthma

Most studies on primary prevention of asthma by allergen avoidance have concentrated on avoidance of perennial allergens such as house-dust mite and have produced disappointing results (44,45). One possible reason for this is that clinically relevant avoidance of such perennial allergens is not feasible. In the latest Cochrane meta-analysis of 49 trials investigating the effectiveness of house-dust mite avoidance measures for treating asthma (most of these addressed secondary, rather than primary prevention) (46) objectively confirmed mite reduction was achieved in only 13 of these. Even in trials in which house-dust mite reduction was successful (assuming that the measurement of mite concentrations in one geographical location is a reasonable surrogate of total individual exposure), however, the outcome was disappointing (47).

These studies are confounded by the fact that most atopic patients are sensitized to a range of allergens so that, if allergen avoidance really does reduce the risk of asthma, its effects may be diluted if only one allergen is reduced. Whatever the case, there is presently insufficient evidence to date to mandate allergen avoidance as an efficacious and feasible strategy for primary prevention of asthma. There is emerging evidence (48) that multifaceted approaches (combinations of allergen reduction, breast feeding, smoking cessation, etc.) may be more successful in preventing, or at least delaying, asthma in children. This rather detracts, however, from a specific influence of allergen sensitization itself. It is interesting that, in the recent NHANES survey referred to above (5), only four individual allergic sensitizations (cat, white oak, *Alternaria* spp., and ryegrass) contributed to the "population attributable risk" for asthma, ryegrass sensitization actually being protective. Dust mite and cockroach allergy did not appear in this survey to affect the PAR significantly.

IV. Allergen Immunotherapy for Atopic Asthma
A. Overview of Allergen Immunotherapy

The end result of specific allergen immunotherapy is to reduce the clinical sensitivity of the respiratory mucosa of sensitized atopic subjects to acute allergen exposure. Understanding of the mechanism of action of allergen immunotherapy has been hampered by lack of basic understanding of how the immunological features of allergic disease relate to the clinical expression of symptoms. While it is easy to imagine how acute release of histamine and other mediators into the airways of sensitized, atopic subjects may cause the symptoms of allergic rhinitis (rhinorrhea, itching, sneezing, and nasal blockage) and exacerbate asthma, what is not clear is why some subjects mount an IgE response to inhaled aeroallergens and yet develop no symptoms at all on allergen exposure. Other factors that regulate susceptibility to the expression of allergic disease in specific individuals, which are at present entirely unrecognized, must clearly exist. It is reasonable to assume that the allergic response involves sensitized, allergen-specific T cells producing cytokines (IL-4 and IL-13) that are capable of switching allergen-specific B cells to IgE synthesis during cognate interaction. There is evidence that allergen immunotherapy inhibits allergen-specific T cells and their interactions with B cells by various mechanisms (49). Early effects of immunotherapy are probably directed at mast cell and basophil releasability by mechanisms that remain unknown but occur long before alterations in the functions of T cells or B cells (50). Later on, there is evidence that immunotherapy induces allergen-specific T regulatory cells, which suppress proliferation of and cytokine production by allergen-specific effector T cells (51,52). There is some evidence that allergen-specific T regulatory cells predominate in atopic, as compared with nonatopic subjects (53), and increase in atopic subjects with clinical sensitivity to allergens who subsequently lose this sensitivity (54). The mechanisms are unclear since, as emphasized, clinical tolerance to allergens, whether spontaneous or facilitated by immunotherapy, clearly does not depend on the loss of allergen-specific IgE production. Allergen-specific IgG, particularly IgG_4, produced in the course of immunotherapy may also play a role. Some of these IgG antibodies are capable of inhibiting IgE-mediated allergen capture by antigen-presenting cells (which include B cells) (55), which may contribute to the clinical effects of immunotherapy. The cytokine IL-10, which induces and is also produced by T regulatory cells, likely plays an important role as a suppressor of IgE production and an inducer of IgG_4 production by allergen-specific B cells in the course of immunotherapy (51), although the difference in the time courses of development of allergen-specific T regulatory cells (days to weeks) and changes in IgE/IgG_4 concentration ratios (years) in the course of immunotherapy remains to be explained. The effects of immunotherapy on clinical sensitivity to acute allergen exposure in the longer term may also be partly explained by the inhibitory effects of cytokines from T regulatory and Th1-type T cells on effector cells such as basophils (56), as well as by the effects of cytokines such as IL-10 in reducing the production of eosinophil-active, Th2-type cytokines by Th2-type T cells (57). Such effects may partly explain not only the increased threshold for allergen exposure necessary to induce early and late phase reactions to allergen exposure in subjects treated with immunotherapy, but also their decreased sensitivity to nonspecific stimulation, as seen, for example, in patients with seasonal atopic asthma (58).

Because of the risk, albeit extremely low, of systemic anaphylaxis with subcutaneously administered allergen immunotherapy, there has been a recent vogue for sublingual administration. So far this route of administration appears to be safe in terms of not inducing anaphylaxis, but it is not without unwanted effects, particularly local effects of histamine release in the mouth and esophagus. Current meta-analysis (59) suggests that at least for allergic rhinitis sublingual immunotherapy is more efficacious than placebo but not as efficacious as subcutaneously administered immunotherapy. The immunological effects (let alone the mechanisms relevant to its clinical effects) of sublingual immunotherapy are still being defined. It is generally postulated that oral Langerhans cells play a critical role in capture of orally presented allergens, with possible subsequent migration to local lymph nodes. Most studies have reported that sublingual immunotherapy is associated with allergen-specific IgG_4 production, albeit in lower quantities than with subcutaneous immunotherapy. There is no consistent picture so far of changes in T-cell and effector cell responses (60), but early suggestions that T regulatory cells and immune deviation may be observed (61).

B. Allergen Immunotherapy for Asthma

Many controlled studies have shown that subcutaneous and sublingual immunotherapies exert beneficial effects on asthma symptoms in atopic, asthmatic adults and children clinically sensitized to seasonal and perennial allergens (62–64). Meta-analysis (65–67) of placebo-controlled trials suggests a small (very small in the case of sublingual immunotherapy) but significant improvement in symptoms and lung function with active therapy as compared with placebo. This is not surprising, since the overt clinical effect of immunotherapy is to reduce sensitivity of target organs to allergen exposure. It is also not surprising that these effects are most marked in asthmatics where allergen exposure plays a major role in disease exacerbation, such as seasonal asthma associated with allergic rhinitis ("pollen asthma"). The problem is that there are very few studies addressing whether and in what circumstances immunotherapy adds to conventional anti-asthma therapy in terms of reduced drug consumption, improved lung function, or indeed any other outcome measure. One such study (68) using mixtures of allergens in asthmatic children was negative, although the results are difficult to interpret since allergens were administered on the basis of skin prick test positivity and not clinical sensitivity. In a more recent study (69), house-dust mite immunotherapy administered for three years to adult atopic asthmatics sensitized to mite slightly but significantly reduced "as required" bronchodilator usage and increased peak flow as compared with placebo, although cumulative inhaled corticosteroid dosages, symptoms, lung volumes, and bronchial responsiveness to methacholine were unchanged.

Although the incidence of severe systemic reactions with subcutaneous allergen immunotherapy is low, asthmatics are particularly susceptible to severe bronchospasm during such reactions and there remains a steady trickle of deaths from allergen immunotherapy, which occur almost exclusively in moderate/severe or unstable asthmatics (62). In view of this risk and the uncertainty of the benefit of immunotherapy, it is not currently recommended for asthma treatment in the United Kingdom. It has been suggested that immunotherapy may modify the natural history of asthma, particularly in children, but this is difficult to investigate given the high spontaneous remission rate of child asthma and the only supportive data have come from prolonged open studies (70). At present, therefore, this contention must be regarded as speculative.

C. New Approaches to Allergen Immunotherapy

An overview of new approaches to allergen immunotherapy is provided in Table 1. Most of the present new strategies are based (rightly or wrongly) on the perceived need to modify allergen-specific T-cell function (by skewing the cytokine profile of Th2 effector cells or inducing allergen-specific T regulatory cells) while abolishing or reducing binding of the injected substance to IgE. This not only reduces or abolishes the risk of anaphylaxis, but also allows much higher quantities of allergen to be administered safely, which may be an important factor for tolerance induction. Strategies include fusion, polymerization, refolding, or fragmentation of allergens to alter their structure while preserving T-cell epitopes, or immunization with identified T-cell epitopes. This latter strategy is the most problematic since many allergenic substances (such as grass pollen) contain a mixture of many proteins to which most individuals (major allergens) or only a minority of individuals (minor allergens) may respond. It is difficult with complex protein mixtures to identify and retain all T-cell epitopes; furthermore, the range of such epitopes even within a single protein may vary between individuals according to their major histocompatibility class II phenotype. Epitope vaccination has been most successful with substances containing one or a few major allergens, such as cat dander, but even then there will be rare individuals whose MHC haplotype precludes their T cells from recognizing the particular epitopes in the vaccine. A compromise is simply to fragment the allergens into small peptides.

Allergenic proteins are conventionally extracted from their sources by relatively simple procedures such as acid precipitation and chromatography. Consequently, the relative amounts of any protein in each batch extract are not constant and each batch has to be biologically standardized (usually by RAST inhibition with reference sera). Each manufacturer has different reference sera, so that units of "biological activity" of allergens are not compatible between manufacturers. This effectively means that switching between vaccines in the course of immunotherapy is impossible. An obvious solution is to produce recombinant allergens that can be used at defined concentrations and in complete purity to produce vaccines that would then be universally standardized. While this has been achieved successfully for some mixtures of allergens (Table 1), it is still problematic when extracts comprise many major and minor allergens, each of which has to be produced in pure, recombinant form and then added back to the final vaccine in predetermined proportions. This is a relatively expensive procedure. Eventually, it may

Table 1 Novel Approaches to Allergen Immunotherapy

New approach	Rationale	Reference
Strategies to alter the shape of intact allergens		
Fusion of major allergens	Several major allergens are fused and expressed as a recombinant protein, thus altering the shape of the individual allergens and reducing IgE binding while preserving T-cell epitopes.	71
Chimeric allergens	Fragments of major allergens are fused and expressed as a single protein, thus reducing IgE binding but preserving T-cell epitopes (provided the fragments are sufficiently large).	72
Polymeric allergens	Major allergens are polymerized, reducing IgE binding but preserving T-cell epitopes.	73
Unrefolded allergens	Major recombinant allergens are denatured and then allowed to refold but in a manner different to the native conformation, reducing or abolishing IgE binding but preserving T-cell epitopes.	74
Strategies to fragment allergens		
Allergen fragments	Major allergens are divided into fragments, thus abolishing IgE binding but preserving T-cell epitopes.	73
Allergen peptides	Treatment is with a mixture of allergen-derived peptides covering the entire molecule or identified T-cell epitopes, thus abolishing IgE binding.	75
Conjugation of allergens to immune response modifiers		
Conjugation to CpG oligonucleotide	Major allergen is bound to a Toll-like receptor ligand (in this case TLR9), thus skewing the induced innate and adaptive immune responses away from the Th2 phenotype.	76
Conjugation to virus-like particles	Allergens or allergen-derived peptides are coupled to virus capsid-like recombinant proteins, thus skewing the adaptive immune response and enhancing immunogenicity.	77
Miscellaneous strategies		
Mixtures of recombinant allergens	An attempt to rationalize allergen concentrations in vaccines by using mixtures of recombinant allergens of complete purity and known concentrations.	78
Combination immunotherapy with anti-IgE therapy	The rationale is to improve the safety of allergen immunotherapy by pretreatment with anti-IgE, thus reducing or abolishing the possibility of anaphylaxis; safety and efficacy are still under investigation.	79,80
Intralymphatic vaccination	Administration of immunotherapy vaccines directly into lymph nodes under ultrasound guidance, the aim being to deliver high concentrations of allergen directly into the secondary lymphoid system; safety and efficacy are still being explored.	81

be possible to "tailor make" vaccines for individuals according to their particular patterns of recognition of major and minor allergens from a source as determined by in vitro, extended IgE measurement. Although attractive in terms of allergen standardization, this strategy is again likely to be expensive and not necessarily of therapeutic advantage.

Immunotherapy has been used (Table 1) in conjunction with anti-IgE therapy. The clearest rationale for this is to improve safety, particularly in asthmatic patients. In addition, removal of allergen-specific IgE by anti-IgE therapy prior to immunotherapy results in its no longer being available to facilitate "capture" of injected allergens when bound to the surface of antigen-processing cells such as B cells and dendritic cells, which could result in alternative processing and presentation of the allergen to T cells and, in theory, improved efficacy of the immunotherapy. This remains to be investigated thoroughly. Furthermore, any such improvement would have to be considerable to justify the high additional cost.

Immunotherapy vaccines are conventionally injected adsorbed to adjuvants such as aluminum hydroxide (alum) that enhances their immunogenicity. Attempts have been made to improve these adjuvants so as to enhance the therapeutic effects of vaccination. Most of these approaches have involved chemical conjugation of the allergen to so-called "immune response modifiers" (Table 1), which typically target Toll-like receptors on the surface of antigen-presenting cells, thus increasing the immunogenicity of the allergen and, at least in theory, skewing the balance of the resulting T-cell response away from the Th2 phenotype. As an alternative to chemically modifying the allergen, another approach is to inject it adsorbed onto a modified conventional adjuvant containing bacterial cell wall analogs such as monophosphoryl lipid A, which is again postulated to act as an immune response modifier (82). Time will tell whether or not these approaches are safe, more efficacious, and more cost-effective.

V. Anti-IgE Therapy for Asthma
A. Neutralizing IgE Without Causing Anaphylaxis

High-affinity antibodies that bind to the constant (Fc) region of human IgE (or more precisely the CHε3 domain) compete for the binding of IgE to both its high-affinity receptor FcεRI (expressed on mast cells and basophils and some antigen-presenting cells) and its lower-affinity receptor FCεRII (or CD23, expressed mainly on B cells, but also T cells, monocytes, eosinophils, and platelets) without binding to and activating these receptors or cross-linking cell surface–bound IgE, which would cause anaphylaxis. Two humanized murine monoclonal anti-CHε3 antibodies, omalizumab and TNX-901, have been developed for clinical use. At the time of writing only omalizumab is commercially available.

Omalizumab forms trimers and hexamers, too small to cause immune complex disease, with free IgE in the circulation. With sufficient dosages, <1% of total serum IgE is left unbound in the circulation. Since the high-affinity IgE receptor FcεRI must bind IgE ligand to escape internalization, expression of this receptor on mast cells, basophils, and dendritic cells is markedly reduced (>90%) on basophils within 7 days and on mast cells within 70 days (83,84). This reduces the potential for mast cell and basophil degranulation by surface IgE cross-linking, and may also impair capture and presentation of allergens and other antigens by dendritic cells. It is not clear whether the expression and function of CD23 are similarly affected, although some speculate (85) that B-cell differentiation and IgE synthesis may be impaired. As an IgG_1 molecule, the half-life of omalizumab in the circulation (26 days) greatly exceeds that of IgE (2 days), so that omalizumab binds to and retains IgE in the circulation for weeks, making conventional measurements of serum IgE concentrations uninterpretable. The "therapeutic" dosage of omalizumab was established, somewhat paradoxically, from a study in seasonal allergic rhinitis (86,87), the symptoms of which are far more clearly related to acute, IgE-mediated mast cell degranulation than is the case in asthma. Maximal clinical efficacy was observed when serum total free IgE concentrations were reduced to <90% of the normal threshold (which is 100 IU/mL or 240 ng/mL). This required a dosage of omalizumab of 0.016 mg/kg per IU/mL of baseline serum total IgE. The effect is observed within one hour with intravenous infusion, and within four weeks with subcutaneous injection. Stopping of therapy causes recovery of FcεRI expression such that basophil releasability is back to baseline within 2 to 10 months (88). In atopic subjects, total serum IgE concentrations may or may not be above the normal threshold and IgE against any given aeroallergen may comprise anything from a tiny fraction to up to 50% or more of this total IgE. The requirement for omalizumab to block essentially all free circulating IgE to be efficacious in allergic rhinitis probably reflects the fact that basophil and mast cell degranulation can be triggered by cross-linking of only a very few FcεRI molecules on the cell surface (83). Other potential actions of anti-IgE, such as impaired IgE-dependent antigen capture and presentation by dendritic cells and B cells, or hypothetical alteration of allergen processing by uptake of IgE/anti-IgE/allergen complexes from the circulation by binding to Fcγ receptors on antigen-processing cells (85) may not require complete blockade of free IgE.

B. Clinical Effects of Anti-IgE

As might be expected, anti-IgE therapy attenuates the clinical effects of acute allergen exposure in appropriately IgE-sensitized subjects. In experimental allergen challenge, it reduces both early (associated with mast cell degranulation) and late (associated with inflammatory cell influx) phase responses in the bronchi, nose, and skin (89–91), and also reduces bronchial mucosal and sputum inflammatory cells in atopic asthmatics in the absence of challenge (92), although it has not been shown to alter bronchial hyperresponsiveness to methacholine, which is regarded by some as a clinical surrogate of the degree of bronchial inflammation. It also reduces nasal inflammation in allergic rhinitis (93). It is not clear if these anti-inflammatory effects of anti-IgE are the result of blockade of IgE-induced mast cell/basophil degranulation or interference with T cell, B cell, or antigen-presenting cell function as discussed above, or both or neither.

In addition to its effects in experimental asthma, anti-IgE also exerted beneficial clinical effects in allergic rhinitis (94,95) and very significantly increased the exposure threshold for systemic reactions in peanut allergic patients (96). Owing to its high production cost, however, Novartis' development of omalizumab for clinical use has so far been confined to asthma, where costs might be recouped through decreased requirements of treated patients for health care services and medications, implying a focus on patients with severe, unstable disease despite a lot of treatment. Randomized, placebo-controlled, double-blinded trials of the efficacy of omalizumab in a total of 3143 patients with mild-to-severe atopic asthma were subjected to Cochrane meta-analysis (97). Compared with placebo, omalizumab therapy reduced asthma exacerbations by 40%, a conclusion concordant with the manufacturer's own estimation (98). The "flagship" of these studies, INNOVATE (99), included nonsmoking asthmatics aged 12 and above with serum total IgE concentration 50 to 700 IU/mL and a positive skin prick test to at least one perennial allergen who remained symptomatic despite receiving GINA step 4 treatment or more. These criteria (somewhat arbitrarily) shaped the licensed indications for omalizumab. Even in these more severe patients, omalizumab reduced disease exacerbations by 26%. On the other hand, meta-analysis showed that airways obstruction was not clinically significantly affected by omalizumab, while symptomatic improvement was small and mean Juniper asthma quality of life (AQOL) scores did not improve by more than 0.5 points, which is the minimum considered to be clinically significant (actual change 0.32, 95% confidence interval 0.22 to 0.43, compared with placebo), although a greater proportion of omalizumab treated patients did experience an improvement in AQOL score of ≥ 0.5 as compared with those treated with placebo (73/126 vs. 46/120, respectively; $p = 0.002$), which presumably largely reflects fewer disease exacerbations and particularly hospitalizations. Omalizumab, compared with placebo therapy, also allowed a modest reduction of inhaled (mean 118 µg/day beclometasone equivalent) but not oral corticosteroid dosages, although none of the trials subjected to analysis was powered specifically to detect an oral corticosteroid sparing effect. Approximately 16% of the treated patients showed no useful response to omalizumab therapy at all. This effect of omalizumab in reducing asthma exacerbations is a challenge to explain given that the drug has such modest effects on lung function and symptomatology, and that the vast majority of exacerbations are caused by colds and not acute exposure to allergens. As emphasized, there is much to be learned about its mechanism of action.

Omalizumab is administered by subcutaneous injection either every two or four weeks according to the required calculated dosage. A maximum of 1.2 mL may be given at a single injection site, so that up to three injections may have to be given at each visit. It is supplied as a lyophilized powder, which must be reconstituted prior to use. The shelf life of the reconstituted drug is eight hours at 4°C. It appears to be very safe and overall withdrawal rates because of adverse events have been very small (0.8%) (97). Pain, induration, and irritation at the injection site(s) are common. A few patients have developed delayed "anaphylactic" reactions (localized or generalized edema, urticaria, and breathlessness): in general, these have been mild. A recent report (100) from the American Academy of Allergy, Asthma, and Immunology suggested that these reactions occur with low frequency (0.09% of injections), usually within two hours of injection and not necessarily following the first three injections. Their etiology is unknown. There was a small, nonsignificant increase in malignancies in patients treated with omalizumab as compared with placebo in the trials surveyed for licensing of the drug. As a result, Genentech has started the Outcomes and Treatment Regimens (TENOR) study (101) and other surveillance programs to document the natural medical history of severe asthmatics, including their proneness to cancer. It is not known to be harmful in pregnancy and breast feeding, although data are limited, and in trials it was usually stopped as soon as pregnancy was noted. It crosses the placenta freely and appears at low concentrations in the breast milk of treated nursing mothers. For this reason it is probably best avoided in pregnant or nursing women unless considered absolutely essential, although on the other hand, one might hypothesize that anti-IgE treatment at this early age might protect against IgE-mediated diseases.

C. Controversies with Anti-IgE Therapy

A major controversy with omalizumab therapy relates to its cost effectiveness. The U.S. Food and Drug Administration has approved omalizumab, according to the Xolair® package insert, for the treatment of "adults and adolescents (12 years of age and above) with moderate-to-severe persistent asthma who have a positive skin prick test or in vitro reactivity to a perennial allergen and whose symptoms are inadequately controlled with inhaled corticosteroids." This means effectively that it could technically be given to all asthmatics who remain symptomatic on high dosages of inhaled corticosteroids, yet its principal clinical effectiveness appears to be reducing unexpected disease exacerbations requiring unplanned medical intervention. One estimate of its cost effectiveness made in the United States over a time horizon of 10 years using data valid in 2007 (102) concluded that omalizumab costs in excess of $800,000 per quality-adjusted life year gained, which greatly exceeds the World Health Organization's definition of a cost-effective intervention, which is three times the per capita gross domestic product (approximately $45,000 in the United States in 2007). This has resulted in reservations about its widespread use (103) and attempts in recent asthma guidelines (such as EPR-3) to restrict this to patients in whom maximal medical therapy fails despite removal of all exacerbating factors and documented compliance (104). In the United Kingdom, the National Institute for Health and Clinical Excellence (NICE) has recommended restriction of the use of omalizumab within its licensed indications only for those asthmatics who have a specified number of severe exacerbations requiring hospital attendance or admission in the year prior to commencing therapy despite documented compliance with treatment with high-dosage inhaled corticosteroid, regular oral corti-costeroid, and any other add-on therapy that is deemed effective (105). Another problem is that attempts to identify "responders" to therapy a priori based on retrospective analysis of existing trials have been largely unsuccessful, and the only current guideline for assessment of response is the physician's assessment, based on as yet poorly defined criteria, of the response of the individual patient after 16 weeks of therapy (106), which in unlikely in every patient to pick up a reduction in the frequency of unplanned medical interventions. On the other side of the coin, the restriction of the use of omalizumab to asthmatics with at least one positive skin prick test to a perennial aeroallergen seems arbitrary and hard to justify in view of the mounting evidence, laid out above, that IgE-mediated mechanisms may play a role in asthma regardless of skin prick test positivity. It seems clear that many more studies will be needed, in adults, children, and the elderly, before omalizumab therapy is safely positioned in the algorithm of asthma management.

VI. Management of Anaphylaxis
A. The Problem of Definition

Anaphylaxis has been described as a "severe, life-threatening generalized or systemic hypersensitivity reaction." It is usually caused by IgE-mediated systemic release of mediators (including histamine, leukotrienes, prostaglandins, thromboxane, and brady-kinin) from mast cells and basophils following exposure to an allergen, but in some patients a clear allergic (specific IgE-mediated) etiology cannot be identified, in which case the World Allergy Organization has suggested that the term "nonallergic anaphy-laxis" be used. Non-IgE mechanisms may underlie anaphylactic reactions to blood and blood products, some artificial plasma expanders, radio contrast media, and some drugs such as opiates and intravenous anesthetics. This overarching definition is obviously vague. A collation of recent U.S. and European guidelines (107–109) suggests that anaphylaxis may be diagnosed when any one of the following three criteria is fulfilled:

1. Acute onset of an illness (minutes to hours) with involvement of the skin (pruritus, flushing, urticaria, angioedema) and at least one of the following:

   i. Respiratory compromise (dyspnea, stridor, bronchospasm, hypoxia)

   ii. cardiovascular compromise [collapse, hypotension (systolic blood pressure <90 mmHg)]

2. Two or more of the following occurring rapidly after exposure to a likely allergen:

   i. Involvement of the skin or mucosal tissue with generalized urticaria, angioedema, pruritus

   ii. Respiratory compromise as above

   iii. Cardiovascular compromise as above

   iv. Persistent gastrointestinal symptoms (colic, vomiting, diarrhea)

3. Hypotension after exposure to a relevant allergen within minutes to hours

This diversity of symptomatology in different individuals is one of the reasons why anaphylaxis is difficult to diagnose accurately. On the one hand, it may be missed (e.g., laryngeal edema may be mistaken for asthma). On the other hand, distinct, non-life-threatening conditions such as idiopathic urticaria or angioedema may be inappropriately labeled as "anaphylaxis." Anaphylaxis in the absence of skin manifestations is unusual, but not unheard of. Respiratory tract symptoms tend to predominate with some allergic triggers (such as foods), while hypotension predominates with others (such as insect venoms), but there are no hard and fast rules. Bronchospasm is rarely life threatening unless the patient has asthma, when it may be. It is critical to document the presence/absence of urticaria/angioedema, bowel upset (abdominal pain, vomiting, diarrhea), respiratory compromise (peak flow or high airway pressures in ventilated patients, low blood oxygen saturation, laryngeal edema wherever possible by direct inspection of the vocal cords), and hypotension when assessing anaphylaxis. Many of these items may be neglected in the clamor of the emergency room. An objective test is to measure serum concentrations of mast cell tryptase as soon as possible and at least six hours after the event. A transient rise returning to baseline supports the diagnosis (110).

B. Diagnosis of Anaphylaxis

In an emergency, this is based on what can be learned about the patient's history and rapid clinical assessment as explained above; if the diagnosis is confirmed or strongly suspected, treatment should be commenced immediately; delay may be fatal (111). Other diagnoses to be considered include the following:

1. Isolated angioedema: This may be from congenital or acquired C1 esterase inhibitor deficiency or caused by drugs, most commonly angiotensin converting enzyme inhibitors. There is no associated urticaria and other systemic features vary according to the precise diagnosis. Isolated urticaria is

rarely life threatening although hereditary angioedema may occasionally cause life-threatening laryngeal edema that requires appropriate airway management (112).

2. Severe asthma may present with bronchospasm and stridor but is not usually associated with urticaria and angioedema.

3. Panic/anxiety attacks associated with stridor as a result of vocal cord adduction: There is no urticaria, angioedema, hypoxia, or hypotension.

4. Vasovagal collapse: There are no features of systemic anaphylaxis.

Other rarer differential diagnoses to be considered include flushing syndromes such as metastatic carcinoid, postprandial syndromes such as scombroid poisoning, and systemic mastocytosis, as well as other causes of shock.

C. Management of Anaphylaxis: Acute

There is no consensus "gold standard" of treatment of anaphylaxis, since clinical trials are difficult. Adrenaline (epinephrine) is generally agreed to be the most important drug for any severe anaphylactic reaction. As an α-agonist, it reverses peripheral vaso-dilatation and reduces edema. As a β-agonist, it reverses bronchospasm, increases the force of myocardial contraction, and inhibits mast cell mediator release. Adrenaline is most effective when given as early as possible; when given intramuscularly it is very safe. Rarely, it may fail to reverse the clinical manifestations of anaphylaxis, particularly when given late or to patients taking β-blockers. Other measures, particularly volume replacement, may then assume greater importance. General measures include the following:

1. Remove the cause if possible.

2. Lie the patient flat with the legs elevated if possible: this is good for hypo-tension but not helpful for those with severe breathing difficulties.

3. Consider early intubation if there is laryngeal edema: delay may make intu-bation extremely difficult.

4. Administer high-flow oxygen (10–15 L/min) if available.

5. Intramuscular adrenaline should be given for shock, life-threatening airway swelling, or severe bronchospasm. For adults and children >12 years, give 0.5 mL of 1:1000 adrenaline (500 µg) (or use an adult adrenaline auto-injector). For children 6 to 12 years use 0.25 mL or an adult injector pen. For children 6 months to 6 years give 0.12 mL or use a child autoinjector. For children <6 months use 0.05 mL. The dose may be repeated in five minutes and occasionally more than once if improvement is transient. Intravenous adrenaline is not recommended as it may cause profound local vaso-constriction leading, for example, to myocardial infarction or stroke. It may be used at a dilution of at least 1:10,000 (never 1:1000) by physicians experienced in its use for profound shock that is immediately life threatening. A further dilution to 1:100,000 enables finer titration of the dose.

6. Give an H1-antihistamine such as chlorphenamine (10–20 mg intramuscularly or intravenously according to the circumstances in adults and children >12 years, 5–10 mg in children 6–12 years, and 2.5–5 mg in children under 6 years).

7. Give hydrocortisone (100–500 mg in adults and children >12 years, 100 mg in children 6–12 years, and 50 mg in children <6 years by slow intramuscular or intravenous injection according to the circumstances), especially in asthmatics. Corticosteroids have no effect for at least four to six hours after dosing, but they minimize later bronchospasm and the possibility of "late" reactions sometimes seen four to six hours after the initial event.

8. Give inhaled β2-agonist such as salbutamol (albuterol) to all those with severe bronchospasm and especially asthmatics; additional inhaled ipratropium may be beneficial in patients taking β-blockers.

9. Fluid replacement should be instituted where practicable and where there is profound shock: give 1 to 2 L of crystalloid or more in adults (20 mL/kg in children). Rapid volume replacement through wide bore intravenous lines may be indicated.

10. Less established measures: there are case reports that vasopressin may benefit severely hypotensive patients (113); that there may be a role for atropine if profound bradycardia is present (111); and that glucagon may be useful in patients unresponsive to adrenaline, especially those receiving β-blockers. This agent is short acting (give 1–2 mg every 5 minutes, intravenously or intramuscularly): common unwanted effects include nausea, vomiting, and hyperglycemia.

Patients should be warned about the possibility of early recurrence of symptoms following the initial episode; it is prudent to observe such patients for at least 8 to 24 hours. This is particularly likely in patients with severe reactions, especially if they have asthma, if there is a possibility of continued absorption of allergen (such as with oral drugs), or if there is a history of previous biphasic reactions (114,115). Generally, patients remaining symptom-free for at least four hours after treatment may be discharged (116).

D. Management of Anaphylaxis: After the Event

A full account of the investigation and further management of anaphylaxis is outside the scope of this account but is covered in major guidelines (107,108). The importance of expert further management of the patient, critically by an experienced allergist, cannot be overemphasized. This will include verification or otherwise of the diagnosis and the identification of the possible precipitating allergen or other product. This may be obvious or on the other hand require a very detailed and careful history. Further details of the circumstances (e.g., a detailed chronological history of drugs administered during anesthesia or dentistry, or elucidation of the evolvement of food-induced, exercise-associated anaphylaxis) may be necessary. Patients (or their parents and carers) must be given written instructions as to how to deal with possible future episodes, and must be taught, with periodic refreshment, how to use adrenaline autoinjector devices. Education may also include how to avoid relevant sources of allergens, such as peanuts or latex or stinging insects, should these be identifiable from the history backed up by appropriate testing. Patients may be advised to wear warning bracelets such as MedicAlert to advise of their condition or of relevant allergies, and often benefit from being placed in touch with relevant support groups. Avoidance management should be personalized, taking into consideration factors such as age, occupation, hobbies, social conditions, access to medical care, comorbidity, and amount of personal anxiety. In some cases, desensitization to certain allergens, such as insect venoms and some drugs and vaccines, is highly effective. Successful management of anaphylaxis is thus often a team effort involving the allergist, the patient, and other key professionals such as carers, school nurses, and dieticians.

References

1. Johansson SGO, Hourihane JO'B, Bousquet J. A revised nomenclature for allergy: an EAACI position statement from the EAACI nomenclature task force [position paper]. Allergy 2001; 56:813–824.
2. Simpson BM, Custovic A, Simpson A, et al. Manchester asthma and allergy study: risk factors for asthma and allergic disorders in adults. Clin Exp Allergy 2001; 31:391–399.
3. Pearce N, Pekkanen J, Beasley R. How much asthma is really attributable to atopy? Thorax 1999; 54:268–272.
4. Pearce N, Douwes J, Beasley R. Is allergen exposure the major primary cause of asthma? Thorax 2000; 55:424–431.
5. Arbes SJ, Gergen PJ, Vaughn B, et al. Asthma cases attributable to atopy: results from the Third National Health and Nutrition Survey. J Allergy Clin Immunol 2007; 120:1139–1145.
6. Rackeman FM. A working classification of asthma. Am J Med 1947; 33:601–606.
7. Romanet-Manent S, Charpin D, Magnan A. Allergic vs non-allergic asthma: what makes the difference? Allergy 2002; 57:607–613.
8. Kroegel C, Jager L, Walker C. Is there a place for intrinsic asthma as a distinct immunopathological entity? Eur Respir J 1997; 10:513–515.
9. Bentley AM, Durham SR, Kay AB. Comparison of the immunopathology of extrinsic, intrinsic and occupational asthma. J Investig Allergol Clin Immunol 1994; 4:222–232.
10. Humbert M, Durham SR, Ying S, et al. IL-4 and IL-5 mRNA and protein in bronchial biopsies from patients with atopic and non-atopic asthma: evidence against "intrinsic" asthma being a distinct immunopathologic entity. Am J Respir Crit Care Med 1996; 154:1497–1504.
11. Ying S, Humbert M, Barkans J, et al. Expression of IL-4 and IL-5 mRNA and protein product by CD4+ and CD8+ T cells, eosinophils, and mast cells in bronchial biopsies obtained from atopic and non-atopic (intrinsic) asthmatics. J Immunol 1997; 158:3539–3544.
12. Humbert M, Durham SR, Kimmitt P, et al. Elevated expression of messenger ribonucleic acid encoding interleukin-13 in the bronchial mucosa of atopic and non-atopic asthma. J Allergy Clin Immunol 1997; 99:657–665.
13. Kotsimbos TC, Ghaffar O, Minshall EM, et al. Expression of the IL-4 receptor alpha-subunit is increased in bronchial biopsy specimens from atopic and non-atopic asthma subjects. J Allergy Clin Immunol 1998; 102:859–866.
14. Yasruel Z, Humbert M, Kotsimbos TC, et al. Membrane-bound and soluble alpha IL-5 receptor mRNA in the bronchial mucosa of atopic and non-atopic asthmatics. Am J Respir Crit Care Med 1996; 154:1497–1504.
15. Humbert M, Ying S, Corrigan C, et al. Bronchial mucosal expression of the genes encoding chemokines RANTES and MCP-3 in symptomatic atopic and non-atopic asthmatics: relationship to the eosinophil-active cytokines interleukin (IL)-5, granulocyte macrophage-colony-stimulating factor, and IL-3. Am J Respir Cell Mol Biol 1997; 16:1–8.
16. Ying S, Meng Q, Zeibecoglou K, et al. Eosinophil chemotactic chemokines (eotaxin, eotaxin-2, RANTES, monocyte chemoattractant protein-3 (MCP-3), and MCP-4), and C-C chemokine receptor 3 expression in bronchial biopsies from atopic and non-atopic (intrinsic) asthmatics. J Immunol 1999; 163:6321–6329.

17. Humbert M, Grant JA, Taborda-Barata L, et al. High-affinity IgE receptor (FcepsilonRI)-bearing cells in bronchial biopsies from atopic and non-atopic asthma. Am J Respir Crit Care Med 1996; 153:1931–1937.
18. Ying S, Humbert M, Meng Q, et al. Local expression of epsilon germ line gene transcripts and RNA for the epsilon heavy chain of IgE in the bronchial mucosa in atopic and non-atopic asthma. J Allergy Clin Immunol 2000; 107:686–692.
19. Takhar P, Corrigan CJ, Smurthwaite L, et al. Class switch recombination to IgE in the bronchial mucosa of atopic and non-atopic patients with asthma. J Allergy Clin Immunol 2007; 119:213–218.
20. Takhar P, Smurthwaite L, Coker CA, et al. Allergen drives class switching to IgE in the nasal mucosa in allergic rhinitis. J Immunol 2005; 174:5024–5032.
21. Smurthwaite L, Walker SN, Wilson DR, et al. Persistent IgE synthesis in the nasal mucosa of hay fever patients. Eur J Immunol 2001; 31:3422–3431.
22. Barbee RA, Hallon M, Kaltenborn W. A longitudinal study of serum IgE in a community cohort: correlations with age, sex, smoking and atopic status. J Allergy Clin Immunol 1987; 79:919–927.
23. Burrows B, Martinez FD, Halonen M, et al. Association of asthma with serum IgE levels and skin-test reactivity to allergens. N Engl J Med 1989; 320:271–277.
24. Beeh KM, Ksoll M, Buhl R. Elevation of total serum immunoglobulin E is associated with asthma in non-allergic individuals. Eur Respir J 2000; 16:609–614.
25. Gould HJ, Takhar P, Harries HE, et al. Germinal-centre reactions in allergic inflammation. Trends Immunol 2006; 7:446–450.
26. Welliver RC. Respiratory syncitial virus and other respiratory viruses. Pediatr Infect Dis J 2003; 22(2 suppl):S6–S10.
27. Coker HA, Harries HE, Banfield GK, et al. Biased use of VH5 IgE-positive cells in the nasal mucosa in allergic rhinitis. J Allergy Clin Immunol 2005; 116:445–452.
28. Lee JY, Kim HM, Ye YM, et al. Role of staphylococcal superantigen-specific IgE antibodies in aspirin-intolerant asthma. Allergy Asthma Proc 2006; 27:341–346.
29. Garn H, Mittermann I, Valenta R, et al. Autosensitisation as a pathomechanism in asthma. Ann N Y Acad Sci 2007; 1107:417–425.
30. Kitaura J, Song J, Tsai M, et al. Evidence that IgE molecules mediate a spectrum of effects on mast cell survival and activation by aggregation of the FcεRI. Proc Natl Acad Sci U S A 2003; 100:12911–12916.
31. Kuehr J, Frischer T, Meinert R, et al. Mite allergen exposure is a risk for the incidence of specific sensitization. J Allergy Clin Immunol 1994; 94:44–52.
32. Custovic A, Hallam CL, Simpson BM, et al. Decreased prevalence of sensitization to cats with high exposure to cat allergen. J Allergy Clin Immunol 2001; 108:537–539.
33. Platts-Mills T, Vaughan J, Squillace S, et al. Sensitisation, asthma, and a modified Th2 response in children exposed to cat allergen: a population-based cross-sectional study. Lancet 2001; 357:752–756.
34. Priftis KN, Anthracopoulos MB, Nikolaou-Papanagiotou A, et al. Increased sensitisation in urban vs rural environment—rural protection or an urban living effect? Pediatr Allergy Immunol 2007; 18:209–216.
35. Zock JP, Heinrich J, Jarvis D, et al. Distribution and determinants of house dust mite allergens in Europe: the European Community Respiratory Health Survey II. J Allergy Clin Immunol 2006; 118:682–690.
36. Prescott SL, Macaubas C, Holt BJ, et al. Transplacental priming of the human immune system to environmental allergens: universal skewing of initial T cell responses toward the Th2 cytokine profile. J Immunol 1998; 160:4730–4737.
37. Piccinni MP, Mecacci F, Sampognaro S, et al. Aeroallergen sensitization can occur during fetal life. Int Arch Allergy Immunol 1993; 102:301–303.

38. Smillie FI, Elderfield AJ, Patel F, et al. Lymphoproliferative responses in cord blood and at one year: no evidence for an effect of in utero exposure to dust mite allergens. Clin Exp Allergy 2001; 31:1194–1204.

39. Prescott SL. The significance of immune responses to allergens in early life. Clin Exp Allergy 2001; 31:1167–1169.

40. Szepfalusi Z, Pichler J, Elsasser S, et al. Transplacental priming of the human immune system with environmental allergens can occur early in gestation. J Allergy Clin Immunol 2000; 106:530–536.

41. Platts-Mills TA, Woodfolk JA. Cord blood proliferative responses to inhaled allergens: is there a phenomenon? J Allergy Clin Immunol 2000; 106:441–443.

42. Sears MR, Herbison GP, Holdaway MD, et al. The relative risks of sensitivity to grass pollen, house dust mite and cat dander in the development of childhood asthma. Clin Exp Allergy 1989; 19:419–424.

43. Gergen PJ, Turkeltaub PC. The association of individual allergen reactivity with respiratory disease in a national sample: data from the second National Health and Nutrition Examination Survey, 1976-80 (NHANES II). J Allergy Clin Immunol 1992; 90:579–588.

44. Koopman LP, van Strien RT, Kerkhof M, et al. Placebo-controlled trial of house dust mite impermeable mattress covers: effect on symptoms in early childhood. Am J Respir Crit Care Med 2002; 166:307–313.

45. Woodcock A, Lowe LA, Murray CS, et al. Early life environmental control: effect on symptoms, sensitisation and lung function at age 3 years. Am J Respir Crit Care Med 2004; 170:433–439.

46. Gotzsche PC, Johansen HK, Schmidt LM, et al. House dust mite control measures for asthma. Cochrane Database Syst Rev 2004; 18:CD001187.

47. Cloosterman SG, Schermer TR, Bijl-Hofalnd ID, et al. Effects of house dust mite avoidance measures on Der p1 concentrations and clinical condition of mild adult house dust mite allergic asthmatics patients using no inhaled steroids. Clin Exp Allergy 1999; 29:1336–1346.

48. van Schayck OCP, Maas T, Kaper J, et al. Is there any role for allergen avoidance in the primary prevention of asthma? J Allergy Clin Immunol 2007; 119:1323–1328.

49. Larche M, Akdis CA, Valenta R. Immunological mechanisms of allergen-specific immunotherapy. Nat Rev Immunol 2006; 6:761–771.

50. Jutel M, Muller UR, Fricker M, et al. Influence of bee venom immunotherapy on degranulation and leukotriene generation in human blood basophils. Clin Exp Allergy 1996; 26:1112–1118.

51. Jutel M, Akdis M, Budak F, et al. IL-10 and TGF-β cooperate in the regulatory T cell response to mucosal allergens in normal immunity and specific immunotherapy. Eur J Immunol 2003; 33:1205–1214.

52. Francis JN, Till SJ, Durham SR. Induction of IL-10+CD4+CD25+ T cells by grass pollen immunotherapy. J Allergy Clin Immunol 2003; 111:1255–1261.

53. Akdis M, Verhagen J, Taylor A, et al. Immune responses in healthy and allergic individuals are characterised by a fine balance between allergen-specific T regulatory 1 and T helper 2 cells. J Exp Med 2004; 199:1567–1575.

54. Karlsson MR, Rugtveit J, Brandtzaeg P. Allergen-responsive CD4+CD25+ regulatory T cells in children who have outgrown cow's milk allergy. J Exp Med 2004; 199:1679–1688.

55. Wachholz PA, Durham SR. Mechanisms of immunotherapy: IgG revisited. Curr Opin Allergy Clin Immunol 2004; 4:313–318.

56. Pierkes M, Bellinghausen I, Hultsch T, et al. Decreased release of histamine and sulfidoleukotrienes by human peripheral blood leukocytes after wasp venom immunotherapy is partially due to induction of IL-10 and IFN-gamma production of T cells. J Allergy Clin Immunol 1999; 103:326–332.

57. Schandane L, Alonso-Vega C, Willems F, et al. B7/CD28-dependent IL-5 production by human resting T cells is inhibited by IL-10. J Immunol 1994; 152:4368–4374.

58. Rak S, Lowhagen O, Venge P. The effect of immunotherapy on bronchial hyper-responsiveness and eosinophil cationic protein in pollen-allergic patients. J Allergy Clin Immunol 1988; 82:470–480.

59. Wilson DR, Lima MT, Durham SR. Sublingual immunotherapy for allergic rhinitis: systematic review and meta-analysis. Allergy 2005; 60:4–12.

60. Moingeon P, Batard T, Fadel R, et al. Immune mechanisms of allergen-specific sublingual immunotherapy. Allergy 2006; 61:151–165.

61. Bohle B, Kinaciyan T, Gerstmayr M, et al. Sublingual immunotherapy induces IL-10-producing T regulatory cells, allergen-specific T cell tolerance and immune deviation. J Allergy Clin Immunol 2007; 120:707–713.

62. Bousquet J, Hejjaoui A, Michel FB. Specific immunotherapy in asthma. J Allergy Clin Immunol 1990; 86:292–305.

63. Cantani A, Arcese G, Lucenti P, et al. A three-year prospective study of specific immunotherapy to inhalant allergens: evidence of safety and efficacy in 300 children with allergic asthma. J Invest Allergol Clin Immunol 1997; 7:90–97.

64. Peroni DG, Paicentini GL, Martinati LC, et al. Double-blind trial of house-dust mite immunotherapy in asthmatic children resident at high altitude. Allergy 1995; 50:925–930.

65. Olaguibel JM, Alvarez Puebla MJ. Efficacy of sublingual allergen vaccinations for respiratory allergy in children. Conclusions from one meta-analysis. J Invest Allergol Clin Immunol 2005; 15:9–16.

66. Calamita Z, Saconato H, Pela AB, et al. Efficacy of sublingual immunotherapy in asthma: systematic review of randomised clinical trials using the Cochrane Collaboration method. Allergy 2006; 61:1162–1172.

67. Abramson MJ, Puy RM, Weiner JM. Immunotherapy in asthma: an updated systematic review. Allergy 1999; 54:1022–1041.

68. Adkinson NF, Eggleston PA, Eney D, et al. A controlled trial of immunotherapy for asthma in allergic children. N Engl J Med 1997; 336:324–331.

69. Maestrelli P, Zanolla L, Pozzan M, et al. Effects of specific immunotherapy added to pharmacologic treatment and allergen avoidance in asthmatic patients allergic to house dust mite. J Allergy Clin Immunol 2004; 113:643–649.

70. Jacobsen L, Niggemann B, Dreborg S, et al. Specific immunotherapy has long-term preventive effect of seasonal and perennial asthma: 10 year follow-up on the PAT study. Allergy 2007; 62:943–948.

71. Kussebi F, Karamloo F, Rhymer C, et al. A major allergen gene-fusion protein for potential usage in allergen-specific immunotherapy. J Allergy Clin Immunol 2005; 115:323–329.

72. Karamloo F, Schmid-Grendelmeier P, Kussebi F, et al. Prevention of allergy by a recombinant multi-allergen vaccine with reduced IgE binding and preserved T cell epitopes. Eur J Immunol 2005; 35:3268–3276.

73. Niederberger V, Horak F, Vrtala S, et al. Vaccination with genetically engineered allergens prevents progression of allergic disease. Proc Natl Acad Sci U S A 2004; 101(suppl 2): 14677–14682.

74. Akdis CA, Blaser K. Bypassing IgE and targeting T cells for specific immunotherapy of allergy. Trends Immunol 2001; 22:175–178.

75. Larche M. Immunoregulation by targeting T cells in the treatment of allergy and asthma. Curr Opin Immunol 2006; 18:745–750.

76. Creticos PS, Schroeder JT, Hamilton RG, et al. Immunotherapy with a ragweed-toll-like receptor 9 agonist vaccine for allergic rhinitis. N Engl J Med 2006; 355:1445–1455.

77. Kundig TM, Senti G, Schnetzler G, et al. Der p1 peptide on virus-like particles is safe and highly immunogenic in healthy adults. J Allergy Clin Immunol 2006; 117:1470–1476.

78. Jutel M, Jaeger L, Suck R, et al. Allergen-specific immunotherapy with recombinant grass pollen allergens. J Allergy Clin Immunol 2005; 116:608–613.

79. Casale TB, Busse WW, Kline JN, et al. Omalizumab pre-treatment decreases acute reactions after rush immunotherapy for ragweed-induced seasonal allergic rhinitis. J Allergy Clin Immunol 2006; 117:134–140.

80. Klunker S, Saggar LR, Seyfert-Margolis V, et al. Combination treatment with omalizumab and rush immunotherapy for ragweed-induced allergic rhinitis: inhibition of IgE-facilitated allergen binding. J Allergy Clin Immunol 2007; 120:688–695.

81. Johansen P, Haffner AC, Koch F, et al. Direct intralymphatic injection of peptide vaccines enhances immunogenicity. Eur J Immunol 2005; 35:568–574.

82. Baldrick P, Richardson D, Woroniecki SR, et al. Pollinex Quattro Ragweed: safety evaluation of a new allergy vaccine adjuvanted with monophosphoryl lipid A (MPL) for the treatment of ragweed pollen allergy. J Appl Toxicol 2007; 27:399–409.

83. MacGlashan DW, Bochner BS, Adelman TC, et al. Down-regulation of FcεRI expression on human basophils during in vivo treatment of atopic patients with anti-IgE antibody. J Immunol 1997; 158:1438–1445.

84. Beck LA, Marcotte GV, MacGlashan D, et al. Omalizumab-induced reductions in mast cell Fc epsilon RI expression and function. J Allergy Clin Immunol 2004; 114:527–530.

85. Chang TW. The pharmacological basis of anti-IgE therapy. Nat Biotechnol 2000; 18:157–162.

86. Casale TB, Bernstein IL, Busse WW, et al. Use of an anti-IgE humanised monoclonal antibody in ragweed-induced allergic rhinitis. J Allergy Clin Immunol 1997; 100:110–121.

87. Casale TB. Anti-immunoglobulin E (omalizumab) therapy in seasonal allergic rhinitis. Am J Respir Crit Care Med 2001; 164(suppl):S18–S21.

88. Saini SS, MacGlashan DW, Sterbinsky SA, et al. Down-regulation of human basophil IgE and FcεRI surface densities and mediator release by anti-IgE infusions is reversible in vitro and in vivo. J Immunol 1999; 162:5624–5630.

89. Fahy JV, Fleming HE, Wong HH, et al. The effect of an anti-IgE monoclonal antibody on the early- and late-phase responses to allergen inhalation in asthmatic subjects. Am J Respir Crit Care Med 1997; 155:1828–1834.

90. Lin H, Boesel KM, Griffith DT, et al. Omalizumab rapidly decreases nasal allergic response and FcεRI on basophils. J Allergy Clin Immunol 2004; 113:297–302.

91. Ong YE, Menzies-Gow A, Barkans J, et al. Anti-IgE (omalizumab) inhibits late-phase reactions and inflammatory cells after repeat skin allergen challenge. J Allergy Clin Immunol 2005; 116:558–564.

92. Djukanovic R, Wilson SJ, Kraft M, et al. Effects of treatment with anti-immunoglobulin E antibody omalizumab on airway inflammation in allergic asthma. Am J Respir Crit Care Med 2004; 170:583–593.

93. Bez C, Schubert R, Kopp M, et al. Effect of anti-immunoglobulin E on nasal inflammation in patients with seasonal allergic rhinitis. Clin Exp Allergy 2004; 34:1079–1085.

94. Casale TB, Condemi J, LaForce C, et al. Effect of omalizumab on symptoms of seasonal allergic rhinitis: a randomised controlled trial. JAMA 2001; 286:2956–2967.

95. Chervinsky P, Casale T, Townley R, et al. Omalizumab, an anti-IgE antibody, in the treatment of adults and adolescents with perennial allergic rhinitis. Ann Allergy Asthma Immunol 2003; 91:160–167.

96. Leung DY, Sampson HA, Yunginger JW, et al. Effect of anti-IgE therapy in patients with peanut allergy. N Engl J Med 2003; 348:986–993.

97. Walker S, Monteil M, Phelan K, et al. Anti-IgE for chronic asthma in adults and children. Cochrane Database Syst Rev 2006; Apr 19(2):CD003559.

98. Bousquet J, Cabrera P, Berkman N, et al. The effect of treatment with omalizumab, an anti-IgE antibody, on asthma exacerbations and emergency medical visits in patients with severe persistent asthma. Allergy 2005; 60:302–308.

99. Humbert M, Beasley R, Ayres J, et al. Benefits of omalizumab as add-on therapy in patients with severe persistent asthma who are inadequately controlled despite best available therapy (GINA 2004 step 4 treatment): INNOVATE. Allergy 2005; 60:309–316.

100. Cox L, Platts-Mills TAE, Finegold I, et al. American Academy of Allergy, Asthma & Immunology/American College of Allergy, Asthma and Immunology Joint Task Force report on omalizumab-associated anaphylaxis. J Allergy Clin Immunol 2007; 120:1373–1377.

101. Slavin RG, Haselkorn T, Lee JH, et al. Asthma in older adults: observations from the Epidemiology and Natural History of Asthma: Outcomes and Treatment Regimens (TENOR) study. Ann Allergy Asthma Immunol 2006; 96:406–414.

102. Wu AC, Paltiel AD, Kuntz KM, et al. Cost-effectiveness of omalizumab in adults with severe asthma: results from the Asthma Policy Model. J Allergy Clin Immunol 2007; 120:1146–1152.

103. Krishnan JA, Gould M. Omalizumab for severe allergic asthma: dollars and sense. J Allergy Clin Immunol 2007; 120:1015–1017.

104. National Heart, Lung and Blood Institute and the National Asthma Education and Prevention Program. Expert Panel Report 3: Guidelines for the Diagnosis and management of Asthma. Summary Report 2007. J Allergy Clin Immunol 2007; 120(suppl):S93–S138.

105. National Institute for Health and Clinical Excellence Technology Appraisal Guidance 133 (2007). omalizumab for severe persistent allergic asthma. Available at: www.nice.org.uk/TA133.

106. Bousquet J, Rabe K, Humbert M, et al. Predicting and evaluating response to omalizumab in patients with severe allergic asthma. Respir Med 2007; 101:1483–1492.

107. Muraro A, Roberts G, Clark A, et al. The management of anaphylaxis in childhood: position paper of the European Academy of Allergology and Clinical Immunology. Allergy 2007; 62:857–871.

108. Lieberman P, Kemp SF, Oppenheimer J, et al. The diagnosis and management of anaphylaxis: an updated practice parameter. J Allergy Clin Immunol 2005; 115(suppl):S463–S518.

109. Soar J, Deakin CD, Nolan JP, et al. European Resuscitation Council guidelines for resuscitation 2005. Section 7. Cardiac arrest in special circumstances. Resuscitation 2005; 67 (suppl):S135–S170.

110. Payne V, Kam PC. Mast cell tryptase: a review of its physiology and clinical significance. Anaesthesia 2004; 59:695–703.

111. Brown AF. Anaphylaxis gets the adrenaline going. Emerg Med J 2004; 21:128–129.

112. Ishoo E, Shah UK, Grillone GA, et al. Predicting airway risk in angioedema: staging system based on presentation. Otolaryngol Head Neck Surg 1999; 121:263–268.

113. Kill C, Wranze E, Wulf H. Successful treatment of severe anaphylactic shock with vasopressin. Two case reports. Int Arch Allergy Immunol 2004; 134:260–261.

114. Stark BJ, Sullivan TJ. Biphasic and protracted anaphylaxis. J Allergy Clin Immunol 1986; 78:76–83.

115. Brazil E, MacNamara AF. "Not so immediate" hypersensitivity: the danger of biphasic anaphylactic reactions. J Accid Emerg Med 1998; 15:252–253.

116. Brady WJ, Luber S, Carter CT, et al. Multiphasic anaphylaxis: an uncommon event in the emergency department. Acad Emerg Med 1997; 4:193–197.

10

New Anti-inflammatory Treatments for Asthma and COPD

KIAN FAN CHUNG
National Heart and Lung Institute, Imperial College, and Royal Brompton Hospital, London, U.K.

I. The Need for New Treatments for Asthma and COPD

Asthma and chronic obstructive pulmonary disease (COPD) are diseases in need of new therapies, particularly in the area of anti-inflammatory treatments. The reasons for this will be expounded in this section. There may be different emphasis for either condition, but as the history of the last 20 years has borne out, the development of new drugs for both conditions has evolved in a similar pathway although the primary therapeutic endpoints for these two airway conditions may be considered different. However, while so far the existing therapies for these two conditions are similar and have a broad-spectrum effect, there are bound to be specific therapies emerging for either condition.

A. Asthma

New treatments are also important to have for the general population of asthma for the following reasons. First, although under trial conditions, combination therapy of long-acting β-agonists (LABAs) and inhaled corticosteroids (ICSs) has been shown to be most effective for the treatment of asthma, when used in the real-world setting, the efficacy of these drugs may not be as good as seen under the trial conditions. Recent surveys of the impact of asthma done worldwide indicate that there is still a lot of morbidity of asthma even in countries where there are excellent healthcare systems with easy access to therapies (1). While there may be many reasons underlying the continuing morbidity (and mortality of asthma) such as the problem of adherence to treatments, proper assessment of asthma control, etc., one particular reason is that in terms of response to treatment to ICS, a sizable proportion of patients do not respond (2). Another reason revolves around the fact that these treatments are not curative or do not induce remission of disease, and need to be taken regularly to be effective. This combined with the fear of steroid side effects does not encourage patient adherence.

Current treatments have been established for asthma, and there is general agreement regarding the treatment of mild persistent and moderate persistent asthma, which is backed by double-blind controlled trials (3). Thus, low-dose ICS therapy remains the long-term treatment of choice for mild persistent asthma, in preference to leukotriene receptor antagonists, a class of anti-asthma medications introduced in the last 15 years. The main issue is that of compliance to ICS therapy by patients with mild asthma who may not feel the need for using sustained therapy. It has been suggested that treatment with as-needed short-acting β-agonists and with intermittent courses of oral prednisolone for exacerbations or as-needed treatment with a combined short-acting β-agonist and low-dose ICS may be all that is needed (4). These potential new approaches for treating mild persistent asthma need to be investigated further.

The advantages of treating moderate-to-severe persistent asthma with the addition of a LABA to low-to-medium dose of ICS have now been demonstrated in many controlled studies; these include a better control of asthma with a significant reduction in the rate of exacerbations compared with a greater dose of the ICS (5–7). Other agents such as leukotriene receptor antagonist (LTRA) and theophylline may be considered as partners for ICS for this category of asthma (8), but possibly less effective than LABA as a partner with ICS (9). More recent evidence has indicated that asthma control may be improved by using combined LABA and ICS (formoterol and budesonide) as maintenance therapy and as as-needed therapy, and this has provided another approach.

At the more severe end of the disease are patients with severe or therapy-resistant asthma, in whom asthma control remains poor despite documentation of adherence to high-dose ICSs and often the regular use of oral corticosteroids (10,11). Such patients often demonstrate evidence of persistent airflow obstruction, experience regular exacerbations, and are less responsive to the therapeutic effects of corticosteroids. They are also usually established on other asthma medications such as LABA, LTRA, and theophylline, and despite being insensitive to effects of corticosteroids, they may develop corticosteroid side effects. Therefore, this category of patients, indicated by the step 5 level of the GINA guidelines (12), is in need of novel therapies to control their asthma. One new class of asthma therapy, the humanized anti-immunoglobulin E (anti-IgE) monoclonal antibody, omalizumab, is now available for treating severe allergic asthma (see chap. 9). However, the fact that this treatment is not efficacious in all patients, the search for more effective drugs continues. It is likely that this category of patients with asthma will be the target of new potential therapies, and since these patients form only 5% to 10% of the general asthma population, such studies would be performed in specialized centers where they can be recruited for trial studies. Severe asthma patients may offer distinct targets for drug therapy (e.g., to overcome steroid insensitivity), while representing a heterogeneous group of mechanisms underlying the loss of control. The specific study of severe asthma as compared with nonsevere asthma could provide useful insights into potential targets of specific subgroups.

B. COPD

For COPD, the degree of reversibility of changes in lung function and airway inflammation is limited with the current therapies that comprise combination therapy with ICSs and LABAs, and long-acting anticholinergics, which is not dissimilar to the pharmacological approach to treating moderate-to-severe persistent asthma. The recent studies such as TORCH and UPLIFT have provided a better idea of the overall benefits of these treatments in COPD because of the large adequate cohort sizes of these studies (13,14). In the TORCH study, LABA and high-dose ICS were significantly effective on their own and also when administered together in reducing the yearly decline in forced expiratory volume in one second (FEV_1); however, the combination was more effective than the ICS treatment alone in improving postbronchodilator FEV_1, quality-of-life measures, and rates of exacerbations. For the first time in a COPD trial, the primary endpoint was to examine the effect on mortality, and the combination of ICS and LABA reduced all-cause mortality by 17.5% compared with placebo at $p = 0.052$. However, there was a significant increase in the probability of having pneumonia reported as an adverse event being higher in patients treated with fluticasone or salmeterol and fluticasone compared with placebo. The UPLIFT study examined the effect of tiotropium and reported no effect on the rate of decline in FEV_1 in a cohort in whom ~60% were taking ICS and LABAs. However, there was a significant bronchodilator effect with a reduction in the risk of exacerbations, related hospitalizations, and respiratory failure (14). These studies therefore indicate that a combination of LABA, and long-acting muscarinic antagonists (LAMA) with ICS would be of interest. Indeed, a randomized double-blind placebo-controlled study in Canada showed that the addition of fluticasone and salmeterol to tiotropium therapy improved lung function, quality-of-life measures, and hospital rates in moderate-to-severe COPD, in comparison to tiotropium alone and tiotropium and salmeterol (15). However, there was no effect on rates of COPD exacerbations, a result likely to be confounded by the high discontinuation rates in the tiotropium alone and in the tiotropium plus salmeterol groups.

Progress in this field will be represented by the availability of the 24-hour LABAs, which when combined with a long-acting ICS would provide a truly once-daily combined treatment. The addition of a 24-hour LAMA to the combination may provide further additive benefit.

Other therapies that have been studied in clinical trials include *N*-acetylcysteine that has been considered to have mucolytic properties and more recently antioxidant effects (16). Results of several meta-analyses indicate that *N*-acetylcysteine reduces exacerbations by 22% to 29% in patients described as suffering from chronic bronchitis (17–20). In a randomized controlled trial involving 523 patients, no effect on yearly decline in FEV_1 or in exacerbation rates was found with treatment with *N*-acetylcysteine at the dose of 600 mg/day (21). The related compound carbocisteine has been shown on the other hand to prevent exacerbations of COPD (22), perhaps a reflection of higher equivalent doses of this related compound. This is likely to support the use of effective antioxidants in the treatment of COPD (16).

New therapies based on more specific targets may provide better responses. However, one aspect that is pervasive in COPD and to a segment of the asthma population is the notion that there is a blunted response to existing therapies in particular corticosteroids. Therefore, one potential approach is to improve corticosteroid responsiveness (23) (see chap. 6). The pathogenesis of COPD is now considered to be very complex involving not only lung inflammation but also systemic inflammation, immune responses, and lung tissue repair and destruction (24), such that treatment paradigms may be more than just anti-inflammatories and bronchodilators.

II. Specific Treatments for Specific Subgroups of Airways Disease

There are good reasons to be searching for new treatments, and these two different diseases need different types of new treatments. Those with severe asthma may need specific anti-inflammatory agents that could target specific pathways. As new treatments are going to be likely focused on the more severe end of disease, it is likely that they will be added to maintenance treatments of combination therapy. But will these new treatments be applied to all patients with one disease severity category? There is now some evidences emerging that inflammatory characteristics may determine responsiveness to treatments. One recent example is the difference reported between asthma characterized by a neutrophilic inflammation versus an eosinophilic inflammation, and the potential effectiveness of macrolide treatment in neutrophilic asthma (25). There is some evidences that the presence of sputum eosinophilia in COPD may predict a good response to corticosteroid therapy (26,27), and that the presence of neutrophilic inflammation in sputum or in the airways submucosa may be an indication of severe asthma (28,29). The validity of such sub-phenotypes of disease based on the type of inflammatory response remains to be determined but any therapeutic responses observed in clinical trials of new therapies could indicate whether there are subgroups of patients that respond better or worse to new medications.

III. Improvements in ICS

Currently available combination of ICS and LABAs are usually used on a twice-daily basis, although for mild disease a once-daily use may be sufficient. The development of LABAs that have a once-daily usage and of more potent ICS may pave the way for a once-daily combination therapy for the treatment of asthma of a whole range of severity. More potent ICS may be developed by finding molecules that have even higher affinity for the glucocorticoid receptor with a greater retention in lung tissue such as the development of fluticasone furoate (30). A once-daily ICS or a combination of ICS and LABA may lead to improved patient compliance but it would remain to be seen whether this could also be used as rescue medication in the same way as the combination of formoterol and budesonide, a twice-daily preparation, can be used.

Another way of increasing potency of ICS would be to adapt the side chains of current ICS. For example, the addition of an NO-donating group to prednisolone (compound NCX1015) or budesonide (compound NCX1020) has resulted in improved corticosteroid efficacy compared with the parent compounds in animal models resulting from the donation of the nitric oxide moiety to specific residues within the gluco-corticoid receptor ligand-binding domain (31,32).

Increasing the potency of ICS may be accompanied with an increased risk of side effects (33) because of greater systemic side effects of the systemic absorbed portion from the lungs. Several approaches have been taken to reduce these problems including systemic or local inactivation or administration of an inactive prodrug that is only converted to active drug in the airways. Ciclesonide is such a recent example (34); it is esterified only in the lung to produce the active form des-ciclesonide. There is further scope in introducing even more potent ICS that works by this mechanism of local lung activation. Another approach is based on the concept of dissociated steroids or also called selective glucocorticoid receptor agonists (35). Many, but not all, of the side effects of corticosteroids are due to the DNA binding [glucocorticoid response element (GRE)] effects of the drugs whereas the anti-inflammatory effects may relate predom-inantly to targeting of proinflammatory transcription factors such as nuclear factor κB (NF-κB) and activator protein 1 (AP-1) (36–38). The development of dissociated cor-ticosteroids that can interact with NF-κB, but not with GREs, thereby preserving ther-apeutic anti-inflammatory effects with reduced side effect profiles, has been undertaken by many companies (33). These dissociated corticosteroids may be just as effective as conventional ICS, but may have a better safety profile (35). One of the problems with conventional corticosteroids is that the steroid backbone can also bind to other nuclear hormone receptors such as MR and PR, which also cause side effects. The development of dissociated corticosteroids with a nonsteroidal backbone such as AL-438 and ZK 216348 may further improve the therapeutic index as these drugs (35,39), and also extend their duration of action to a once-a-day therapy.

Other nuclear hormone receptors, for example, LXR, PPARγ, and RXR, have distinct anti-inflammatory patterns in murine macrophages (40), which may be complementary to that seen with corticosteroids. Combination of corticosteroids or possibly more promiscuous drugs that bind to two or more of these receptors may result in an enhanced anti-inflammatory profile than that seen with current corticosteroids particularly in patients with severe disease (41). Several key signaling pathways are involved in the inflammatory response (42,43) and also in the modulation of corticosteroid responsiveness in asthma and COPD (33,44–47). This raises the potential of novel combination therapies utilizing selective p38 mitogen-activated protein kinase (MAPK) or phosphoinositide-kinase 3 (PI3K) pathway inhibitors, which may reverse corticosteroid insensitivity, and new corticosteroids, which reduce the dose of each component necessary to produce a clinically effective response. One could therefore foresee the development of multicombination therapies involving corticosteroids, bronchodilators, pathway inhibitors, and other nuclear hormone receptor ligands as seen in other therapeutic areas such as rheumatoid arthritis (48).

IV. Development of New Anti-inflammatories

The past 10 years has seen the introduction of two new different classes of therapies for asthma, derived from a study of the generation of mediators in asthma. The leukotriene inhibitors introduced in clinical practice in the last 15 years are mainly classed as leukotriene receptor antagonists and 5-lipoxygenase inhibitors, which have found a niche in the treatment of mild-to-moderate asthma (discussed in chap. 8), while the more recently introduced anti-IgE antibody, representing the first treatment using monoclonal antibody approach, is used to treat more severe asthma with an allergic background. Amid these advances, there has also been many failures of anti-inflammatory or antimediator approaches that include small-molecule antagonist at receptors of specific mediators such as platelet-activating factor receptor antagonists, bradykinin receptor antagonists, and tachykinin receptor antagonists. The failure of these compounds is likely to be an attestation of the lack of importance of these mediators or their redundancy in asthma pathophysiology. Other targets have come into existence with increasing understanding of their potential role in asthma (Fig. 1 and Table 1). Current development of new drugs is now focusing particularly on the inhibition of specific cytokines such as those of Th2-cytokines and chemokines through the use of blocking monoclonal antibodies, or the soluble receptors, or through small-molecule receptor blockers, or at the level of their intracellular signaling (33). Other approaches may be considered more broad-based in inhibiting several pathways rather than a single discrete entity such as inhibitors of enzymes including kinases, esterases, particularly illustrated by the development of small-molecule kinase inhibitors such as inhibitors of the p38 MAPK or PI3K, inhibitors of transcription factors, or activation of endogenous anti-inflammatory pathways (49). Antioxidants are other classes of anti-inflammatories that are particularly being considered particularly for COPD, but there has been not sufficiently potent antioxidant for clinical use (16). Immunomodulation and antiallergic approaches are discussed in chapter 9.

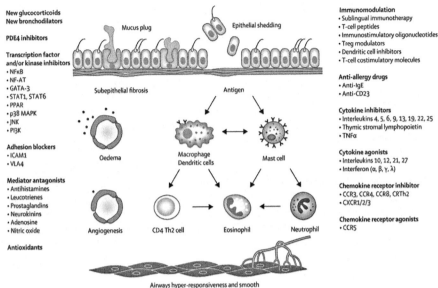

Figure 1 Classes of potential new drugs developed for asthma. Figure shows some of the important inflammatory and structural cells involved in the pathogenesis of asthma. *Source*: From Ref. 33.

For both asthma and COPD, the concept of corticosteroid insensitivity is an important one and development of agents to reverse corticosteroid insensitivity is a very reasonable approach, and to demonstrate such an effect of new agents, specific protocols need to be devised. Theophylline, a medication already in use for asthma and COPD as a bronchodilator, has been shown to reverse corticosteroid resistance in COPD in macrophages through increasing recruitment of histone deacetylase 2 enzyme activity (50), but there has been no clinical trial demonstrating this effect in COPD or in severe asthma. Other mechanisms demonstrated in vitro include activation of p38 MAPK or of c-jun N-terminal kinase (JNK) or of PI3K (37). Reversal of corticosteroid insensitivity should be part of the assessment of new anti-inflammatory agents.

Many of the targets have either not reached the clinical trial stage yet, or there is no information as yet in the public domain (33,51). These potential targets are listed in Figure 1 and Table 1. The rest of the chapter will concentrate on those new agents that have been tried in clinical trials and results publicly reported.

V. Targeting Cytokines and Chemokines

Because cytokines and chemokines are involved in multiple aspects of the inflammatory process of asthma and COPD, they are potentially therapeutic targets (52,53). There has already been some experience of the therapeutic effects of targeting specific cytokines in asthma that will be summarized. One potential drawback for considering these as targets

Table 1 Function of Various Targets, and Drugs Being Developed for These Targets

	Function	Drug development
β₂-Adrenergic receptor	Ultra-long bronchodilation	Indacaterol (phase II), carmoterol (phase II), GSK159797 (phase II)
Glucocorticoid receptor	Anti-inflammatory	GSK685689 (phase II), GSK870086 (phase II), AL-438 (phase I), ZK 216348 (phase I)
PGD2/CRTh2 inhibitors	Th2 cell recruitment and activation	TM30089, ODC9101 (phase II), AZD1981 (phase II), ramatroban (phase II)
BLT1 antagonist	Mononuclear/granulocyte recruitment	CP-105696 (phase I), LY293111 (phase II, no effect against allergen challenge)
CCL11	Blocks eosinophil recruitment/activation	CAT-213 (preclinical)
CCR3	Blocks eosinophil recruitment/activation	Met-RANTES (phase II, moderate/severe asthma)
CXCR4	Blocks Th2 activation	AMD070, AMD3100, SP01A (all preclinical for asthma, all phase II HIV, AMD3100 phase III for multiple myeloma)
CXCR1/2	Blocks neutrophil recruitment/activation	Repertaxin (preclinical, phase II for graft vs. host disease)
Interleukin 5	Blocks eosinophil recruitment/activation	MEDI-563 (phase I, severe asthma), mepolizumab (phase II)
Interleukin 12	–	Interleukin 12 (phase II, no effect on lung function, adverse side effects, not developed further)
Interleukin 10	Endogenous anti-inflammatory agent	Interleukin 10 (preclinical for asthma, approved for psoriasis/Crohn's disease, recruited in 1999 for asthma)
Interferon γ	–	Interferon γ (phase II, no effect on lung function in severe asthma, not developed further)
Interleukin 13	Key driver of asthmatic inflammation	Pitrakinra (interleukin-4/13 mutein), CAT-354, IMA-638 (both in phase II)
VLA4 antagonist	Adhesion molecule blocker	GW-559090, IVL745, CDP323 (CDP323 phase II, not developed)
PDE4	Anti-inflammatory	GSK256066 (phase II)
p38 MAPK	Anti-inflammatory	GSK681323, GSK856553, VX-745, BIRB-796, Ro-320-1195, Scio-469 (all in phase II), SB2439063, RWJ-67657
JNK	Anti-inflammatory	SP600125, CC-401, CNI-1493 (dual JNK/p38 MAPK) (all in preclinical for asthma; CC-401 and CNI-1493 in phase II in rheumatoid arthritis and Crohn's disease)
SYK	Mast cell degranulation, T-cell and B-cell function	Antisense (preclinical), BAY61-3606 (preclinical), R343 (phase I)
IKK2	Anti-inflammatory	AS206868, SC-514, BMS345541, TPCA-1 (all preclinical, MLN0415 [phase I])
CD23	Reduces IgE	Lumiliximab (phase I)
Sphingosine-1 phosphate receptor	Prevents dendritic cell activity	FTY720 (preclinical for asthma, phase II for multiple sclerosis and transplant rejection)
DP1	Prevents dendritic cell activity	BW245C (preclinical)

Abbreviations: JNK, c-jun N-terminal kinase; MAPK, mitogen-activated protein kinase; IgE, immunoglobulin E.
Source: From Ref. 33.

is the wide pleiotropy and element of redundancy in the cytokine family, in that each cytokine has many overlapping functions, with each function potentially mediated by more than one cytokine. Blocking antibodies, soluble receptors, or receptor antagonists have been used to block the effects of a particular cytokine. In cases of anti-inflammatory cytokines, the cytokine itself may be used. More recent general inhibitory approaches include the inhibition of specific signal transduction pathways that are either involved in the generation of many types of cytokines or in the downstream action of many cytokines, such as signaling through kinases.

A. Anti-IL5 Antibody

Two humanized anti-human IL-5 monoclonal antibodies, Sch-55700 and mepolizumab (SB-240563), have been studied in patients with asthma. The effect of mepolizumab was examined against allergen challenge in a double-blind randomized placebo-controlled trial, when a single intravenous infusion of SB-240563 was given at doses of 2.5 mg/kg ($n = 8$) or 10.0 mg/kg ($n = 8$) (54). An immediate fall in circulating eosinophil counts occurred, maximal at 10 mg/kg, and persists for up to three months. After inhaled allergen challenge, nine days after treatment with mepolizumab, sputum eosinophils fell from 12.2% in the placebo group to 0.9% (-1.2 to 3.0; $p = 0.0076$) in the 10 mg/kg mepolizumab-treated group, an effect that persisted at day 30 after the dose. However, the physiological response to allergen, namely, the late asthmatic response or airway hyperresponsiveness (AHR), was unaffected.

In 24 patients with mild asthma receiving three intravenous doses of either 750 mg of mepolizumab or placebo in a randomized, double-blind, parallel-group fashion over 20 weeks, a persistent suppression of blood eosinophils and a greater than 90% reduction in bronchoalveolar lavage (BAL) eosinophilia were observed after mepolizumab, but it decreased mucosal eosinophils in the airways by only 55% (55); there were no effects on bronchial hyperresponsiveness or FEV_1, although the groups studied were small. In another study, mepolizumab has been shown to decrease mature eosinophil numbers in the bone marrow by 70% in comparison with placebo and decreased numbers of eosinophil myelocytes and metamyelocytes by 37% and 44%, respectively (56). However, mepolizumab had no effect on numbers of blood or bone marrow $CD34^+$, $CD34^+$/ $IL-5R\alpha^+$ cells, or eosinophil/basophil colony-forming units. There was a significant decrease in bronchial mucosal $CD34^+$/$IL-5R\alpha^+$ mRNA-positive cell numbers in the anti-IL-5 treated group. These studies indicated that at the doses of mepolizumab used, there was only partial depletion of eosinophils in the airway tissues and of eosinophil progenitors in the bone marrow and in the airway tissues. This raised the possibility that the dose administered was not sufficient, or else IL-5 may not be the only cytokine important in eosinophil recruitment or in eosinophil maturation. Cooperation between IL-5 and eotaxin in these aspects has been previously shown in murine models (57), and therefore blocking the effects of IL-5 and eotaxin simultaneously could be important.

The lack of clinical response observed in the initial studies with mepolizumab was reflected also in clinical studies with anti-IL5 antibody. In a phase II double-blind placebo-controlled study of 362 moderately severe symptomatic patients experiencing persistent symptoms despite ICS therapy, mepolizumab (250 or 750 mg IV) was administered monthly for three months (58). Mepolizumab caused a significant reduction in blood and sputum eosinophils in both treatment groups but there were no

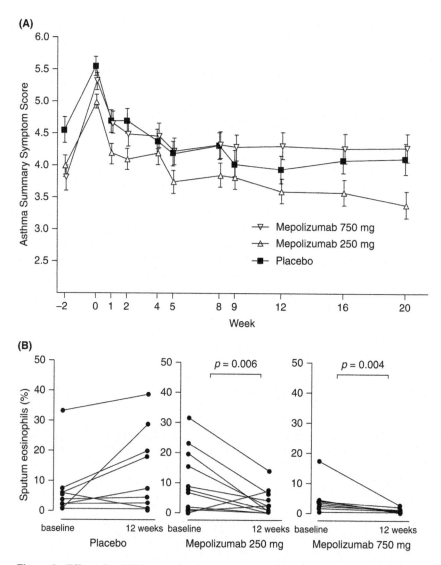

Figure 2 Effect of anti-IL5 monoclonal antibody, mepolizumab, on asthma symptoms. (**A**) No effect of antibody treatment (250 or 750 mg) on asthma symptoms over the 20-week period of observation. (**B**): Inhibition of sputum eosinophils in mepolizumab-treated patients. *Source*: From Ref. 58.

significant changes in clinical endpoints, such as peak expiratory flow, FEV_1, daily β-agonist use, and symptom scores (Fig. 2). There was a nonsignificant decrease in exacerbation rates in the high-dose mepolizumab-treated group.

In a group of patients with severe persistent asthma on oral or high doses of ICSs, the humanized anti-IL5 antibody, Sch-55700, administered as a single dose (0.03, 0.1, 0.3, or

1.0 mg/kg subcutaneously) dose-dependently reduced blood eosinophil counts. A trend toward improvement in baseline FEV_1 was noted and reached significance 24 hours after the 0.3-mg/kg dose, but with no changes in other parameters of asthma activity (59).

Finally, one study with mepolizumab indicated that this compound may have beneficial effects in reversing some of the features of airway wall remodeling (60). In a randomized, double-blind, placebo-controlled study, bronchial biopsies were obtained before and after three infusions of mepolizumab in 24 atopic asthmatics. The anti-IL-5 antibody, which specifically decreased airway eosinophil numbers, significantly reduced the expression of tenascin, lumican, and procollagen III in the bronchial mucosal reticular basement membrane when compared with placebo. Anti-IL-5 treatment was associated with a significant reduction in the numbers and percentage of airway eosinophils expressing mRNA for TGF-β1 and the concentration of TGF-β1 in BAL fluid. This study indicated that eosinophils may be important effectors of extracellular matrix deposition, perhaps through the production of TGFβ.

In a study of patients with the hypereosinophilic syndrome (without asthma) requiring 20 to 60 mg prednisolone/day to maintain clinical status and blood eosinophil count $<1000/\mu$L, mepolizumab significantly reduced the maintenance dose of prednisolone, demonstrating corticosteroid-sparing effects. Therefore, it may particularly help patients with asthma who have an eosinophil predominant disease with high levels of circulating eosinophil counts (61). In patients with hypereosinophilic syndrome, mepolizumab caused a reduction in eosinophil counts and in the percentage of CCR3+ cells (62).

In these studies in asthma patients with either Sch-55700 or mepolizumab, no serious adverse events were observed, in particular the potential problem of antibody generation or anaphylaxis.

It is possible that the asthma patients that were chosen for study were not those who would respond to anti-IL-5 approach. Several studies are recruiting asthma patients with sputum eosinophilia and high circulating eosinophil counts for their studies. Such approach is of interest since high sputum eosinophil counts have been associated with loss of control of asthma (63). A recent study showed that mepolizumab therapy reduced exacerbations and improved quality of life scores in asthmatics with refractory eosinophilic asthma without improving symptoms, lung function (FEV_1) or airway hyperresponsiveness (64).

B. Soluble IL-4 Receptor

IL-4 and IL-13 share the α-chain of the IL-4 receptor (IL-4Rα). The IL-4R is a cell surface heterodimeric complex consisting of a specific, high-affinity α-chain and a second chain that could be either the common β-chain or the γ-chain of the IL-13 receptor. IL-4 binds to IL-4Rα alone, but both chains are necessary for cellular activation. On engagement of the ligand with IL-4Rα, signal transducer and activator of transcription 6 (STAT6) translocates to the nucleus and germline ε mRNA transcription is initiated together with class-switching of immunoglobulin genes. Secreted forms of IL-4Rα occur naturally, and soluble IL-4R can bind to IL-4, without leading to cellular activation. Therefore, soluble IL-4R can bind and sequester IL-4, and therefore acts as an antagonist for IL-4. Soluble recombinant human IL-4 receptor (Nuvance) is the extracellular portion of human IL-4Rα and is nonimmunogenic.

In the first study of Nuvance, mild or moderate asthmatics were withdrawn from ICS therapy and received either placebo or rhuIL-4R (0.5 or 1.5 mg by nebulizer) (65).

No adverse events were observed and no patients developed any antibodies. The serum half-life was approximately five days. Two out of eight patients in the placebo group and three out of eight in the rhuIL-4R 0.5-mg group had exacerbations, while none of the patients in the rhuIL-4R 1.5-mg group experienced exacerbations. The latter group also demonstrated an improvement in FEV_1 at two hours, and on days 2, 4, and 15 after treatment, with improved symptom scores and reduction in β_2-agonist use. Improvement was also reflected in the improved scores on the asthma quality-of-life questionnaire in the rhuIL-4R 1.5-mg group, while these scores worsened in the placebo-treated group. An anti-inflammatory effect was supported by the reduction in exhaled nitric oxide levels in the patients receiving rhuIL-4R.

In the second phase I/II double-blind, placebo-controlled study, 62 moderate persistent asthmatics were randomized to receive 12 weekly nebulizations of 0.75, 1.5, or 3.0 mg of rhuIL4R or placebo (66); inhaled steroids were discontinued. A significant decline in FEV_1 and an increase in symptom score were observed in the placebo group, but this was not seen in the 3.0-mg treatment group. Although these results were promising, further development of Nuvance as a therapy for asthma was suspended because the clinical response observed was sufficiently important.

C. Inhibition of IL-13

The extensive properties of IL-13 in regulating IgE production, eosinophilic inflammation, airway smooth muscle hyperplasia, and induction of goblet cell hyperplasia with mucus production make it an interesting mediator in asthma (67). Acute administration of IL-13 into naïve mice reproduces many features of asthma such as AHR, eosinophilic inflammation, and mucus cell hyperplasia (68,69). Targeted overexpression of IL-13 also reproduces these features, in addition to subepithelial fibrosis and the presence of Charcot-Leyden particles (70). Specific blockade of IL-13 was achieved in the mouse by using a soluble form of the IL-13Rα2 chain, which binds only to IL-13 but not to IL-4, and this led to the reversal of AHR and mucus production in the allergen-exposed sensitized mouse (68). IL-13 facilitates the recruitment of eosinophils, monocytes/macrophages, and T cells into the airway spaces through the induction of vascular cell adhesion molecule 1 (71), and can also cause the upregulation of many chemokines such as MCP-1, MCP-3, eotaxin, and MIP-1α (72). IL-13 can also induce and activate TGFβ, thus contributing to subepithelial fibrosis (73). IL-13 may induce proliferation of airway smooth muscle cells indirectly via LTD4 receptors (74) and can directly induce increased intracellular calcium fluxes in isolated smooth muscle strips induced by histamine, bradykinin, and acetylcholine, and increased contractile responses to carbachol (75).

IL-13 binds to a low-affinity binding chain, IL-13Rα1, and a high-affinity complex made up of IL-13Rα1 and IL-4R. Binding to the latter complex leads to phosphorylation-dependent activation of JAK1 and JAK2 and STAT6 proteins. IL-13, and not IL-4, binds also to another receptor IL-13Rα2 that may inhibit the activity of IL-13, therefore not contributing to IL-13 signaling. Antagonizing IL-13 may be achieved by administering soluble IL-13 receptors (as for IL-4 targeting), anti-IL-13 monoclonal antibodies, and antireceptor antibodies. sIL-13R has an extended half-life and high-affinity binding to IL-13 using a fully humanized peptide. These agents are currently undergoing clinical trials in asthma.

Inhibition of both IL-4 and IL-13 has been achieved by an interleukin-4 variant that potently inhibits the binding of IL-4 and IL-13 to the interleukin-4Ra receptor complexes. Pitrakinra was studied in two randomized double-blind placebo-controlled parallel-group phase 2a studies (76). In one study, pitrakinra was administered subcutaneously once daily (1.25 mg), and in a second study, by nebulization twice daily (2.6 mg). Pitrakinra inhibited significantly the late-phase response to allergen with minimal effect on the early-phase response in the second study but not in the first study. Therefore, topical administration was found to be more efficient against late-phase than subcutaneous administration at the doses used. There were no significant effects of pitrakinra on AHR associated with allergen challenge, but this could have been due to a type-1 error. Pitrakinra is now undergoing a phase II study.

Anti-IL-13 antibodies have also been developed and are undergoing clinical trials.

D. Inhibition of Eotaxin

Eotaxin is a chemokine with selective actions on eosinophils (77). The importance of eotaxin in allergic eosinophilic inflammation has been underlined in models using CCR3 knockout mice (78,79). Eotaxin selectively mediates its effects through the CCR3 receptor, and allergen-sensitized CCR3 knockout mice were protected against allergen challenge induced AHR. This was accompanied by a reduction in CCR3 positive cells in the lungs, usually eosinophils and epithelial mast cells. The CCR3 receptor is a member of the G protein–coupled receptor superfamily, and both peptide-derived and small-molecule CCR3 antagonists have been developed (80). A novel way of measuring the activity of these antagonists in whole blood using white blood cell shape change and chemokine receptor internalization can be used to assess the activity of these molecules in vivo (81).

Small-molecule inhibitors of CCR3 have been effective in inhibiting eosinophilic inflammation, AHR, and goblet cell hyperplasia in the ovalbumin mouse model (82,83). In asthmatics, antisense oligonucleotides that inhibit CCR3 led to a reduction in sputum eosinophilia following allergen challenge associated with inhibition of the early response but only a trend for a reduced late response (84). CCR3 receptor antagonists are undergoing clinical trials, but there are no results published (85,86).

E. Inhibition of TNFα

Inhibition of tumor necrosis factor (TNF)α either by using monoclonal antibodies, anti-TNFα, or recombinant soluble TNF receptors has been successful in modifying the activity of rheumatoid arthritis. TNFα may be involved in asthma (87) and COPD. TNFα stored in granules of mast cells can be released through IgE-mediated mechanisms (88), and other cellular sources include epithelial cells, eosinophils, macrophages, neutrophils, and T cells. An excess expression of TNFα mRNA in asthmatic airways has been demonstrated (89), and following allergen challenge, TNFα levels in BAL fluid of asthmatic subjects is increased. In severe asthma, TNFα levels in BAL fluid were increased compared with mild asthmatics, together with an increase in TNFα-positive cells in the airway submucosa (90). Patients with refractory asthma have an increased expression of membrane-bound TNF-α, TNF-α receptor 1, and TNF-α-converting enzyme in peripheral-blood monocytes (91).

TNFα has been implicated in facilitating the migration of eosinophils and neutrophils since it can upregulate the expression of adhesion molecules and can induce the release of chemotactic factors such as chemokines from a variety of cells including airway epithelium, macrophages, vascular endothelium, and muscle cells. In addition,

TNFα can modulate the levels of various proteolytic enzymes such as MMP-9 and extracellular matrix proteins such as tenascin and collagen; TNFα may also induce the proliferation and activation of subepithelial myofibroblasts and fibroblasts. These properties place TNFα as being important for airway wall remodeling. TNFα can also induce goblet cell hyperplasia in the mouse through the expression of gob-5 and MUC-5AC (92), in addition to its direct mucus secretagogue role. TNFα has direct effects on airway smooth muscle cells such as enhancing calcium signaling pathways leading to hypercontractility (93). TNFα increases maximal isotonic contraction to methacholine in guinea-pig tracheal preparations (94). In an allergen exposure model, a TNF receptor fusion protein that blocked the effects of TNFα prevented allergen-induced BHR in sensitized guinea-pigs (95). Direct administration of TNFα induces BHR in sensitized rats (96). Similarly, healthy volunteers or asthmatics develop BHR when inhaling rh-TNFα (97). TNFα has been implicated in inducing muscle loss in the cachexia often seen in COPD.

Therapeutic blockade of TNFα has been successful in the treatment of severe refractory rheumatoid arthritis, and there are several clinically available TNFα blockers. These are infliximab, a chimeric mouse/human monoclonal anti-TNFα antibody, etanercept, a soluble fusion protein made of TNF-receptor with an Fc fragment of human IgG1, and adalimumab, a human monoclonal anti-TNFα antibody. The major side effects of TNFα blockade have been reactivation of tuberculosis, demyelination, and an increased risk of lymphoma and cancers.

In an open uncontrolled study, 17 patients with corticosteroid-dependent asthma were treated with etanercept 25 mg twice daily for 12 weeks. At the end of 12 weeks, there was a significant improvement in symptom scores, a 12% improvement in FEV_1 and bronchial responsiveness improved by 2.5 doubling doses (90). In a clinical trial of 10 patients with refractory asthma, 10 patients with mild-to-moderate asthma, and 10 control subjects, treatment with a soluble TNF receptor, etanercept, for 10 weeks was associated with a significant increase in PC_{20}, an improvement in the asthma-related quality-of-life score, and a 0.32-L increase in postbronchodilator FEV_1 (91). These results are in sharp contrast to those of a similar study performed with a similar design using etanercept at the higher dose of 50 mg/wk for 12 weeks in corticosteroid-dependent asthmatics: a small but significant reduction in asthma control questionnaire score was reported but no improvements in asthma-related quality-of-life (AQLQ), lung function, bronchial hyperresponsiveness, or exacerbation rates, despite a reduction in sputum macrophages, serum CRP, and increases in serum TNFα (98).

A more recent randomized double-blind placebo-controlled parallel-group trial of etanercept in 39 patients with severe corticosteroid refractory asthma showed a small significant reduction in Asthma Control questionnaire scores but without any significant improvement in AQLQ scores, lung function, peak expiratory flow rates, bronchial hyperresponsiveness, or exacerbation rates (93). Inflammatory markers such as sputum serum C-reactive protein and macrophages were reduced.

Using a monoclonal antibody to TNF-α, infliximab (5 mg/kg) given intravenously at weeks 0, 2, and 6 in 38 patients with moderate asthma treated with ICS, Erin et al. showed that infliximab had no significant effect on changes in morning peak expiratory flow but decreased mean diurnal variation of peak expiratory flow at week 8 (99) (Fig. 3). There was a decrease in the number of patients with exacerbations of asthma. Infliximab decreased the levels of TNFα and other cytokines in sputum supernatants.

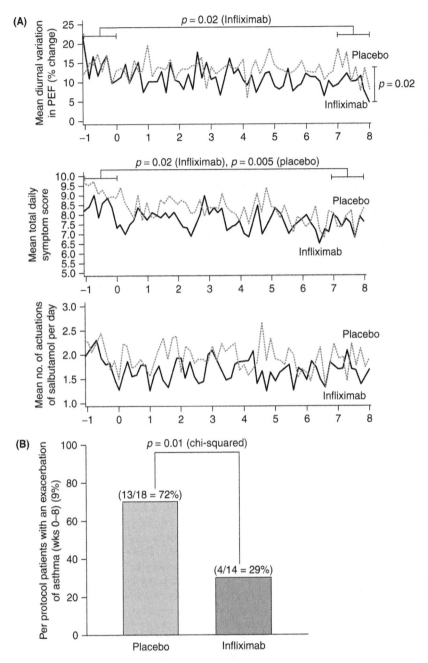

Figure 3 Effect of anti-TNFα monoclonal antibody, infliximab, in symptomatic asthma. **(A)** Electronic diary lung function, symptom score, and β_2-agonist use are shown over the eight-week period of treatment. Infliximab-treatment caused an improvement in mean diurnal variation in peak expiratory flows and in mean total daily symptom score. **(B)** Incidence of exacerbations of asthma during treatment period, with a significant reduction in infliximab-treated group. *Source*: From Ref. 99.

Finally, the largest study so far in this field has been the recently completed study with golimumab, a human monoclonal antibody to TNFα, involving uncontrolled, severe persistent asthmatic patients, which showed no beneficial clinical outcomes (100). Thus, golimumab did not improve FEV_1 or reduced the number of severe exacerbations. Importantly, up to 19.5% of patients treated with golimumab discontinued therapy because of serious adverse events with serious infections being the more frequent side effects. Also, one death and eight malignancies occurred in the golimumab-treated group. Overall, the more recent studies using TNFα approach in asthma have not confirmed the encouraging responses in initial studies.

COPD

In a multicenter, randomized, double-blind, placebo-controlled, parallel-group study, patients with moderate-to-severe COPD received infliximab (3 mg/kg or 5 mg/kg) or placebo at weeks 0, 2, 6, 12, 18, and 24 (101). Those treated with infliximab showed no treatment benefit as measured by chronic respiratory questionnaire total score and by secondary measures, including prebronchodilator FEV_1, six-minute walk distance, SF-36 physical score, transition dyspnea index (TDI), or moderate-to-severe COPD exacerbations. Post hoc analysis revealed that subjects who were younger or cachectic showed improvement in the 6-minute walk distance. Although the treatment was well-tolerated, malignancies were diagnosed during the study in 9 of 157 infliximab-treated subjects versus 1 of 77 placebo-treated subjects. The incidence of pneumonia was higher in infliximab-treated subjects but no infection-related mortality was observed.

The more recent results of the studies with TNF-α blocking approaches so far in asthma have been conflicting, and any beneficial effect would be small considering the potential serious side effects reported particularly the excess malignancies in COPD patients and the potential for reactivation of tuberculosis are worrying.

F. Inhibition of IL-8 in COPD

In a randomized, double-blind, parallel-group, placebo-controlled trial, three intravenous infusions of either human monoclonal antibody recognizing IL-8 or active buffer solution were administered monthly over a three-month period to patients with COPD (102). There was a significant improvement in the TDI total score between anti-IL-8 antibody and placebo at week 2 and months 1 to 3. At all time points, the proportion of patients achieving ≥ 1 point improvement in the TDI was greater for the monoclonal antibody group compared with the placebo group: 28% versus 11% at week 2 ($p = 0.028$). There were no significant differences observed for lung function, health status, 6-minute walking distance, and adverse events between groups. Thus, the anti-IL-8 antibody may provide some relief of dyspnea in COPD, but the basis for this observation remains unclear.

This approach has not been tried in asthma, although they could be considered in asthma associated with sputum neutrophilia. Receptor antagonists of the chemokine receptors, CXCR-1 and CXR-2, through which IL-8 mediates its effects, are under development for both asthma and COPD.

G. IL-12 Injections

In a small study, IL-12 subcutaneous injections in patients with mild asthma inhibited circulating blood eosinophils following allergen challenge but not sputum eosinophilia, but with no effect on late-phase response or bronchial hyperresponsiveness (103). The most notable feature of this study was the incidence of side effects with flu-like symptoms, abnormal liver function tests, and cardiac arrhythmias. This study illustrates the limitations of using anti-inflammatory cytokines as a form of therapy in asthma. Such therapies will require systemic administration, as aerosol administration may not allow for sufficient tissue penetration with tight epithelial airway and alveolar barriers to large molecules. In addition, systemic administration is associated with significant systemic side effects, as each specific cytokine usually possesses a plethora of effects.

H. IL-10 Injections

Administration of IL-10 to normal volunteers induced a fall in circulating CD2, CD3, CD4, and CD8 lymphocytes with a suppression of mitogen-induced T-cell proliferation and reduction of TNFα and IL-1β production from whole blood stimulated with endotoxin ex vivo (104). There have been no reports of IL-10 administration in asthma, although IL-10 therapy has been studied in rheumatoid arthritis, inflammatory bowel disease, and psoriasis (105). However, endogenous release of IL-10 can be achieved by boosting regulatory T cells using allergen-specific immunotherapy (106).

I. IFNγ Administration

IFNγ, a Th1 cytokine, may inhibit Th2-mediated allergic inflammation (107), but studies of administration of IFNγ to asthmatics have been disappointing (108,109). Daily subcutaneous injections of 0.05 mg/M2 of r-IFNγ in nine patients with steroid-dependent asthma for 90 days did not lead to any changes in the maintenance dose of prednisone or in lung function. There was a greater fall in blood eosinophil count after IFNγ, compared with the effect of placebo in a parallel group of patients, but this did not achieve statistical significance (109). In a later study, incremental doses of nebulized r-IFNγ were administered in five mild atopic asthmatics. No changes in symptoms or lung function or bronchial responsiveness were noted. In four of the five patients, there was a fall in eosinophil count measured in bronchoalveolar lavage fluid, but overall statistical significance was not achieved (108).

VI. PDE4 Inhibitors

The phosphodiesterases (PDEs) are a group of 11 families of metallophosphohydrolases that hydrolyses adenosine $3'5'$-cyclic AMP (cAMP) and guanosine $3'5'$-cyclic monophosphate (cGMP) to their inactive $5'$ monophosphates (110). cAMP and cGMP bind to specific intracellular regulatory proteins such as protein kinase A, cyclic nucleotide gated ion channels, and cAMP/cGMP stimulated guanyl triphosphatase exchange factors. Inhibition of cyclic nucleotide PDEs allows cAMP/cGMP to elevate within cells. Therefore, inhibition of PDE is a useful way of causing a variety of cellular effects and can influence inflammatory cell activation, immune cell activation, and smooth muscle contractile responses. The family of PDE4 enzymes is encoded by four distinct genes (PDE4A, PDE4B, PDE4C, PDE4D), and specifically hydrolyses cAMP. Each of the four PDE4 genes encodes splice variants that share similar highly conserved catalytic and C-terminal domains.

A. PDE4 Inhibitors and Anti-inflammatory Effects

PDE4 inhibitors have been developed for the treatment of asthma and COPD. Rolipram is a highly selective first generation PDE4 inhibitor that has been used to investigate the role of PDE4. Rolipram possesses anti-inflammatory and anti-immunomodulatory effects (111). It inhibits neutrophilic and eosinophilic inflammation, and the release of cytokines from activated T-helper (Th)-1 and Th-2 cells, and airway epithelial cells, basophils, and monocytes and macrophages. New second generation PDE4 inhibitors have now been developed with the hope of a wider therapeutic ratio, particularly with respect to nausea and vomiting. Roflumilast reduced accumulation of eosinophils and chronic inflammatory cells, subepithelial collagen, thickening of the airway epithelium, goblet cell hyperplasia and only slightly decreased AHR (112). Rolipram inhibits IL-5 production induced by antigen in an antigen-driven system of splenocytes from ovalbumin-sensitized mice (113). Cilomilast inhibits the release of TNFα from epithelial cells of patients with COPD (114). PDE4 inhibitors can also inhibit the release of proinflammatory cytokines such as TNFα (115). Incubation of whole blood or blood monocytes from healthy subjects or from COPD patients with cilomilast or rolipram inhibits the release of TNFα induced by lipopolysaccharide (116,117).

Cilomilast and rolipram inhibit fibroblast chemotaxis and fibroblast-mediated collagen contraction; cilomilast also inhibited TNF-α induced release of MMP-1 and MMP-9 from a fibroblast cell line (118,119). Roflumilast partially prevented the increase in BAL neutrophils after acute exposure of mice to cigarette smoke, the increase in lung macrophages partially, and airspace enlargement indicating protective effect against cigarette-induced emphysema (120). The mechanism of this effect on emphysema is unknown. PDE4 inhibitors may interfere with the process of airway wall remodeling.

Rolipram caused high levels of nausea and vomiting, and this side effect is an important cause for drug unacceptability among patients, particularly for a long-term medication. Inhibition of PDE4 at the low-affinity rolipram binding site may transduce anti-inflammatory effects while the high-affinity rolipram binding site may be related to emesis (116,121). Cilomilast and roflumilast have similar potency at both high-affinity and low-affinity rolipram binding sites, and have lesser degrees of nausea and vomiting, seemingly supporting the hypothesis initially set out. Another approach to improving the therapeutic ratio is to reduce penetration into the central nervous system or to deliver to the airways directly by aerosol.

B. PDE4 Inhibitors in Asthma

Roflumilast had a small inhibitory effect on the early response to allergen challenge in patients with mild-to-moderate asthma, and a bigger effect in inhibiting the late response at the dose of 500 μg daily given for 7 to 10 days prior to allergen challenge (122); a single dose of 1000 μg of roflumilast attenuated allergen-induced bronchial hyperrresponsiveness but had no effect on the early or late response (123). Both roflumilast and cilomilast attenuate exercise-induced bronchoconstriction (124).

Studies analyzed after 6 weeks and after 12 months of cilomilast treatment showed small improvements in FEV$_1$ in patients with asthma already on ICS therapy (125,126). After 6 weeks with 15 mg twice daily of cilomilast, there was a significant increase in FEV$_1$ of 0.21 L after 2 weeks when compared with placebo, but no significant improvements in FEV$_1$ were observed during the 12-month studies. Studies with roflumilast showed more convincing benefits, most likely related to their greater potency. In a three-month study of patients with asthma, there was a dose-dependent improvement in FEV_1 and mean morning peak flow rates, with a 16% improvement (400 mL) in FEV_1 at the 500 µg once-daily dose, which was greater than that produced by the 100 µg/day dose (11% increase; 260 mL) (127), and maintained over a 12-month treatment period. In a comparative study of 500 µg/day of roflumilast with inhaled beclomethasone propionate 200 µg twice daily over 12 weeks in 499 asthma patients, equivalent effects were observed in terms of improvement in FEV_1 (0.27 L for roflumilast and 0.32 L with beclomethasone), morning peak expiratory flows, reduction in asthma symptoms, and reduction in use of rescue medications (128).

C. PDE4 Inhibitors and COPD

In moderately severe COPD, cilomilast at 15 mg twice daily caused a significant increase in prebronchodilator and in postbronchodilator FEV_1 compared with placebo (0.16 L and 0.10 L, respectively) (126). Significant improvements in postbronchodilator forced vital capacity and peak expiratory flows were also observed. There were no significant differences in quality-of-life measures. In a six-month study, more positive effects were observed with cilomilast at 15 mg twice daily, with an improvement in FEV_1 by 0.08 L, a decrease in risk of exacerbations by 39%, and improvements in St Georges respiratory questionnaire of 4.1 units (129). A bronchial biopsy study showed that cilomilast 15 mg twice daily for 12 weeks reduced $CD8^+$ T cells, $CD-68^+$ macrophages, and also $CD4^+$ T cells and neutrophils. However, in induced sputum, there were no changes in neutrophils or macrophages, or levels of IL-8 or neutrophil elastase in supernatants (130). By contrast, roflumilast after four weeks reduced the number of eosinophils and neutrophils in sputum, and also reduced levels of IL-8, neutrophil elastase, ECP in sputum (131).

The experience with roflumilast is similar to that of cilomilast with small increases in FEV_1. In a six-month phase III multicenter double-blind randomized placebo-controlled study of 1411 patients with moderate COPD, postbronchodilator FEV_1 improved significantly with once daily 500 µg roflumilast by 0.097 L and 250 µg roflumilast by 0.074 L compared with placebo (132) (Fig. 4). There were significant reductions in the number of exacerbations of COPD per patient with a mean of 1.13 for placebo versus 1.03 for 250 µg roflumilast and 0.75 for 500 µg roflumilast. There were significant improvements in St Georges' respiratory questionnaire score of -3.5 units at the 500 µg/day dose and of -3.4 units at the 250 µg/day dose, but there were no significant differences at these two doses. By contrast, in a more severe group of COPD patients (GOLD stages III and IV), postbronchodilator FEV_1 increased by 39 mL compared with placebo, without effect on exacerbation rates or health status (133) (Fig. 4).

More recent studies with roflumilast have reported results in COPD patients already treated with long-acting bronchodilates Thus roflumilast was shown to improve mean prebronchodilator FEV_1 by 49 mL in patients treated with salmeterol, and 80 mL in those treated with tiotropium (134). The effect of roflumilast on exacerbations has also been reported in COPD patients with more severe airflow obstruction and a history of exacerbations. Roflumilast increased prebronchodilator FEV_1 by 48 ml and reduced moderate to severe exacerbations rates from 1.37 per patient per year to 1.14 (reduction of 17%; $p < 0.0003$) (135).

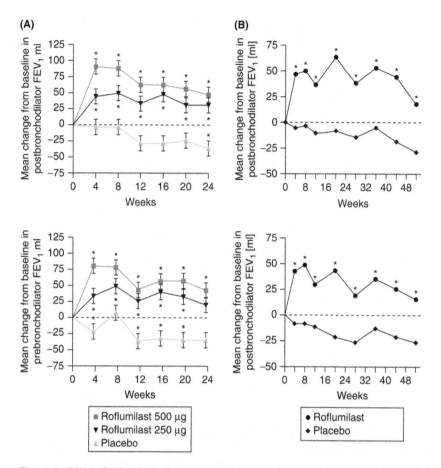

Figure 4 Effect of roflumilast on prebronchodilator and postbronchodilator FEV$_1$ in COPD in two separate studies: (**A**) Patients with moderate-to-severe COPD in response to 250- and 500-μg roflumilast/day; (**B**) Patients with severe COPD responding to 500-μg roflumilast/day. There was a sustained improvement in FEV$_1$ over the 24- and 52-week period of observation, respectively. SEM bars are shown in (A). *Abbreviations*: FEV$_1$, forced expiratory volume in one second; COPD, chronic obstructive pulmonary disease. *Source*: From Refs. 132 and 133.

VII.   Side effects

The most frequent side effect recorded in these studies is that of nausea. With cilomilast 15 mg twice daily over six months of treatment, diarrhea was reported as 12.7% versus 6.0% for placebo; nausea 12.5% versus 4.1%; these were described as mild-to-moderate and self-limiting (126). For roflumilast, the side effects appeared less frequent; over six-month period, with the 500 μg/day dose, nasopharyngitis was reported as 8% versus 7% for placebo; diarrhea was 9% versus 2%; and nausea was 5% versus 1% (132).

Currently, only roflumilast is undergoing phase III clinical trials. The problem of nausea and vomiting, and the low efficacy of the compound are issues that need to be resolved, and administration of these compounds by aerosol may be a way forward.

VIII. Bronchial Thermoplasty

Bronchial thermoplasty represents a new approach to the treatment of asthma (136). Although this does not represent an anti-inflammatory approach and although its efficacy has yet to be demonstrated, its approach designed to reduce the contractile ability of airway smooth muscle by directly reducing smooth muscle mass using the delivery of radiofrequency heat energy to the airway wall is unique. One would expect a decreased potential for bronchoconstriction and possibly decreased frequency and severity of asthma symptoms. In an open controlled study of bronchial thermoplasty in patients with moderate or severe persistent asthma, this treatment led to greater improvements in morning peak flows, asthma quality-of-life scores, the percentage of symptom-free days, and symptom scores (137). However, the results of double-blind, sham-controlled studies are currently awaited. Whether this procedure can also impact on airway inflammation is not known.

IX. Summary and Conclusions

There is a need for new treatments particularly with anti-inflammatory properties since not all patients with asthma respond adequately to current anti-asthma treatments, and the response of patients with advanced COPD to steroids and bronchodilators is less than adequate. More specific anti-inflammatory targets are provided by the range of cytokines and chemokines that may contribute to the chronic inflammatory processes in asthma and COPD. For asthma, the targeted inhibition of IL-4, IL-5, and IL-13 in asthma is currently being investigated, while the data with an anti-TNFα antibody in COPD has been negative. Similarly, anti-TNFα approaches although shown initially to be effective in small group of severe asthma patients have proven to be less positive in larger studies of asthma and COPD patients. In addition, anti-TNFα approaches may be associated with higher incidence of cancer and reactivation of tuberculosis. Specific antiallergic approach with anti-IgE humanized monoclonal antibody has been approved for use in severe allergic asthma. PDE4 inhibitors are under study for asthma and COPD, but their efficacy is limited by side effects such as nausea and vomiting, and headaches. Other approaches target corticosteroid insensitivity in severe asthma and COPD, such as devising small-molecule inhibitors of kinases that could improve corticosteroid actions.

The treatment of asthma and COPD is evolving rapidly with increasing understanding of their pathophysiologies. While the current best treatments for both conditions rest on a combination of agents that have a wide range of effects on the inflammatory process found in the airways of these diseases, the focus has been to target specific targets in these diseases. Of the new anti-inflammatories described in detail, none are yet licensed for treatment of asthma or COPD. It may be likely that these agents would benefit a particular subgroup of patients, and such subgroups need to be identified. This would make drug development more hazardous particularly for pharmaceutical establishments since they would be treating a smaller proportion of the diseased population and the costs of development of new drugs are ever increasing.

References

1. Rabe KF, Vermeire PA, Soriano JB, et al. Clinical management of asthma in 1999: the Asthma Insights and Reality in Europe (AIRE) study. Eur Respir J 2000; 16:802–807.
2. Israel E, Chervinsky PS, Friedman B, et al. Effects of montelukast and beclomethasone on airway function and asthma control. J Allergy Clin Immunol 2002; 110:847–854.
3. O'Byrne PM, Parameswaran K. Pharmacological management of mild or moderate persistent asthma. Lancet 2006; 368:794–803.
4. Boushey HA, Sorkness CA, King TS, et al. Daily versus as-needed corticosteroids for mild persistent asthma. N Engl J Med 2005; 352:1519–1528.
5. Pauwels RA, Lofdahl C, Postma D, et al. Effect of inhaled formoterol and budesonide on exacerbations of asthma. N Engl J Med 1997; 337:1405–1411.
6. Greening AP, Ind PW, Northfield M, et al. Added salmeterol versus higher-dose corticosteroid in asthma patients with symptoms on existing inhaled corticosteroid. Lancet 1994; 344:219–224.
7. Bateman ED, Boushey HA, Bousquet J, et al. Can guideline-defined asthma control be achieved? The Gaining Optimal Asthma ControL study. Am J Respir Crit Care Med 2004; 170:836–844.
8. Ram FS, Cates CJ, Ducharme FM. Long-acting beta-2-agonists versus anti-leukotrienes as add-on therapy to inhaled corticosteroids for chronic asthma. Cochrane Database Sys Rev 2005; 1:CD003137.
9. Kankaanranta H, Lahdensuo A, Moilanen E, et al. Add-on therapy options in asthma not adequately controlled by inhaled corticosteroids: a comprehensive review. Respir Res 2004; 5:17.
10. Chung KF, Godard P, Adelroth E, et al. Difficult/therapy-resistant asthma: the need for an integrated approach to define clinical phenotypes, evaluate risk factors, understand pathophysiology and find novel therapies. ERS Task Force on Difficult/Therapy-Resistant Asthma. European Respiratory Society [in process citation]. Eur Respir J 1999; 13: 1198–1208.
11. Proceedings of the ATS workshop on refractory asthma: current understanding, recommendations, and unanswered questions. American Thoracic Society. Am J Respir Crit Care Med 2000; 162:2341–2351.
12. Bateman ED, Hurd SS, Barnes PJ, et al. Global strategy for asthma management and prevention: GINA executive summary. Eur Respir J 2008; 31:143–178.
13. Calverley PM, Anderson JA, Celli B, et al. Salmeterol and fluticasone propionate and survival in chronic obstructive pulmonary disease. N Engl J Med 2007; 356:775–789.
14. Celli BR, Thomas NE, Anderson JA, et al. Effect of pharmacotherapy on rate of decline of lung function in chronic obstructive pulmonary disease: results from the TORCH study. Am J Respir Crit Care Med 2008; 178:332–338.
15. Aaron SD, Vandemheen KL, Fergusson D, et al. Tiotropium in combination with placebo, salmeterol, or fluticasone-salmeterol for treatment of chronic obstructive pulmonary disease: a randomized trial. Ann Intern Med 2007; 146:545–555.
16. Rahman I, Adcock IM. Oxidative stress and redox regulation of lung inflammation in COPD. Eur Respir J 2006; 28:219–242.
17. Grandjean EM, Berthet P, Ruffmann R, et al. Efficacy of oral long-term N-acetylcysteine in chronic bronchopulmonary disease: a meta-analysis of published double-blind, placebo-controlled clinical trials. Clin Ther 2000; 22:209–221.
18. Stey C, Steurer J, Bachmann S, et al. The effect of oral N-acetylcysteine in chronic bronchitis: a quantitative systematic review. Eur Respir J 2000; 16:253–262.
19. Poole PJ, Black PN. Oral mucolytic drugs for exacerbations of chronic obstructive pulmonary disease: systematic review. BMJ 2001; 322:1271–1274.

20. Gerrits CM, Herings RM, Leufkens HG, et al. N-acetylcysteine reduces the risk of re-hospitalisation among patients with chronic obstructive pulmonary disease. Eur Respir J 2003; 21:795–798.

21. Decramer M, Rutten-van Molken M, Dekhuijzen PN, et al. Effects of N-acetylcysteine on outcomes in chronic obstructive pulmonary disease (Bronchitis Randomized on NAC Cost-Utility Study, BRONCUS): a randomised placebo-controlled trial. Lancet 2005; 365:1552–1560.

22. Zheng JP, Kang J, Huang SG, et al. Effect of carbocisteine on acute exacerbation of chronic obstructive pulmonary disease (PEACE Study): a randomised placebo-controlled study. Lancet 2008; 371:2013–2018.

23. Adcock IM, Ford PA, Bhavsar P, et al. Steroid resistance in asthma: mechanisms and treatment options. Curr Allergy Asthma Rep 2008; 8:171–178.

24. Chung KF, Adcock IM. Multifaceted mechanisms in COPD: inflammation, immunity, and tissue repair and destruction. Eur Respir J 2008; 31:1334–1356.

25. Simpson JL, Powell H, Boyle MJ, et al. Clarithromycin targets neutrophilic airway inflammation in refractory asthma. Am J Respir Crit Care Med 2008; 177:148–155.

26. Brightling CE, Monteiro W, Ward R, et al. Sputum eosinophilia and short-term response to prednisolone in chronic obstructive pulmonary disease: a randomised controlled trial. Lancet 2000; 356:1480–1485.

27. Chanez P, Vignola AM, O'Shaugnessy T, et al. Corticosteroid reversibility in COPD is related to features of asthma. Am J Respir Crit Care Med 1997; 155:1529–1534.

28. Jatakanon A, Uasuf C, Maziak W, et al. Neutrophilic inflammation in severe persistent asthma. Am J Respir Crit Care Med 1999; 160:1532–1539.

29. Wenzel SE, Schwartz LB, Langmack EL, et al. Evidence that severe asthma can be divided pathologically into two inflammatory subtypes with distinct physiologic and clinical characteristics. Am J Respir Crit Care Med 1999; 160:1001–1008.

30. Valotis A, Hogger P. Human receptor kinetics and lung tissue retention of the enhanced-affinity glucocorticoid fluticasone furoate. Respir Res 2007; 8:54.

31. Paul-Clark MJ, Roviezzo F, Flower RJ, et al. Glucocorticoid receptor nitration leads to enhanced anti-inflammatory effects of novel steroid ligands. J Immunol 2003; 171: 3245–3252.

32. Nevin BJ, Broadley KJ. Comparative effects of inhaled budesonide and the NO-donating budesonide derivative, NCX 1020, against leukocyte influx and airway hyperreactivity following lipopolysaccharide challenge. Pulm Pharmacol Ther 2004; 17:219–232.

33. Adcock IM, Caramori G, Chung KF. New targets for drug development in asthma. Lancet 2008; 372:1073–1087.

34. Derendorf H. Pharmacokinetic and pharmacodynamic properties of inhaled ciclesonide. J Clin Pharmacol 2007; 47:782–789.

35. Schacke H, Berger M, Rehwinkel H, et al. Selective glucocorticoid receptor agonists (SEGRAs): novel ligands with an improved therapeutic index. Mol Cell Endocrinol 2007; 275:109–117.

36. Ito K, Chung KF, Adcock IM. Update on glucocorticoid action and resistance. J Allergy Clin Immunol 2006; 117:522–543.

37. Schacke H, Schottelius A, Docke WD, et al. Dissociation of transactivation from trans-repression by a selective glucocorticoid receptor agonist leads to separation of therapeutic effects from side effects. Proc Natl Acad Sci U S A 2004; 101:227–232.

38. Schacke H, Docke WD, Asadullah K. Mechanisms involved in the side effects of gluco-corticoids. Pharmacol Ther 2002; 96:23–43.

39. Miner JN, Ardecky B, Benbatoul K, et al. Antiinflammatory glucocorticoid receptor ligand with reduced side effects exhibits an altered protein-protein interaction profile. Proc Natl Acad Sci U S A 2007; 104:19244–19249.

40. Ogawa S, Lozach J, Benner C, et al. Molecular determinants of crosstalk between nuclear receptors and toll-like receptors. Cell 2005; 122:707–721.

41. Farrow SN. Nuclear receptors: doubling up in the lung. Curr Opin Pharmacol 2008; 8:275–279.

42. Renda T, Baraldo S, Pelaia G, et al. Increased activation of p38 MAPK in COPD. Eur Respir J 2008; 31:62–69.

43. Ito K, Caramori G, Adcock IM. Therapeutic potential of phosphatidylinositol 3-kinase inhibitors in inflammatory respiratory disease. J Pharmacol Exp Ther 2007; 321:1–8.

44. Marwick JA, Stevenson CS, Barnes PJ, et al. Cigarette smoke reduces steroid sensitivity by reducing glucocorticoid receptor (GR) and GR co-repressor expression. Proc Am Thorac Soc 2008; 5:A333.

45. Irusen E, Matthews JG, Takahashi A, et al. p38 Mitogen-activated protein kinase-induced glucocorticoid receptor phosphorylation reduces its activity: role in steroid-insensitive asthma. J Allergy Clin Immunol 2002; 109:649–657.

46. Kent L, Smyth L, Plumb J, et al. Inhibition of LPS stimulated COPD macrophage inflammatory gene expression by dexamethasone and the p38 MAPK inhibitor SB706504. J Pharmacol Exp Ther 2009; 328:458–468.

47. Bhavsar P, Hew M, Khorasani N, et al. Relative corticosteroid insensitivity of alveolar macrophages in severe asthma compared to non-severe asthma. Thorax 2008; 63(9):784–790.

48. Rothschild BM. Review: individual DMARDs have similar efficacy for RA, but combination therapy improves response. Evid Based Med 2008; 13:76.

49. Adcock IM, Chung KF, Caramori G, et al. Kinase inhibitors and airway inflammation. Eur J Pharmacol 2006; 533:118–132.

50. Ito K, Yamamura S, Essilfie-Quaye S, et al. Histone deacetylase 2-mediated deacetylation of the glucocorticoid receptor enables NF-kappaB suppression. J Exp Med 2006; 203:7–13.

51. Holgate ST, Polosa R. Treatment strategies for allergy and asthma. Nat Rev Immunol 2008; 8:218–230.

52. Chung KF, Barnes PJ. Cytokines in asthma. Thorax 1999; 54:825–857.

53. Chung KF. Cytokines in chronic obstructive pulmonary disease. Eur Respir J Suppl 2001; 34:50s–59s.

54. Leckie MJ, Ten BA, Khan J, et al. Effects of an interleukin-5 blocking monoclonal antibody on eosinophils, airway hyper-responsiveness, and the late asthmatic response. Lancet 2000; 356(9248):2144–2148.

55. Flood-Page PT, Menzies-Gow AN, Kay AB, et al. Eosinophil's role remains uncertain as anti-interleukin-5 only partially depletes numbers in asthmatic airway. Am J Respir Crit Care Med 2003; 167:199–204.

56. Menzies-Gow A, Flood-Page P, Sehmi R, et al. Anti-IL-5 (mepolizumab) therapy induces bone marrow eosinophil maturational arrest and decreases eosinophil progenitors in the bronchial mucosa of atopic asthmatics. J Allergy Clin Immunol 2003; 111:714–719.

57. Hisada T, Hellewell PG, Teixeira MM, et al. alpha4 integrin-dependent eotaxin induction of bronchial hyperresponsiveness and eosinophil migration in interleukin-5 transgenic mice. Am J Respir Cell Mol Biol 1999; 20:992–1000.

58. Flood-Page P, Swenson C, Faiferman I, et al. A study to evaluate safety and efficacy of mepolizumab in patients with moderate persistent asthma. Am J Respir Crit Care Med 2007; 176:1062–1071.

59. Kips JC, O'Connor BJ, Langley SJ, et al. Effect of SCH55700, a humanized anti-human interleukin-5 antibody, in severe persistent asthma: a pilot study. Am J Respir Crit Care Med 2003; 167:1655–1659.

60. Flood-Page P, Menzies-Gow A, Phipps S, et al. Anti-IL-5 treatment reduces deposition of ECM proteins in the bronchial subepithelial basement membrane of mild atopic asthmatics. J Clin Invest 2003; 112:1029–1036.
61. Rothenberg ME, Klion AD, Roufosse FE, et al. Treatment of patients with the hypereosinophilic syndrome with mepolizumab. N Engl J Med 2008; 358:1215–1228.
62. Stein ML, Villanueva JM, Buckmeier BK, et al. Anti-IL-5 (mepolizumab) therapy reduces eosinophil activation ex vivo and increases IL-5 and IL-5 receptor levels. J Allergy Clin Immunol 2008; 121(6):1473–1483, 1483.e1–e4.
63. Green RH, Brightling CE, McKenna S, et al. Asthma exacerbations and sputum eosinophil counts: a randomised controlled trial. Lancet 2002; 360:1715–1721.
64. Haldar P, Brightling CE, Hargadon B, et al. Mepolizumab and exacerbations of refractory eosinophilic asthma. N Engl J Med 2009; 360:973–984.
65. Borish LC, Nelson HS, Lanz MJ, et al. Interleukin-4 receptor in moderate atopic asthma. A phase I/II randomized, placebo-controlled trial. Am J Respir Crit Care Med 1999; 160:1816–1823.
66. Borish LC, Nelson HS, Corren J, et al. Efficacy of soluble IL-4 receptor for the treatment of adults with asthma. J Allergy Clin Immunol 2001; 107:963–970.
67. Wills-Karp M. Interleukin-13 in asthma pathogenesis. Immunol Rev 2004; 202:175–190.
68. Wills-Karp M, Luyimbazi J, Xu X, et al. Interleukin-13: central mediator of allergic asthma [in process citation]. Science 1998; 282:2258–2261.
69. Gr nig G, Warnock M, Wakil AE, et al. Requirement for IL-13 independently of IL-4 in experimental asthma [in process citation]. Science 1998; 282:2261–2263.
70. Zhu Z, Homer RJ, Wang Z, et al. Pulmonary expression of interleukin-13 causes inflammation, mucus hypersecretion, subepithelial fibrosis, physiologic abnormalities, and eotaxin production. J Clin Invest 1999; 103:779–788.
71. Bochner BS, Klunk DA, Sterbinsky SA, et al. IL-13 selectively induces vascular cell adhesion molecule-1 expression in human endothelial cells. J Immunol 1995; 154:799–803.
72. Zhu Z, Ma B, Zheng T, et al. IL-13-induced chemokine responses in the lung: role of CCR2 in the pathogenesis of IL-13-induced inflammation and remodeling. J Immunol 2002; 168:2953–2962.
73. Lee CG, Homer RJ, Zhu Z, et al. Interleukin-13 induces tissue fibrosis by selectively stimulating and activating transforming growth factor beta(1). J Exp Med 2001; 194:809–821.
74. Espinosa K, Bosse Y, Stankova J, et al. CysLT1 receptor upregulation by TGF-beta and IL-13 is associated with bronchial smooth muscle cell proliferation in response to LTD4. J Allergy Clin Immunol 2003; 111:1032–1040.
75. Tliba O, Deshpande D, Chen H, et al. IL-13 enhances agonist-evoked calcium signals and contractile responses in airway smooth muscle. Br J Pharmacol 2003; 140(7):1159–1162.
76. Wenzel S, Wilbraham D, Fuller R, et al. Effect of an interleukin-4 variant on late phase asthmatic response to allergen challenge in asthmatic patients: results of two phase 2a studies. Lancet 2007; 370:1422–1431.
77. Williams TJ, Jose PJ. Role of eotaxin and related CC chemokines in allergy and asthma. Chem Immunol 2000; 78:166–177.
78. Humbles AA, Lu B, Friend DS, et al. The murine CCR3 receptor regulates both the role of eosinophils and mast cells in allergen-induced airway inflammation and hyperresponsiveness. Proc Natl Acad Sci U S A 2002; 99:1479–1484.
79. Ma W, Bryce PJ, Humbles AA, et al. CCR3 is essential for skin eosinophilia and airway hyperresponsiveness in a murine model of allergic skin inflammation. J Clin Invest 2002; 109:621–628.
80. Elsner J, Escher SE, Forssmann U. Chemokine receptor antagonists: a novel therapeutic approach in allergic diseases. Allergy 2004; 59:1243–1258.

81. Bryan SA, Jose PJ, Topping JR, et al. Responses of leukocytes to chemokines in whole blood and their antagonism by novel CC-chemokine receptor 3 antagonists. Am J Respir Crit Care Med 2002; 165:1602–1609.

82. Das AM, Vaddi KG, Solomon KA, et al. Selective inhibition of eosinophil influx into the lung by small molecule CC chemokine receptor 3 antagonists in mouse models of allergic inflammation. J Pharmacol Exp Ther 2006; 318:411–417.

83. Wegmann M, Goggel R, Sel S, et al. Effects of a low-molecular-weight CCR-3 antagonist on chronic experimental asthma. Am J Respir Cell Mol Biol 2007; 36:61–67.

84. Gauvreau GM, Boulet LP, Cockcroft DW, et al. Antisense therapy against CCR3 and the common beta chain attenuates allergen-induced eosinophilic responses. Am J Respir Crit Care Med 2008; 177:952–958.

85. Wacker DA, Santella JB III, Gardner DS, et al. CCR3 antagonists: a potential new therapy for the treatment of asthma. Discovery and structure-activity relationships. Bioorg Med Chem Lett 2002; 12:1785–1789.

86. De Lucca GV, Kim UT, Vargo BJ, et al. Discovery of CC chemokine receptor-3 (CCR3) antagonists with picomolar potency. J Med Chem 2005; 48:2194–2211.

87. Russo C, Polosa R. TNF-alpha as a promising therapeutic target in chronic asthma: a lesson from rheumatoid arthritis. Clin Sci (Lond) 2005; 109:135–142.

88. Bradding P, Roberts JA, Britten KM, et al. Interleukin-4, -5 and -6 and tumor necrosis factor-α in normal and asthmatic airways: evidence for the human mast cell as a source of these cytokines. Am J Respir Cell Mol Biol 1994; 10:471–480.

89. Ying S, Robinson DS, Varney V, et al. TNF-α mRNA expression in allergic inflammation. Clin Exp Allergy 1991; 21:745–750.

90. Howarth PH, Babu KS, Arshad HS, et al. Tumour necrosis factor (TNFalpha) as a novel therapeutic target in symptomatic corticosteroid dependent asthma. Thorax 2005; 60: 1012–1018.

91. Berry MA, Hargadon B, Shelley M, et al. Evidence of a role of tumor necrosis factor alpha in refractory asthma. N Engl J Med 2006; 354:697–708.

92. Busse PJ, Zhang TF, Srivastava K, et al. Chronic exposure to TNF-alpha increases airway mucus gene expression in vivo. J Allergy Clin Immunol 2005; 116:1256–1263.

93. Amrani Y, Krymskaya V, Maki C, et al. Mechanisms underlying TNF-alpha effects on agonist-mediated calcium homeostasis in human airway smooth muscle cells. Am J Physiol 1997; 273:L1020–L1028.

94. Pennings HJ, Kramer K, Bast A, et al. Tumour necrosis factor-alpha induces hyperreactivity in tracheal smooth muscle of the guinea-pig in vitro. Eur Respir J 1998; 12:45–49.

95. Renzetti LM, Paciorek PM, Tannu SA, et al. Pharmacological evidence for tumor necrosis factor as a mediator of allergic inflammation in the airways. J Pharmacol Exp Ther 1996; 278:847–853.

96. Kips JC, Tavernier J, Pauwels RA. Tumor necrosis factor causes bronchial hyper-responsiveness in rats. Am Rev Respir Dis 1992; 145:332–336.

97. Thomas PS, Yates DH, Barnes PJ. Tumor necrosis factor-alpha increases airway responsiveness and sputum neutrophilia in normal human subjects. Am J Respir Crit Care Med 1995; 152:76–80.

98. Morjaria JB, Chauhan AJ, Babu KS, et al. The role of a soluble Tnf-A receptor fusion protein (Etanercept) in corticosteroid-refractory asthma: a double blind, randomised placebo-controlled trial. Thorax 2008; 63(7):584–591.

99. Erin EM, Leaker BR, Nicholson GC, et al. The effects of a monoclonal antibody directed against tumor necrosis factor-alpha in asthma. Am J Respir Crit Care Med 2006; 174: 753–762.

100. Wenzel SE, Barnes PJ, Bleecker ER, et al. A randomized, double-blind, placebo-controlled study of tumor necrosis factor-alpha blockade in severe persistent asthma. Am J Respir Crit Care Med 2009; 179:549–558.

101. Rennard SI, Fogarty C, Kelsen S, et al. The safety and efficacy of infliximab in moderate to severe chronic obstructive pulmonary disease. Am J Respir Crit Care Med 2007; 175: 926–934.

102. Mahler DA, Huang S, Tabrizi M, et al. Efficacy and safety of a monoclonal antibody recognizing interleukin-8 in COPD: a pilot study. Chest 2004; 126:926–934.

103. Bryan SA, O'Connor BJ, Matti S, et al. Effects of recombinant human interleukin-12 on eosinophils, airway hyper-responsiveness, and the late asthmatic response. Lancet 2000; 356:2149–2153.

104. Chernoff AE, Granowitz EV, Shapiro L, et al. A randomized, controlled trial of IL-10 in humans. Inhibition of inflammatory cytokine production and immune responses. J Immunol 1995; 154:5492–5499.

105. Asadullah K, Sterry W, Volk HD. Interleukin-10 therapy–review of a new approach. Pharmacol Rev 2003; 55:241–269.

106. James LK, Durham SR. Update on mechanisms of allergen injection immunotherapy. Clin Exp Allergy 2008; 38:1074–1088.

107. Huang TJ, Macary PA, Eynott P, et al. Allergen-specific Th1 cells counteract efferent Th2 cell-dependent bronchial hyperresponsiveness and eosinophilic inflammation partly via IFN-gamma. J Immunol 2001; 166:207–217.

108. Boguniewicz M, Martin RJ, Martin D, et al. The effects of nebulized recombinant interferon-gamma in asthmatic airways. J Allergy Clin Immunol 1995; 95:133–135.

109. Boguniewicz M, Schneider LC, Milgrom HN, et al. Treatment of steroid-dependent asthma with recombinant interferon-gamma. J Allergy Clin Immunol 1992; 89:288.

110. Beavo JA. Cyclic nucleotide phosphodiesterases: functional implications of multiple isoforms. Physiol Rev 1995; 75:725–748.

111. Sanz MJ, Cortijo J, Morcillo EJ. PDE4 inhibitors as new anti-inflammatory drugs: effects on cell trafficking and cell adhesion molecules expression. Pharmacol Ther 2005; 106: 269–297.

112. Kumar S, Boehm J, Lee JC. p38 MAP kinases: key signalling molecules as therapeutic targets for inflammatory diseases. Nat Rev Drug Discov 2003; 2:717–726.

113. Foissier L, Lonchampt M, Coge F, et al. In vitro down-regulation of antigen-induced IL-5 gene expression and protein production by cAMP-specific phosphodiesterase type 4 inhibitor. J Pharmacol Exp Ther 1996; 278:1484–1490.

114. Profita M, Chiappara G, Mirabella F, et al. Effect of cilomilast (Ariflo) on TNF-alpha, IL-8, and GM-CSF release by airway cells of patients with COPD. Thorax 2003; 58:573–579.

115. Griswold DE, Webb EF, Badger AM, et al. SB 207499 (Ariflo), a second generation phosphodiesterase 4 inhibitor, reduces tumor necrosis factor alpha and interleukin-4 production in vivo. J Pharmacol Exp Ther 1998; 287:705–711.

116. Souness JE, Griffin M, Maslen C, et al. Evidence that cyclic AMP phosphodiesterase inhibitors suppress TNF alpha generation from human monocytes by interacting with a 'low-affinity' phosphodiesterase 4 conformer. Br J Pharmacol 1996; 118:649–658.

117. Gonçalves de Moraes VL, Singer M, Vargaftig BB, et al. Effects of rolipram on cyclic AMP levels in alveolar macrophages and lipopolysaccharide-induced inflammation in mouse lung. Br J Pharmacol 1998; 123:631–636.

118. Kohyama T, Liu X, Zhu YK, et al. Phosphodiesterase 4 inhibitor cilomilast inhibits fibroblast-mediated collagen gel degradation induced by tumor necrosis factor-alpha and neutrophil elastase. Am J Respir Cell Mol Biol 2002; 27:487–494.

119. Kohyama T, Liu X, Wen FQ, et al. PDE4 inhibitors attenuate fibroblast chemotaxis and contraction of native collagen gels. Am J Respir Cell Mol Biol 2002; 26:694–701.

120. Martorana PA, Beume R, Lucattelli M, et al. Roflumilast fully prevents emphysema in mice chronically exposed to cigarette smoke. Am J Respir Crit Care Med 2005; 172(7):848–853.

121. Barnette MS, Bartus JO, Burman M, et al. Association of the anti-inflammatory activity of phosphodiesterase 4 (PDE4) inhibitors with either inhibition of PDE4 catalytic activity or competition for [3H]rolipram binding. Biochem Pharmacol 1996; 51:949–956.

122. van Schalkwyk E, Strydom K, Williams Z, et al. Roflumilast, an oral, once-daily phosphodiesterase 4 inhibitor, attenuates allergen-induced asthmatic reactions. J Allergy Clin Immunol 2005; 116:292–298.

123. Louw C, Williams Z, Venter L, et al. Roflumilast, a phosphodiesterase 4 inhibitor, reduces airway hyperresponsiveness after allergen challenge. Respiration 2007; 74:411–417.

124. Timmer W, Leclerc V, Birraux G, et al. The new phosphodiesterase 4 inhibitor roflumilast is efficacious in exercise-induced asthma and leads to suppression of LPS-stimulated TNF-alpha ex vivo. J Clin Pharmacol 2002; 42:297–303.

125. Compton C, Cedar E, Nieman RB, et al. Ariflo improves pulmonary function in patients with asthma: results of a study in patients taking inhaled corticosteroids. Am J Respir Crit Care Med 1999; 195:A624.

126. Compton CH, Gubb J, Nieman R, et al. Cilomilast, a selective phosphodiesterase-4 inhibitor for treatment of patients with chronic obstructive pulmonary disease: a randomised, dose-ranging study. Lancet 2001; 358:265–270.

127. Bateman ED, Izquierdo JL, Harnest U, et al. Efficacy and safety of roflumilast in the treatment of asthma. Ann Allergy Asthma Immunol 2006; 96:679–686.

128. Bousquet J, Aubier M, Sastre J, et al. Comparison of roflumilast, an oral anti-inflammatory, with beclomethasone dipropionate in the treatment of persistent asthma. Allergy 2006; 61:72–78.

129. Rennard SI, Schachter N, Strek M, et al. Cilomilast for COPD: results of a 6-month, placebo-controlled study of a potent, selective inhibitor of phosphodiesterase 4. Chest 2006; 129:56–66.

130. Gamble E, Grootendorst DC, Brightling CE, et al. Antiinflammatory effects of the phosphodiesterase-4 inhibitor cilomilast (Ariflo) in chronic obstructive pulmonary disease. Am J Respir Crit Care Med 2003; 168:976–982.

131. Grootendorst DC, Gauw SA, Verhoosel RM, et al. Reduction in sputum neutrophil and eosinophil numbers by the PDE4 inhibitor roflumilast in patients with COPD. Thorax 2007; 62:1081–1087.

132. Rabe KF, Bateman ED, O'Donnell D, et al. Roflumilast—an oral anti-inflammatory treatment for chronic obstructive pulmonary disease: a randomised controlled trial. Lancet 2005; 366:563–571.

133. Calverley PM, Sanchez-Toril F, McIvor A, et al. Effect of 1-year treatment with roflumilast in severe chronic obstructive pulmonary disease. Am J Respir Crit Care Med 2007; 176:154–161.

134. Fabbri LM, Calverley PM, Izquierdo-Alonso JL, et al. Roflumilast in moderate-to-severe chronic obstructive pulmonary disease treated with long-acting bronchodilators: two randomised clinical trials. Lancet 2009; 374:695–703.

135. Calverley PM, Rabe KF, Goehring UM, et al. Roflumilast in symptomatic chronic obstructive pulmonary disease: two randomised clinical trials. Lancet. 2009; 374:685–694.

136. Cox G, Miller JD, McWilliams A, et al. Bronchial thermoplasty for asthma. Am J Respir Crit Care Med 2006; 173:965–969.

137. Cox G, Thomson NC, Rubin AS, et al. Asthma control during the year after bronchial thermoplasty. N Engl J Med 2007; 356:1327–1337.

11

Airway Wall Remodeling as a Concept for Airway Disease Therapeutics

E. HAYDN WALTERS and DAVID P. JOHNS
Menzies Research Institute, University of Tasmania, Tasmania, Australia

CHRIS WARD
Institute of Cellular Medicine, Freeman Road Hospital, Newcastle University, Newcastle-upon-Tyne, U.K.

I. Introduction

Airway remodeling is the term given to the structural changes and gross thickening that occur in the airway wall as part of the pathological processes in inflammatory chronic obstructive airway diseases, most studied in asthma and smoking-related chronic obstructive pulmonary disease (COPD). The much asked questions of whether remodeling is part of the inflammatory process, or whether it occurs as a consequence of inflammatory damage, or whether it is a separate but parallel process are probably somewhat rhetorical. All these concepts are likely to be correct to some extent in what is a complex process, involving the whole tracheobronchial tree and all layers of the airway wall. Furthermore, inevitably with such a multifaceted pathology, there will be marked individual and temporal variation as the disease progresses, with strong genetic influences (1,2).

Some aspects of remodeling, for example, epithelial changes and subepithelial reticular basement membrane (Rbm) thickening in asthma, may occur early in the disease process or even well before there are clinical manifestations (3–11), and are presumed to lead to early loss of lung function (12–14).

In smokers, in contrast, physiologically compromising remodeling with the development of COPD may occur only after many years of "dedicated" self-harm and induced airway inflammation (15), but earlier and more significant loss of airflow may be greater in those with some asthma-type features such as airway hyperreactivity (16–18) and in those with frequent exacerbations, presumably as an index of the intensity of recurrent insults to the airway and ongoing inflammation (19,20). Smoking in asthmatic patients also predisposes to excessive loss of lung function, presumed related to an additive intensity of the remodeling process (14,21–23). Other factors leading to excessive lung function loss in asthma include more severe disease of longer duration, with worse underlying inflammation, and more intense airway hyperresponsiveness (24–29). Later onset asthma also tends to remodel and lose airflow more aggressively (24,25), but even in childhood-onset asthma about 25% of individuals lose maximal airflow excessively and being male and less atopic seems to be risk factors (30), for reasons which are, as yet, unclear.

There has been substantial renewed interest over the past year or so in the area of airway structural remodeling, which has led to a number of excellent reviews and a whole review series in the European Respiratory Journal in 2007 (31). Most reviews have emphasized changes in asthma, since most research has focused on this, and have dealt in detail with likely basic mechanisms of these disease processes (32–36) and/or emphasized the possibilities for therapeutic interventions (32,33,37) targeting these processes.

Given this background, with so many recent and well-referenced review articles, in this chapter we will deal only in relative outline with the basic description of remodeling changes in asthma and COPD, and the etiological mechanisms thought to be involved from animal models and bronchoscopic sampling in humans. We will focus more on the means by which remodeling can be best assessed and followed clinically, whether physiologically or with imaging and with the uncertainties and current debates in these areas. Given the nature of this monograph we will also outline what is known about how current therapies may affect and benefit airway remodeling and what future developments there might be in therapeutics from what we understand about the basic mechanisms of disease process. Finally, we will introduce some relatively new findings from research in the area of bronchiolitis obliterans syndrome (BOS), thought to represent a manifestation of chronic airway rejection post–lung transplant, because it is a process that seems to resemble remodeling that occurs in COPD but with a much shorter time scale and may give clues to how this much commoner but underresearched illness may be better dealt with in the future.

II. Components of Airway Remodeling in Asthma and COPD
A. Epithelium

In asthma, the luminal surface epithelium is thickened (38) with hyperplasia of goblet cells (39) (Figs. 1 and 2). Mucus plugging of the airways may be a significant part of airflow limitation in critical life-threatening attacks (40,41), but such plugs consist not only of glandular mucins but also of extravasated proteins and inflammatory cells (42). These luminal components may also disrupt normal function of surfactant in small airways causing wall instability (34). The epithelium in asthma is more friable than normal, with increased epithelial cell numbers in bronchoalveolar lavage (BAL) and sputum (43), and frequently almost complete denudation of the epithelium in airway wall biopsies, since the epithelium literally falls off because of the trauma of harvesting, which is an artifact present quite substantially even in normals (44,45). Ultrastructurally, there is evidence for disruption of desmosomes maintaining contact between epithelial cells themselves and between them and the basement membrane (46).

In COPD, the epithelium is also thicker than normal, metaplastic, has loss of cilia, and increased goblet cells (47) (Fig. 3). Submucosal glands empty through ducts, which pass to the surface through the epithelium, and increased volume of these glands was possibly the first aspect of remodeling to be quantified in the Reid index (48). The index correlated with symptoms of cough and phlegm, though central airway inflammation is even better correlated with chronic bronchitis (49,50).

B. Lamina Propria and Its Extracellular Matrix

The lamina propria is the area between the epithelium and the muscle layer—all three layers together constituting the mucosa (although some authors rather confusingly refer

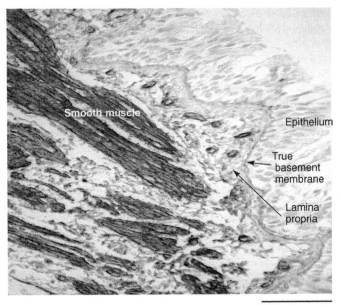

100 micrometer

Figure 1 Normal: Airway biopsy section in a normal subject (200×, hematoxylin and anti-collagen IV antibody staining). Epithelium is intact and reticular basement membrane is not prominent. Blood vessels in lamina propria are relatively large.

to the subepithelial structures as synonymous with "submucosal"—but in traditional nomenclature this area is deep to the smooth muscle layer).

The "true" epithelial basement membrane consists of collagen IV, fibronectin, and elastin (51). Condensation of extracellular matrix (ECM) in the Rbm just below this true basement membrane gives rise to Rbm thickening (commonly referred to simply as "basement membrane thickening"). It is a distinctive feature of asthma airway pathology emphasized in what are now classic studies (52,53). The ECM consists of a complex mixture of proteoglycans and glycosaminoglycans, and has complex functions including "sticking" the tissues together, controlling hydration and osmotic pressure, modulating cell motility and cell activation through cell-surface integrin ligand receptors, and storage of cytokines and growth factors. The asthmatic Rbm thickening includes increases in especially "scar" collagens (types I, III, and V) and laminin but also is decorin, tenascin, versican, biglycan, perlican, and hyaluronan (35,54), but decreases in lumican (55) and elastin (56). It has been suggested that in asthma ECM is generally abnormal throughout the lamina propria (57), but this has not been confirmed.

It is fortuitous that not only is Rbm thickness easily quantified in airway biopsies but it also seems to be a good surrogate for all other changes including airway smooth muscle thickening, glandular enlargement, and gross wall thickening (58,59), which are much more difficult to assess in clinical biopsy studies.

Collagens are produced in the lamina propria by myofibroblasts, which are a specialized fibroblast, forming a network via long cytoplasmic extensions, predominantly in

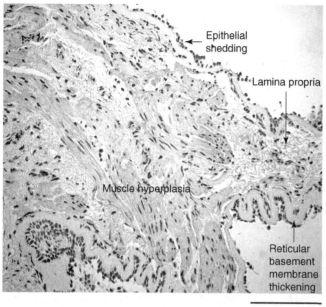

100 micrometer

Figure 2 Asthma: Airway biopsy section in asthma (200×, hematoxylin and anti-collagen IV antibody staining). Epithelium is denuded, reticular basement membrane is thickened, lamina propria is narrow but contains increased small blood vessels and cells, and smooth muscle layer is thickened.

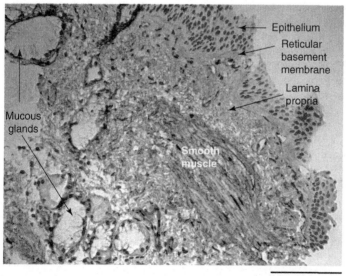

100 micrometer

Figure 3 COPD: Airway biopsy section in COPD (200×, hematoxylin and anti-collagen IV antibody staining). Epithelium is metaplastic. Reticular basement membrane thickening is variable. Mucous glands are prominent in submucosa.

the immediate subepithelial layer of the lamina propria (60). They are increased in asthma and correlate with Rbm thickening (60,61). They also produce proinflammatory cytokines, and can induce proliferation of fibroblasts and airway smooth muscle cells (32).

Fibronectin is a fibrillary glycoprotein produced by epithelial cells that can also induce fibroblast and airway smooth muscle proliferation and fibroblast chemotaxis (62,63). It is increased in concentration in BAL fluid in asthma (64) and its receptor expression on bronchial epithelial cells is increased (63), suggesting a general upregulation on this system. The balance of ECM degradation to accumulation is controlled by the enzymic equilibrium between destructive matrix metalloproteinases (MMPs) and this inhibitor, tissue inhibitor of MMP-1 (TIMP-1). MMP-1 and -13 are collagenases, MMP-2 and -9 are gelatinases that degrade especially fibronectin and elastin, and MMP-3, -10, and -11 are stromelysins with a broad spectrum of ECM degradation (32). MMP-9 is thought to be the predominant MMP relevant to asthma (65,66). In chronic stable asthma TIMP-1 predominates over MMP-9, which leads to ECM accumulation, the ratio correlating with airway wall thickening (67–69). Paradoxically, there was reversal of this ratio in a model of acute allergen challenge (70,71), as well as in acute asthma (72) suggesting a burst of ECM breakdown.

Much less is known about ECM deposition in COPD and its control. This is a major gap in knowledge given the importance of these tissue constituents in tissue integrity and physical character, as well as that influence on acute and chronic inflammation and remodeling.

C. Airway Smooth Muscle Layer

This layer is especially thickened in asthma and probably contributes most to airway thickening in this condition (73). In asthma, there is convincing evidence for hyperplasia of airway smooth muscle cells, notably in peripheral small airways, but also in central airways where it may be a marker for exceptionally severe and potentially fatal disease (35,74–77). Evidence that significant hypertrophy of airway smooth muscle cells occurs is less certain (35,75), because there is also a marked increase in ECM between muscle cells (78), which may have confounded calculations of cell volume based on the total area of smooth muscle in sections, divided by number of nuclei that could be counted. Functionally, this excess ECM in the muscle layer has been suggested as a braking mechanism to limit exaggerated muscle concentration in asthma. Phenotypically and functionally, airway smooth muscle cells themselves may also be altered in asthma: they may participate in the inflammatory and remodeling asthmatic pathology through production of cytokines, chemokines, and ECM proteins and be hypercontractile (35,76,79–81).

In COPD, although early studies suggested increased airway smooth muscle in peripheral airways, especially in the individuals physiologically most obstructed and in older, heavier smokers (15), subsequent reports have been equivocal on this issue (35). There is less airway smooth muscle than in asthma (82,83), and in general, airway thickness in COPD is intermediate between asthmatic and normal. As can be said so frequently for COPD, further clinical studies are required in a variety of well-phenotyped individuals.

D. Airway Blood Vessels

The potential for airway vascularity, and especially the plexus of capillaries and venules in the lamina propria to be a critical part of remodeling and the pathophysiology chronic airway diseases, has recently been reviewed (36,84). There is strong evidence that these vessels are increased in number and volume in asthma through endothelial proliferation, and that these changes have physiological consequences in terms of contributing to airway obstruction, especially when muscle contracts, and therefore to airway hyper-responsiveness (85–89). In addition, the airway vascular system demonstrates considerable plasticity in acute blood flow, which may be accompanied by increased permeability and fluid exudation with major potential effects almost immediately on airway wall thickness (90,91). Further, theoretical modeling has convincingly suggested that increase in volume of the airway tissue inside the muscle layer will have markedly exaggerated effects on narrowing of the airway lumen when the muscle contracts (92–94).

Although there are a substantial number of potential angiogenic mediators that can be generated in asthmatic airways, the likely most strategic mediator in this respect is thought to be vascular endothelial growth factor (VEGF) (36,85,95,96).

Compared with asthma studies, there are considerably fewer data on airway blood vessels available in COPD. However, angiogenesis does seem to be a feature at least of smokers' airways, though whether vessels are further upregulated as a feature of COPD seems more equivocal (84,96–98).

E. Cartilage

Cartilage is present throughout the airways in humans, and is a major feature in larger airways. It has major function in limiting the effective shortening of airway smooth muscle (35,99). Cartilage may be reduced in thickness in COPD (100), which could be one factor that could make the airway more collapsible (35).

III. Basic Pathogenic Mechanisms

Airway remodeling is likely to occur in the context not only of airway inflammation with activation of resident or recruited inflammatory cells (of both the innate and the adaptive immune systems) but also with a focal or generalized activation of structural cells (epithelium, endothelium, fibroblasts, airway smooth muscle cells, etc.). The purpose of this section is to summarize the range of mediators and their sources that have been implicated in remodeling, so as to emphasize potential therapeutic targets for antiremodeling strategies.

A. Epithelial Cells and ECM

Epithelial cells can produce growth factors as well as a range of proinflammatory mediators (34) and the concept of the epithelial-mesenchymal unit (EMU) has arisen, through which epithelial activation can occur by both allergic and nonallergic means (100,101) (e.g., microbial products, oxidants/cigarette smoke, physico/mechanical stimulation) to stimulate remodeling process beneath the epithelium (102). Indeed, an extension of this concept is the hypothesis that the epithelium in asthma is inherently abnormal and fixed in a damage-repair phenotype so as to be continually activated and stimulating airway inflammation and remodeling. Markers of this are upregulation of epidermally derived growth factor receptors and production of transforming growth factor beta (TGFβ)-1 and -2, basic fibroblast growth factor (bFGF), endothelin, and IGF (103,104), which stimulate subepithelial myofibroblasts to increase deposition of ECM in the lamina propria. However, there is a contrasting biopsy study suggesting that epithelial TGFβ-1 staining was decreased in asthma compared with normal (105).

Activated epithelial cells and myofibroblasts show increased expression of integrins that facilitates subepithelial accumulation of fibronectin and other ECM proteins, plus migration and differentiation of fibroblasts (45,106,107). In severe asthma, epithelial and subepithelial cell (eosinophil) expression of IL-11 also correlated with lamina propria collagen deposition (108). Hoshino et al. (109) in a human biopsy study indicated that subepithelial collagen deposition correlated moderately but significantly with both epithelial and submucosal MMP-9 expression (109). However, in animal models of allergic "asthmatic" remodeling the strongest temporal relationship between collagen deposition was with airway TGFβ-1 production (110,111), assessed in the epithelium and BAL fluid.

Airway smooth muscle cells can be induced to proliferate by a number of mitogens produced in the inflammatory milieu, including PDGF and bFGF acting through cell receptors with kinase activity, and thrombin via G protein–coupled receptors (32). Proinflammatory cytokines such as tumor necrosis factor alpha (TNFα) can also induce muscle cell proliferation (112). The ECM components fibronectin and vitronectin can enhance airway smooth muscle proliferation while laminin is antimuscle proliferative (32,113). In a murine model, the expression of TGFβ-1 and its intracellular effectors pSMAD-2 and -3 were markedly elevated in bronchial epithelium and endothelium, inflammatory cells, and airway smooth muscle cells, concomitantly with the increase in airway smooth muscle thickness (114).

Activated T cells can adhere to smooth muscle cells via integrin-CD44 cell-cell interactions and induce muscle proliferation (115,116). T-cell products including TH2 interleukins IL-4, IL-5 and IL-13, IL-11, IL-17, as well as endothelin and cysteinyl leukotrienes (117–122), are likely to be important in airway smooth muscle proliferation as well as other aspects of remodeling and repeated allergen challenges including T-cell activation may be a major driver of remodeling in allergic asthma (32).

Mast cells may also have an important role in remodeling. One of the particular features of asthma, which differentiates it pathologically from eosinophilic bronchitis (where there are many of the other features of asthma but not bronchospasm or airway hyperresponsiveness), is that there is a prominent infiltration of the airway smooth muscle layer with mast cells, which produce IL-4 and IL-13 (123,124) and are likely to be linked to airway muscle cell hyperplasia (125). Mast cell tryptase increased myocyte proliferation as well as collagen production from fibroblasts (126) and mast cell-derived plasminogen activator inhibitor-1 decreased MMP activity to alter the MMP/TIMP balance in the airway toward fibrosis (127,128).

Eosinophils are another prominent "asthma" cell implicated in the process of airway remodeling. They can produce TGFβ-1 and activate fibroblasts and ECM deposition (129,130).

Angiogenesis is likely to be driven predominantly in the asthmatic airway by VEGF and upregulation of its receptor system (84,88,89,131,132). VEGF in asthma is produced by endothelial cells, macrophages, eosinophils, mast cells, and potentially by epithelial cells and airway smooth muscle cells (84,133).

In COPD, conclusions about vasculogenic mediators are more difficult to draw, generally because of lack of data and the mixed phenotypes usually studied (84). However, upregulation of VEGF and its receptors in the airways seems to be a result of cigarette smoking (in contrast to opposite changes in the lung parenchyma), and it is probable but not certain that this occurs to an even greater extent where the fixed airway obstruction of COPD is present (98,134,135).

B. Summary: Which Mediators Are Likely to Make Best Targets?

As applies to inflammation, there is an alarmingly complex array of cells and mediators potentially involved in remodeling, with an apparently absurd degree of inbuilt redundancy. However, two growth factors stand out as potentially core mediators: VEGF and TGFβ-1. TH2-type cytokines probably act in remodeling at least partly via TGFβ (136,137). A pro-TGFβ-1 mouse model demonstrated increased airway myofibroblast and airway smooth muscle cell hyperplasia and epithelial apoptosis (138) and topical application of TGFβ-1 to the airways induced collagen synthesis, increased Rbm thickness, and airway hyperresponsiveness (139). TGFβ-1 is the main stimulator of the important intracellular SMAD transcription factor pathway (140) with SMAD-2, -3, and -4 activating transcription of ECM components such as collagen. At the same time, TGFβ-1 inhibits SMAD-7 that is the transcription factor for decorin. If decorin decreases then ECM may be weak even if it looks thick. In contrast to this emphasis on TGFβ-1, Lee et al. (141) have shown that overexpression of VEGF in the airways induced the full panoply of asthma pathology including remodeling changes and cellular inflammation, and it is likely that there are important mutually stimulating interactions between TGFβ-1 and VEGF at a high level in the remodeling mediator cascade.

IV. Clinically Assessing Airway Remodeling
A. Radiological Imaging and Clinical Correlates

The availability of high-resolution CT scanning in the 1990s with "thin slice," that is, 1 to 2 mm lung axial slices and an edge-enhancing software algorithm, allowed attempts to visualize airways in sufficient detail to obtain quantitative assessments of airway thickness/volume. There were usually 10-mm gaps between the images, and so the focus was usually on a single right upper lobe bronchus, which fortuitously tended to present at right angles to the plane of imaging. The acquisition protocol usually involved a brief breath hold at a set lung volume to obtain the image. The technique relied on manual tracing of the airway images (142,143).

Fortunately, technology and software updates over the past five years or so have transformed the situation (144,145), with introduction of multidetector row CT (MDCT), for example, 16-channel GE LightSpeed 16. These provide "volumetric" image data and submillimeter spatial resolution in both axial and longitudinal directions. The fully automated software (e.g., BronCare in France) allows for the tendency of CT scans to overestimate airway wall area (WA) relative to lumen area (LA) because of difficulties with "edge" discrimination. Much work with experimental modeling in phantoms and animals has gone into developing these complex algorithms. They now allow high-resolution images of cross sections of the bronchi to be reformatted in the precise axis of a particular airway, which replaces the need for manual evaluation of a single airway. Indeed, several bronchi can be evaluated in each subject, although data acquisition is currently much more consistent with segmental rather than subsegmental airways.

Specific predetermined criteria have been developed to aid accuracy with MDCT and lung volume is controlled by a pneumotachograph to trigger the acquisitions at 60% to 90% of total lung capacity during a slow expiration following a deep inspiration (146). Volumetric imaging allows true isotropic voxels where slice thickness is the same as the resolution of the system that allows true cross sectioning of airways using retrospective reconstruction. The acquisition volume in practice is currently limited to the right lung base with reconstructions centered on the middle and lower lobes, with an 18 to 20 cm field of view and 512×512 pixel matrix, 0.6-mm slice thickness, and reconstruction interval of just 0.3 mm. One quality criterion is that 10 contiguous airway slices are needed to validate WA and LA for each airway, allowing 3D reconstruction and analysis of bronchial cross section at 90° of true axis of the airway. Currently, WA and LA dimensions for segmental airways can be obtained for almost 100% of subjects (98% and 96%, respectively). The main limitation for smaller airways is contact of the airway with accompanying artery for >55% of its circumference, which precludes accurate reconstruction.

Overall the goal of MDCT is to compare airways at the same or closely comparable lung volumes, at which airways will be assumed to be maximally dilated (145). However, in reality, and especially in pathological conditions, airway area-lung volume-pressure curves may be different or more heterogeneous than normal, and also the relationships may change after a therapeutic intervention. Thus, stiffer airways or more compliant lungs or both could change the effect of lung inflation on airway diameter and so, WA and LA at a given volume may not be comparable between individuals or over time. Sufficient physiology-radiology correlations have not yet been done to address such issues.

The major limitation to CT scanning is radiation exposure and cancer risk (144), which is greater in young people rather than older individuals. It has been advised that research should be restricted to individuals over the age of 55 years whose risk is very low (147). This would imply that CT-based research studies of airway disease should largely be restricted to COPD and not "classic" asthma. Specific guidelines for the use of modern methods is urgently required and are not dealt with even in current reviews or even working protocol papers (145,146,148).

In spite of these unresolved technical reservations, provisional but useful and informative data from a number of studies have already been published over the past five years:

In asthma, airway CT has consistently demonstrated wall thickening compared with normal, with variable results for the airway lumen, although it is signally more heterogeneous in caliber (144,149–151). Acute bronchodilation and bronchoconstriction have been demonstrable (146,152). Wall thickening has been identified even in mild disease and children (144) but in general the degree of wall thickening is related to duration and severity of clinical disease, and also level of airway obstruction (149,153,154). However, and perhaps tellingly, there is no obvious relationship between LA of segmental airways on CT and clinical severity (154).

Some researchers have been able to relate imaged airway wall thickening in asthma to airway hyperresponsiveness (155) but others have not (149), while yet others have suggested that estimated wall thickening protects against induced bronchoconstriction (156). A major problem with such studies is that CT images are unable to differentiate which layer(s) within the airway wall are thickened in any particular individual or condition, and differential changes anatomically inside or outside the smooth muscle layer could potentially be responsible for such variable findings. Vignola et al. (68) reported a significant relationship between elastase levels and MMP-9/TIMP-1 ratio in sputum and airway thickness in asthma and suggested their data demonstrated that biomarkers can reflect remodeling. This may well be true, but thickening of the airway wall on CT scans is also currently unable to differentiate inflammatory/edematous thickening from true remodeling structural changes. Thus, although inhaled corticosteroid (ICS) could be demonstrated to reduce airway thickness (157), this change is unable to separate inflammatory from structural improvement. In this study there was residual thickening after 12 months, which presumably is then indeed largely because of corticosteroid-unresponsive remodeling.

In COPD, although the main physiological defect causing airflow limitation is thought to be at the small airway level, CT scans of airways show thickening of both large and small airways with significant correlation between these regional changes (158). Larger airways are better imaged than small airways, so these relationships are potentially very useful for clinical investigation, that is, CT images of larger airways may give a good assessment of general airway changes. The WA of smokers with COPD is greater than that of smokers without COPD and both are greater than normal although WA is intermediate in COPD between normal and asthma. However, and in contrast to asthma, LA and "normalized" WA (ratio of WA to LA) may be more reflective of airflow limitation than WA itself in COPD (159) perhaps because of the confounding effect of submucosal gland hyperplasia in chronic bronchitis (160). In an earlier study, Nakano et al. (161) found that WA did relate to forced expiratory volume in one second (FEV_1), and low attenuation areas (LAA) in the lung parenchyma to both FEV_1 and diffusing capacity. In this study some individuals with COPD had only WA thickening and some only LAA abnormality suggesting extreme "airway" versus "emphysema" COPD phenotypes. However, it is difficult to know how much of LAA changes reflect emphysema per se, and how much of it is caused by air trapping from small airway disease (162). Whether LAA and a "mosaic" appearance radiologically are as sensitive or specific for early emphysema as a measurement of diffusing capacity or whether these CT changes are potential confounders need clarification, and before CT imaging becomes adopted as any sort of "standard" for emphysema in research studies.

B. Pathophysiological Correlations

The consequences of airway remodeling are reasonably assumed to be airway hyperresponsiveness, which is a pathognomonic feature of asthma but occurring variably in COPD, and fixed (nonbronchodilator responsive airflow limitation) and progressive loss of maximal airflow. This is first observed in small airways and then becomes more generalized; it is pathognomonic of COPD but also common in asthma (32). Some of this discussion, especially relating to clinical airflow obstruction and accelerated loss of airflow, has already been dealt with. Here we will deal mainly with human airway biopsy studies.

The various remodeling and inflammatory changes in the airway wall in these airway diseases are, of course, multiple, probably pathogenetically linked and somewhat inseparable. However, different studies have frequently tried to link just one aspect of pathology, or sometimes more than one, with a particular physiological index but since one change may be a surrogate of another there may be a circular or tautological element to such studies. Dissecting the system so as to give a percentage attribution of more than one pathological change to one or a set of physiological changes has been attempted in a human airway biopsy study, as well as in an animal model, albeit to an inevitably limited extent (43,111,163,164). Ward et al. (163) performed multiple regression analysis of relationships between inflammatory and structural changes in the airway wall and found that 55% of the variability in airway hyperresponsiveness in asthma could be explained on the basis of airway eosinophils, desquamated epithelial cells, and Rbm thickness, with inflammatory changes and remodeling changes contributing about 50% each. This was borne out in a longitudinal intervention study with fluticasone. Generally, confirmatory data were recently published by Southam et al. (111) using an allergic mouse model: early increases in airway responsiveness were associated with inflammation while a later sustained further increase was related to airway fibrosis. Deposition of collagen was related to a surge in TGFβ-1 production. In an earlier mouse study (164), some of the results were similar including a late phase of fibrosis associated with TGFβ-1 upregulation, but airway hyperresponsiveness was related to early acute inflammation only and, indeed, reduced somewhat in the later fibrotic/remodeling phase.

There are a number of endobronchial biopsy pathophysiological correlation studies or remodeling in human volunteers that have included, independently, epithelial changes, Rbm thickening, or airway epithelial hypervascularity in the analysis. By their superficial position in biopsies changes in these layers can be reasonably easily assessed. Almost all such studies have so far been in asthma subjects and, although not completely consistent, there is certainly majority support for airway hyperresponsiveness being significantly associated with epithelial changes and denudation (32,35,44) and Rbm thickening (44,103,165–168). In general, these pathological changes have not been associated with much, if any, derangement in conventional measurement of ventilatory function, that is, FEV_1. Airway hypervascularity in asthma, in contrast, has been associated with airflow obstruction as well as airway hyperresponsiveness (36,84,140,168–170).

In COPD, although the airways are generally less thickened than in asthma it is accepted that it is thickening and obliteration of the small airways that leads to airway obstruction (171). However, these changes may be physiologically subtle for some time in the natural history of the disease and, as emphasized in the last section, there is good evidence that the pathological airway changes in COPD are, in reality, generalized. There is a paucity of studies in COPD using endobronchial biopsies, making it difficult to relate specific changes of remodeling to physiological derangement. Where airway hyperresponsiveness is present it is usually assumed to be secondary to the geometric effect of baseline airway narrowing, though the relationship to remodeling is likely to be considerably more complex than this.

An area of increasing interest, which gives enhanced insights into structure-function relationships, is how the changes in remodeling, and perhaps especially different combinations of ECM (deposition vs. denudation), may lead to relative alterations in normal airway stiffness or collapsibility. The methods for measuring such physiological indices are as yet not fully developed and may be confounded by issues such as heterogeneity of peripheral airway emptying, but do suggest that in asthma at least, the airways are abnormally stiff (172,173). This may be related to reticular basement thickening and be associated with airway hyperresponsivenss (43,163). It has been suggested that the increased stiffness of the airway and factors such as the increased ECM deposition in the airway smooth muscle layer may provide a brake in asthmatics on bronchoconstriction through elastic impedance to muscle contraction, so as to oppose dynamic compression of the airways (32,35). As a result airways in asthma may also be less easy to dilate.

In COPD, on the other hand, the evidence suggests that the airways are more collapsible than normal. This may be why even with less thickened walls compared with asthma the effects of the disease process on the airway lumen and airflow limitation are greater. The influence of inherent cholinergic tone in COPD on airway caliber may, as a result, be exaggerated, perhaps explaining why anticholinergic agents have more clinical success in COPD than in chronic stable asthma. Further investigations are needed in COPD to define the changes in ECM, which could be undermining the mechanical strength of the airways and their resistance to bronchoconstriction. This requires means to directly measure airway stiffness/compliance, and technology is now becoming available to allow this to occur with relative ease (174,175).

Summary: The Physiological Consequences of Remodeling in Asthma Vs. COPD

In asthma, remodeling is associated with thicker and stiffer airway walls but they encroach only minimally on the lumen, at least in mild-to-moderate disease. The airways resist distension and also probably contraction, but when the latter effect is overcome by intense muscle shortening this leads to exaggerated airway narrowing because of the mechanical effect of the expanded tissue mass within the muscle ring, so obliterating the lumen.

In COPD, in contrast, the remodeled thickness (WA) of the airway tends to be less marked than in asthma but encroachment on the airway lumen is relatively greater. Dilatation is restricted but collapsibility is increased. Even effects of normal vagal cholinergic tone are exaggerated on luminal size, and so anticholinergics are especially effective. If emphysema coexists, then loss of supportive lung recoil forces is an added jeopardy to collapsibility.

V. Pharmacology of Airway Remodeling in Asthma and COPD
A. Animal Studies: "Allergic Models"

Because of the design of these studies it is more coherent to review the literature by drug type, while for human studies (next section) we will overview therapies by their effects on each layer of the remodeled airway. We will focus on studies where effects on remodeling have been significant; recent reviews of therapy in remodeling also reviewed negative studies (33,37).

Corticosteroid

Corticosteroid given concurrently with allergen challenge in rats could prevent remodeling changes comprehensively, but timing and high dose were important factors. Changes were not reversed once established. At a lower dose effects were more limited: fibronectin deposition was reduced but not goblet cell hyperplasia or overall airway wall thickness (176,177).

In a mouse model, fluticasone topically to the airway for three months inhibited airway smooth muscle thickening, and decreased elevated TGFβ-1 expression and its intracellular stimulatory signals pSMAD-2 and -3, while upregulating pSMAD-7 (177). In a similar mouse model, dexamethasone given with allergen prevented the observed general increase in laminin in the airways, probably produced by inflammatory cells. Laminin receptors (integrin α6β1) increased on inflammatory and vessel endothelial cells were also downregulated by treatment, but it is difficult to know how much of these changes were primarily antiremodeling, and how much secondary to an anti-inflammatory effect on the cell infiltrate (178). Budesonide also decreased collagen deposition, which was related to inhibition of TGFβ-1, but again there was a wide spectrum of anti-inflammatory effects, as a potential confounder including decrease in eosinophils and TH2 cytokines (179).

β-Agonists
In the rat, adding a long-acting β-agonist to ICS may have the paradoxical effect of increasing rather than decreasing fibronectin deposition (177). Similarly, regular short-acting β-agonist therapy may enhance goblet cell hyperplasia and worsen airway hyperresponsiveness (180), but this was prevented with concomitant corticosteroid. Fortunately, such apparently negative effects of β-agonists in animal models does not seem to translate into negative clinical outcomes in asthma (181), which rather limits their usefulness.

Phosphodiesterase Inhibitors
The selective phosphodiesterase inhibitor PDEI-4, roflumilast, decreased collagen deposition and epithelial thickening in a mouse model (182). There was no effect on TGFβ-1 accumulation in the ECM, which contrasted with the effect of corticosteroid and suggests that PDEIs may work through a different mechanism.

Anticholinergics
Given their widespread use in airway disease, there have been hardly any studies investigating possible effects on airway structure. However, in a guinea-pig ovalbumin allergy model, the long-acting M3-antagonist tiotropium inhibited airway smooth muscle hyperplasia, as well as inhibiting the increased myosin expression and enhanced muscle contractility seen in this model (183). This suggests that allergen challenge may cause changes in airway muscle modulated by vagal cholinergic stimulation.

Leukotriene Modulators
In the mouse, the cysteinyl leukotriene receptor antagonist (LTRA) montelukast somewhat remarkably almost completely abrogated the effects of allergen challenge on muscle hyperplasia and collagen deposition (184). It had a greater effect on remodeling than airway inflammation. In a subsequent mouse allergy study by the same authors, montelukast decreased airway smooth muscle mass and leukotriene receptors and collagen more effectively than corticosteroid (185). At a low dose, montelukast had more effect on goblet cells and fibrosis than airway muscle (186). Leukotrienes seem less important in rat models where LTRA have more modest effects (37). Even so, in a rat allergic asthma model some very interesting comparative data on this system was obtained (122). A LTRA (pranlukast), 5-lipoxygenase inhibition, and a LTB_4 receptor antagonist all attenuated muscle thickness and all but the LTB_4 blocker downregulated muscle DNA synthesis—suggesting that LTB_4 may affect the muscle layer ECM deposition rather than muscle cell hyperplasia. None of the drugs affected the increased epithelial DNA synthesis, nor airway hyperresponsiveness seen in the model, although all three agents had an antieosinophilic action. These data suggest that hyper-responsiveness in the allergic mouse is more related to remodeling than inflammation, but leukotrienes seem involved in both processes.

Chromones

In the rat, nedocromil was more effective than an LTRA on airway smooth muscle remodeling (187).

Immunostimulatory Sequences—Oligodeoxynucleotides

These methylated DNA sequences are rich in CpG dinucleotides and have flanking palindromic nucleotide sequences, which together simulate microbial DNA. They activate Toll-like receptor-9. They are anti-TH2 cytokine production, and pro-TH1 cytokines. There is evidence that such sequences can act in both primary prevention and secondary suppression of remodeling in mouse allergy/asthma models (collagen deposition, mucus production, muscle thickening, myofibroblast accumulation, and also TGFβ-1 production) (188,189), and are also effective in the monkey (epithelial and Rbm thickening) (37,190).

Anti-TGFβ-1 Neutralizing Antibodies

Given the potential importance of TGFβ-1 as a growth factor for driving remodeling, these studies are of crucial interest. However, the outcomes have been contradictory and confusing, which perhaps puts into perspective the usefulness of animal models: they should be best regarded as raising hypotheses for testing in human clinical studies but can never be definitive.

McMillan et al. (191) initially seemed to confirm the centrality of TGFβ-1. They suggested apparently convincingly that TGFβ-1 suppression during the chronic allergen challenge phase in their mouse model substantially inhibited remodeling of airway smooth muscle, fibrosis, and goblet cell hyperplasia. There was no effect on TH2 cytokines or inflammatory cell infiltration. TGFβ-1 receptors and SMAD signaling pathways were downregulated. However, subsequent studies from other laboratories with similar mouse models have suggested: a different source for TGFβ-1 (epithelium and not inflammatory cells), with no effect on fibrosis or inflammation but a paradoxical increase in airway hyperresponsiveness (192), or even more paraxodically that anti-TGFβ-1 antibodies cause no change in remodeling but increases in eosinophilic inflammation as well as an increase in airway hyperresponsiveness (193). To make matters even more uncertain, a study using pirfenidone as an antifibrotic agent in sensitized allergen challenged mice, apparently working through TGFβ-1 inhibition, suppressed all aspects of asthma-type pathology both inflammatory and remodeling (194).

All the animal studies on therapy of remodeling that we are aware of are relevant only to asthma. There seems to have been a paucity of corresponding work focusing primarily on COPD models.

B. Human Airway Biopsy Studies

Epithelium

Studies consistent with the "EMU" hypothesis have suggested that epithelial receptor activation and enhanced epithelial cell tumor in asthma are not corticosteroid responsive (195,196). In marked contrast, there are corticosteroid intervention studies that demonstrated resolution of epithelial friability (43) and long-term follow-up clinical studies showing restoration of normal epithelial structure with corticosteroid therapy (197,198).

Rbm Thickening and the ECM

Short-term oral corticosteroid for two weeks did not affect airway collagen or TGFβ deposition in asthma although it did suppress two other potential pro-remodeling cytokines, IL-11 and IL-17 (199). However, elevated tenascin deposition below the true basement membrane was decreased by just six weeks or less of medium-dose budesonide (200). Sont et al. in the AMPUL study (201) showed that Rbm thickening was decreased by "optimizing" inhaled steroid therapy titrated against airway hyperresponsiveness rather than symptoms—thus needing higher doses than would otherwise have been conventional. It does seem that long and aggressive therapy may be required to reverse this asthma hallmark Rbm remodeling change. Using such a strategy, our group showed that with 2000 μg of fluticasone per day, it took more than three months, possibly as much as 12 months, to obtain normalization of Rbm thickening even in relatively mild (but symptomatic) asthma (43,163). These studies also allowed some "dissection' of the effects of corticosteroid on methacholine airway hyperresponsiveness, with inflammation (and possibly other changes such as hypervascularity) contributing about 50% and Rbm thickness (and perhaps other unmeasured related changes) the rest.

A two-week placebo controlled study of lower dose ICS (budesonide) 400 μg per day, given with five times per week low-dose allergen challenge in allergic asthma subjects, focused on proteoglycan changes in the lamina propria. At baseline in asthma, there was a suggestive increase in biglycan and decrease in decorin. In the steroid limb, biglycan and versican seemed to increase, probably irrespective of the allergen challenges, that is, as an effect of the budesonide, but the number of individuals involved was small and the data rather variable, so firm conclusions are difficult to draw (202).

The LTRA montelukast for two weeks may have had a beneficial effect on accumulation of subepithelial myofibroblasts after allergen challenge in mild allergic asthma, but the data were neither biologically nor statistically strong or compelling (203). Regular short-acting β-agonist over 12 months decreased tenascin density in the subepithelial ECM condensation (204).

There have been very few clinical studies in asthma involving immune or cytokine modulation, at least with remodeling outcomes. An exception was the study by Flood-Page et al. (205) using anti-IL-5 monoclonal antibody therapy. There was a decrease in airway eosinophils by about 50%, but also decreased Rbm tenascin, lumicam, and procollagen III staining in airway biopsies. There was accompanying decreased BAL TGFβ-1 levels and eosinophil TGFβ-1 mRNA expression. However, there was no obvious clinical benefit that puts the relevance of these changes into doubt.

Blood Vessels

A number of intervention studies have indicated that airway hypervascularity in asthmatic airways can be downregulated by ICS therapy (206,207). Again initial data suggested that relatively high doses and/or protracted periods of therapy may be required for effect (206,208), but the antivascular dose of corticosteroid may be less if a long-acting β-agonist is used in combination (209). The study by Hoshino et al. (207) indicated that the decrease in vascularity was proportional to improvement in FEV_1 and hyperresponsiveness. However, the change in vessels was also related to thinning of Rbm, so it is not completely clear from the study which aspect of remodeling was physiologically most relevant.

Using again a high dose of fluticasone, our group recently showed that hyper-vascularity in asthma lamina propria resolved in a shorter time scale than Rbm thickening (210). Furthermore, there was a decrease in VEGF staining in biopsies and a normalization of the VEGF receptor system. Elevated BAL VEGF levels did not fall, however, but there was loss of the close statistical relationship between BAL VEGF and vessel numbers found in untreated asthma. It was suggested that the BAL VEGF may reflect an exit system for removing VEGF from the airways, and that this may have been enhanced by corticosteroid. Newly described angiogenic sprouts in the vessel walls were markedly decreased with therapy (210).

Immunomodulation

In addition to the anti-IL-5 study already mentioned (205), the only other relevant published study of cytokine manipulation we are aware of in humans that had a possible effect on remodeling used an intravenous soluble TNFα receptor (TNF-antagonist). In severe asthma patients airway hyperresponsiveness was ameliorated but without anti-inflammatory changes (211). Whether the effect observed on responsiveness was at the level of remodeling changes needs further directed investigation.

C. Human Airway Biopsy Studies—COPD and BOS

As yet, there are few data available from therapeutic studies on remodeling in COPD. Some lessons, however, can probably be learned from BOS, thought to be a manifestation of chronic lung rejection post–lung transplantation. This shares a number of pathological similarities to COPD, albeit with a more subacute time scale of progression (212).

Uncontrolled trials of azithromycin have shown a reversal of BOS in some patients, essentially the only agent shown to do so (213), probably through an anti-neutrophil system effect (214).

It is increasingly recognized that statins are more than simply lipid-lowering agents. They seem to possess wide-ranging anti-inflammatory effects including anti-neutrophil effects and a lowering of C-reactive protein in COPD, accompanied by a lowering of all-cause mortality. The six-year survival of lung transplant recipients taking simvastatin was 90% compared with 50% in control patients (215). Statins have recently been shown to reduce the annual decline in smoking-related lung function loss (216), possibly through an effect on airway remodeling, as simvastatin can decrease the stimulated release of IL-8 and MMPs from bronchial epithelial cells (217). Such an attenuation of MMP-2 and MMP-9 production from epithelial cells in vivo would be consistent with attenuation of the process known as epithelial-mesenchymal transition, in which epithelial cells become myofibroblasts under the influence of TGFβ-1. This has been described in the airways of the transplanted lung (218).

VI. Conclusions

We have reviewed the biology, physiology, and clinical relevance of airway remodeling, especially in asthma where most data have been collected. There are both differences and similarities in remodeling in COPD compared with asthma and in both airways are thickened. However, physiologically remodeling in COPD may be the "mirror image" of asthma with decreased rather than increased airway wall stiffness. Consequences of remodeling on airflow are, if anything, more profound in COPD. New physiology measuring methods are now close to unlocking a great deal more understanding of these issues.

Most of the commonly used medications in airway disease have effects on remodeling, although they are relatively understudied in this context, and especially in COPD. We have nominated TGFβ-1 and VEGF as particular mediators of strategic interest in remodeling and clinical studies directed against these agents are urgently needed in chronic airway disease. Given its apparently remarkable anti-asthma actions in animal studies (194), a study of pirfenidone in asthma (and COPD) is now indicated.

References

1. Van Eerdewegh P, Little RD, Dupuis J, et al. Association of the ADAM 33 gene with asthma and bronchial hyperresponsiveness. Nature 2002; 418:426–430.
2. Jongepier H, Boezen HM, Dijkstra A, et al. Polymorphisms of the ADAM 33 gene are associated with accelerated lung function decline in asthma. Clin Exp Allergy 2004; 150: 629–634.
3. Roche WR, Beasley R, Williams JH, et al. Subepithelial fibrosis in the bronchi of asthmatics. Lancet 1989; 1:520–524.
4. Saetta M, DiStefano A, Maestrelli P, et al. Airway mucosal inflammation in occupational asthma induced by toluene diisocyanate. Am Rev Respir Dis 1992; 145:160–168.
5. Djukanovic R, Lai CK, Wilson JW, et al. Bronchial mucosal manifestations of atopy: asthmatics, atopic non-asthmatics and healthy controls. Eur Respir J 1992; 5:538–544.
6. Chakir J, Laviolette M, Boutet M, et al. Lower airways remodelling in non-asthmatic subjects with allergic rhinitis. Lab Invest 1996; 75:735–744.
7. Laprise C, Boulet LP. Asymptomatic airway hyperresponsiveness: a three year follow-up. Am J Respir Crit Care Med 1997; 156:403–409.
8. Payne DN, Rogers AV, Adelroth E, et al. Early thickening of the reticular basement membrane in children with difficult asthma. Am J Respir Crit Care Med 2003; 167:78–82.
9. Warner JO, Pohunek P, Marguet C, et al. Progression from allergic sensitization to asthma. Pediatric Allergy Immunol 2000; 11(suppl 13):12–14.
10. Pohunek P, Warner JO, Turzikova J, et al. Markers of eosinophilic inflammation and tissue remodelling in children before clinically diagnosed bronchial asthma. Pediatr Allergy Immunol 2005; 16:43–51.
11. Saglani S, Malmstrom K, Pelkonen AS, et al. Airway remodelling and inflammation in symptomatic infants with reversible airflow obstruction. Am J Respir Crit Care Med 2005; 171: 722–727.
12. Rasmussen F, Taylor DR, Flannery EM, et al. Risk factors for airway remodelling in asthma manifested by a low post bronchodilator FEV1/vital capacity ratio: a longitudinal population study from childhood to adulthood. Am J Respir Crit Care Med 2002; 165:1480–1488.
13. Phelan PD, Robertson CF, Olinksy A. The Melbourne Asthma Study: 1964–1999. J Allergy Clin Immunol 2002; 109:189–194.
14. James AL, Palmer LJ, Kicic E, et al. Decline in lung function in the Busselton health study: the effects of asthma and cigarette smoking. Am J Respir Crit Care Med 2005; 171:109–114.
15. Hogg JC, Macklem PT, Thurlbeck WM. Site and nature of airway obstruction in chronic obstructive lung disease. N Engl J Med 1968; 278:1355–1360.
16. O'Connor GT, Sparrow D, Weiss ST. A prospective longitudinal study of methacholine airway responsiveness as a predictor of pulmonary-function decline: the Normative Ageing Study. Am J Respir Crit Care Med 1995; 152:87–92.
17. Tracey M, Villar A, Dow L, et al. The influence of increased bronchial responsiveness, atopy and serum IgE on decline in FEV1. A longitudinal study in the elderly. Am J Respir Crit Care Med 1995; 151:656–662.
18. Rijcken B, Schouten JP, Xu X, et al. Airway hyperresponsiveness to histamine associated with accelerated decline in FEV1. Am J Respir Crit Care Med 1995; 151:1377–1382.

19. Seemungal TA, Donaldson GC, Bhowmik A, et al. Time course and recovery of exacerbations in patients with chronic obstructive pulmonary disease. Am J Respir Crit Care Med 2000; 161:1608–1613.
20. Donaldson GC, Seemungal TA, Patel IS, et al. Airway and systemic inflammation and decline in lung function in patients with COPD. Chest 2005; 128:1995–2004.
21. Lange P, Parner J, Vestbo J, et al. A 15 year follow-up study of ventilatory function in adults with asthma. N Engl J Med 1998; 339:1194–1200.
22. Peat JK, Woolcock AJ, Cullen K. Decline of lung function and development of chronic airflow limitation: a longitudinal study of non-smokers and smokers in Busselton, Western Australia. Thorax 1990; 45, 32–37.
23. Ulrik CS, Lange P. Decline of lung function in adults with bronchial asthma. Am J Respir Crit Care Med 1994; 150:629–634.
24. Ulrik CS. Outcome of asthma: longitudinal changes in lung function. Eur Respir J 1999; 13: 904–918.
25. ten Brinke A, Zwinderman AH, Sterk PJ, et al. Factors associated with persistent airflow limitation in severe asthma. Am J Respir Crit Care Med 2001; 164:744–748.
26. Vonk JM, Jongepier H, Panhuysen CI, et al. Risk factors associated with the presence of irreversible airflow limitation and reduced transfer coefficient in patients with asthma after 26 years of follow-up. Thorax 2003; 58:322–327.
27. ten Brinke A, Zwinderman AH, Sterk PJ, et al. "Refractory" eosinophilic airway inflammation in severe asthma: effect of parentaeral corticosteroids. Am J Respir Crit Care Med 2004; 170:601–605.
28. Stachan DP, Butland BK, Anderson HR. Incidence and prognosis of asthma and wheezing illness from early childhood to age 33 in a national British cohort. BMJ 1996; 312:1195–1199.
29. Brown PJ, Greville HW, Finucane KE. Asthma and irreversible airflow obstruction. Thorax 1984; 39:131–136.
30. Covar RA, Spahn JD, Murphy JR, et al. Progression of asthma measured by lung function in the childhood asthma management program. Am J Respir Crit Care Med 2004; 170:234–241.
31. Boulet LP, Sterk PJ. Airway remodelling: the future. Eur Respir J 2007; 30:831–834.
32. Tang ML, Wilson JW, Stewart AG, et al. Airway remodelling in asthma: current understanding and implications for future therapies. Pharmacol Ther 2006; 112:474–488.
33. Mauad T, Bel EH, Sterk PJ. Asthma therapy and airway remodeling. J Allergy Clin Immunol 2007; 120:997–1009.
34. Fixman ED, Stewart A, Martin JG. Basic mechanisms of development of airway structural changes in asthma. Eur Respir J 2007; 29:379–389.
35. James AL, Wenzel S. Clinical relevance of airway remodelling in airway diseases. Eur Respir J 2007; 30:134–155.
36. Walters EH, Soltani A, Reid DW, et al. Vascular remodelling in asthma. Curr Opin Allergy Clin Immunol 2008; 8:39–43.
37. Walters EH, Reid DW, Johns DP, et al. Non pharmacological and pharmacological interventions to prevent or reduce airway remodelling. Eur Respir J 2007; 30:574–588.
38. Carroll N, Elliot J, Morton A, et al. The structure of large and small airways in non-fatal and fatal asthma. Am Rev Respir Dis 1993; 147:405–410.
39. Ordonez CL, Khashayar R, Wong HH, et al. Mild and moderate asthma is associated with airway goblet cell hyperplasia and abnormalities in mucin gene expression. Am J Respir Crit Care Med 2001; 163:517–523.
40. Aikawa T, Shimura S, Sasaki H, et al. Marked goblet cell hyperplasia with mucus accumulation in the airways of patients who died of severe acute asthma attack. Chest 1992; 101: 916–921.
41. James AL, Elliot JG, Abramson MJ, et al. Time to death, airway wall inflammation and remodeling in fatal asthma. Eur Respir J 2005; 26:429–434.

42. Kuyper LM, Pare PD, Hogg JC, et al. Characterization of airway plugging in fatal asthma. Am J Med 2003; 115:6–11.

43. Ward C, Pais M, Bish R, et al. Airway inflammation, basement membrane thickening and bronchial hyperresponsiveness in asthma. Thorax 2002; 57:309–316.

44. Jeffery PK, Wardlaw AJ, Nelson FC, et al. Bronchial biopsies in asthma. An ultrastructural, quantitative study and correlation with hyperreactivity. Am Rev Respir Dis 1989; 140:1745–1753.

45. Knight DA, Holgate ST. The airway epithelium: Structural and functional properties in health and disease. Respirology 2003; 8:432–446.

46. Shahana S, Bjornsson E, Ludviksdottir D, et al. Ultrastructure of bronchial biopsies from patients with allergic and non-allergic asthma. Respir Med 2005; 99:429–443.

47. Saetta M, Turato G, Baraldo S, et al. Goblet cell hyperplasia and epithelial inflammation in peripheral airways of smokers with both symptoms of chronic bronchitis and chronic airflow limitation. Am J Respir Crit Care Med 2000; 161:1016–1021.

48. Reid L. Measurement of the bronchial mucous gland layer: a diagnostic yardstick in chronic bronchitis. Thorax 1960; 15:132–141.

49. Mullen JB, Wright JL, Wiggs BR, et al. Reassessment of inflammation of airways in chronic bronchitis. BMJ 1985; 291:1235–1239.

50. Saetta M, Turato G, Facchini FM, et al. Inflammatory cells in the bronchial glands of smokers with chronic bronchitis. Am J Respir Crit Care Med 1997; 156:1633–1639.

51. Merker HJ. Morphology of the basement membrane. Microsc Res Tech 1994; 28:95–124.

52. Huber H, Koessler KK. The pathology of bronchial asthma. Arch Intern Med 1992; 30: 689–760.

53. Houston JC, De Navasquez S, Trounce JR. A clinical and pathological study of fatal cases of status asthmaticus. Thorax 1953; 8:207–213.

54. Huang J, Olivenstein R, Taha R, et al. Enhanced proteoglycan deposition in the airway wall of atopic athmatics. Am J Respir Crit Care Med 1999; 160:725–729.

55. de Medeiros Matsushita M, da Silva LF, dos Santos MA, et al. Airway proteoglycans are differentially altered in fatal asthma. J Pathol 2005; 207:102–110.

56. Bousquet J, Lacoste JY, Chanez P, et al. Bronchial elastic fibres in normal subjects and asthmatic patients. Am J Respir Crit Care Med 1996; 153:1648–1654.

57. Wilson JW, Li X. The measurement of reticular basement membrane and submucosal collagen in the asthmatic airway. Clin Exp Allergy 1997; 27:363–371.

58. James AL, Maxwell PS, Pearce-Pinto G, et al. The relationship of reticular basement membrane thickness to airway wall remodeling in asthma. Am J Respir Crit Care Med 2001; 166:1590–1595.

59. Kasahara K, Shiba K, Ozawa T, et al. Correlation between the bronchial subepithelial layer and whole airway wall thickness in patients with asthma. Thorax 2002; 57:242–246.

60. Brewster CE, Howarth PH, Djukanvic R, et al. Myofibroblasts and subepithelial fibrosis in bronchial asthma. Am J Respir Cell Mol Biol 1990; 3:507–511.

61. Gizycki MJ, Adelroth E, Rogers AV, et al. Myofibroblast involvement in the allergen-induced late response in mild atopic asthma. Am J Respir Cell Mol Biol 1997; 16:664–673.

62. Shoji S, Rickard KA, Ertl RF, et al. Bronchial epithelial cells produce lung fibroblast chemotactic factor: fibronectin. Am J Respir Cell Mol Biol 1989; 1:13–20.

63. Lobb RR, Pepinsky B, Leone DR, et al. The role of alpha4 integrins in lung pathophysiology. Eur Respir J 1996; (suppl 22):104–108.

64. Meerschaert J, Kelly EA, Mosher DF, et al. Segmental allergen challenge increases fibronectin in bronchoalveolar lavage fluid. Am J Respir Crit Care Med 1999; 159:619–625.

65. Lee YC, Lee HB, Rhee YK, et al. The involvement of matrix metalloproteinase-9 in airway inflammation of patients with acute asthma. Clin Exp Allergy 2001; 31:1623–1630.

66. Ohbayashi H, Shimokata K. Matrix metalloproteinase-9 and airway remodeling in asthma. Curr Drug Targets Inflamm Allergy 2005; 4:177–181.

67. Mautino G, Henriquet C, Jaffuel D, et al. Tissue inhibitor of metalloproteinase-1 levels in bronchoalveolar lavage fluid from asthmatic subjects. Am J Respir Crit Care Med 1999,160:324–330.

68. Vignola AM, Paganin F, Capieu L, et al. Airway remodelling assessed by sputum and high-resolution computed tomography in asthma and COPD. Eur Respir J 2004; 24:910–917.

69. Matsumoto H, Niimi A, Takemura M, et al. Relationship of airway wall thickening to an imbalance between matrix metalloproteinase-9 and its inhibitor in asthma. Thorax 2005; 60: 277–281.

70. Cataldo DD, Bettiol J, Noel A, et al. Matrix metalloproteinase-9, but not tissue inhibitor of matrix metalloproteinase-1, increases in sputum from allergic asthmatic patients after allergen challenge. Chest 2002; 122:1553–1559.

71. Cataldo DD, Tournoy KG, Vermaelen K, et al. Matrix metalloproteinase-9 deficiency impairs cellular infiltration and bronchial hyperresponsiveness during allergen-induced airway inflammation. Am J Pathol 2002; 161:491–498.

72. Tanaka H, Miyazaki N, Oashi K, et al. Sputum matrix metalloproteinase-9: tissue inhibitor of metalloproteinase-1 ratio in acute asthma. J Allergy Clin Immunol 2000; 105:900–905.

73. James AL. Relationship between airway wall thickness and airway hyperresponsiveness. In: Stewart AG, ed. Airway Wall Remodelling in Asthma. New York: CRC Press Inc, 1997: 1–28.

74. Heard BE, Hossain S. Hyperplasia of bronchial muscle in asthma. J Pathol 1973; 110: 319–331.

75. Ebina M, Takahashi T, Chiba T, et al. Cellular hypertrophy and hyperplasia or airway smooth muscle underlying bronchial asthma. A 3-D morphometric study. Am Rev Respir Dis 1993; 148:720–726.

76. Woodruff PG, Dolganov GM, Ferrando RE, et al. Hyperplasia of smooth muscle in mild to moderate asthma without changes in cell size or gene expression. Am J Respir Crit Care Med 2004; 169:1001–1006.

77. Johnson PR, Roth M, Tamm M, et al. Airway smooth muscle cell proliferation is increased in asthma. Am J Respir Crit Care Med 2001; 164:474–477.

78. Thomson RJ, Bramley AM, Schellenberg RR. Airway muscle stereology: implications for increased shortening in asthma. Am J Respir Crit Care Med 1996; 154:749–757.

79. Panettieri RA. Airway smooth muscle: an immunomodulatory cell. J Allergy Clin Immunol 2002; 110(suppl 6):269–274.

80. Hakonarson H, Maskeri N, Carter C, et al. Regulation of TH1- and TH2-type cytokine expression and action in atopic asthmatic sensitized airway smooth muscle. J Clin Invest 1999; 103:1077–1087.

81. Johnson PR. Role of human airway smooth muscle in altered extracellular matrix production in asthma. Clin Exp Pharmacol Physiol 2001; 28:233–236.

82. Dunnill MS, Massarella GR, Anderson JA. A comparison of the quantitative anatomy of the bronchi in normal subjects, in status asthmatics, in chronic bronchitis, and in emphysema. Thorax 1969; 24:176–179.

83. Kuwano K, Bosken CH, Pare PD, et al. Small airways dimensions in asthma and in chronic obstructive pulmonary disease. Am Rev Respir Dis 1993; 148:1220–1225.

84. Walters EH, Reid D, Soltani A, et al. Angiogenesis: a potentially critical part of remodelling in chronic airway diseases? Pharmacol Ther 2008; 118:128–137.

85. Dunnill MS. The pathology of asthma, with special reference to changes in the bronchial mucosa. J Clin Pathol 1960; 13:27–33.

86. Charan NB, Baile EM, Pare PD. Bronchial vascular congestion and angiogenesis. Eur Respir J 1997; 10:1173–1180.

87. Li X, Wilson JW. Increased vascularity in the bronchial mucosa in mild asthma. Am J Respir Crit Care Med 1997; 156:229–233.

88. Hoshino M, Takahashi M, Aoike N. Expression of vascular endothelial growth factor, basic fibroblast growth factor, and angiogenin immunoreactivity in asthmatic airways and its relationship to angiogenesis. J Allergy Clin Immunol 2001; 107:295–301.

89. Hoshino M, Nakamura Y, Hamid QA. Gene expression of vascular endothelial growth factor and its receptors and angiogenesis in bronchial asthma. J Allergy Clin Immunol 2001; 107:1034–1038.

90. Gilbert IA, Winslow CJ, Lenner KA, et al. Vascular volume expansion and thermally induced asthma. Eur Respir J 1993; 6:189–197.

91. Mitzner W, Wagner E, Browns RH. Is asthma a vascular disorder? Chest 1995; 107(suppl 3): 97–102.

92. Moreno RH, Hogg JC, Pare PD. Mechanics of airway narrowing. Am Rev Respir Dis 1986; 133:1171–1180.

93. Hogg JC, Pare PD, Moreno R. The effect of submucosal oedema in airway resistance. Am Rev Respir Dis 1987; 135:S54–S56.

94. James AL, Pare PD, Hogg JC. The mechanics of airway narrowing in asthma. Am Rev Respir Dis 1989; 139:242–246.

95. Salvato G. Quantitative and morphological analysis of the vascular bed in bronchial biopsy specimens from asthmatic and non-asthmatic subjects. Thorax 2001; 56:902–906.

96. Hiroshima K, Iyoda A, Shibuya K, et al. Evidence of neoangiogenesis and an increase in the number of proliferating cells within the bronchial epithelium of smokers. Cancer 2002; 95: 1539–1545.

97. Hashimoto M, Tanaka H, Abe S. Quantitative analysis of bronchial wall vascularity in the medium and small airways of patients with asthma and COPD. Chest 2005; 127:965–972.

98. Calabrese C, Bocchino V, Vatrella A, et al. Evidence of angiogenesis in bronchial biopsies of smokers with and without airway obstruction. Respir Med 2006; 100:1415–1422.

99. James AL, Pare PD, Moreno RH, et al. Quantitative measurement of smooth muscle shortening in isolated pig trachea. J Appl Physiol 1987; 63:1360–1365.

100. Hogg JC, Eggleston PA. Is asthma an epithelial disease? Am Rev Respir Dis 1984; 129: 207–208.

101. Comhair SA, Xu W, Ghosh S, et al. Superoxide dismutase inactivation in pathophysiology of asthmatic airway remodeling and reactivity. Am J Pathol 2005; 166:663–674.

102. Holgate ST, Holloway J, Wilson S, et al. Epithelial-mesenchymal communication in the pathogenesis of chronic asthma. Proc Am Thorac Soc 2004; 1:93–98.

103. Holgate S, Lackie P, Davies DE, et al. The bronchial epithelium as a key regulator of airway inflammation and remodeling in asthma. Clin Exp Allergy 1999; 29:90.

104. Holgate ST. Genetic and environmental interaction in allergy and asthma. J Allergy Clin Immunol 1999; 104:1139–1146.

105. Magnan A, Retornaz F, Tsicopoulos A, et al. Altered compartimentalization of transforming growth factor-β in asthmatic airways. Clin Exp Allergy 1997; 27:389–395.

106. Shepherd D. Airway epithelial integrins: why so many? Am J Respir Cell Mol Biol 1998; 19: 349–351.

107. Knight D. Epithelium-fibroblast interactions in response to airway inflammation. Immunol Cell Biol 2001; 79:160–164.

108. Minshall E, Chakir J, Laviolette M, et al. IL-11 expression is increased in severe asthma: association with epithelial cells and eosinophils. J Allergy Clin Immunol 2000; 105:232–238.

109. Hoshino M, Takahashi M, Takai Y, et al. Inhaled corticosteroids decrease subepithelial collagen deposition by modulation of the balance between matrix metalloproteinase-9 and tissue inhibitor of metalloproteinase-1 expression in asthma. J Allergy Clin Immunol 1999; 104:356–363.

110. Kumar RK, Herbert C, Foster PS. Expression of growth factors by airway epithelial cells in a model of chronic asthma: regulation and relationship to subepithelial fibrosis. Clin Exp Allergy 2004; 34:567–575.

111. Southam DS, Ellis R, Wattie J, et al. Components of airway hyperresponsivness and their associations with inflammation and remodeling in mice. J Allergy Clin Immunol 2007; 119:848–854.

112. Stewart AG, Tomlinson PR, Fernandes DJ, et al. Tumour necrosis factor alpha modulates mitogenic responses of human cultured airway smooth muscle. Am J Respir Cell Mol Biol 1995; 12:110–119.

113. Hirst SJ, Twort CH, Lee TH, et al. Differential effects of extracellular matrix proteins on human airway smooth muscle cell proliferation and phenotype. Am J Respir Cell Mol Biol 2000; 23:335–344.

114. Lee SY, Kim JS, Lee JM, et al. Inhaled corticosteroid prevents the thickening of airway smooth muscle in murine model of chronic asthma. Pulm Pharmacol Ther 2008; 21:14–19.

115. Lazaar AL, Albelda SM, Pilewski JM, et al. T lymphocytes adhere to airway smooth muscle cells via integrins and CD44 and induce smooth muscle cell DNA synthesis. J Exp Med 1994; 180:807–816.

116. Ramos-Barbon D, Presley JF, Hamid QA, et al. Antigen-specific CD4+ T cells drive airway smooth muscle remodeling in experimental asthma. J Clin Invest 2005; 115:1580–1589.

117. Cho JY, Miller M, Baek KJ, et al. Inhibition of airway remodeling in IL-5-deficient mice. J Clin Invest 2004; 113:551–560.

118. Leigh R, Ellis R, Wattie JN, et al. Type 2 cytokines in the pathogenesis of sustained airway dysfunction and airway remodeling in mice. Am J Respir Crit Care Med 2004; 169: 860–867.

119. Tang W, Geba GP, Zheng T, et al. Targeted expression of IL-11 in the murine airway causes lymphocytic inflammation, bronchial remodeling and airway obstruction. J Clin Invest 1996; 98:2845–2853.

120. Molet S, Hamid Q, Davoine F, et al. IL-17 is increased in asthmatic airways and induces human bronchial fibroblasts to produce cytokines. J Allergy Clin Immunol 2001; 108:430–438.

121. Salmon M, Liu YC, Mak JC, et al. Contribution of upregulated airway endothelin-1 expression to airway smooth muscle and epithelial cell DNA synthesis after repeated allergen exposure of sensitized Brown-Norway rats. Am J Respir Cell Mol Biol 2000; 23:618–625.

122. Salmon M, Walsh DA, Huang TJ, et al. Involvement of cysteinyl leukotrienes in airway smooth muscle cell DNA synthesis after repeated allergen exposure in sensitized Brown Norway rats. Br J Pharmacol 1999; 127:1151–1158.

123. Brightling CE, Bradding P, Symon FA, et al. Mast-cell infiltration of airway smooth muscle in asthma. N Engl J Med 2002; 346:1699–1705.

124. Brightling CE, Symon FA, Holgate ST, et al. Interleukin-4 and -13 expression is co-localised to mast cells within the airway smooth muscle in asthma. Clin Exp Allergy 2003; 33:1711–1716.

125. Johnson PR, Burgess JK, Underwood PA, et al. Extracellular matrix proteins modulate asthmatic airway smooth muscle cell proliferation via an autocrine mechanism. J Allergy Clin Immunol 2004; 113:690–696.

126. Akers IA, Parsons M, Hill MR, et al. Mast cell tryptase stimulates human lung fibroblast proliferation via protease-activated receptor-2. Am J Physiol Lung Cell Mol Physiol 2000; 278:L193–L201.

127. Cho SH, Tam SW, Demissie-Sanders S, et al. Production of plasminogen activator inhibitor-1 by human mast cells and its possible role in asthma. J Immunol 2000; 165:3154–3161.

128. Oh CK, Ariue B, Alban RF, et al. PAI-1 promotes extracellular matrix deposition in the airways of a murine asthma model. Biochem Biophys Res Commun 2002; 294:1155–1160.

129. Minshall EM, Leung DY, Martin RJ, et al. Eosinophil-associated TGF-β1 mRNA expression and airways fibrosis in bronchial asthma. Am J Respir Cell Mol Biol 1997; 17:326–333.
130. Humbles AA, Lloyd CM, McMillan SJ, et al. A critical role for eosinophils in allergic airways remodeling. Science 2004; 305:1776–1779.
131. Chetta A, Zanini A, Foresi A, et al. Vascular endothelial growth factor up-regulation and bronchial wall remodelling in asthma. Clin Exp Allergy 2005; 35:1437–1442.
132. Feltis BN, Wignarajah D, Zheng L, et al. Increased vascular endothelial growth factor and receptors: relation to angiogenesis in asthma. Am J Respir Crit Care Med 2006; 173: 1201–1207.
133. Alagappan VK, McKay S, Widyastuti A, et al. Pro-inflammatory cytokines upregulate mRNA expression and secretion of vascular endothelial growth factor in cultured human airway smooth muscle cells. Cell Biochem Biophys 2005; 43:119–129.
134. Kanazawa A, Asai K, Hirata K, et al. Possible effects of vascular endothelial growth factor in the pathogenesis of chronic obstructive pulmonary disease. Am J Med 2003; 114:354–358.
135. Kranenburg AR, de Boer WI, Alagappan VKT, et al. Enhanced bronchial expression of vascular endothelial growth factor and receptors (Flk-1 and Flt-1) in patients with chronic obstructive pulmonary disease. Thorax 2005; 60:106–113.
136. Elias JA, Lee CG, Zheng T, et al. New insights into the pathogenesis of asthma. J Clin Invest 2003; 111:291–297.
137. Wills-Karp M, Chiaramonte M. Interleukin-13 in asthma. Curr Opin Pulm Med 2003; 9:21–27.
138. Lee JJ, Dimina D, Macias MP, et al. Defining a link with asthma in mice congenitally deficient in eosinophils. Science 2004; 305:1773–1776.
139. Kenyon NJ, Ward RW, McGrew G, et al. TGF-beta 1 causes airway fibrosis and increased collagen I and III mRNA in mice. Thorax 2003; 58:772–777.
140. Postma DS, Timens W. Remodeling in asthma and chronic obstructive pulmonary disease. Proc Am Thorac Soc 2006; 3:434–439.
141. Lee CG, Link H, Baluk P, et al. Vascular endothelial growth factor (VEGF) induces remodeling and enhances TH2–mediated sensitization and inflammation in the lung. Nat Med 2004; 10:1095–1103.
142. Seneterre E, Paganin F, Bruel JM, et al. Measurement of the internal size of bronchi using high resolution computed tomography (HRCT). Eur Respir J 1994; 7:596–600.
143. Bankier AA, Fleischmann D, Mallek R, et al. Bronchial wall thickness: appropriate window settings for thin-section CT and radiologic-anatomic correlation. Radiology 1996; 199:831–836.
144. de Jong PA, Muller NL, Pare PD, et al. Computed tomographic imaging of the airways: relationship to structure and function. Eur Respir J 2005; 26:140–152.
145. Brillet PY, Fetita CI, Beigelman-Aubry C, et al. Quantification of bronchial dimensions at MDCT using dedicated software. Eur Radiol 2007; 17:1483–1489.
146. Beigelman-Aubry C, Capderou A, Grenier PA, et al. Mild intermittent asthma CT assessment of bronchial cross-sectional area and lung attenuation at controlled lung volume. Radiology 2002; 223:181–187.
147. Mayo JR, Aldrich J, Muller NL. Radiation exposure at chest CT: a statement of the Fleischner Society. Radiology 2003; 228:15–21.
148. Bergeron C, Tulic MK, Hamid Q. Tools used to measure airway remodelling in research. Eur Respir J 2007; 29:596–604.
149. Little SA, Sproule MW, Cowan MD, et al. High resolution computed tomographic assessment of airway wall thickness in chronic asthma: reproducibility and relationship with lung function and severity. Thorax 2002; 57:247–253.
150. Silva CI, Colby TV, Muller NL. Asthma and associated conditions high resolution CT and pathologic findings. Am J Roentgenol 2004; 183:817–824.
151. King GG, Carroll JD, Muller NL, et al. Heterogeneity of narrowing in normal and asthmatic airways measured by HRCT. Eur Respir J 2004; 24:211–218.

152. Goldin JG, McNitt-Gray MF, Sorenson SM, et al. Airway hyperreactivity: assessment with helical thin-section CT. Radiology 1998; 208:321–329.
153. Awadh N, Muller NL, Park CS, et al. Airway wall thickness in patients with near fatal asthma with or without fixed airflow obstruction. Thorax 1998; 53:248–253.
154. Niimi A, Matsumoto H, Amitani R, et al. Airway wall thickness in asthma assessed by computed tomography. Relation to clinical studies. Am J Respir Crit Care Med 2000; 162: 1518–1523.
155. Boulet L, Belanger M, Carrier G. Airway responsiveness and bronchial-wall thickness in asthma with or without fixed airflow obstruction. Am J Respir Crit Care Med 1995; 152:865–871.
156. Niimi A, Matsumoto H, Takemura M, et al. Relation of airway sensitivity and airway reactivity in asthma. Am J Respir Crit Care Med 2003; 168:983–988.
157. Niimi A, Matsumoto H, Amitani R, et al. Effects of short term treatment with inhaled corticosteroid on airway wall thickening in asthma. Am J Med 2004; 116:725–731.
158. Nakano Y, Wong JC, de Jong PA, et al. The prediction of small airway dimensions using computed tomography. Am J Respir Crit Care Med 2005; 171:142–146.
159. Berger P, Perot V, Desbarats P, et al. Airway wall thickness in cigarette smokers: quantitative thin-section CT assessment. Radiology 2005; 235:1055–1064.
160. Orlandi I, Moroni C, Camiciottoli G, et al. Chronic obstructive pulmonary disease: thin-section CT measurement of airway wall thickness and lung attenuation. Radiology 2005; 234: 604–610.
161. Nakano Y, Muro S, Sakai H, et al. Computed tomographic measurements of airway dimensions and emphysema in smokers. Correlation with lung function. Am J Respir Crit Care Med 2000; 162:1102–1108.
162. Goldin JG, Tashkin DP, Kleerup EC, et al. Comparative effects of hydrofluoroalkane and chlorofluorocarbon beclomethasone dipropionate inhalation on small airways: assessment with functional helical thin-section computed tomography. J Allergy Clin Immunol 1999; 104:S258–S267.
163. Ward C, Reid DW, Orsida BE, et al. Inter-relationships between airway inflammation, reticular basement membrane thickening and bronchial hyper-reactivity to methacholine in asthma; a systemic bronchoalveolar lavage and airway biopsy analysis. Clin Exp Allergy 2005; 35:1565–1571.
164. McMillan SJ, Lloyd CM. Prolonged allergen challenge in mice leads to persistent airway remodelling. Clin Exp Allergy 2004; 34:497–507.
165. Ohashi Y, Motojma S, Fukuda T, et al. Airway hyperresponsiveness, increased intracellular spaces of bronchial epithelium and increased infiltration of eosinophils and lymphocytes in bronchial mucosa in asthma. Am Rev Respir Dis 1992; 145:1469–1476.
166. Boulet LP, Laviolette M, Turcotte H, et al. Bronchial subepithelial fibrosis correlates with airway responsiveness to methacholine. Chest 1997; 112:45–52.
167. Chetta A, Foresi A, Del Donno M, et al. Bronchial responsiveness to distilled water and methacholine and its relationship to inflammation and remodeling of the airways in asthma. Am J Respir Crit Care Med 1996; 153:910—917.
168. Lee SY, Sim SJ, Kwon SS, et al. Relation of airway reactivity and sensitivity with bronchial pathology in asthma. J Asthma 2002; 39:537–544.
169. Makinde T, Murphy RF, Agrawal DK. Immunomodulatory role of vascular endothelial growth factor and angiopoietin-1 in airway remodeling. Curr Mol Med 2006; 6:831–841.
170. Knox AJ, Deacon K, Clifford R. Blanching the airways: steroid effects in asthma. Thorax 2007; 62:283–285.
171. Berend N, Woolcock AJ, Marlin GE. Correlation between the function and structure of the lung in smokers. Am Rev Respir Dis 1979; 119:695–705.
172. Ward C, Johns DP, Bish R, et al. Reduced airway distensibility, fixed airflow limitation, and airway remodeling in asthma. Am J Respir Crit Care Med 2001; 164:1718–1721.

173. Johns DP, Burns G, Reid DW, et al. Airway distensibility in normal and asthmatic subjects and partitioning of the Fowler dead space. Appl Physiol Nutr Metab 2006; 31:460—466.

174. Brown NJ, Salome CM, Berend N, et al. Airway distensibility in adults with asthma and healthy adults, measured by forced oscillation technique. Am J Respir Crit Care Med 2007; 176:129–137.

175. Chan JH, Walls JT, Walters EH, et al. Flow dependence of anatomical dead space and relationship to spirometry in healthy subjects. Respirology 2007; 12(suppl 4) P2–169.

176. Vanacker NJ, Palmans E, Kips JC, et al. Fluticasone inhibits but does not reverse allergen-induced structural airway changes. Am J Respir Crit Care Med 2001; 163:674–679.

177. Vanacker NJ, Palmans E, Pauwels RA, et al. Dose-related effect of inhaled fluticasone on allergen induced airway changes in rats. Eur Respir J 2002; 20:873–879.

178. Christie PE, Jonas M, Tsai CH, et al. Increase in laminin expression in allergic airway remodelling and decrease by dexamethasone. Eur Respir J 2004; 24:107–115.

179. McMillan SJ, Xanthou G, Lloyd CM. Therapeutic administration of Budesonide ameliorates allergen-induced airway remodelling. Clin Exp Allergy 2005; 35:388–396.

180. Kamachi A, Munakata M, Nasuhara Y, et al. Enhancement of goblet cell hyperplasia and airway hyperresponsiveness by salbutamol in a rat model of atopic asthma. Thorax 2001; 56: 19–24.

181. Walters EH, Walters J. Inhaled short-acting β_2-agonist use in chronic asthma: regular versus as needed treatment. Cochrane Database Syst Rev 2003; CD001285.

182. Kumar RK, Herbert C, Thomas PS, et al. Inhibition of inflammation and remodeling by roflumilast and dexamethasone in murine chronic asthma. J Pharmacol Exp Ther 2003; 307: 349–355.

183. Gosens R, Bos IS, Zaagsma J, et al. Protective effects of tiotropium bromide in the progression of airway smooth muscle remodeling. Am J Respir Crit Care Med 2005; 171:1096–1102.

184. Henderson WR, Tang LO, Chu SJ, et al. A role for cysteinyl leukotrienes in airway remodeling in a mouse asthma model. Am J Respir Crit Care Med 2002; 165:108–116.

185. Henderson WR, Chiang GK, Tien Y, et al. Reversal of allergen-induced airway remodeling by CysLT$_1$ receptor blockage. Am J Respir Crit Care Med 2006; 173:718–728.

186. Muz MH, Deveci F, Bulut Y, et al. The effects of low dose leukotriene receptor antagonist therapy on airway remodeling and cysteinyl leukotriene expression in a mouse asthma model. Exp Mol Med 2006; 38:109–118.

187. Du T, Sapienza S, Wang CG, et al. Effect of nedocromil sodium on allergen-induced airway responses and changes in the quantity of airway smooth muscle in rats. J Allergy Clin Immunol 1996; 98:400–407.

188. Jain VV, Kitagaki K, Businga T, et al. CpG-oligodeoxynucleotides inhibit airway remodeling in a murine model of chronic asthma. J Allergy Clin Immunol 2002; 110:867–872.

189. Cho JY, Miller M, Baek KJ, et al. Immunostimulatory DNA inhibits transforming growth factor-beta expression and airway remodeling. Am J Respir Cell Mol Biol 2004; 30:651–661.

190. Fanucchi MV, Schelegle ES, Baker GL, et al. Immunostimulatory oligonucleotides attenuate airways remodeling in allergic monkeys. Am J Respir Crit Care Med 2004; 170:1153–1157.

191. McMillan SJ, Xanthou G, Lloyd CM. Manipulation of allergen-induced airway remodelling by treatment with anti-TGF-β antibody: effect on the SMAD signalling pathway. J Immunol 2005; 174:5774–5780.

192. Alcorn JF, Rinaldi LM, Jaffe EF, et al. Transforming growth factor-beta-1 suppresses airway hyperresponsiveness in allergic airway disease. Am J Respir Crit Care Med 2007; 176:974–982.

193. Fattouh R, Midence G, Arias K, et al. TGF-β regulates house dust mite induced allergic airway inflammation but not airway remodelling. Am J Respir Crit Care Med 2008; 177: 593–603.

194. Hirano A, Kanehiro A, Ono K, et al. Pirfenidone modulates airway responsiveness, inflammation and remodeling after repeated challenge. Am J Respir Crit Care Med 2006; 35:366–377.

195. Polosa R, Puddicombe SM, Krishna MT, et al. Expression of c-erb receptors and ligands in the bronchial epithelium of asthmatic subjects. J Allergy Clin Immunol 2002; 109:75–81.

196. Puddicombe SM, Torres-Lozano C, Richter A, et al. Increased expression of p21(waf) cyclin-dependent kinase inhibitor in asthmatic bronchial epithelium. Am J Respir Cell Mol Biol 2003; 28:61–68.

197. Lundgren R, Soderberg M, Horstedt P, et al. Morphological studies of bronchial mucosal biopsies from asthmatics before and after ten years of treatment with inhaled steroids. Eur Respir J 1988; 1:883–889.

198. Laitinen LA, Laitinen A, Haahtela T. A comparative study of the effects of an inhaled corticosteroid, budesonide, and a beta-2-agonist, terbutaline, on airway inflammation in newly diagnosed asthma: a randomised double-blind, parallel-group controlled trial. J Allergy Clin Immunol 1992; 90:32–42.

199. Chakir J, Shannon J, Molet S, et al. Airway remodeling-associated mediators in moderate to severe asthma: effect of steroids on TGF-β, IL-11, IL-17 and type I and type III collagen expression. J Allergy Clin Immunol 2003; 111:1293–1298.

200. Laitinen A, Altraja A, Kampe M, et al. Tenascin is increased in airway basement membrane of asthmatics and decreased by an inhaled steroid. Am J Respir Crit Care Med 1997; 156:951–958.

201. Sont JK, Willems LN, Bel EH, et al. Clinical control and histopathologic outcome of asthma when using airway hyperresponsiveness as an additional guide to long-term treatment. The AMPUL Study Group. Am J Respir Crit Care Med 1999; 159:1043–1051.

202. de Kluijver J, Schrumpf JA, Evertse CE, et al. Bronchial matrix and inflammation respond to inhaled steroids despite ongoing allergen exposure in asthma. Clin Exp Allergy 2005; 35: 1361–1369.

203. Kelly MM, Chakir J, Vethanayagam D, et al. Montelukast treatment attenuates the increase in myofibroblasts following low-dose allergen challenge. Chest 2006; 130:741–753.

204. Altraja A, Laitinen A, Meriste S, et al. Regular albuterol or nedocromil sodium-effects on airway subepithelial tenascin in asthma. Respir Med 1999; 93:445–453.

205. Flood-Page P, Menzies-Gow A, Phipps S, et al. Anti-IL-5 treatment reduces deposition of ECM proteins in the bronchial subepithelial basement membrane of mild atopic asthmatics. J Clin Invest 2003; 112:1029–1036.

206. Chetta A, Zanini A, Foresi A, et al. Vascular component of airway remodeling in asthma is reduced by high dose of fluticasone. Am J Respir Crit Care Med 2003; 167:751–757.

207. Hoshino M, Takahashi M, Takai Y, et al. Inhaled corticosteroids decrease vascularity of the bronchial mucosa in patients with asthma. Clin Exp Allergy 2001; 31:722—730.

208. Orsida BE, Li X, Hickey B, et al. Vascularity in asthmatic airways: relation to inhaled steroid dose. Thorax 1999; 54:289–295.

209. Orsida BE, Ward C, Li X, et al. Effect of a long-acting β2-agonist over 3 months on airway wall vascular remodeling in asthma. Am J Respir Crit Care Med 2001; 164:117–121.

210. Feltis BN, Wignarajah D, Zheng L, et al. Effects of inhaled fluticasone on angiogenesis and vascular endothelial growth factor in asthma. Thorax 2007; 62:314–319.

211. Howarth PH, Babu KS, Arshad HS, et al. Tumour necrosis factor (TNFα) as a novel therapeutic target in symptomatic corticosteroid asthma. Thorax 2005; 60:1012–1018.

212. Nicod LP. Mechanisms of airway obliteration after lung transplantation. Proc Am Thorac Soc 2006; 3:444–449.

213. Yates B, Murphy DM, Forrest IA, et al. Azithromycin reverses airflow obstruction in established bronchiolitis obliterans syndrome. Am J Respir Crit Care Med 2005; 172:772–775.

214. Verleden GM, Vanaudenaerde BM, Dupont LJ, et al. Azithromycin reduces airway neu-
      trophilia and interleukin-8 in patients with bronchiolitis obliterans syndrome. Am J Respir
      Crit Care Med 2006; 174:566–570.
215. Johnson BA, Iacono AT, Zeevi A, et al. Statin use is associated with improved function and
      survival of lung allografts. Am J Respir Crit Care Med 2003; 167:1271–1278.
216. Alexeef SE, Litonjua AA, Sparrow D, et al. Statin use reduces decline in lung function. VA
      normative Ageing Study. Am J Respir Crit Care Med 2007; 176:742–747.
217. Murphy DM, Forrest IA, Corris PA, et al. Simvastatin attenuates release of neutrophilic and
      remodeling factors from primary bronchial epithelial cells derived from stable lung trans-
      plant recipients. Am J Physiol Lung Cell Mol Physiol 2008; 294:L592–L599.
218. Ward C, Forrest IA, Murphy DM, et al. Phenotype of airway epithelial cells suggests
      epithelial to mesenchymal cell transition in clinically stable lung transplant recipients.
      Thorax 2005; 60:865–871.

12
Acute Exacerbations of COPD

J. A. WEDZICHA and J. R. HURST
Academic Unit of Respiratory Medicine, UCL Medical School, University College, London, U.K.

I. Epidemiology of COPD Exacerbations

There has been considerable interest in the causes and mechanisms of exacerbations of chronic obstructive pulmonary disease (COPD) as exacerbations are an important cause of the considerable morbidity and mortality associated with COPD (1). COPD exacerbations increase in frequency and severity with increasing severity of the underlying disease. Some patients are prone to frequent exacerbations that are an important cause of hospital admission and readmission, and these "frequent exacerbations" experience a particular burden on quality of life, disease progression, and mortality (2) (Fig. 1). COPD exacerbations are also associated with physiological deterioration and increased airway inflammation (3). These events are caused by a variety of factors such as viruses, bacteria, and probably common pollutants. COPD exacerbations are commoner in the winter months and there may be important interactions between cold temperature and exacerbations caused by viruses or pollutants (4).

Earlier descriptions of COPD exacerbations had concentrated mainly on studies of hospital admission, though most COPD exacerbations are treated in the community and are not associated with hospital admission. A cohort of moderate-to-severe COPD patients was followed in East London, United Kingdom (London COPD Study) with daily diary cards and peak flow readings, and these patients were asked to report exacerbations as soon as possible after symptomatic onset (2). The diagnosis of COPD exacerbation was based on criteria modified from those initially described by Anthonisen and colleagues (5), which require two symptoms for diagnosis, one of which must be a "major" symptom of increased dyspnea, sputum volume, or sputum purulence. Minor exacerbation symptoms include cough, wheeze, sore throat, nasal discharge, or fever (Table 1). The study found that about 50% of exacerbations went unreported to the research team, despite considerable encouragement provided, and were only diagnosed from diary cards. Interestingly, there were no differences in major symptoms or physiological parameters between reported and unreported exacerbations (2). Patients with COPD are accustomed to frequent symptom changes and thus may tend to underreport exacerbations to physicians. These patients have high levels of anxiety and depression and may accept their situation (6,7). The tendency of patients to underreport exacerbations may explain the higher total rate of exacerbation at 2.7 per patient per year, which is higher than previously reported by Anthonisen and coworkers at 1.1 per patient

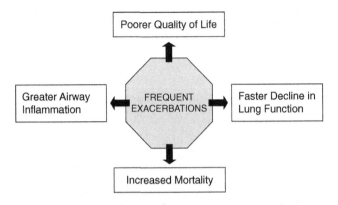

Figure 1 Impact of COPD Exacerbations. *Abbreviation*: COPD, chronic obstructive pulmonary disease.

Table 1 Causes of COPD Exacerbations

Viruses	Rhinovirus (common cold)
	Influenza
	Parainfluenza
	Coronavirus
	Adenovirus
	RSV
	Chlamydia pneumoniae
Bacteria	*Haemophilus influenzae*
	Streptococcus pneumoniae
	Moraxella catarrhalis
	Staphylococcus aureus
	Pseudomonas aeruginosa
Common pollutants	Nitrogen dioxide
	Particulates
	Sulfur dioxide
	Ozone

Abbreviations: COPD, chronic obstructive pulmonary disease; RSV, respiratory syncytial virus.

per year (5). However, in the latter study, exacerbations were diagnosed from patients' recall of symptoms.

Using the median number of exacerbations as a cut-off point, COPD patients in the London Study were classified as frequent and infrequent exacerbators. Quality-of-life scores measured using a validated disease specific scale—the St George's Respiratory Questionnaire—were significantly worse in all of the three component scores (symptoms, activities, and impacts) in the frequent, compared with the infrequent exacerbators. This suggests that exacerbation frequency is an important determinant of health status in COPD and should therefore be an important outcome measure in COPD. Factors predictive of frequent exacerbations included daily cough and sputum, and frequent exacerbations in the previous year. A previous study of acute infective exacerbations of chronic bronchitis found that one of the factors predicting exacerbation was also the number in the previous year (8), though this study was limited to exacerbations presenting with purulent sputum and no physiological data was available during the study.

In a further prospective analysis of 504 exacerbations, where daily monitoring was performed, there was some deterioration in symptoms, though no significant peak flow changes (9). Falls in peak flow and forced expiratory volume in one second (FEV_1) at exacerbation were generally small and not useful in predicting exacerbations, but larger falls in peak flow were associated with symptoms of dyspnea, the presence of coryzal symptoms, and were also related to longer recovery time from exacerbations. Symptoms of dyspnea, common colds, sore throat, and cough increased significantly during the prodromal phase, and this suggests that respiratory viruses may have early effects at exacerbations. The median time to recovery of peak flow was six days, and seven days for symptoms. However, at 35 days peak flow had returned to normal in only 75% of exacerbations, while at 91 days, 7.1% of exacerbations had still not recovered to baseline lung function. Recovery was longer in the presence of increased dyspnea or symptoms of a common cold at exacerbation. The changes observed in lung function at exacerbation were smaller than those observed in other studies during exacerbations of asthma, though the average duration of an asthma exacerbation was longer at 9.6 days (10,11).

The reasons for the incomplete recovery of symptoms and lung function are not clear, but may involve inadequate treatment or persistence of the causative agent. The incomplete physiological recovery after an exacerbation could also contribute to the decline in lung function with time in patients with COPD. However, to date, there is no evidence that patients with incomplete recovery of their exacerbation have a greater decline in lung function and further studies on the natural history of COPD exacerbations are required. Data from a U.K. audit has shown that approximately 30% of patients seen at hospital with an index exacerbation will be seen again (and possibly readmitted) with a recurrent exacerbation within eight weeks (12). In a cohort of moderate-to-severe COPD patients, 22% of patients had a recurrent exacerbation within 50 days of the first (index) exacerbation and this event can be separated discretely from the index exacerbation (13). This concept of exacerbation "clustering" is deserving of further study, and may relate to the persistence of the inflammatory response as discussed further below. In summary, exacerbations are complex events and careful follow up is essential to ensure complete recovery.

The association of the symptoms of increased dyspnea and of the common cold at exacerbation with a prolonged recovery suggests that viral infections may lead to more prolonged exacerbations. As colds are associated with longer exacerbations, COPD patients who develop a cold may be prone to more severe exacerbations and should be considered for therapy early at onset of symptoms. Approximately 50% of colds in patients with COPD are associated with exacerbations.

II. Inflammatory Changes at Exacerbation

COPD exacerbations are associated with rises in airway (both upper and lower airways) and systemic inflammation (2,14). Increases in systemic markers seen at exacerbations are most likely driven by increases in airway inflammation with exacerbation as the changes in airway and systemic inflammation at exacerbation are correlated (14). Biopsy studies are difficult to perform at exacerbation in COPD patients, and much data comes from analysis of sputum. However, in one study, where biopsies were performed at exacerbation in patients with chronic bronchitis, increased airway eosinophilia was found, though the patients studied had only mild COPD (15). With exacerbation, there were modest increases observed in neutrophils, T lymphocytes (CD3), and TNF-α positive cells, while there were no changes in CD4 or CD8 T cells, macrophages, or mast cells. Qiu and coworkers have studied biopsies from COPD patients who were intubated (and therefore experiencing more severe exacerbations) and showed that there was considerable airway neutrophilia, neutrophil elastase expression with upregulation of neutrophil chemokine expression (16). However, intubated COPD patients may have secondary airway infection and thus results may be difficult to interpret. Oxidative stress also plays an important role in the development of airway inflammation at COPD exacerbation. Markers of oxidative stress have been shown to rise in the airways during exacerbations such as hydrogen peroxide and 8-isoprostane, and these markers may take some time to recover to baseline stable levels (16). Patients with severe exacerbations associated with hospitalization and assisted ventilation have evidence of increased oxidative stress (17,18).

Most studies on airway inflammatory markers at exacerbation have been performed using sputum samples, either spontaneous or induced. Sputum inflammatory markers such as IL-6, IL-8, and myeloperoxidase rise at the start of the exacerbation and usually recover to normal by 14 days, though in some cases higher airway inflammatory markers may persist for some time, suggesting incomplete recovery of exacerbations. Perera and colleagues also showed that systemic inflammation may persist after the exacerbation and those patients with an elevated C-reactive protein (CRP) two weeks after the onset of an exacerbation were more likely to develop an early recurrent exacerbation (13). Patients with a history of frequent exacerbations also have increased airway inflammation in the stable state, compared with patients with infrequent exacerbations (2,19).

III. Etiology of COPD Exacerbation

COPD exacerbations have been associated with a number of etiological factors, including infection and pollution episodes (Table 1). COPD exacerbations are frequently triggered by upper respiratory tract infections (20) and these are commoner in the winter months, when there are more respiratory viral infections in the community. Patients may also be more prone to exacerbations in the winter months as lung function in COPD patients shows small but significant falls with reduction in outdoor temperature during the winter months (4). COPD patients have been found to have increased hospital admissions, suggesting increased exacerbation when increasing environmental pollution occurs. During the December 1991 pollution episode in the United Kingdom, COPD mortality was increased together with an increase in hospital admission in elderly COPD patients (21). However, common pollutants especially oxides of nitrogen and particulates may interact with viral infection to precipitate exacerbation rather than acting alone (22).

A. Viral Infections

Viral infections are an important trigger for COPD exacerbations (20,23,24). Studies have shown that at least one-third of COPD exacerbations were associated with viral infections, and that the majority of these were due to human rhinovirus, the cause of the common cold (20,23,24). Viral exacerbations were associated with symptomatic colds and prolonged recovery of the exacerbation (9). Using molecular techniques, Seemungal and colleagues also showed that rhinovirus can be recovered from induced sputum more frequently than from nasal aspirates at exacerbation, suggesting that wild-type rhinovirus can infect the lower airway and contribute to inflammatory changes at exacerbation (23). They also found that exacerbations associated with the presence of rhinovirus in induced sputum had larger increases in airway IL-6 levels (23), suggesting that viruses increase the severity of airway inflammation at exacerbation. This finding is in agreement with data that respiratory viruses produce longer and more severe exacerbations, and therefore have a major impact on health care utilization (9,25). Other viruses may trigger COPD exacerbation. Coronavirus has been associated with only a small proportion of asthmatic exacerbations and is unlikely to play a major role in COPD (26). Influenza, parainfluenza, and adenovirus can all trigger exacerbations. Influenza has become a less prominent cause of exacerbation with the introduction of immunization, though this is still likely to be an important factor at times of influenza epidemics. While respiratory syncytial virus (RSV) infection has been found at COPD exacerbation (27), it is not clear if RSV can cause exacerbation as RSV can be as frequently detected in the airways of COPD patients when the patient is stable (28).

B. Bacterial Infection

Over the past years, the role of bacterial infection at COPD exacerbation has been somewhat controversial as airway bacterial colonization is often found when patients are stable state and the same organisms are isolated exacerbations. These include *Haemophilus influenzae, Streptococcus pneumoniae, Moraxella catarrhalis, Staphylococcus aureus,* and *Pseudomonas aeruginosa* (29). In a study in patients with moderate-to-severe COPD, bacteria were found in 48.2% of patients in the stable state and at exacerbation, bacterial detection rose to 69.6%, with an associated rise in airway bacterial load (30). The case for involvement of bacteria has come from studies of antibiotic therapy as exacerbations often present with increased sputum purulence and volume and antibiotics have traditionally been used as first-line therapy in such exacerbations. Anthonisen and colleagues in a classical paper investigating the benefit of antibiotics in over 300 acute exacerbations demonstrated a greater treatment success rate in patients treated with antibiotics, especially if their initial presentation was with all three of the symptoms of increased dyspnea, sputum volume, and purulence (5). Patients with mild COPD obtained less benefit from antibiotic therapy. A meta-analysis of trials of antibiotic therapy in COPD has concluded that antibiotic therapy offered a small but significant benefit in outcome in exacerbations (31). Sethi and colleagues have suggested that isolation of a new bacterial strain in COPD patients who were regularly sampled was associated with an increased risk of an exacerbation (32), though this also does not conclusively prove that bacteria are direct causes of exacerbations as not all exacerbations were associated with strain change, and not all strain changes resulted in exacerbation.

At COPD exacerbations both respiratory viruses and bacteria may be isolated. A greater systemic inflammatory response has been reported in those exacerbations associated with both *H. influenzae* and rhinovirus isolation, and if the isolation of

Haemophilus was associated with new or worsening coryzal symptoms (a surrogate of viral infection). Such infections were also more severe as assessed by changes in symptoms and lung function at exacerbation onset (30). This has been confirmed in a further study demonstrating greater lung function impairment and longer hospitalizations in exacerbations associated with viral and bacterial coinfection (33). It has also been suggested that atypical microorganisms such as *Chlamydia* and *Mycoplasma* may cause COPD exacerbations, though evidence on their role is conflicting and these infective agents may interact with other bacteria and viruses in the airways (34,35).

IV. Pathophysiological Changes at COPD Exacerbation

In patients with moderate and severe COPD, the mechanical performance of the respiratory muscles is reduced. The airflow obstruction leads to hyperinflation, with the respiratory muscles acting at a mechanical disadvantage and generating reduced inspiratory pressures. The load on the respiratory muscles is also increased in patients with airflow obstruction by the presence of intrinsic positive end-expiratory pressure. With an exacerbation of COPD, the increase in airflow obstruction will further increase the load on the respiratory muscles and increase the work of breathing, precipitating respiratory failure in more severe cases. The minute ventilation may be normal, but the respiratory pattern will be irregular with increased frequency and decreased tidal volume. The resultant hypercapnia and acidosis will also then decrease inspiratory muscle function, contributing to further deterioration of the respiratory failure.

Hypoxemia at exacerbation of COPD usually occurs due to a combination of ventilation-perfusion mismatch and hypoventilation, although arteriovenous shunting can also contribute in the acute setting. This causes increases in pulmonary artery pressure, which can lead to salt and water retention and the development of peripheral edema. The degree of ventilation-perfusion abnormalities increases during acute exacerbations and then resolves over the following few weeks. Acidosis is an important prognostic factor in survival from respiratory failure during a COPD exacerbation and thus early correction of acidosis is an essential goal of therapy.

V. Treatment
A. Inhaled Bronchodilator Therapy

β_2-Agonists and anticholinergic agents are the inhaled bronchodilators most frequently used in the treatment of acute exacerbations of COPD. An increase in the dose or frequency of these drugs is the cornerstone of exacerbation therapy, and may be all that is required in the mildest exacerbations. In patients with stable COPD, symptomatic benefit can be obtained with bronchodilator therapy in COPD, even without significant changes in spirometry. This is probably due to a reduction in dynamic hyperinflation that is characteristic of COPD and hence leads to a decrease in the sensation of dyspnea especially during exertion (36). In stable COPD, greater bronchodilatation has been demonstrated with anticholinergic agents than with β_2-agonists, which may be due to the excessive cholinergic neuronal bronchoconstrictor tone (37). However, studies investigating bronchodilator responses in acute exacerbations of COPD have shown no differences between agents used and no significant additive effect of the combination therapy, even though combination of an anticholinergic and β-agonist bronchodilator has benefits in the stable state (38,39). This difference in effect between the acute and the stable states may be due to the fact that the larger doses of drug delivered in the acute setting produce maximal bronchodilatation, whereas the smaller doses administered in the stable condition may be having a submaximal effect.

B. Corticosteroids

Corticosteroids are indicated in those exacerbations failing to respond to an increase in bronchodilators alone. Only about 10% to 15% of patients with stable COPD show a spirometric response to oral corticosteroids (40) and, unlike the situation in asthma, steroids have little effect on airway inflammatory markers in patients with COPD (41,42). A number of early studies have investigated the effects of corticosteroid therapy at COPD exacerbation. In an early controlled trial in patients with COPD exacerbations and acute respiratory failure, Albert and coworkers found that there were larger improvements in pre- and postbronchodilator FEV_1 when patients were treated for the first three days of the hospital admission with intravenous methylprednisolone compared with placebo (43). Another trial found that a single dose of methylprednisolone given within 30 minutes of arrival in the accident and emergency department produced no improvement after five hours in spirometry, and also had no effect on hospital admission, though in another readmission was reduced (44,45). A retrospective study comparing patients treated with steroids at exacerbation compared with those not treated showed that the steroid group had a reduced chance of relapse after therapy (46).

Thompson and colleagues gave a nine-day course of prednisolone or placebo in a randomized manner to outpatients presenting with acute exacerbations of COPD (47). Unlike the previous studies, these patients were either recruited from outpatients or from a group that were preenrolled and self-reported the exacerbation to the study team. In this study, patients with exacerbations associated with acidosis or pneumonia were excluded, so exacerbations of moderate severity were generally included. Patients in the steroid treated group showed a more rapid improvement in PaO_2, alveolar-arterial oxygen gradient, FEV_1, peak expiratory flow rate, and a trend toward a more rapid improvement in dyspnea in the steroid-treated group.

In a recent cohort study by Seemungal and colleagues, the effect of therapy with prednisolone on COPD exacerbations diagnosed and treated in the community was studied (9). Exacerbations treated with steroids were more severe and associated with larger falls in peak flow rate. The treated exacerbations also had a longer recovery time to baseline for symptoms and peak flow rate. However, the rate of peak flow rate recovery was faster in the prednisolone-treated group, although not the rate of symptom score recovery. An interesting finding in this study was that steroids significantly prolonged the median time from the day of onset of the initial exacerbation to the next exacerbation from 60 days in the group not treated with prednisolone to 84 days in the patients treated with prednisolone. In contrast, antibiotic therapy had no effect on the time to the next exacerbation. If short-course oral steroid therapy at exacerbation does prolong the time to the next exacerbation, then this could be an important way to reduce exacerbation frequency in COPD patients, which is an important determinant of health status (2).

Davies and colleagues randomized patients admitted to hospital with COPD exacerbations to prednisolone or placebo (48). In the prednisolone group, the FEV_1 rose faster until day 5, when a plateau was observed in the steroid treated group. Changes in the prebronchodilator and postbronchodilator FEV_1 were similar suggesting that this is not just an effect on bronchomotor tone, but involves faster resolution of airway inflammatory changes or airway wall edema with exacerbation. Length of hospital stay analysis showed that patients treated with prednisolone had a significantly shorter length of stay. Six weeks later, there were no differences in spirometry between the patient groups and health status was similar to that measured at five days after admission. Thus, the benefits of steroid therapy at exacerbation are most obvious in the early course of the exacerbation. A similar proportion of the patients, approximately 32% in both study groups, required further treatment for exacerbations within six weeks of follow up, emphasizing the high exacerbation frequency in these patients.

Niewoehner and colleagues performed a randomized controlled trial of either a two- or eight-week prednisolone course at exacerbation compared with placebo, in addition to other exacerbation therapy (49). The primary end point was a first treatment failure, including death, need for intubation, readmission, or intensification of therapy. There was no difference in the results using the two- or eight-week treatment protocol. The rates of treatment failure were higher in the placebo group at 30 days, compared with the combined two- and eight-week prednisone groups. As in the study by Davies and colleagues, the FEV_1 improved faster in the prednisolone treated group, though there were no differences by two weeks. In contrast, Niewoehner and colleagues performed a detailed evaluation of steroid complications and found considerable evidence of hyperglycemia in the steroid-treated patients. Thus, steroids should be used at COPD exacerbation in short courses of no more than two-week duration to avoid risk of complications.

C. Antibiotics

Acute exacerbations of COPD often present with increased sputum purulence and volume, and antibiotics have traditionally been used as a first-line therapy in such exacerbations. However, viral infections may be the triggers in a significant proportion of acute infective exacerbations in COPD and antibiotics used for the consequences of secondary infection. As discussed above, antibiotic therapy at exacerbations is most useful if patients present with symptoms of increased dyspnea, sputum volume, and purulence (5). A randomized placebo controlled study investigating the value of antibiotics in patients with mild obstructive lung disease in the community concluded that antibiotic therapy did not accelerate recovery or reduce the number of relapses, though patients had mixed pathologies (50).

D. Methylxanthines

Methylxanthines such as theophylline are sometimes used in the management of acute exacerbations of COPD. There is some evidence that theophyllines are useful in COPD, though the main limiting factor is the frequency of toxic side effects. The therapeutic action of theophylline is thought to be due to its inhibition of phosphodiesterase that breaks down cyclic AMP, an intracellular messenger, thus facilitating bronchodilatation. However, studies of intravenous aminophylline therapy in acute exacerbations of COPD have shown no significant beneficial effect over and above conventional therapy (51,52). There are some reports of beneficial effects of methylxanthines upon dia-phragmatic and cardiac function, though these mechanisms require further study in patients with COPD exacerbations.

E. Management of Respiratory Failure

Hypoxemia occurs with more severe exacerbations and usually requires hospital admission. Caution should always be taken in providing supplemental oxygen to patients with COPD, particularly during acute exacerbations, when respiratory drive and muscle strength can be impaired leading to significant increases in carbon dioxide tension at relatively modest oxygen flow rates. However, in the vast majority of cases, the administration of supplemental oxygen increases arterial oxygen tension sufficiently without clinically significant rises in carbon dioxide. It is suggested that supplemental oxygen is delivered at an initial flow rate of 1 to 2 L/min via nasal cannulae or 24% to 28% inspired oxygen via Venturi mask, with repeat blood gas analysis after 30 to 45 minutes of oxygen therapy.

Historically, hypercapnia during COPD exacerbations was managed initially with the use of respiratory stimulants. The most commonly used was doxapram, which acts centrally to increase respiratory drive and respiratory muscle activity. The effect is probably only appreciable for 24 to 48 hours; the main factor limiting use being side effects that can lead to agitation and are often not tolerated by the patient. There are only a few studies of the clinical efficacy of doxapram, and short-term investigations suggest that improvements in acidosis and arterial carbon dioxide tension can be attained (53). A small study comparing doxapram with noninvasive ventilation (NIV) in acute exacerbations of COPD suggested that noninvasive positive pressure ventilation (NPPV) was superior with regard to correction of blood gases during the initial treatment phase (54). Increases in pulmonary artery pressure during acute exacerbations of COPD can result in right-sided cardiac dysfunction and development of peripheral edema. Diuretic therapy may thus be necessary if there is edema or a rise in jugular venous pressure.

Noninvasive Ventilation

The introduction of noninvasive ventilation (NIV) using nasal or face masks has had a major impact on the management of acute exacerbations and has enabled acidosis to be corrected at an early stage. Studies have shown that NIV can produce improvements in pH relatively rapidly, at one hour after instituting ventilation (55,56). This will allow time for other conventional therapies to work, such as oxygen therapy, bronchodilators, steroids, and antibiotics, and thus reverses the progression of respiratory failure and reduces mortality. With NIV, there are improvements in minute ventilation and reductions in respiratory rate and in transdiaphragmatic activity. Thus, NIV can improve gas exchange and allows respiratory muscle rest in respiratory failure.

With the use of NIV, patient comfort is improved; there is also no requirement for sedation with preservation of speech and swallowing (in contrast to endotracheal intubation and invasive mechanical ventilation). The technique can be applied in a general ward, though a high dependency area is preferable. Patient cooperation is important in application of NIV. The main advantage of the use of NIV is avoidance of tracheal intubation and the ability to offer ventilatory support to patients with respiratory failure due to severe COPD, who would be considered unsuitable for intubation. A lower incidence of nosocomial pneumonia has been also reported with the use of NIV compared with conventional intubation and ventilation.

Following a number of uncontrolled studies, randomized controlled trials have shown benefit of NIV in acute COPD exacerbations. A U.K. study showed that with the use of NIV in exacerbations of respiratory failure, earlier correction of pH can be achieved, together with reduction in breathlessness over the initial three days of ventilation, compared with a control standard therapy group (55). A study from the United States showed a significant reduction in intubation rates with NIV from 67% in a group receiving conventional therapy to 9% in the NIV group (56). A third study showed convincingly that in patients with exacerbations of respiratory failure, the use of NIV with pressure support ventilation reduces the need for intubation and mortality was significantly reduced from 29% in the conventionally treated group to 9% in the NIV group (57). Complications, which were specifically associated with the use of mechanical ventilation, were also reduced. The difference in mortality disappeared after adjustment for intubation, suggesting that the benefits with NIV are due to fewer patients requiring intubation. This was also the first study to show that hospital length of stay can be reduced with the use of NIV. A recent study showed that NIV can be applied on general wards, though patients with more severe acidosis had a worse outcome (58).

These studies have treated patients where the pH was below 7.35, rather than just below 7.26, when the prognosis of COPD worsens. A number of these patients may have improved without NIV, though it seems that the major effect of NIV is the earlier correction of acidosis and thus avoidance of tracheal intubation, with all its associated complications. Studies have shown that NIV can be successfully implemented in up to 80% of cases (59,60). NIV is less successful in patients who have worse blood gases at baseline before ventilation, are underweight, have a higher incidence of pneumonia, have a greater level of neurological deterioration, and where compliance with the ventilation is poor (59). Moretti and colleagues have shown that "late treatment failure" (after an initial 48 hours of therapy with NIV) is up to 20% and that patients with late failure were more likely to have severe functional and clinical disease with more complications at the time of admission (61). Identification of patients with a potentially poor outcome is important as delay in intubation can have serious consequences for the patient.

Indications for Invasive Ventilation

If NIV fails, or is unavailable in the hospital, invasive ventilation may be required in the presence of increasing acidosis. It may be considered in any patient when the pH falls below 7.26. Decisions to ventilate these patients may be difficult, though with improved modes of invasive ventilatory support and better weaning techniques, the outlook for the COPD patient is better.

Patients will be suitable for tracheal intubation if this is the first presentation of COPD exacerbation or respiratory failure, or there is a treatable cause of respiratory failure, such as pneumonia. Information will be required on the past history and quality of life, especially the ability to perform daily activities. Patients with severe disabling and progressive COPD may be less suitable, but it is important that adequate and appropriate therapy has been used in these patients, with documented disease progression. The patient's wishes and those of any close relatives should be considered in any decision to institute or withhold life supporting therapy.

F. Supported Discharge

Many hospital admissions are related to exacerbations of COPD and thus reductions of admissions especially during the winter months when they are most frequent are particularly desirable. Over recent years a number of different models of supported discharge have been developed and some evaluated (62–64). Patients have been discharged early with an appropriate package of care organized, including domiciliary visits made to these patients after discharge by trained respiratory nurses.

Cotton and colleagues randomized patients to discharge on the next day or usual management and found that there were no differences in mortality or readmission rates between the two groups (62). There was a reduction in hospital stay from a mean of 6.1 days to 3.2 days. In another larger study by Skwarska and colleagues, patients were randomized to discharge on the day of assessment or conventional management (63). Again there were no differences in readmission rates and no differences in visits to primary care physicians and health status measured eight weeks after discharge was similar in the two groups. The authors also demonstrated that there were significant cost savings of around 50% for the home support group, compared with the admitted group. However, other considerations need to be taken into account in organizing an assisted discharge service, in that resources have to be released for the nurses to follow the patients and the benefits may be seasonal, as COPD admissions are a particular problem in the winter months. Further work is required on the different models of supported discharge available and the cost effectiveness of these programs.

VI. Prevention of COPD Exacerbation

There has been much recent emphasis on prevention of exacerbations in patients with COPD. As respiratory tract infections are common factors in causing exacerbation, influenza, and pneumococcal vaccinations are recommended for all patients with significant COPD. A study that reviewed the outcome of influenza vaccination in a cohort of elderly patients with chronic lung disease found that influenza vaccination is associated with significant health benefits with fewer outpatient visits, fewer hospitalizations, and a reduced mortality (65).

Long-term antibiotic therapy has been used in the past in patients with very frequent exacerbations, though the evidence was not strong for benefit. However, with the advent of novel and more specific antibiotics against airway organisms, the topic of long-term antibiotic therapy in COPD is currently being revisited. A recently reported long-term trial of the macrolide antibiotic erythromycin, for example, reported a significant reduction in exacerbation frequency in those patients on the active drug (66). Recently, there has been a report of the effects of an immunostimulatory agent in patients with COPD exacerbations, with reduction in severe complications and hospital admissions in the actively treated group (67). However, the mechanisms of benefit are not clear and further studies on the effects of these agents in the prevention of COPD exacerbation are required.

Long-acting bronchodilators (LABA) have been shown to reduce exacerbations. In the recently reported TORCH study, salmeterol, a long-acting β-agonist, reduced the frequency of exacerbations (68), while a number of other studies have shown that the long-acting anticholinergic tiotropium reduces the exacerbation rate and also a trend to hospital admission (69–72). However, there is no good evidence at present that long-acting anticholinergic agents possess anti-inflammatory activity (73) and it is likely that tiotropium reduces exacerbations by reducing dynamic hyperinflation and thus dyspnea. Combinations of long-acting β-agonists and inhaled corticosteroids have been also evaluated and reduced exacerbations more than the individual components (68). A direct comparison of inhaled tiotropium with the salmeterol/fluticasone (SFC) combination in the recently reported INSPIRE study in moderate-to-severe COPD patients showed that both interventions had an equal effect exacerbation rates (74). However, patients taking tiotropium required more courses of oral corticosteroids with exacerbations while patients on the SFC combination required more courses of antibiotics (74). For the first time, it has been shown that different interventions have different effects on exacerbations.

The optimal study recently evaluated the combination of tiotropium with inhaled LABA (salmeterol) and inhaled steroids (fluticasone) (75). The triple combination reduced hospitalization as a result of exacerbation, but not the total number of exacerbations. In addition a trend was observed in the reduction of the number of exacerbations with the triple combination, which did not reach statistical significance due to the relatively small size of the study and the high dropout rate. Triple therapy may be more effective than other therapies and further studies of these combinations are now required with adequately powered studies.

VII. Conclusion

COPD exacerbations are important events and affect quality of life, disease progression, and mortality. They are often triggered by airway infection and are an important cause of morbidity, impairment of health status, and mortality. A number of pharmacological and nonpharmacological interventions have been shown to prevent exacerbations. However, the degree of reduction in exacerbation frequency is still limited and newer interventions need to be studied in well-designed and adequately powered trials. It is most likely that combinations of interventions will be most effective. Thus, we will be able to meet one of the main objectives of therapy for COPD is to reduce the morbidity associated with COPD exacerbations.

References

1. Wedzicha JA, Seemungal TAR. COPD exacerbations: defining their cause and prevention. Lancet 2007; 370:786–796.
2. Seemungal TAR, Donaldson GC, Paul EA, et al. Effect of exacerbation on quality of life in patients with chronic obstructive pulmonary disease. Am J Respir Crit Care Med 1998; 151:1418–1422.
3. Bhowmik A, Seemungal TAR, Sapsford RJ, et al. Relation of sputum inflammatory markers to symptoms and physiological changes at COPD exacerbations Thorax 2000; 55:114–200.
4. Donaldson GC, Seemungal T, Jeffries DJ, et al. Effect of environmental temperature on symptoms, lung function and mortality in COPD patients. Eur Respir J 1999; 13:844–849.
5. Anthonisen NR, Manfreda J, Warren CP, et al. Antibiotic therapy in exacerbations of chronic obstructive pulmonary disease. Ann Intern Med 1987; 106:196–204.
6. Okubadejo AA, Jones PW, Wedzicha JA. Quality of life in patients with COPD and severe hypoxaemia. Thorax 1996; 51:44–47.
7. Okubadejo AA, O'Shea L, Jones PW, et al. Home assessment of activities of daily living in patients with severe chronic obstructive pulmonary disease on long term oxygen therapy. Eur Respir J 1997; 10:1572–1575.
8. Ball P, Harris JM, Lowson D, et al. Acute infective exacerbations of chronic bronchitis. Q J Med 1995; 88:61–68.

9. Seemungal TAR, Donaldson GC, Bhowmik A, et al. Time course and recovery of exacerbations in patients with chronic obstructive pulmonary disease. Am J Respir Crit Care Med 2000; 161:1608–1613.

10. Reddel HS, Ware S, Marks G, et al. Differences between asthma exacerbations and poor asthma control. Lancet 1999; 353:364–369.

11. Tattersfield AE, Postma DS, Barnes PJ, et al. Exacerbations of asthma. Am J Respir Crit Care Med 1999; 160:594–599.

12. Roberts CM, Lowe D, Bucknall CE, et al. Clinical audit indicators of outcome following admission to hospital with acute exacerbation of chronic obstructive pulmonary disease. Thorax 2002; 57:137–141.

13. Perera WR, Hurst JR, Wilkinson TMA, et al. Inflammatory changes and recurrence at COPD exacerbations. Eur Respir J 2007; 29:527–534.

14. Hurst JR, Perera WR, Wilkinson TMA, et al. Systemic and upper and lower airway inflammation at exacerbation of chronic obstructive pulmonary disease. Am J Respir Crit Care Med 2006; 173:71–78.

15. Saetta M, Di Stefano A, Maestrelli P, et al. Airway eosinophilia in chronic bronchitis during exacerbations. Am J Respir Crit Care Med 1994; 150:1646–1652.

16. Qiu Y, Zhu J, Bandi V, et al. Biopsy neutrophilia, neutrophil chemokin and receptor gene expression in severe exacerbations of chronic obstructive pulmonary disease. Am J Respir Crit Care Med 2003; 168:968–975.

17. Biernacki W, Kharitonov SA, Barnes PJ. Increased leukotriene B4 and 8-isprostane in exhaled breath condensate of patients with exacerbations of COPD. Thorax 2003; 58:294–298.

18. Drost EM, Skwarski KM, Sauleda KM, et al. Oxidative stress and airway inflammation in severe exacerbations of COPD. Thorax 2005; 60:293–300.

19. Donaldson GC, Seemungal TAR, Patel IS, et al. Airway and systemic inflammation and decline in lung function, in chronic obstructive pulmonary disease. Chest 2005; 128:1995–2004.

20. Seemungal TAR, Harper-Owen R, Bhowmik A, et al. Respiratory viruses, symptoms and inflammatory markers in acute exacerbations and stable chronic obstructive pulmonary disease. Am J Respir Crit Care Med 2001; 164:1618–1623.

21. Anderson HR, Limb ES, Bland JM, et al. Health effects of an air pollution episode in London, December 1991. Thorax 1995; 50:1188–1193.

22. Linaker CH, Coggon D, Holgate ST, et al. Personal exposure to nitrogen dioxide and risk of airflow obstruction in asthmatic children with upper respiratory infection. Thorax 2000; 55:930–933.

23. Seemungal TAR, Harper-Owen R, Bhowmik A, et al. Detection of rhinovirus in induced sputum at exacerbation of chronic obstructive pulmonary disease. Eur Respir J 2000; 16:677–683.

24. Rohde G, Wiethege A, Borg I, et al. Respiratory viruses in exacerbations of chronic obstructive pulmonary disease requiring hospitalisation: a case-control study. Thorax 2003; 58:37–42.

25. Greenberg SB, Allen M, Wilson J, et al. Respiratory viral infections in adults with and without chronic obstructive pulmonary disease. Am J Respir Crit Care Med 2000; 162:167–173.

26. Johnston SL, Pattemore PK, Sanderson G, et al. Community study of the role of viral infections in exacerbations of asthma in 9–11 year old children. Br Med J 1995; 310:1225–1229.

27. Falsey AR, Formica MA, Hennessey PA, et al. Detection of respiratory syncytial virus in adults with chronic obstructive pulmonary disease. Am J Respir Crit Care Med 2006; 173: 639–643.

28. Wilkinson TM, Donaldson GC, Johnston SL, et al. respiratory syncytial virus, airway inflammation and FEV1 decline in patients with COPD. Am J Respir Crit Care Med 2006; 173:871–876.

29. Sapey E, Stockley RA. COPD exacerbations. 2: Aetiology. Thorax 2006; 61:250–258.

30. Wilkinson TMA, Hurst JR, Perera WR, et al. Interactions between lower airway bacterial and rhinoviral infection at exacerbations of chronic obstructive pulmonary disease. Chest 2006; 129:317–324.

31. Antibiotics for exacerbations of chronic obstructive pulmonary disease. Cochrane Database Syst Rev 2006; (2):CD004403. DOI: 10.1002/14651858.CD004403.pub2.

32. Sethi S, Evans N, Grant BJ, et al. New strains of bacteria and exacerbations of chronic obstructive pulmonary disease. N Engl J Med 2002; 347:465–471.

33. Papi A, Bellettato CM, Braccioni F, et al. Infections and airway inflammation in chronic obstructive pulmonary disease severe exacerbations. Am J Respir Crit Care Med 2006; 173:1114–1121.

34. Blasi F, Damato S, Consentini R, et al. *C. Pneumoniae* and chronic bronchitis: association with severity and bacterial clearance following treatment. Thorax 2002; 57:672–676.

35. Seemungal TAR, Wedzicha JA, MacCallum PK, et al. *C. Pneumoniae* and COPD exacerbation. Thorax 2002; 57:1087–1088.

36. Belman MJ, Botnick WC, Shin JW. Inhaled bronchodilators reduce dynamic hyperinflation during exercise in patients with chronic obstructive pulmonary disease. Am J Respir Crit Care Med 1996; 153:967–975.

37. Braun SR, McKenzie WN, Copeland C, et al. A comparison of the effect of ipratropium and albuterol in the treatment of chronic obstructive airway disease. Arch Intern Med 1989; 149:544–547.

38. Combivent Inhalation Aerosol Study Group. In chronic obstructive pulmonary disease, a combination of ipratropium and albuterol is more effective than either agent alone. Chest 1994; 105:1411–1419.

39. Rebuck AS, Chapman KR, Abboud R, et al. Nebulized anticholinergic and sympathomimetic treatment of asthma and chronic obstructive airways disease in the emergency room. Am J Med 1987; 82:59–64.

40. Callahan CM, Cittus RS, Katz BP. Oral corticosteroid therapy for patients with stable chronic obstructive pulmonary disease: a meta-analysis. Ann Intern Med 1991; 114:216–223.

41. Keatings VM, Jatakanon A, Worsdell Y, et al. Effects of inhaled and oral glucocorticoids on inflammatory indices in asthma and COPD. Am J Respir Crit Care Med 1997; 155:542–548.

42. Culpitt SV, Maziak W, Loukidis S, et al. Effects of high dose inhaled steroids on cells, cytokines and proteases in induced sputum in chronic obstructive pulmonary disease. Am J Respir Crit Care Med 1999; 160:1635–1639.

43. Albert RK, Martin TR, Lewis SW. Controlled clinical trial of methylprednisolone in patients with chronic bronchitis and acute respiratory insufficiency. Ann Intern Med 1980; 92:753–758.

44. Emerman CL, Connors AF, Lukens TW, et al. A randomised controlled trial of methylprednisolone in the emergency treatment of acute exacerbations of chronic obstructive pulmonary disease. Chest 1989; 95:563–567.

45. Bullard MJ, Liaw SJ, Tsai YH, et al. Early corticosteroid use in acute exacerbations of chronic airflow limitation. Am J Emerg Med 1996; 14:139–143.

46. Murata GH, Gorby MS, Chick TW, et al. Intravenous and oral corticosteroids for the prevention of relapse after treatment of decompensated COPD. Chest 1990; 98:845–849.

47. Thompson WH, Nielson CP, Carvalho P, et al. Controlled trial of oral prednisolone in outpatients with acute COPD exacerbation. Am J Respir Crit Care Med 1996; 154:407–412.

48. Davies L, Angus RM, Calverley PMA. Oral corticosteroids in patients admitted to hospital with exacerbations of chronic obstructive pulmonary disease: a prospective randomised controlled trial. Lancet 1999; 354:456–460.

49. Niewoehner DE, Erbland ML, Deupree RH, et al. Effect of systemic glucocorticoids on exacerbations of chronic obstructive pulmonary disease. N Engl J Med 1999; 340:1941–1947.

50. Sachs APE, Koeter GH, Groenier KH, et al. Changes in symptoms, peak expiratory flow and sputum flora during treatment with antibiotics of exacerbations in patients with chronic obstructive pulmonary disease in general practice. Thorax 1995; 50:758–763.

51. Rice KL, Leatherman JW, Duane PG, et al. Aminophylline for acute exacerbations of chronic obstructive pulmonary disease. A controlled trial. Ann Intern Med 1987; 107:305–309.

52. Duffy N, Walker P, Diamantea P, et al. Intravenous aminophylline in patients admitted to hospital with non-acidotic exacerbations of chronic obstructive pulmonary disease: a prospective randomised controlled trial. Thorax 2005; 60:713–717.

53. Moser KM, Luchsinger PC, Adamson JS, et al. Respiratory stimulation with intravenous doxapram in respiratory failure. N Engl J Med 1973; 288:427–431.

54. Angus RM, Ahmed AA, Fenwick LJ, et al. Comparison of the acute effects on gas exchange of nasal ventilation and doxapram in exacerbations of chronic obstructive pulmonary disease. Thorax 1996; 51:1048–1050.

55. Bott J, Carroll MP, Conway JH, et al. Randomised controlled trial of nasal ventilation in acute ventilatory failure due to chronic obstructive airways disease. Lancet 1993; 341:1555–1557.

56. Kramer N, Meyer TJ, Meharg J, et al. Randomized prospective trial of noninvasive positive pressure ventilation in acute respiratory failure. Am J Respir Crit Care Med 1995; 151:1799–1806.

57. Brochard L, Mancebo J, Wysocki M, et al. Non-invasive ventilation for acute exacerbations of chronic obstructive pulmonary disease. N Engl J Med 1995; 333:817–822.

58. Plant PK, Owen JL, Elliott MW. A multicentre randomised controlled trial of the early use of non-invasive ventilation for acute exacerbations of chronic obstructive pulmonary disease on general respiratory wards. Lancet 2000; 355:1931–1935.

59. Ambrosino N, Foglio K, Rubini F, et al. Non-invasive mechanical ventilation in acute respiratory failure due to chronic obstructive pulmonary disease: correlates for success. Thorax 1995; 50:755–757.

60. Brown JS, Meecham Jones DJ, Mikelsons C, et al. Outcome of nasal intermittent positive pressure ventilation when used for acute-on-chronic respiratory failure on a general respiratory ward. J R Coll Physicians Lond 1998; 32:219–224.

61. Moretti M, Cilione C, Tampieri A, et al. Incidence and causes of non-invasive mechanical ventilation failure after initial success. Thorax 2000; 55:819–825.

62. Gravil JH, Al-Rawas OA, Cotton MM, et al. Home treatment of exacerbations of COPD by an acute respiratory assessment service. Lancet 1998; 351:1853–1855.

63. Cotton MM, Bucknall CE, Dagg KD, et al. Early discharge for patients with exacerbations of COPD: a randomised controlled trial. Thorax 2000; 55:902–906.

64. Skwarska E, Cohen G, Skwarski KM, et al. A randomised controlled trial of supported discharge in patients with exacerbations of COPD. Thorax 2000; 55:907–912.

65. Nichol KL, Baken L, Nelson A. Relation between influenza vaccination and out patient visits, hospitalisation and mortality in elderly patients with chronic lung disease. Ann Intern Med 1999; 130:397–403.

66. Seemungal TA, Wilkinson TM, Hurst JR, et al. Long term erythromycin therapy is associated with decreased COPD exacerbations. Am J Respir Crit Care Med 2008; 178:1139–1147.

67. Collet JP, Shapiro S, Ernst P, et al. Effect of an immunostimulating agent on acute exacerbations and hospitalization in COPD patients. Am J Respir Crit Care Med 1997; 156:1719–1724.

68. Calverley PM, Anderson JA, Celli B, et al. Salmeterol and fluticasone propionate and survival in chronic obstructive pulmonary disease. N Engl J Med 2007; 356:775–789.

69. Vincken W, van Noord JA, Greefhorst APM. Improved health outcomes in patients with COPD during 1 yr's treatment with tiotropium. Eur Respir J 2002; 19:209–216.

70. Casaburi R, Mahler DA, Jones PA, et al. A long-term evaluation of once-daily inhaled tiotropium in chronic obstructive pulmonary disease. Eur Respir J 2002; 19:217–224.

71. Niewoehner DE, Rice K, Cote C, et al. Prevention of exacerbations of chronic obstructive pulmonary disease with tiotropium, a once daily inhaled anticholinergic bronchodilator: a randomised trial. Ann Intern Med 2005; 143:317–326.

72. Tashkin DP, Celli B, Senn S, et al.; UPLIFT Study Investigators. A 4-year trial of tiotropium in chronic obstructive pulmonary disease. N Engl J Med 2008; 359(15):1543–1554.

73. Powrie DJ, Wilkinson TMA, Donaldson GC, et al. Effect of tiotropium on inflammation and exacerbations in chronic obstructive pulmonary disease Eur Respir J 2007; 30:472–478.

74. Wedzicha JA, Calverley PMA, Seemungal TA, et al.; for the INSPIRE Investigators. The prevention of chronic obstructive pulmonary disease exacerbations by salmeterol/fluticasone propionate or tiotropium bromide. Am J Respir Crit Care Med 2008; 177:19–26.

75. Aaron SD, Vandemheen KL, Fergusson D, et al.; Canadian Thoracic Society/Canadian Respiratory Clinical Research Consortium. Tiotropium in combination with placebo, salmeterol, or fluticasone-salmeterol for treatment of chronic obstructive pulmonary disease: a randomized trial. Ann Intern Med 2007; 146:545–555.

13
Treatment of Stable COPD

STEPHEN I. RENNARD and WILLIAM PEASE
University of Nebraska Medical Center, Omaha, Nebraska, U.S.A.

PETER J. BARNES
National Heart and Lung Institute, Imperial College, London, U.K.

I. Introduction

The medications used to treat chronic obstructive pulmonary disease (COPD) are reviewed in detail in other chapters in this volume (chaps. 6 and 7). Effective management of the patient with COPD, however, requires implementation of an overall disease management strategy that integrates these medications with nonpharmacologic interventions as well as the treatment of concurrent conditions, which are frequently present in COPD patients. Currently available medications that treat COPD can improve patient well-being and prognosis in important ways. Unfortunately, the available therapies are often underused and when prescribed are often not used in ways that optimize their effectiveness. The current chapter will review the strategies of COPD management.

Several sets of guidelines that provide recommendations for COPD management have been developed by a number of local, national, and international societies. The most widely referenced are those prepared jointly by the American Thoracic Society and the European Respiratory Society (1), and the guidelines of the Global Initiative for Chronic Obstructive Lung Disease (GOLD), which originated as a collaboration of the World Health Organization and the National Heart, Lung, and Blood Institute, NIH, U.S.A., and these are updated regularly (2). These guidelines define seven broad treatment goals in the management of COPD. Each of these goals can be addressed, at least in part, by available therapies (Table 1).

Current guidelines also provide a general stepwise approach to the COPD patient, gauged roughly to disease severity (Fig. 1). This approach is truly a "guideline" to be used as a suggestion to clinicians as a basis from which a management plan can be adapted to achieve best care. COPD patients are extremely heterogeneous in clinical presentation and in response to therapeutic interventions. Thus, management must be individualized. This requires careful diagnostic testing of individual patients. In addition, ideal management will often require a series of individual clinical trials in which therapeutic modalities are tested against individual patient goals. Even in this setting, however, optimal care requires an approach that carefully integrates pharmacologic and nonpharmacologic interventions to assure ideal therapeutic benefit.

Table 1 Treatment Goals and Available Therapies for COPD

Goals	Effective therapy[a]	Possibly effective therapy[b]
1. Relieve symptoms	Smoking cessation, β-agonist and anticholinergic bronchodilators, rehabilitation	Inhaled glucocorticoids, theophylline
2. Prevent disease progression	Smoking cessation	β-Agonist bronchodilators, inhaled glucocorticoids
3. Improve exercise tolerance	β-Agonist and anticholinergic bronchodilators, rehabilitation	
4. Improve health status	Rehabilitation	β-Agonist and anticholinergic bronchodilators, inhaled glucocorticoids
5. Prevent and treat complications	Many	Many
6. Prevent and treat exacerbations	Inhaled glucocorticoids, β-agonist, and anticholinergic bronchodilators	Theophylline
7. Reduce mortality	Oxygen	Inhaled glucocorticoids, β-agonist, and anticholinergic bronchodilators

Therapy that may be appropriate for highly selected individuals with severe disease, for example, volume reduction surgery and transplantation are not listed.
[a]Supported by large (often multiple) studies.
[b]Supported by fewer and/or smaller studies or demonstrating effects that may not achieve a consensus "Minimum Clinically Important Difference."

A. Underdiagnosis and Undertreatment

The clinical assessment of the COPD patient is surprisingly difficult. COPD is readily diagnosed and staged with simple spirometry (2). With modern equipment, spirometry is easy and inexpensive to perform. Nevertheless, COPD is underdiagnosed, with two-thirds or more of cases being undetected (3–6). In addition, a "diagnosis" of COPD is often made without spirometry, and this is more often wrong than right (3,6,7). This diagnostic inaccuracy, which can be readily addressed by the performance of spirometry, has led to both failure to treat individuals who could benefit and to overtreatment of those who are unlikely to benefit. Management of COPD, therefore, requires diagnostic use of spirometry. "Screening" spirometry in unselected populations is not currently recommended (8), although this has been questioned (9). At a minimum, individuals with symptoms of cough and sputum or with dyspnea either at rest or on exertion should have spirometry. In addition, individuals over the age of 40 with risk factors, including family history of COPD, current or past cigarette smoking, or exposure to dusts or fumes should also be considered for spirometry (9).

While spontaneously reported symptoms of dyspnea should always lead to a consideration of COPD and performance of spirometry, they are not a sensitive indicator of disease. Similarly, casually reported symptoms are not a good gauge of therapeutic response (10). In this context, dyspnea in COPD stems from dynamic

Therapy at Each Stage of COPD

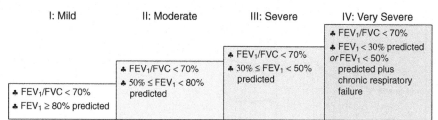

I: Mild	II: Moderate	III: Severe	IV: Very Severe
			♣ FEV₁/FVC < 70%
		♣ FEV₁/FVC < 70%	♣ FEV₁ < 30% predicted *or* FEV₁ < 50% predicted plus chronic respiratory failure
	♣ FEV₁/FVC < 70% ♣ 50% ≤ FEV₁ < 80% predicted	♣ 30% ≤ FEV₁ < 50% predicted	
♣ FEV₁/FVC < 70% ♣ FEV₁ ≥ 80% predicted			

Active reduction of risk factor(s); influenza vaccination
Add short-acting bronchodilator (when needed)

Add regular treatment with one or more long-acting bronchodilators (when needed); ***Add*** rehabilitation

Add inhaled glucocorticosteroids if repeated exacerbations

Add long term oxygen if chronic respiratory failure. Consider surgical treatments

Figure 1 Therapeutic strategy for the management of COPD based on severity as assessed by airflow (FEV₁). *Abbreviations*: FEV₁, forced expiratory volume in one second; COPD, chronic obstructive pulmonary disease. *Source*: From Ref. 2.

hyperinflation (Fig. 2) (11,12). Because expiratory airflow is limited, the lungs empty slowly. If respiratory rate is low, this poses relatively little problem. If respiratory rate increases, however, inadequate emptying of the lungs will occur. This will result in retention of air and progressive hyperinflation. Hyperinflation is partially adaptive as it increases airway diameters and thus increases flows, so that a new equilibrium can be reached. However, this is achieved at a cost of increased work of breathing, which is thought to be the major driver of dyspnea. Symptomatic dyspnea, therefore, can be avoided by minimizing tachypnea, which most commonly means restricting activity. COPD patients progressively decrease their level of activity. This is reflected not only in conventional activities associated with exertion, such as climbing stairs, but also in decreased amount of time spent ambulating or standing (13).

COPD patients may overestimate their level of activity (14), although they recognize their limitations. However, there appears to be a "response shift" in terms with respect to expectations. In one survey, one-quarter of COPD patients who were housebound because of dyspnea rated their disease as mild or moderate (15). Similarly, one-third of respondents who experienced dyspnea with speech rated their disease as completely or well controlled. The clinician managing the COPD patient, therefore, is faced with a difficult dilemma: patients often have significant limitations, which do not generate patient complaint and which may affect patients more than they realize. As a consequence, the clinician may significantly underestimate disease impact. The insidious development of symptoms, together with the associated response shift in patient expectations, likely accounts for the difficulty in clinically identifying COPD patients by

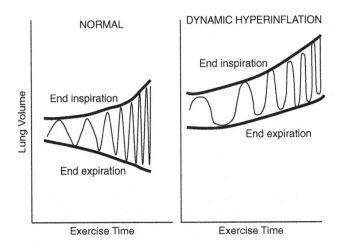

Figure 2 Schematic representation of dynamic hyperinflation. Vertical axes represent lung volumes. Horizontal axes represent time during an exertion. The thin lines indicate the volume of air in the lungs. A normal individual (*left*) increases total ventilation by increasing both the frequency of ventilation and the size of each breath. The latter is accomplished by both inhaling to a larger volume and exhaling to a smaller volume. In contrast, in an individual with expiratory airflow limitation, dynamic hyperinflation may develop (*right*). As the reduced airflow prevents lung emptying, air is progressively retained in the lung as rate increases. This results in an increase in the volume of the lung at the end of each breath. This results in increased work of breathing, which causes dyspnea, and can limit breath size and ventilation. Note that the COPD patient may have hyperinflation at baseline as well. *Abbreviation*: COPD, chronic obstructive pulmonary disease.

routine history. It can also compromise management of the diagnosed patient by masking the need for more aggressive interventions.

B. Extrapulmonary Disease

COPD patients frequently have problems outside the lungs (16–18). Many of these concurrent problems may be chance associations that increase as individuals age. However, a number of clinically important extrapulmonary problems appear to be more common among COPD patients than in similarly aged individuals with similar risk factors, including smoking (Table 2). This suggests that COPD represents one manifestation of a systemic disorder, a concept that is currently being actively investigated. Whether these comorbidities reflect a shared pathogenesis or not, they are important clinical problems. Thus, the key issue for the clinician is that appropriate management of the COPD patient must include the accurate diagnosis and management of these conditions.

C. Cigarette Smoking

Cigarette smoking is the most common cause of COPD, and smoking cessation is a major therapeutic goal. In the United States, about 80% of COPD patients are smokers (3) and, in general, cigarette smoking accounts for about 50% of the attributable risk (19). Appropriate interventions aimed at smoking are key. However, it is important to separate the

Table 2 Common Comorbidities Associated with COPD

Cardiac
Myocardial infarction
Arrhythmia
Failure
Aortic aneurysm
Hypercoagulability
Stroke
Pulmonary embolism
Deep vein thrombosis
Atrophy
Weakness/cachexia
Osteoporosis
Skin wrinkling
Anemia
Fluid retention
Depression
Lung cancer
Metabolic syndrome

problems of smoking and of COPD. Linking them can lead to underdiagnosis of COPD in the nonsmoker. It has also led to diagnostic and therapeutic nihilism in the approach to COPD in current or former smokers. This attitude was cited by Fletcher and colleagues on the dust jacket of their classic monograph (20) where they quoted Williams:

> Chronic bronchitis with it accompanying emphysema is a disease on which a good deal of wholly unmerited sympathy is frequently wasted. It is a disease of the gluttonous, bibulous, otiose, and obese and represents a well-deserved nemesis for these unlovely indulgences ... the majority of cases are undoubtedly due to surfeit and self-indulgence.

Unfortunately, this attitude persists and is reflected in the behavior of many health care practitioners and providers.

Current therapy offers many benefits to patients with COPD. Its effective implementation, however, requires a careful and individualized approach.

II. Smoking Cessation

Cigarette smoking is recognized as a primary disorder in which addiction to nicotine plays a primary role (21,22). Like most complex disorders, smoking has both genetic and environmental determinants, and these complex factors contribute to both smoking initiation and persistence (23). Addiction is not the only reason for smoking. Most smokers also smoke for a variety of "benefits" derived from their smoking (24). In this context, smoking is associated with a sensation of euphoria (25); has an antidepressant effect (26), which may be due to nicotine or other substances in cigarette smoke (27); can measurably improve cognition, especially when attention is required to tedious, repetitive tasks (28,29); and can result in a modest weight loss (30). Smoking is often integrated into social activities, and smoking behaviors within social networks are often relatively

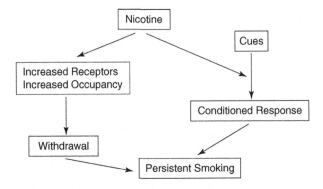

Figure 3 Conceptual basis for persistent smoking. Nicotine unlike most agonists induces increased expression of its own receptors. In the absence of ligand, withdrawal symptoms develop and contribute to persistent smoking. In addition, smoking behavior is linked to environmental cues resulting in conditioned responses. Nicotine can potentiate the development and intensity of conditioning, which can lead to persistent smoking by other mechanisms than "withdrawal."

homogeneous (31). Smoking, therefore, can be an important part of participation in social activities. Individuals giving up smoking will lose these benefits from smoking.

Nicotine affects many pathways in the brain, and the biological basis for addiction is complex (32,33). Smoking behavior, moreover, is more complex than "simple" addiction. Smoking is often linked to other stimuli resulting in powerful conditioned responses. Interestingly, nicotine can potentiate the acquisition and strength of cue-conditioned responses (34), suggesting a multifactorial pathogenesis (Fig. 3). The combined pathogenesis of biological addiction and conditioned responses is consistent with the clinical observation that a combination of pharmacologic and nonpharmacologic interventions is the most effective approach to achieve smoking cessation.

A. Nonpharmacologic Support

Nonpharmacologic interventions include behavioral, cognitive, and motivational support (35). The benefits of these interventions have been assessed in many studies and have been the subject of systematic review (21,22,36). In general, cessation rates increase with increasing intervention. Increases in duration and frequency of visits both increase success. The most intensive programs generally report quit rates of about 20% with behavioral support alone, although it is likely that those who participate in such programs are more highly motivated than the average smoker (37). In addition, increasing the number of providers and types of providers who assist with smoking cessation within a practice improves success. Thus, smoking cessation should be structurally integrated into clinical practices.

Intensive nonpharmacologic therapy will be appropriate for some individuals, and is most commonly provided by specialists. For smokers willing to participate in intensive programs, referrals should be made. However, the majority of smokers will decline to participate in an intense program. For these individuals, brief counseling is both appropriate and cost effective. Most clinicians should be able to provide this type of support in most

Table 3 The Five A's and R's

The five A's: For smokers willing to quit
  Ask: about tobacco use
  Advise: to quit
  Assess: willingness to make a quit attempt
  Assist: in quit attempt
  Arrange: for follow-up
The five R's: To motivate smokers unwilling to make a quit attempt at the present time
  Relevance: tailor advice and discussion to each smoker
  Risks: outline risks of continued smoking
  Rewards: outline the benefits of quitting
  Roadblocks: identify barriers to quitting
  Repetition: reinforce the motivational message at every visit

clinical settings. Simple advice to quit, coming from a physician, can increase quit rates over one year from 2% to 4–6% (38,39). The five A's and the five R's (Table 3) have been developed to serve as a basis for simple clinician intervention in both the primary and the secondary care settings. The five A's guide the identification of smokers and provide the key components for those individuals willing to make a quit attempt. The five R's help to provide brief motivation for the smoker unwilling to make a quit attempt with the understanding that the issue will be revisited in the future.

It is important for each clinician to provide a level of nonpharmacologic intervention within each practice and, in addition, to be aware of the resources for additional support within the community. These include not only intense support programs, but also readily accessible and often fully subsidized resources such as telephone quitlines (1-800-QUITNOW, e.g., is available for free within the United States). Importantly, telephone quitlines have a high degree of acceptance among smokers and have well-demonstrated efficacy (22,40,41).

B. Pharmacologic Support

Pharmacologic support can further improve the likelihood of achieving abstinence by two- to four-fold, depending on the medication, when compared with placebo (21,22,36). The added benefits of pharmacologic treatment have been observed when added to both minimal and intensive nonpharmacologic support programs. Current recommendations are that each serious quit attempt be given the best chance for success. Thus, each quit attempt should be supported with the most aggressive nonpharmacologic support program combined with pharmacologic support, unless contraindicated. Interestingly, aggressive therapy appears to be more cost effective than less aggressive therapy, as the increased success rates easily justify the marginal increases in costs (22,42,43).

Several pharmacologic support modalities are available. First-line therapies include nicotine replacement therapy, which is available in a number of formulations, bupropion and varenicline. Second-line therapies include nortriptyline and clonidine (Table 4). Detailed reviews of the clinical trial experience of these compounds are available (21,22,36).

Table 4 Pharmacotherapy for Smoking Cessation

First-line therapy
  Nicotine replacement therapy
    Transdermal nicotine systems
    Nicotine polacrilex
      Gum
      Lozenge
    Nicotine inhaler
    Nicotine nasal spray
  Bupropion
  Varenicline
Second-line therapy
  Clonidine
  Nortriptyline

C. Nicotine Replacement Therapy

Nicotine replacement therapy is probably the most commonly used pharmacologic treatment to assist with smoking cessation. Of the pharmacotherapies approved for use in smoking cessation, it has been available longest. The apparent paradox of using nicotine to treat nicotine addiction is best explained by the pharmacokinetics of nicotine delivery on which its addictive effects likely depend (44,45). In this context, the psychoactive effects of most addicting drugs depend not only on the amount of drug delivered to the brain, but also on the kinetics. Rapid, bolus-like delivery greatly increases the "hit" associated with the euphoric effects and likely contributes to the cellular changes that lead to addiction. Following peak levels, drug is redistributed and metabolized, resulting in gradually declining levels. Withdrawal symptoms are believed to develop with time following decreasing levels. Drug replacement therapy to treat drug addiction, therefore, is based on the concept that replacement can maintain levels to mitigate withdrawal symptoms without providing peak levels that reinforce addiction. This pharmacologic approach, of course, must be combined with nonpharmacologic interventions in which the smoker deals with the social aspects of smoking, the many cues that may condition smoking and the loss of the psychoactive benefits that may come from smoking.

    Several formulations of nicotine replacement have been evaluated in clinical trials and are available for use either over the counter or by prescription. While they differ in their pharmacokinetics, all appear to have similar efficacy, approximately doubling quit rates compared with placebo (21,22,36). All are used with the same general approach: pharmacotherapy is combined with nonpharmacologic support to achieve abstinence. After achieving abstinence and after having confidence in having become an ex-smoker, the smoker either gradually weans or discontinues nicotine replacement. The availability of multiple formulations allows the practitioner to tailor therapy to individual patient needs.

Transdermal Nicotine Systems

Transdermal nicotine systems (nicotine patches) deliver nicotine with the slowest and the steadiest pharmacokinetics among the available nicotine formulations. Nicotine is contained in a reservoir that is directly applied to the skin. Because nicotine is highly lipid-soluble, it is absorbed directly through the skin into the venous circulation. A fresh patch is applied once daily and removed the next day. This makes its administration relatively convenient and may improve compliance compared with formulations that require multiple dosing throughout the day. Because of the slow pharmacokinetics, addiction potential is low. Patches may be worn at night, thus providing nicotine levels early in the morning, when cravings for cigarettes may be particularly intense. On the other hand, nicotine delivery during sleep may lead to insomnia and/or highly vivid dreams. If a problem, the patch may be removed at night, although craving for a morning cigarette may increase. To prevent skin irritation, the site of application should be varied (46).

Nicotine Polacrilex
Nicotine bound to a polacrilex resin is available both as a gum and as a lozenge. The lozenge is kept in the mouth and releases nicotine as it slowly dissolves. The gum releases nicotine only upon chewing. With both formulations, nicotine is absorbed across the buccal mucosa into the venous circulation. Since nicotine will be ionized at low pH, eating acidic foods or drinking acidic beverages before using nicotine polacrilex will result in ionization of nicotine and decrease its absorption (47–49). Nicotine released into the mouth should not be swallowed. It may cause local irritation of the stomach and is absorbed through the gastrointestinal tract (46,48,49). Unfortunately, it is then metabolized with relative efficiency first pass in the liver, resulting in minimal therapeutic efficacy.

Nicotine polacrilex is available over the counter, and a range of doses of both the lozenge and the gum are available. Major advantages of this formulation are its ease of use and the ability of smokers to adjust dosing as needed.

Nicotine Inhaler
The nicotine inhaler contains nicotine bound to a cotton pledget contained in a tubular plastic holder. Sucking on the device results in inhalation of an aerosol of nicotine. The currently available device generates an aerosol that does not reach the lungs. Nicotine is deposited in the mouth and pharynx from which it is absorbed into the venous circulation. The device permits individual dosing, and a number of smokers find that the mechanics of using the device, which partially recapitulates the mechanics of smoking a cigarette, can be helpful during a quit attempt. Local irritation of the pharynx may preclude use (46,50).

Nicotine Nasal Spray
The nicotine nasal spray delivers 1 mg of nicotine to the nasal mucosa from which it is absorbed into the venous circulation. Of the currently available nicotine formulations, it has the most rapid pharmacokinetics. Consistent with the concept that pharmacokinetics are related to addiction, prolonged use is reported in 3% to 15% (51). It is highly irritating, but is tolerated by many despite the local effects (52). Nevertheless, a number of smokers find it a highly desirable formulation, as its rapid delivery of nicotine helps with acute cravings. Combined with the ability to dose as needed, it may have significant advantages in selected smokers.

Choice of and Combinations of Nicotine Formulations

Smokers are exceedingly heterogeneous in the amount smoked and the patterns of smoking. Which nicotine replacement formulation will be most effective for a given individual must be determined empirically. Most formulations result in only partial nicotine replacement. These agents, therefore, do not eliminate nicotine withdrawal symptoms. The intensity of symptoms, however, can be reduced (21,22,36). While some studies have suggested that increasing the dose of nicotine replacement therapy may increase quit rates (53,54), it has not been possible to relate this clearly to baseline smoking behavior (55,56). Thus, while practitioners have recommended use of higher doses for refractory individuals, this represents an "off-label" use that is not currently supported by guidelines (53). Cotinine, which is the major metabolite of nicotine in most individuals, may be used to individualize forms of nicotine replacement therapy (57,58).

Simultaneous use of two formulations of nicotine replacement therapy has some rationale. Specifically, use of a nicotine transdermal system can provide steady-state levels. This can be combined with a formulation that permits additional dosing as needed for cravings. Studies utilizing this strategy have demonstrated improved efficacy (22). While this represents an off-label use, this strategy has been supported for use in selected individuals in guidelines (22).

Bupropion

The antidepressant bupropion was empirically observed to lead to smoking cessation among depressed individuals. This led to a series of clinical trials demonstrating that bupropion is an effective aid in smoking cessation (59,60), approximately doubling quit rates compared with placebo. A number of additional clinical trials have consistently confirmed the efficacy of bupropion, including one specifically evaluating COPD patients (61). Bupropion may be particularly effective among individuals with a past history of depression (62,63). Among these individuals, bupropion appears to approximately double quit rates compared with placebo, while nicotine replacement therapy may be ineffective. Bupropion can lower seizure thresholds and is, therefore, contraindicated in individuals with an increased seizure risk. In addition, as bupropion is available under several trade names, care must be taken to avoid dual prescription.

Varenicline

Varenicline is a partial agonist of the $\alpha 2\beta 4$ nicotinic receptor, which is believed to play a key role in nicotine addiction (64,65). As a partial agonist, varenicline can mitigate symptoms of nicotine withdrawal. In addition, as partial agonists can block the activity of full agonists, varenicline may reduce the reinforcing effects of nicotine. Both of these psychoactive effects have been reported in clinical trials (66). When compared with placebo, varenicline improves quit rates three- to four-fold (22). Superiority to bupropion therapy has been demonstrated in direct comparison trials (22,67). Extended use of varenicline, over six months, may help reduce relapse rates (68).

Reports of behavioral disturbance, including agitation and suicidal ideation, have been associated with varenicline. Whether this represents a true adverse effect of the drug or an association due to smoking cessation in susceptible individuals remains to be determined at the present time. However, when used, patients and their relatives should be cautioned about the potential for behavioral disturbances, and they should be advised to contact health care providers immediately should they be observed (69).

Second-Line Therapies

Two second-line therapies, which are not specifically approved for use in smoking cessation, have been evaluated in a number of trials and are listed for consideration in current guidelines (22). These include clonidine, an antihypertensive, and the tricyclic antidepressant nortriptyline. The majority of clinical trials evaluating clonidine have demonstrated trends toward statistical significance. Meta-analyses suggest its potential efficacy (70). Similarly, nortriptyline has been evaluated in several studies. These include its use both alone and in combination with nicotine replacement therapy. Statistically significant efficacy was observed both in individual studies and in combined analyses (71). Both clonidine and nortriptyline have potential for serious adverse events. Nevertheless, for practitioners comfortable with their use, they can be considered as aids in smoking cessation in selected individuals.

Combination Therapy

There are limited data on combinations of pharmacotherapeutics to achieve smoking cessation. Combinations of various formulations of nicotine replacement therapy (NRT) have been suggested to increase efficacy in selected individuals as discussed above. Similarly, data evaluating combination of NRT with bupropion demonstrates increased efficacy (63), and its use is supported in guidelines (22). Other combinations are currently being evaluated.

Ineffective Agents

A number of other psychoactive agents have been assessed and have been found to be without benefit for smoking cessation (22). In particular, selective serotonin reuptake inhibitors have been found to be without benefit. They should not be used for the purpose of smoking cessation. Benzodiazepines similarly are without benefit. Interestingly, haloperidol has been demonstrated to increase smoking (72). Studies done with naltrexone, propranolol, silver acetate, and mecamylamine failed to demonstrate efficacy (22).

D. Overall Approach to Smoking Cessation

Many clinicians are often discouraged about smoking cessation interventions. Quit rates reported in clinical trials are substantially higher than those observed in clinical practice. This is due, without doubt, to the significant selection bias: individuals volunteering to participate in a smoking cessation trial are much more motivated to quit than those seen in routine practice. Nevertheless, clinicians can have a substantial impact on smoking during routine practice.

The current approach to smoking is to regard it as a chronic relapsing disease (22). The most appropriate "model" might be lymphoma. In this regard, each smoking cessation attempt can be regarded as an attempt to induce a remission. As with lymphoma, the most aggressive appropriate therapy that maximizes the likelihood of inducing a remission is the most appropriate clinical choice. Once induced, it is important to achieve as "durable" a remission as possible. Many smokers will relapse at times of stress, particularly in combination with alcohol use or in situations previously associated with cues for smoking. If forewarned, relapse may be forestalled. Pharmacotherapy has not been developed to prevent relapse. However, several studies suggest that this may be possible.

When considered as a chronic relapsing disorder, smoking cessation attempts should not be regarded as "successes" and "failures." Rather, if an attempt does not succeed, it should be carefully evaluated so that subsequent attempts can be modified to increase success. There is no interval that is required before a subsequent attempt. Thus, additional smoking cessation attempts should be undertaken as soon as a smoker is willing to try.

Benefits in the COPD Patient
Smoking cessation, at least early in the course of COPD, reduces the rate at which lung function declines (73,74). Smoking cessation is also associated with a reduction in symptoms of cough and sputum production and an improvement in heath status (75). In addition, smoking cessation improves many comorbidities associated with COPD, in particular heart disease (76). Ex-smokers with COPD, however, have persistent lower respiratory tract inflammation (77,78). Depression may worsen following smoking cessation and suicide has been reported (79). As depression is common in COPD and is often undiagnosed (80,81), COPD patients should be monitored for the presence of this comorbidity and treated as appropriate. Thus, smoking cessation is an essential goal in the management of COPD, but represents only one among many goals of management.

III. Treatment of Symptomatic COPD
Current management of symptomatic COPD, if successfully implemented, can reduce patient symptoms and improve patient performance. In addition, bronchodilators, which are the first-line mainstay for symptomatic COPD management, and inhaled corticosteroids (ICS) not only improve airflow and reduce symptoms but can also prevent exacerbations and may have beneficial effects in slowing disease progression and improving mortality. Successful use of these medications, however, requires more than simply their prescription. They must be integrated into a comprehensive disease management program.

As noted above, the natural history of COPD complicates clinical management. COPD patients generally lose lung function slowly and gradually over a period of decades (20,82). As lung function is lost, expiratory airflow progressively declines. This results in increasing dynamic hyperinflation, particularly with exertion, which is believed to be the key driver of dyspnea (11). COPD patients often control their symptoms by gradually restricting their level of exertion. As a result, COPD patients may be relatively "asymptomatic" despite having severely limited activity. In addition, perhaps because of the insidious nature of disease progression, COPD patients often have exceedingly modest expectations (15). This not only delays diagnosis but also complicates management of symptomatic disease.

Available therapies can modestly improve airflow, a response of 100 to 300 mL generally being regarded as very good (83). As a consequence of improved expiratory flow, dynamic hyperinflation is reduced, and exercise performance can be improved (11,84). Even in the absence of an improvement in airflow as assessed by the FEV_1

(forced expiratory volume in one second), however, lung deflation and improved exercise performance may occur (11,85,86). Thus, bronchodilators should be empirically assessed whether the FEV_1 improves acutely or not. Unfortunately, for an individual who is asymptomatic because activity is sufficiently restricted to prevent symptoms, no improvement in symptoms results from improving physiology. Such individuals will only perceive benefits of therapy if a concurrent attempt to increase activity is made. This complicates the clinical assessment of an empiric trial of bronchodilators.

A. Bronchodilators

Three major classes of bronchodilators are currently available. These include agonists active on the β_2-adrenergic receptor, which relaxes airway smooth muscle; antagonists of the M3 muscarinic cholinergic receptor, which induces contraction of airway smooth muscle; and theophylline, which has a modest bronchodilator effect and may improve airflow by other mechanisms. The pharmacology of these agents is reviewed in chapter 7.

β_2-Adrenergic Agonists

Activation of β_2-adrenergic receptors results in relaxation of airway smooth muscle and improves airflow. A number of compounds are available and can be roughly classified based on the kinetics of their onset and duration of action (see chap. 7). When administered via inhalation, rapidly acting β_2-adrenergic agonists, such as albuterol, improve airflow measurably within five minutes. Maximal bronchodilation is achieved shortly after. Albuterol and other rapidly acting agents can be used for "rescue" therapy to improve acute symptoms. In general, however, these agents have relatively short duration of action, making them less desirable for the management of patients who are always physiologically limited (10). Longer-acting agents, which include formoterol (87) and salmeterol (88), are appropriate for twice-daily use. This is not only more convenient than more frequent dosing but also results in more prolonged improvement in airflow both throughout the day and throughout the night. It is believed that persistent airflow improvement can increase habitual activity and prevent the development of symptoms and may contribute to reduction in exacerbation frequency. Formoterol is also rapid in its onset of action (89), although it is not recommended for rescue therapy, as the long duration of action may cause accumulation of drug with repeated dosing.

Currently available β-adrenergic agonists used to treat COPD are highly selective for the β_2-receptor. This selectivity minimizes side effects mediated through the β_1-receptor, which is present in the heart and is the major mechanism leading to the side effects of tachycardia and palpitations. The heart, however, also contains β_2-receptors (90). Thus, β_2 selective agonists are not entirely free of risk for these side effects, and these agents must be used with caution in patients at significant risk for ventricular arrhythmias. β_2-Agonists may also cause hypokalemia, hyperglycemia, and tremor. β_2-Adrenergic agonists are available for inhalation via metered-dose inhalers, dry powder inhalers, and as nebulized solutions. In addition, oral formulations are available. In general, oral administration results in more systemic side effects. For this reason, the inhaled route is preferred. Currently, dry powder inhalers are generally regarded as easier to use than metered-dose inhalers that deliver a spray of medication, but with both types of device, patient compliance with proper technique is poor and deteriorates significantly with time (91–94). Administration of drug via inhalation does not result in complete deposition within the lung. Significant amounts of drug may be deposited in the pharynx and swallowed. This is particularly the case with drug administered via conventional metered-dose inhalers. Since swallowed drug can result in systemic side effects, use of a spacer, which decreases oral deposition without compromising delivery to the lung (95), can reduce these side effects.

A large study in poorly treated asthmatics suggested that there could be increased mortality when long-acting β_2-agonists were used without concurrent ICS therapy (96). This has led to a "black box" warning in the FDA approved labeling for all β_2-agonists. In asthma, β_2-agonists are not currently recommended for use without concurrently administered ICS (97). A meta-analysis that included four studies that followed subjects for 4 to 12 months suggested that there may be similar concerns in COPD as there were 21 deaths in 1320 subjects treated with β_2-agonist compared with 8 deaths in 1084 treated with placebo ($p = 0.03$) (98). However, the TORCH study, a three-year study, demonstrated numerically fewer deaths in the β_2-agonist (salmeterol) treated group, 205 of 1521 subjects, compared with placebo, 231 in 1524 subjects, a difference that was not statistically significant ($p = 0.18$) (99). Thus, current guidelines do not recommend against using β_2-agonist therapy without the use of ICS for patients with COPD (2).

Many patients with COPD and concurrent heart disease may also be treated with β_1-adrenergic antagonists. Several studies support the use of these agents in COPD patients, as they can improve mortality and appear to have little if any adverse effect on lung function (100). This can result in the interesting situation of patients being treated with a β_1-antagonist and a β_2-agonist.

β_2-Adrenergic receptors are present on many cells in addition to airway smooth muscle. As a result, β_2-adrenergic agonists have the potential for nonbronchodilator effects, a number of which may be of clinical benefit (101). In this regard, salmeterol, which has been best studied in this regard, has been demonstrated to reduce inflammatory cell activation, edema formation, and epithelial damage caused by bacteria, and to enhance clearance of edema from the lung (101). The clinical relevance of these nonbronchodilator effects, however, remains to be established. Nevertheless, these may contribute clinically beneficial effects of these medications such as reduction in exacerbations or slowing the rate at which lung function is lost (see below).

Anticholinergics

Anticholinergic bronchodilators (see also chap. 7) are believed to mediate their effects by blocking M3 muscarinic receptors present on airway smooth muscle. Activation of these receptors is thought to contribute to a basal smooth muscle tone that is present in normal individuals and in patients with COPD. Inhibition of this "tone" can improve airflow. The variable "bronchodilator" response in COPD patients has been suggested to reflect variable baseline tone (102). While the effects are modest, they can be highly meaningful in patients with COPD. Both short- and long-acting medications are available. Ipratropium, the most widely used short-acting agent, induces measurable bronchodilation within 10 to 15 minutes and has an effect that lasts for 4 to 6 hours. Tiotropium, in contrast, has an onset of action of one to two hours, but dissociates from the receptor extremely slowly. It has a half-life of approximately 36 hours and is quite effective with once-a-day usage (103,104). Clinical trials with both ipratropium and tiotropium have demonstrated efficacy of these agents as bronchodilators. In addition, reduction in exacerbation frequency has been demonstrated, particularly for tiotropium (105–107).

The currently available anticholinergics are quaternary amines. As a result, there is very little absorption of these drugs into the central nervous system so that the well-described anticholinergic side effects of other antimuscarinics, such as atropine, are generally not observed. Systemic anticholinergic effects, however, may be observed. The most common adverse effect observed with tiotropium is dry mouth, which occurs in 10% or so of subjects. Urinary retention and ocular problems appear to be rare.

A meta-analysis suggested that anticholinergic agents may be associated with adverse cardiovascular effects, particularly stroke (108). A number of concerns have been raised regarding this analysis. More definitely, in the prospective UPLIFT trial, 5993 individuals were randomized to receive either tiotropium or placebo in addition to other medications (107); 1887 of the tiotropium and 1648 of the placebo-treated subjects completed the four-year treatment period. There were numerically fewer deaths and numerically fewer cardiovascular events and strokes among subjects treated with tiotropium compared with placebo. Thus, concerns regarding potential cardiovascular adverse effects with tiotropium have not been substantiated (2).

As with β_2-adrenergic receptors, muscarinic receptors are also present on many cell types within the lung. In this context, in vitro studies suggest the potential for muscarinic antagonists to have an anti-inflammatory effect (109,110). Whether such effects are observed in vivo and whether they are of any clinical relevance remain to be determined.

Theophylline

Theophylline is a modest bronchodilator that may also have additional therapeutic effects. These include anti-inflammatory effects (111,112), as well as inotropic and diuretic effects and augmentation of skeletal muscle strength. Any of these have the potential to result in clinical benefit in COPD patients (see chap. 6). Clinical trials of theophylline in COPD patients have demonstrated modest bronchodilator effects (113,114). Interestingly, subjective responses appear to be much greater than the responses in FEV_1 (115). Whether these subjective responses reflect a disproportionate effect on dynamic hyperinflation or nonbronchodilator effects of theophylline remains to be determined. If used, target blood levels of 5 to 10 mg/mL are currently recommended (2). These appear to achieve adequate clinical response and provide a much greater margin of safety than the higher levels previously recommended. Theophylline has a number of dose-related adverse effects, including nausea and vomiting, seizures, and arrhythmias. In addition, its use is complicated by many drug-drug interactions that can be particularly problematic for COPD patients who are often taking many medications.

B. Use of Bronchodilators

All of the available bronchodilators discussed above may be used as first-line therapy for the treatment of COPD (2). The GOLD guidelines suggest that inhaled therapy is the preferred route but, in the absence of head-to-head data, initiation of therapy with either

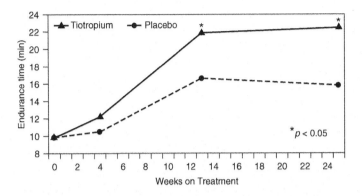

Figure 4 Effect of bronchodilation and rehabilitation on exercise performance. Subjects were randomly assigned to treatment with tiotropium or placebo. After four weeks there was a trend toward improved exercise time in the tiotropium-treated subjects. All subjects then underwent rehabilitation, which included exercise training. Both groups had a significant improvement in exercise time that was greater than achieved with tiotropium alone. The improvement in the tiotropium group was significantly greater than achieved in the placebo group, despite starting at a higher level. The benefits were still present three months following the rehabilitation program. *Source*: From Ref. 117.

a β_2-adrenergic agonist or an anticholinergic is acceptable (2). In some settings, oral agents are highly preferred. Thus, therapy with theophylline (at "low" doses designed to achieve blood levels of 5–10 mg/mL) has been popular in some countries, such as Japan (116).

The choice of agent with which to initiate therapy is likely of much less importance than the overall therapeutic plan. This is the case as bronchodilators improve airflow, which decreases dynamic hyperinflation and increases the potential for exertion. However, in the absence of exertion, a patient may fail to note any benefits. In addition, synergies between increased activity and bronchodilation are likely to be obtained. In this context, Casaburi (117) randomized a group of subjects to receive either tiotropium or placebo (Fig. 4). Tiotropium treatment, consistent with its bronchodilator effect and reduction in dynamic hyperinflation, demonstrated a trend toward improved exercise capacity as reflected by endurance time. After four weeks of treatment, all subjects underwent rehabilitation with exercise training. This resulted in substantial improvement in exercise performance. Individuals being treated with placebo had improvements with exercise training that greatly exceeded those obtained from tiotropium alone. Individuals treated with tiotropium, however, also experienced improvements in performance with exercise training. Importantly, the further improvement experienced by tiotropium-treated individuals with exercise training was even greater than that achieved in placebo-treated individuals despite their already having improved with drug treatment alone. This, therefore, represents a true synergy. Since the benefits of exercise training depend, at least in part, on the intensity of the training and since bronchodilator treatment allows exercise to a higher level of intensity, this synergy is highly plausible.

In clinical practice, therefore, bronchodilator therapy needs to be initiated together with a program increasing activity, ideally as part of a pulmonary rehabilitation program (118). Participation in such a program requires active participation of the patient. Thus, careful attention to individual patient goals and concurrent medical problems is essential. In particular, depression and conditions that compromise exercise, such as heart disease and skeletal muscular problems, must be addressed (118).

Combination Therapy with Bronchodilators

It is rational to begin bronchodilator therapy with a single agent. However, all patients with COPD, by definition, will continue to have physiologic limitation despite bronchodilator therapy. Most will also continue to have symptoms or exercise limitation. As a result, additional bronchodilator benefit is most often desirable. Addition of a second or third bronchodilator can result in both improved airflow and clinical benefit. A large series of clinical trials have demonstrated that combinations of β-agonists and anticholinergics, both long- and short-acting, can result in additional therapeutic benefits (2,119–121). Addition of theophylline to a regimen with other bronchodilators can also result in further clinical benefit (113,120).

The mechanisms by which multiple bronchodilators lead to increased benefits are not fully established. It is possible that they have actions at distinct sites within the lung. Alternatively, interactions among the diverse pathways through which these agents act raise the possibility of true pharmacologic synergies. While the mechanisms remain to be established, the use of bronchodilators in combination is well supported by clinical observations and is encouraged by current guidelines (2). Whether the increased costs and complexity of multiple medications are desirable must be assessed on an individualized basis. When multiple medications are to be used, preparations containing bronchodilators in combination may have a number of advantages. Combination products containing the short-acting β$_2$-agonist albuterol (salbutamol) and the short-acting antimuscarinic ipratropium are available in metered-dose inhaler and nebulized solution formulations. These have been extremely popular. Additional combination products that will contain long-acting agents are in development.

Inhaled Corticosteroids

ICS have been extensively evaluated as therapeutic agents in COPD (see chap. 6). Inhaled glucocorticoids have very modest effects on lung function or symptoms when used alone, although they do reduce the frequency of exacerbations (122). More importantly, when added to long-acting β-agonist bronchodilators, several ICS preparations have been demonstrated to result in further physiologic and symptomatic benefit (99,122–124). The benefits of these agents taken in combination include improved "trough" airflow, which is the airflow observed immediately prior to taking medication. As currently available, fixed-dose combinations are appropriate for twice-daily use; this means that a COPD patient upon awakening will have better airflow. Often, patients with COPD have particular difficulty with activities of personal hygiene in the early morning, and the ability of ICS in combination with β$_2$-agonists to improve airflow at this time may be particularly important. ICS, in addition, reduce the frequency of COPD exacerbations (122). As a consequence of these added benefits, combinations of ICS/LABA have been approved for use and are recommended for the treatment of patients with COPD who have frequent exacerbations (2).

ICS may cause local side effects in the pharynx and larynx, including thrush and dysphonia. Inhaled glucocorticoids may also cause systemic effects, including adverse effects on bone density. Systemic effects may be minimized by reducing the amount of medication that is swallowed through the use of a spacer (125). In addition, agents that are rapidly cleared or metabolized also have the potential for reduced systemic effects. An increased incidence of pneumonia has been reported in several COPD clinical trials with ICS (126). In general, these events are not well characterized and often were diagnosed in the absence of chest X ray or other confirmatory testing. In addition, while associated with increased incidence of pneumonia, ICS were associated with reduced COPD exacerbations and numerically reduced mortality (99). The clinical importance of these events remains to be determined.

Chronic use of systemically administered glucocorticoids is currently discouraged in the management of COPD (2). Short-term use during acute exacerbations has consistently demonstrated benefits (2,127). However, therapy beyond two weeks is without added benefit (128), and long-term therapy with systemic glucocorticoids is associated with increased mortality (129).

C. Other Therapeutic Effects
Mortality
As noted above, long-acting β-agonist bronchodilators, anticholinergic bronchodilators, and inhaled glucocorticoids have all been demonstrated to reduce COPD exacerbations. A number of retrospective studies suggested that there may also be an associated reduction in mortality, which is reasonable as exacerbations are times at which COPD patients are at hazard for fatal events (130,131). These observations led to the TORCH trial that was designed to determine if the combination of fluticasone (500 μg)/salmeterol (50 μg) reduced mortality compared with placebo (99). Although a numerical reduction in mortality was observed, this did not achieve statistical significance ($p = 0.052$) by the prespecified statistical analysis plan. Interestingly, there were far more dropouts in the placebo group, consistent with a lack of benefit in this group, which may have biased against detecting a beneficial drug effect. Thus, while TORCH failed to show a beneficial effect on mortality, such a benefit remains highly likely.

The UPLIFT trial was a similarly sized study evaluating tiotropium compared with placebo (107). It was designed primarily to determine if tiotropium slowed the rate of progression of lung function, but mortality was also assessed. A statistically significant benefit was observed in the tiotropium group compared with placebo at the end of treatment. However, the primary prespecified analysis was based on follow-up four weeks after completing treatment. While there were fewer deaths in the tiotropium-treated group at this time, the difference was no longer statistically significant both because of increased deaths in the group discontinuing tiotropium compared with those discontinuing placebo and because of loss of subjects to follow-up. Thus, while UPLIFT also failed to show a benefit in mortality, it also remains possible that tiotropium does, in fact, have such a benefit. Whether there is increased mortality upon tiotropium discontinuation, however, remains undetermined.

Disease Progression

Several studies have assessed the ability of inhaled glucocorticoids either alone or in combination with long-acting β_2-agonist bronchodilators to slow the rate of lung function loss in patients with COPD. While a number of these studies failed to show a statistically significant difference, meta-analyses suggested a significant benefit of approximately 5 mL of FEV_1 per year (122,132). While the rate of FEV_1 loss was not the primary endpoint in the TORCH study, significant benefits in the rate of lung function loss were observed in all three treatment groups compared with placebo (a difference of 13 mL/yr for the salmeterol group and for the fluticasone group and a difference of 16 mL/yr for the fluticasone/salmeterol combination group) (133).

The UPLIFT trial was specifically designed to determine if tiotropium would slow the rate of decline in lung function, and no therapeutic benefit compared with placebo was observed (107). However, the majority of patients treated with placebo were also being treated with either a long-acting β_2-agonist or a long-acting β-agonist inhaled glucocorticoid combination. It is possible, therefore, that the failure of tiotropium to affect the rate of decline in lung function was masked by the concurrent administration of these other agents. Importantly, tiotropium did have a significant added benefit, despite concurrent therapy, in improving airflow, reducing exacerbations, and improving health status.

Influenza Vaccination

Viral infections, including infections with influenza, are a major cause of COPD exacerbations. These are associated with increased morbidity and mortality (134,135). Influenza vaccination has been reported to reduce serious illness and death by 50% in COPD patients (136). COPD increases both in prevalence and severity with age. Many COPD patients would qualify on age alone. Vaccination is reasonable for all with COPD (2,137,138). The virus strain used, of course, must be appropriate for the individual year. The vaccination should be given once in the autumn or twice in the autumn and winter. As vaccination provides only partial protection, careful monitoring of COPD patients for influenza with the appropriate introduction of influenza-specific antibiotics is still warranted.

Pneumococcus

The utility of pneumococcal vaccination in the COPD patient population is not unequivocally demonstrated. However, its use is recommended similar to that in other elderly populations (2,138). Use among individuals younger than age 65 may also prevent the development of community-acquired pneumonia (2).

Oxygen

Two trials completed in the late 1970s demonstrated improved survival among hypoxic COPD patients treated with oxygen (139,140). The MRC trial demonstrated that oxygen administered primarily at night-time improved survival compared with no oxygen therapy (139). The nocturnal oxygen therapy trial further demonstrated that oxygen administered throughout the day resulted in improved survival compared with nocturnal oxygen alone (140). On the basis of these two trials, oxygen therapy for hypoxic COPD patients (PA O_2 < 55 mmHg, 7.3 kPa, or <89% saturated) is now standard of care.

Several subsequent trials have assessed mortality in COPD patients treated with oxygen. Interestingly, there appears to be a steady improvement in survival among these subjects (141). All, of course, have been treated with oxygen, as lack of treatment would be regarded as malpractice and unethical. Whether the improved survival reflects a change in the nature of the hypoxic COPD patient or in therapeutic benefits from concurrently administered medications, either for COPD or for comorbid conditions, remains to be determined.

The mechanism(s) by which oxygen therapy improves survival is undetermined. Beneficial effects on pulmonary hypertension may play a role. Alternatively, hypoxemia is a prominent systemic effect of COPD. Hypoxia leads to activation of many genes in a variety of cell types (142). It is possible, therefore, that correction of hypoxemia has beneficial effects on the systemic manifestations of COPD.

Whether oxygen should be used for patients with less severe or with intermittent hypoxia is less well established (143). However, intermittent hypoxia can lead to secondary problems, including pulmonary hypertension and polycythemia and may compromise exercise performance and predispose to cardiac events. Use of oxygen for individuals with intermittent hypoxemia who have clinical indications is currently recommended (2). Interestingly, normoxic COPD patients who undergo exercise training do better with supplemental oxygen (144). This may be due to a reduction in respiratory rate and reduced dynamic hyperinflation, which permits exercise to a higher level of intensity. The clinical benefits of oxygen in this setting, however, are not established.

Mucoactive Agents
Cough and sputum production can be major problems for COPD patients and are likely related to increased risk of exacerbation and lung function decline (145). Despite a very long history of empiric use of agents to alleviate these symptoms (146), no agents are currently approved and recommended for use for this purpose (2). A large trial evaluated *N*-acetyl cysteine, which has both antioxidant and mucoactive actions. The primary outcomes were COPD exacerbations and FEV_1, and clinical benefits were observed (147). Centrally acting agents, particularly opiates, can suppress cough (148). As these agents may impair clearance of secretions, they may increase risk for infection and are not routinely recommended (2).

D. Pharmacotherapy of Comorbidities
It is becoming increasingly clear that patients with COPD have a high prevalence of co-morbid conditions (16,149,150). Often these are major problems facing individual patients and, very frequently, they complicate the management of the COPD. Unfortunately, there are few studies of patients with complex comorbidities. Available guidelines, moreover, have almost uniformly been prepared with single disease focus, and often provide conflicting recommendations for patients with commonly associated problems (151). This often leaves the clinician faced with making decisions that must be based on a relative paucity of data and guidance. Several comorbid conditions create specific issues.

Among the comorbid conditions, anxiety and depression are likely more common among COPD patients than among the general population (152–155). Psychiatric dysfunction may complicate participation in rehabilitation programs, and even sub-clinical psychiatric disorders have been associated with increased morbidity among COPD patients (156). The prevalence of concurrent depression, moreover, is associated with increased mortality among COPD patients (157,158). Progressive diagnosis and appropriate treatment of depression in COPD patients, therefore, is essential for optimal patient management. In some cases, this may require referral to specialists (159).

Which psychotherapeutics to use in COPD patients has not been specifically assessed. Benzodiazepines have the potential to suppress ventilatory drive and, if possible, should be avoided (160). Treatment with nortriptyline (161), sertraline (152), and buspirone (162) have all been reported to reduce anxiety in COPD patients. Buspirone also reduced dyspnea without adversely affecting ventilatory drive or blood gases in one small trial (162). Psychotherapy may also provide symptomatic benefit for anxiety and depression in COPD patients (163,164). Pulmonary rehabilitation has also been demonstrated to improve psychiatric well-being among COPD patients.

Heart disease is a common cause of death among patients with COPD (165). Appropriate diagnosis and management of concurrent heart disease, therefore, are essential. Interestingly, agents used to treat heart disease may have additional benefits in COPD patients. In this context, Mancini evaluated the effect of statins, angiotensin-converting enzyme inhibitors, and angiotensin-receptor blockers in COPD patients (166). These agents were found to reduce both hospitalizations and mortality from respiratory causes in a large health care database review. Most of the individuals prescribed these medications, as might be expected, had cardiovascular risk factors that accounted for their being prescribed these medications. Interestingly, 5344 individuals who were not at increased risk for cardiovascular events were prescribed these medications. These individuals also demonstrated reduced respiratory morbidity. This has led to the suggestion that these agents may have direct benefit in the management of COPD, perhaps through an anti-inflammatory effect.

The possibility that statins may have a therapeutic benefit by controlling inflammation in COPD is currently under investigation. Whether these cardiovascular drugs are beneficial for COPD per se or not, however, they should certainly be used appropriately for the large number of COPD patients who have concurrent cardiovascular disease risk factors.

E. Nonpharmacologic Treatments

Several nonpharmacologic interventions can have important benefits for COPD patients. As noted above, pulmonary rehabilitation and, in particular, exercise training can be of substantial benefit (118). While rehabilitation does not improve lung function, it improves exercise performance. This likely results from improving the efficiency at which exercise is performed and by decreasing the tachypnea associated with exercise because of a "training" effect. A smaller increase in respiratory rate results in less dynamic hyperinflation and, in turn, less dyspnea upon exertion. Exercise training is currently recommended for all COPD patients with moderate disease or worse (118). The limited availability of rehabilitation programs should not discourage the clinician from recommending exercise training.

F. Surgical Interventions

Surgical interventions may also benefit selected patients with COPD. These have been reviewed in detail elsewhere (167). Removal of large bullae is of benefit for the rare individuals in whom these are present. Volume reduction surgery may have similar benefits for individuals with localized disease who do not respond well to aggressive medical management. Similarly, transplantation may be of benefit in highly selected individuals.

G. α-1 Antitrypsin Deficiency

Deficiency in the serum protein α-1 antitrypsin is a recessive genetic disorder that predisposes to the development of emphysema (168). The relevant protein can be purified from human blood and is available for replacement therapy. The drug was approved in the United States as an "orphan drug" based on biochemical measures. A randomized controlled trial is in progress in Europe. Several observational registry trials, however, suggest that its use can slow the development of emphysema among selected individuals with α-1 antitrypsin deficiency (169). Among individuals with normal lung function, there is little benefit, as lung function is not being lost or is being lost very slowly. Similarly, among individuals with very poor lung function, it is difficult to demonstrate benefits. The maximum benefit appears to be among individuals with FEV_1 about 50% predicted, in whom the rate of lung function loss may slow decline from about 100 mL/yr to about 80 mL/yr (170). Replacement therapy must be given intravenously, although inhaled formulations are being investigated. It is a blood product prepared from a pool of donors and, while treated and evaluated for potential pathogens, is not entirely risk free. It should not be used among concurrent smokers, as smoking inactivates the α-1 proteinase inhibitor. In addition, it should not be used following liver transplantation, as transplantation with a normal liver restores α-1 levels. Not all individuals with diagnosed deficiency, therefore, may be appropriate for therapy. Thus, careful monitoring with lung function testing and/or CT scanning is important to help in the decision of whether replacement therapy is warranted.

IV. Summary

Pharmacotherapy of COPD can contribute to all the therapeutic goals listed in the GOLD guidelines. None can be achieved completely with existing agents, so additional treatments are needed. Nevertheless, use of the currently available medications can improve lung function, reduce symptoms, lower the incidence of exacerbations, reduce mortality, and slow disease progression. To achieve the best effect from the medications available, the clinician must integrate their use into a personalized comprehensive disease management program.

References

1. Celli BR, MacNee W. Standards for the diagnosis and treatment of patients with COPD: a summary of the ATS/ERS position paper. Eur Respir J 2004; 23(6):932–946.
2. Global Strategy for Diagnosis. Management and Prevention of COPD, 2008. Available at: http://www.goldcopd.com.

3. Mannino DM, Gagnon RC, Petty TL, et al. Obstructive lung disease and low lung function in adults in the United States: data from the National Health and Nutrition Examination Survey, 1988–1994. Arch Intern Med 2000; 160(11):1683–1689.
4. Mannino DM, Homa DM, Akinbami LJ, et al. Chronic obstructive pulmonary disease surveillance—United States, 1971–2000. MMWR Surveill Summ 2002; 51(6):1–16.
5. Schirnhofer L, Lamprecht B, Vollmer WM, et al. COPD prevalence in Salzburg, Austria: results from the Burden of Obstructive Lung Disease (BOLD) Study. Chest 2007; 131(1): 29–36.
6. Talamo C, de Oca MM, Halbert R, et al. Diagnostic labeling of COPD in five Latin American cities. Chest 2007; 131(1):60–67.
7. Tinkelman DG, Price DB, Nordyke RJ, et al. Misdiagnosis of COPD and asthma in primary care patients 40 years of age and over. J Asthma 2006; 43(1):75–80.
8. Qaseem A, Snow V, Shekelle P, et al. Diagnosis and management of stable chronic obstructive pulmonary disease: a clinical practice guideline from the American College of Physicians. Ann Intern Med 2007; 147(9):633–638.
9. Petty TL, Mannino DM. Will recommendations against spirometry make chronic obstructive pulmonary disease harder to treat? Ann Intern Med 2008; 149(7):512–513; author reply 513.
10. Rennard SI, Calverley P. Rescue! Therapy and the paradox of the Barcalounger. Eur Respir J 2003; 21(6):916–917.
11. O'Donnell DE. Hyperinflation, dyspnea, and exercise intolerance in chronic obstructive pulmonary disease. Proc Am Thorac Soc 2006; 3(2):180–184.
12. O'Donnell DE, Lam M, Webb KA. Measurement of symptoms, lung hyperinflation, and endurance during exercise in chronic obstructive pulmonary disease. Am J Respir Crit Care Med 1998; 158(5 pt 1):1557–1565.
13. Pitta F, Troosters T, Spruit MA, et al. Characteristics of physical activities in daily life in chronic obstructive pulmonary disease. Am J Respir Crit Care Med 2005; 171(9):972–977.
14. Pitta F, Troosters T, Spruit MA, et al. Activity monitoring for assessment of physical activities in daily life in patients with chronic obstructive pulmonary disease. Arch Phys Med Rehabil 2005; 86(10):1979–1985.
15. Rennard S, Decramer M, Calverley PM, et al. Impact of COPD in North America and Europe in 2000: subjects' perspective of Confronting COPD International Survey. Eur Respir J 2002; 20(4):799–805.
16. Fabbri LM, Luppi F, Beghé B, et al. Complex chronic comorbidities of COPD. Eur Respir J 2008; 31(1):204–212.
17. Barr RG, Celli BR, Mannino DM, et al. Comorbidities, patient knowledge, and disease management in a national sample of patients with COPD. Am J Med 2009; 122(4):348–355.
18. Decramer M, Rennard S, Troosters T, et al. COPD as a lung disease with systemic consequences—clinical impact, mechanisms, and potential for early intervention. COPD 2008; 5(4):235–256.
19. Mannino DM, Buist AS. Global burden of COPD: risk factors, prevalence, and future trends. Lancet 2007; 370(9589):765–773.
20. Fletcher C, Peto R, Tinker C, et al. The natural history of chronic bronchitis and emphysema. New York: Oxford University Press, 1976:272.
21. Fiore MC. US public health service clinical practice guideline: treating tobacco use and dependence. Respir Care 2000; 45(10):1200–1262.
22. Fiore MC. Treating Tobacco Use and Dependence: 2008 Update. Rockville, MD: U.S. Department of Health and Human Services, Public Health Service, 2008:257.
23. Rennard SI, Daughton DM. Cigarette smoking and disease. In: Elias JA, Fishman JA, Grippi MA, et al., eds. Pulmonary Diseases and Disorders. New York: McGraw Hill, 1998:697–708.

24. Heishman SJ. Behavioral and cognitive effects of smoking: relationship to nicotine addiction. Nicotine Tob Res 1999; 1(suppl 2):S143–S147; discussion S165–S166.

25. Henningfield JE, Miyasato K, Jasinski DR. Abuse liability and pharmacodynamic characteristics of intravenous and inhaled nicotine. J Pharmacol Exp Ther 1985; 234:1–12.

26. Salin-Pascual RJ. Relationship between mood improvement and sleep changes with acute nicotine administration in non-smoking major depressed patients. Rev Invest Clin 2002; 54(1): 36–40.

27. Kay AB, Austen KF. The IgE-mediated release of an eosinophil leukocyte chemotactic factor from human lung. J Immunol 1971; 107(3):899–902.

28. Mumenthaler MS, Taylor JL, O'Hara R, et al. Influence of nicotine on simulator flight performance in non-smokers. Psychopharmacology (Berl) 1998; 140(1):38–41.

29. Huang SK, Wettlaufer SH, Hogaboam CM, et al. Variable prostaglandin E2 resistance in fibroblasts from patients with usual interstitial pneumonia. Am J Respir Crit Care Med 2008; 177(1):66–74.

30. Jo YH, Talmage DA, Role LW. Nicotinic receptor-mediated effects on appetite and food intake. J Neurobiol 2002; 53(4):618–632.

31. Christakis NA, Fowler JH. The collective dynamics of smoking in a large social network. N Engl J Med 2008; 358(21):2249–2258.

32. Balfour DJ. The neuronal pathways mediating the behavioral and addictive properties of nicotine. Handb Exp Pharmacol 2009; (192):209–233.

33. Benowitz NL. Neurobiology of nicotine addiction: implications for smoking cessation treatment. Am J Med 2008; 121(4 suppl 1):S3–S10.

34. Olausson P, Jentsch JD, Taylor JR. Repeated nicotine exposure enhances responding with conditioned reinforcement. Psychopharmacology (Berl) 2004; 173(1–2):98–104.

35. Niaura R. Nonpharmacologic therapy for smoking cessation: characteristics and efficacy of current approaches. Am J Med 2008; 121(4 suppl 1):S11–S19.

36. Fiore MC, Bailey WC, Cohen SJ. Smoking Cessation. Guideline Technical Report No. 18. Rockville, MD: U.S. Department of Health and Human Services, Public Health Service, Agency for Health Care Policy and Research. Publication No. AHCPR 97-Noo4, October 1997.

37. Schwartz JL. Review and Evaluation of Smoking Cessation Methods: The United States and Canada, 1978–1985. Bethesda, MD: National Cancer Institute, 1987.

38. Gilpin EA, Pierce JP, Johnson M, et al. Physician advice to quit smoking: results from the 1990 California Tobacco Survey. J Gen Intern Med 1993; 8(10):549–553.

39. Silagy C, Stead LF. Physician advice for smoking cessation. Cochrane Database Syst Rev 2001; (2):CD000165.

40. Miguez MC, Vazquez FL, Becona E. Effectiveness of telephone contact as an adjunct to a self-help program for smoking cessation: a randomized controlled trial in Spanish smokers. Addict Behav 2002; 27(1):139–144.

41. Zhu SH, Anderson CM, Tedeschi GJ, et al. Evidence of real-world effectiveness of a telephone quitline for smokers. N Engl J Med 2002; 347(14):1087–1093.

42. Cornuz J, Gilbert A, Pinget C, et al. Cost-effectiveness of pharmacotherapies for nicotine dependence in primary care settings: a multinational comparison. Tob Control 2006; 15(3): 152–159.

43. Bolin K, Mörk AC, Willers S, et al. Varenicline as compared to bupropion in smoking-cessation therapy—cost-utility results for Sweden 2003. Respir Med 2008; 102(5): 699–710.

44. Benowitz NL. Pharmacokinetics and pharmadynamics of nicotine. In: Rand MJ, Thurau K, eds. The Pharmacology of Nicotine. Washington, D.C.: IRL Press, 1987:3–18.

45. Benowitz NL. Pharmacodynamics of nicotine: Implications for rational treatment of nicotine addiction. Br J Addict 1991; 86:495–499.

46. Silagy C, Lancaster T, Stead L, et al. Nicotine replacement therapy for smoking cessation. Cochrane Database Syst Rev 2004; (3):CD000146.
47. Henningfield JE, Radzius A, Cooper TM, et al. Drinking coffee and carbonated beverages blocks absorption of nicotine from nicotine polacrilex gum. JAMA 1990; 264(12):1560–1564.
48. Healthcare GC. Product information: Commit oral lozenge, nicotine polacrilex oral lozenge. Pittsburgh, 2003.
49. Healthcare GC. Product information: Nicorette gum, nicotine polacrilex gum. Moon Township, 2005.
50. Healthcare PC. Product information: Nicotrol inhalation solution, nicotine inhalation solution. Morris Plains, 2005.
51. Hajek P, McRobbie H, Gillison F. Dependence potential of nicotine replacement treatments: effects of product type, patient characteristics, and cost to user. Prev Med 2007; 44(3): 230–234.
52. Healthcare PC. Product information: Nicotrol vs nicotine nasal spray. Morris Plains, 2005.
53. Tonnesen P, Paoletti P, Gustavsson G, et al. Higher dosage nicotine patches increase one-year smoking cessation rates: results from the European CEASE trial. Collaborative European Anti-Smoking Evaluation. European Respiratory Society. Eur Respir J 1999; 13(2): 238–246.
54. Hurt RD, Krook JE, Croghan IT, et al. Nicotine patch therapy based on smoking rate followed by bupropion for prevention of relapse to smoking. J Clin Oncol 2003; 21(5):914–920.
55. Hughes JR, Lesmes GR, Hatsukami DK, et al. Are higher doses of nicotine replacement more effective for smoking cessation? Nicotine Tobacco Res 1999; 1:169–174.
56. Glover ED, Dachs DPL, Stitzer ML, et al. Smoking cessation in highly dependent smokers with 4 mg nicotine polacrilex. Am J Health Behav 1996; 20:319–332.
57. Sachs DP, Benowitz NL. Individualizing medical treatment for tobacco dependence. Eur Respir J 1996; 9(4):629–631.
58. Lawson GM, Hurt RD, Dale LC, et al. Application of serum nicotine and plasma cotinine concentrations to assessment of nicotine replacement in light, moderate, and heavy smokers undergoing transdermal therapy. J Clin Pharmacol 1998; 38(6):502–509.
59. Bluemke DA, Soyer P, Fishman EK. Nontumorous low-attenuation defects in the liver on helical CT during arterial portography: frequency, location, and appearance. AJR Am J Roentgenol 1995; 164(5):1141–1145.
60. DeMeo DL, Campbell EJ, Brantly ML, et al. Heritability of lung function in severe alpha-1 antitrypsin deficiency. Hum Hered 2009; 67(1):38–45.
61. Tashkin D, Kanner R, Bailey W, et al. Smoking cessation in patients with chronic obstructive pulmonary disease: a double-blind, placebo-controlled, randomised trial. Lancet 2001; 357(9268):1571–1575.
62. Hurt RD, Sachs DP, Glover ED, et al. A comparison of sustained-release bupropion and placebo for smoking cessation. N Engl J Med 1997; 337:1195–1202.
63. Jorenby DE, Leischow SJ, Nides MA, et al. A controlled trial of sustained-release bupropion, a nicotine patch, or both for smoking cessation. New Engl J Med 1999; 340:685–691.
64. Glover ED, Rath JM. Varenicline: progress in smoking cessation treatment. Expert Opin Pharmacother 2007; 8(11):1757–1767.
65. Arneric SP, Holladay M, Williams M. Neuronal nicotinic receptors: a perspective on two decades of drug discovery research. Biochem Pharmacol 2007; 74(8):1092–1101.
66. Gonzales D, Rennard SI, Nides M, et al. Varenicline, an alpha4beta2 nicotinic acetylcholine receptor partial agonist, vs sustained-release bupropion and placebo for smoking cessation: a randomized controlled trial. JAMA 2006; 296(1):47–55.
67. Jorenby DE, Hays JT, Rigotti NA, et al. Efficacy of varenicline, an alpha4beta2 nicotinic acetylcholine receptor partial agonist, vs placebo or sustained-release bupropion for smoking cessation: a randomized controlled trial. JAMA 2006; 296(1):56–63.

68. Tonstad S, Tønnesen P, Hajek P, et al. Effect of maintenance therapy with varenicline on smoking cessation: a randomized controlled trial. JAMA 2006; 296(1):64–71.
69. Available at: www.fda.gov/Drugs/DrugSafety/PostmarketDrugSafetyInformationfor-PatientsandProviders/DrugSafetyInformationforHeathcareProfessionals/ucm169986.htm.
70. Gourlay SG, Stead LF, Benowitz NL. Clonidine for smoking cessation. Cochrane Database Syst Rev 2004; (3):CD000058.
71. Hughes J, Stead L, Lancaster T. Antidepressants for smoking cessation. Cochrane Database Syst Rev 2004; (4):CD000031.
72. McEvoy JP, Freudenreich O, Levin ED, et al. Haloperidol increases smoking in patients with schixophrenia. Psychopharmacology (Berl) 1995; 119:124–126.
73. Anthonisen NR, Connett JE, Kiley JP, et al. Effects of smoking intervention and the use of an inhaled anticholinergic bronchodilator on the rate of decline of FEV1. JAMA 1994; 272:1497–1505.
74. Anthonisen NR, Connett JE, Murray RP. Smoking and lung function of Lung Health Study participants after 11 years. Am J Respir Crit Care Med 2002; 166(5):675–679.
75. Buist AS, Sexton GJ, Nagy JM, et al. The effect of smoking cessation and modification on lung function. Am Rev Respir Dis 1976; 114:115–122.
76. U.S. Department of Health and Human Services, The health benefits of smoking cessation. A report of the Surgeon General, Washington, D.C.: Department of Health and Human Services (US), Publication No. (CDC) 90-8416. 1990.
77. Rutgers SR, Postma DS, ten Hacken NH, et al. Ongoing airway inflammation in patients with COPD who do not currently smoke. Thorax 2000; 55(1):12–18.
78. Willemse BW, ten Hacken NH, Rutgers B, et al. Effect of 1-year smoking cessation on airway inflammation in COPD and asymptomatic smokers. Eur Respir J 2005; 26(5):835–845.
79. Hughes JR. Smoking and suicide: a brief overview. Drug Alcohol Depend 2008; 98(3): 169–178.
80. Schane RE, Walter LC, Dinno A, et al. Prevalence and risk factors for depressive symptoms in persons with chronic obstructive pulmonary disease. J Gen Intern Med 2008; 23(11): 1757–1762.
81. Lewis KE, Annandale JA, Sykes RN, et al. Prevalence of anxiety and depression in patients with severe COPD: similar high levels with and without LTOT. COPD 2007; 4(4):305–312.
82. Rennard SI, Vestbo J. Natural histories of chronic obstructive pulmonary disease. Proc Am Thorac Soc 2008; 5(9):878–883.
83. Donohue JF. Minimal clinically important differences in COPD lung function. COPD 2005; 2(1):111–124.
84. Belman MJ, Botnick WC, Shin JW. Inhaled bronchodilators reduce dynamic hyperinflation during exercise in patients with chronic obstructive pulmonary disease. Am J Respir Crit Care Med 1996; 153:967–975.
85. Di Marco F, Milic-Emili J, Boveri B, et al. Effect of inhaled bronchodilators on inspiratory capacity and dyspnoea at rest in COPD. Eur Respir J 2003; 21(1):86–94.
86. Corsico A, Fulgoni P, Beccaria M, et al. Effects of exercise and beta 2-agonists on lung function in chronic obstructive pulmonary disease. J Appl Physiol 2002; 93(6):2053–2058.
87. Jarvis B, Markham A. Inhaled salmeterol: a review of its efficacy in chronic obstructive pulmonary disease. Drugs Aging 2001; 18(6):441–472.
88. Devine SM, Cobbs C, Jennings M, et al. Mesenchymal stem cells distribute to a wide range of tissues following systemic infusion into nonhuman primates. Blood 2003; 101(8): 2999–3001.
89. Cazzola M, Di Marco F, Santus P, et al. The pharmacodynamic effects of single inhaled doses of formoterol, tiotropium and their combination in patients with COPD. Pulm Pharmacol Ther 2004; 17(1):35–39.
90. Xiao RP. Beta-adrenergic signaling in the heart: dual coupling of the beta2-adrenergic receptor to G(s) and G(i) proteins. Sci STKE 2001; 2001(104):RE15.

91. van Beerendonk I, Mesters I, Mudde AN, et al. Assessment of the inhalation technique in outpatients with asthma or chronic obstructive pulmonary disease using a metered-dose inhaler or dry powder device. J Asthma 1998; 35(3):273–279.

92. Dompeling E, Van Grunsven PM, Van Schayck CP, et al. Treatment with inhaled steroids in asthma and chronic bronchitis: long-term compliance and inhaler technique. Fam Pract 1992; 9(2):161–166.

93. Gray SL, Williams DM, Pulliam CC, et al. Characteristics predicting incorrect metered-dose inhaler technique in older subjects. Arch Intern Med 1996; 156(9):984–988.

94. Tan NC, Ng CJ, Goh S, et al. Assessment of metered dose inhaler technique in family health service patients in Singapore. Singapore Med J 1999; 40(7):465–467.

95. Ullman A, Lofdahl CG, Melander B, et al. Formoterol inhaled as dry powder or via pressurized metered-dose inhaler in a cumulative dose-response study. Allergy 1996; 51(10): 745–748.

96. Nelson HS, Weiss ST, Bleecker ER, et al. The Salmeterol Multicenter Asthma Research Trial: a comparison of usual pharmacotherapy for asthma or usual pharmacotherapy plus salmeterol. Chest 2006; 129(1):15–26.

97. Global Initiative for Asthma (GINA). Available at: http://www.ginasthma.com/.

98. Salpeter SR, Buckley NS, Salpeter EE. Meta-analysis: anticholinergics, but not beta-agonists, reduce severe exacerbations and respiratory mortality in COPD. J Gen Intern Med 2006; 21(10):1011–1019.

99. Calverley PM, Anderson JA, Celli B, et al. Salmeterol and fluticasone propionate and survival in chronic obstructive pulmonary disease. N Engl J Med 2007; 356(8):775–789.

100. Salpeter S, Ormiston T, Salpeter E. Cardioselective beta-blockers for chronic obstructive pulmonary disease. Cochrane Database Syst Rev 2005; (4):CD003566.

101. Johnson M, Rennard S. Alternative mechanisms for long-acting beta(2)-adrenergic agonists in COPD. Chest 2001; 120(1):258–270.

102. Calverley PM, Burge PS, Spencer S, et al. Bronchodilator reversibility testing in chronic obstructive pulmonary disease. Thorax 2003; 58(8):659–664.

103. Hansel TT, Barnes PJ. Tiotropium bromide: a novel once-daily anticholinergic broncho-dilator for the treatment of COPD. Drugs Today (Barc) 2002; 38(9):585–600.

104. On LS, Boonyongsunchai P, Webb S, et al. Function of pulmonary neuronal M(2) mus-carinic receptors in stable chronic obstructive pulmonary disease. Am J Respir Crit Care Med 2001; 163(6):1320–1325.

105. Casaburi R, Mahler DA, Jones PW, et al. A long-term evaluation of once-daily inhaled tiotropium in chronic obstructive pulmonary disease. Eur Respir J 2002; 19(2):217–224.

106. Donohue JF, van Noord JA, Bateman ED, et al. A 6-month, placebo-controlled study comparing lung function and health status changes in COPD patients treated with tio-tropium or salmeterol. Chest 2002; 122(1):47–55.

107. Tashkin DP, Celli B, Senn S, et al. A 4-year trial of tiotropium in chronic obstructive pulmonary disease. N Engl J Med 2008; 359(15):1543–1554.

108. Singh S, Loke YK, Furberg CD. Inhaled anticholinergics and risk of major adverse car-diovascular events in patients with chronic obstructive pulmonary disease: a systematic review and meta-analysis. JAMA 2008; 300(12):1439–1450.

109. Koyama S, Rennard SI, Robbins RA. Acetylcholine stimulates bronchial epithelial cells to release neutrophil and monocyte chemotactic activity. Am J Physiol 1992; 262: L466–L471.

110. Buhling F, Lieder N, Kühlmann UC, et al. Tiotropium suppresses acetylcholine-induced release of chemotactic mediators in vitro. Respir Med 2007; 101(11):2386–2394.

111. Rennard SI, Thompson A, Daughton D, et al. Theophylline reduces neutrophil recruitment in vitro and lowers airway neutrophilia in chronic bronchitis in vivo. Eur Respir J 1990; 3: 116S.

112. Barnes PJ. Theophylline in chronic obstructive pulmonary disease: new horizons. Proc Am Thorac Soc 2005; 2(4):334–339; discussion 340–341.

113. ZuWallach RL, Mahler DA, Reilly D, et al. Salmeterol plus theophylline combination therapy in the treatment of COPD. Chest 2001; 119(6):1661–1670.

114. Rossi A, Kristufek P, Levine BE, et al. Comparison of the efficacy, tolerability, and safety of formoterol dry powder and oral, slow-release theophylline in the treatment of COPD. Chest 2002; 121(4):1058–1069.

115. Taylor DR, Buick B, Kinney C, et al. The efficacy of orally administered theophylline, inhaled salbutamol, and a combination of the two as chronic therapy in the management of chronic bronchitis with reversible air-flow obstruction. Am Rev Respir Dis 1985; 131: 747–751.

116. Ohta K, Fukuchi Y, Grouse L, et al. A prospective clinical study of theophylline safety in 3810 elderly with asthma or COPD. Respir Med 2004; 98(10):1016–1024.

117. Casaburi R, Kukafka D, Cooper CB, et al. Improvement in exercise tolerance with the combination of tiotropium and pulmonary rehabilitation in patients with COPD. Chest 2005; 127(3):809–817.

118. Ries AL, Bauldoff GS, Carlin BW, et al. Pulmonary Rehabilitation: Joint ACCP/AACVPR Evidence-Based Clinical Practice Guidelines. Chest 2007; 131(5 suppl):4S–42S.

119. Rennard SI. Treatment of stable chronic obstructive pulmonary disease. Lancet 2004; 364(9436):791–802.

120. Rennard SI. Anticholinergics in combination bronchodilator therapy in COPD. In: Spector SL, ed. Anticholinergic Agents in the Upper and Lower Airways. New York: Marcel Dekker, Inc., 1999:119–136.

121. van Noord JA, Aumann JL, Janssens E, et al. Effects of tiotropium with and without formoterol on airflow obstruction and resting hyperinflation in patients with COPD. Chest 2006; 129(3):509–517.

122. Yang IA, Fong KM, Sim EH, et al. Inhaled corticosteroids for stable chronic obstructive pulmonary disease. Cochrane Database Syst Rev 2007; (2):CD002991.

123. Nannini L, Cates CJ, Lasserson TJ, et al. Combined corticosteroid and long-acting beta-agonist in one inhaler versus placebo for chronic obstructive pulmonary disease. Cochrane Database Syst Rev 2007; (4):CD003794.

124. Tashkin DP, Rennard SI, Martin P, et al. Efficacy and safety of budesonide and formoterol in one pressurized metered-dose inhaler in patients with moderate to very severe chronic obstructive pulmonary disease: results of a 6-month randomized clinical trial. Drugs 2008; 68(14):1975–2000.

125. Dolovich MB, Ahrens RC, Hess DR, et al. Device selection and outcomes of aerosol therapy: Evidence-based guidelines: American College of Chest Physicians/American College of Asthma, Allergy, and Immunology. Chest 2005; 127(1):335–371.

126. Drummond MB, Dasenbrook EC, Pitz MW, et al. Inhaled corticosteroids in patients with stable chronic obstructive pulmonary disease: a systematic review and meta-analysis. JAMA 2008; 300(20):2407–2416.

127. Walters JA, Gibson PG, Wood-Baker R, et al. Systemic corticosteroids for acute exacerbations of chronic obstructive pulmonary disease. Cochrane Database Syst Rev 2009; (1):CD001288.

128. Niewoehner DE, Erbland ML, Deupree RH, et al. Effect of systemic glucocorticoids on exacerbations of chronic obstructive pulmonary disease. N Engl J Med 1999; 340:1941–1947.

129. Schols AM, Wesseling G, Kester AD, et al. Dose dependent increased mortality risk in COPD patients treated with oral glucocorticoids. Eur Respir J 2001; 17(3):337–342.

130. Sin DD, Tu JV. Inhaled corticosteroids and the risk of mortality and readmission in elderly patients with chronic obstructive pulmonary disease. Am J Respir Crit Care Med 2001; 164(4):580–584.

131. Sin DD, Wu L, Anderson JA, et al. Inhaled corticosteroids and mortality in chronic obstructive pulmonary disease. Thorax 2005; 60(12):992–997.
132. Sutherland ER, Allmers H, Ayas NT, et al. Inhaled corticosteroids reduce the progression of airflow limitation in chronic obstructive pulmonary disease: a meta-analysis. Thorax 2003; 58(11):937–941.
133. Celli BR, Thomas NE, Anderson JA, et al. Effect of pharmacotherapy on rate of decline of lung function in chronic obstructive pulmonary disease: results from the TORCH study. Am J Respir Crit Care Med 2008; 178(4):332–338.
134. Griffin MR, Coffey CS, Neuzil KM, et al. Winter viruses: influenza- and respiratory syncytial virus-related morbidity in chronic lung disease. Arch Intern Med 2002; 162(11): 1229–1236.
135. Nichol KL, Baken L, Nelson A. Relation between influenza vaccination and outpatient visits, hospitalization, and mortality in elderly persons with chronic lung disease. Ann Intern Med 1999; 130(5):397–403.
136. Nichol KL, Margolis KL, Wuorenma J, et al. The efficacy and cost effectiveness of vaccination against influenza among elderly persons living in the community. N Engl J Med 1994; 331(12):778–784.
137. Edwards KM, Dupont WD, Westrich MK, et al. A randomized controlled trial of cold-adapted and inactivated vaccines for the prevention of influenza A disease. J Infect Dis 1994; 169(1):68–76.
138. Global Strategy for the Diagnosis, Management, and Prevention of Chronic Obstructive Pulmonary Disease [cited 2003]. Available at: http://www.goldcopd.com.
139. Council MR. Long term domiciliary oxygen therapy in chronic hypoxic cor pulmonale complicating chronic bronchitis and emphysema. Report of the Medical Research Council Working Party. Lancet 1981; 1(8222):681–686.
140. Kvale PA, Cugell DW, Athonisen NR, et al. Continuous or nocturnal oxygen therapy in hypoxemic chronic obstructive lung disease. Ann Intern Med 1980; 93:391–398.
141. Rennard S, Carrera M, Agusti AG. Management of chronic obstructive pulmonary disease: are we going anywhere? Eur Respir J 2000; 16(6):1035–1036.
142. Walmsley SR, McGovern NN, Whyte MK, et al. The HIF/VHL pathway: from oxygen sensing to innate immunity. Am J Respir Cell Mol Biol 2008; 38(3):251–255.
143. Cranston JM, Crockett AJ, Moss JR, et al. Domiciliary oxygen for chronic obstructive pulmonary disease. Cochrane Database Syst Rev 2005; (4):CD001744.
144. Emtner M, Porszasz J, Burns M, et al. Benefits of supplemental oxygen in exercise training in nonhypoxemic chronic obstructive pulmonary disease patients. Am J Respir Crit Care Med 2003; 168(9):1034–1042.
145. Vestbo J, Prescott E, Lange P. Association of chronic mucus hypersecretion with FEV_1 decline and chronic obstructive pulmonary disease morbidity. Am J Respir Crit Care Med 1996; 153:1530–1535.
146. Ziment I. Historic overview of mucoactive drugs. In: Braga PC, Allegra L, eds. Drugs in Bronchial Mucology. New York: Raven Press, 1989:1–33.
147. Decramer M, Rutten-van Mölken M, Dekhuijzen PN, et al. Effects of N-acetylcysteine on outcomes in chronic obstructive pulmonary disease (Bronchitis Randomized on NAC Cost-Utility Study, BRONCUS): a randomised placebo-controlled trial. Lancet 2005; 365(9470): 1552–1560.
148. Irwin RS, Curley FJ, Pratter MR. The effects of drugs on cough. Eur J Respir Dis Suppl 1987; 153:173–181.
149. Fabbri LM, Rabe KF. From COPD to chronic systemic inflammatory syndrome? Lancet 2007; 370(9589):797–799.
150. Wouters EF. Chronic obstructive pulmonary disease. 5: systemic effects of COPD. Thorax 2002; 57(12):1067–1070.

151. Boyd CM, Darer J, Boult C, et al. Clinical practice guidelines and quality of care for older patients with multiple comorbid diseases: implications for pay for performance. JAMA 2005; 294(6):716–724.
152. Brenes GA. Anxiety and chronic obstructive pulmonary disease: prevalence, impact, and treatment. Psychosom Med 2003; 65(6):963–970.
153. Singer HK, Ruchinskas RA, Riley KC, et al. The psychological impact of end-stage lung disease. Chest 2001; 120(4):1246–1252.
154. Yohannes AM, Baldwin RC, Connolly MJ. Depression and anxiety in elderly outpatients with chronic obstructive pulmonary disease: prevalence, and validation of the BASDEC screening questionnaire. Int J Geriatr Psychiatry 2000; 15(12):1090–1096.
155. Borson S, Claypoole K, McDonald GJ. Depression and chronic obstructive pulmonary disease: treatment trials. Semin Clin Neuropsychiatry 1998; 3(2):115–130.
156. Yohannes AM, Baldwin RC, Connolly MJ. Prevalence of sub-threshold depression in elderly patients with chronic obstructive pulmonary disease. Int J Geriatr Psychiatry 2003; 18(5):412–416.
157. Fan VS, Ramsey SD, Giardino ND, et al. Sex, depression, and risk of hospitalization and mortality in chronic obstructive pulmonary disease. Arch Intern Med 2007; 167(21): 2345–2353.
158. de Voogd JN, Wempe JB, Koëter GH, et al. Depressive symptoms as predictors of mortality in patients with COPD. Chest 2009; 135(3):619–625.
159. Jordan N, Lee TA, Valenstein M, et al. Effect of depression care on outcomes in COPD patients with depression. Chest 2009; 135(3):626–632.
160. Franco-Bronson K. The management of treatment-resistant depression in the medically ill. Psychiatr Clin North Am 1996; 19(2):329–350.
161. Borson S, McDonald GJ, Gayle T, et al. Improvement in mood, physical symptoms, and function with nortriptyline for depression in patients with chronic obstructive pulmonary disease. Psychosomatics 1992; 33(2):190–201.
162. Argyropoulou P, Patakas D, Koukou A, et al. Buspirone effect on breathlessness and exercise performance in patients with chronic obstructive pulmonary disease. Respiration 1993; 60(4):216–220.
163. Rose C, Wallace L, Dickson R, et al. The most effective psychological-based treatments to reduce anxiety and panic in patients with chronic obstructive pulmonary disease (COPD): a systematic review. Patient Educ Couns 2002; 47(4):311–318.
164. de Godoy DV, de Godoy RF. A randomized controlled trial of the effect of psychotherapy on anxiety and depression in chronic pulmonary disease. Arch Phys Med Rehabil 2003; 84(8):1154–1157.
165. McGarvey LP, John M, Anderson JA, et al. Ascertainment of cause-specific mortality in COPD: operations of the TORCH Clinical Endpoint Committee. Thorax 2007; 62(5): 411–415.
166. Mancini GB, Etminan M, Zhang B, et al. Reduction of morbidity and mortality by statins, angiotensin-converting enzyme inhibitors, and angiotensin receptor blockers in patients with chronic obstructive pulmonary disease. J Am Coll Cardiol 2006; 47(12):2554–2560.
167. Martinez FJ, Chang A. Surgical therapy for chronic obstructive pulmonary disease. Semin Respir Crit Care Med 2005; 26(2):167–191.
168. Ioachimescu OC, Stoller JK. A review of alpha-1 antitrypsin deficiency. COPD 2005; 2(2): 263–275.
169. Heresi GA, Stoller JK. Augmentation therapy in alpha-1 antitrypsin deficiency. Expert Opin Biol Ther 2008; 8(4):515–526.
170. The Alpha-1-Antitrypsin Deficiency Registry Study Group. Survival and FEV1 decline in individuals with severe deficiency of alpha1-antitrypsin. Am J Respir Crit Care Med 1998; 158:49–59.

14
Management of Chronic Asthma in Adults

KIAN FAN CHUNG
National Heart and Lung Institute, Imperial College, and Royal Brompton Hospital, London, U.K.

I. Introduction

The setting up of consensus national guidelines, later culminating in the setting up of the global initiative for asthma (GINA) in collaboration with NHLBI and WHO, has probably been the most important progress in the management of asthma over the last two decades. These have helped to disseminate a uniform approach to asthma management nationally and internationally, and allow many sections of health care professionals and patients themselves to be involved in management of asthma. GINA has developed a global strategy for asthma management and prevention in 1995, with several revisions with a later update in 2007. It was the increasing concern about the worldwide increasing trends in morbidity and mortality of asthma that had triggered the establishment under the WHO of the GINA group that sets up a consensus- and evidenced-based set of guidelines for the management of asthma in 1989. The goals of asthma management were to control chronic and nocturnal symptoms, maintain normal activity, prevent acute episodes of asthma, minimize the need for reliever medication, maintain near-normal lung function, and avoid adverse effects of asthma medications. Key objectives of the document were that to improve outcomes of asthma worldwide the process of asthma care must be improved through education of both patient and carer. It was advocated that asthma management consists of an objective assessment, physician/patient partnership, control of environmental influences, and pharmacological therapy.

This chapter will discuss the management of asthma as recommended by GINA, since this is perhaps the most influential document that has and continues to shape the management of asthma worldwide.

A. Morbidity and Mortality of Asthma

The prevalence of asthma has increased over the last decades globally by approximately 50% every decade according to data from the International Study of Asthma and Allergies in Childhood (ISAAC) and the European Community Respiratory Health Survey (ECRHS) (1). Countries with the highest prevalences are mainly the developed countries such as United Kingdom, New Zealand, Australia, Canada, and the United States, with values of 11% to 15%. However, the prevalence is also increasing in developing countries. There is also significant morbidity and mortality on a worldwide scale. Internationally, there are an increased number of hospital admissions for asthma, most pronounced in young children. However, there has been a decreasing trend in some countries of hospital-treated asthma episodes. In Europe, The Asthma Insights and

Reality in Europe (AIRE) study conducted interviews with members of 3000 households with asthma patients in France, Germany, Italy, the Netherlands, Spain, Sweden, and the United Kingdom, and found that only 5.3% met the GINA criteria for asthma control (2). In addition, 18% of children and 11% of adults reported at least one emergency room visit, and 7% had required hospitalization in the past 12 months. Additional AIRE studies conducted in Central and Eastern Europe, the United States, and Asia indicate that suboptimal asthma control is also a global phenomenon (3). All participating regions performed equally poorly on the different GINA goals and the frequency of hospital admissions and emergency visits were similarly high across regions. However, there is some evidence that asthma deaths and hospital admissions for acute severe asthma may be showing a downward trend, perhaps because of the more widespread use of anti-inflammatory treatments, particularly inhaled corticosteroids (ICSs). Therefore, there is still ongoing significant international burden for asthma and there is an important task to try and reduce this burden significantly. The most important approach is to apply the management guidelines for asthma as widely as possible, which needs mobilization at the highest level of the health care system. Indeed, the Finnish National program to tackle asthma as a national priority has been successful in reducing the morbidity (4). It is possible that clinicians may not be adequately connecting with patients and the message of gaining control may not be communicated to patients. Therefore, there should be more emphasis on developing good relationships between caregiver and patient, and asthma educational programs.

II. Aims of Management

The aims of management are to control disease and to prevent episodes of worsening (exacerbations of asthma) and long-term consequences of asthma. The principles of management include the following: (*i*) minimizing or if possible eliminating symptoms completely; (*ii*) achieving the best possible lung function, and normal lung function if possible, which is possible in less severe asthma and if asthma is treated with controller medication as early as possible; (*iii*) preventing asthma exacerbations; (*iv*) using the least amount of medication to achieve best control of asthma, which is part of the step-down part of management; (*v*) minimizing short-term and long-term side effect, which is the idea behind step-down aspect of management, although in severe asthma, one has to accept that side effects will occur, but measures to combat these are needed; (*vi*) educating each patient about his disease and about the goals of management; and (*vii*) finally, overall, asthma management should lead to a reduction in mortality from the disease. While these objectives are all commendable, it is not clear to what degree these are achieved at.

III. Avoiding Causes and Triggers of Asthma

While it is possible to avoid certain triggers that are known to induce asthma episodes or attack in certain patients (Table 1), it remains more difficult to recommend measures to prevent the development of asthma (primary prevention). This is because many of the factors that lead to the development of asthma remain unclear and are not well understood. There are certain factors that are preventable such as certain indoor pollutants, occupational exposures, drugs, and food and food additives.

Table 1 Triggers of Asthma

1. Indoor allergens
   House-dust mites
   Furred animals
   Cockroaches
   Fungi
2. Outdoor allergens
   Plant pollens
   Fungi
   Moulds
3. Indoor air pollutants
   Cigarette smoke
   Gas combustion products (nitrogen dioxide etc)
   Wood combustion fumes
   Formaldehyde
   Endotoxin
4. Outdoor air pollutants
   Nitrogen dioxide, ozone, acid aerosols, particulates
   Thunderstorms
   Changes in temperature
5. Occupational exposure
   High molecular weight agents, for example, enzymes, latex, seafoods, and cereals
   Low molecular weight agents, for example, isocyanates, anhydrides, and wood dusts
6. Food and food additives
   Food allergies
   Preservatives (e.g., metabisulfite) or coloring agents (e.g., tartrazine)
7. Drugs
   Aspirin
   Nonsteroidal antiallergic compounds
   β-blockers
   Cholinergic agents (e.g., pilocarpine)
8. Infections
9. Stress factors
   Emotions
   Life events
   Hyperventilation
   Concomitant ME
10. Exacerbating factors
    Rhinosinusitis
    Gastroesophageal reflux disease
    Menstrual periods
    Pregnancy
    Obesity

A. Primary Prevention of Development of Asthma

While allergic sensitization has been demonstrated to occur prenatally, it remains unclear what intervention can be recommended to prevent its occurrence since the critical time window for exposure or levels of allergenic exposures has not been worked out. In addition, other environmental exposures such as smoking, air pollution, diet, microbial exposures and day care, pet keeping, moisture and dampness, and chemicals at the workplace have been related to the new onset of asthma (5,6).

Early exposure to house-dust mite allergen in infant's mattress was associated with an increased risk of asthma by seven years of age (7), indicating that primary prevention may be important. However, longitudinal studies of house-dust mite avoidance have provided disappointing results as a primary prevention strategy. One reason may be that the reduction in exposure to house-dust mite was inadequate as indicated in the latest meta-analysis of 49 trials (8). However, even in the one study that had significant reduction in house-dust mite exposure, there was no significant improvement in asthma control or lung function (9). Use of chemical and physical methods aimed at reducing exposure to house-dust mite was not recommended (8). Postnatally, there is some evidence regarding the use of breast-feeding being associated with lesser wheezing episodes than compared with cow milk or soya milk protein feeds, and also with lower asthma prevalence in childhood. Exposure to tobacco smoke either prenatally or postnatally is associated with a greater likelihood of wheezing in childhood together with potential harmful effects on the development of the lung. Combined reduction in house-dust mite exposure, breast-feeding, and smoking cessation of parents has led to a small reduction in current wheezing symptoms at the age of two (10) and to secondary prevention of asthma symptoms (11), indicating that a multifaceted approach rather than just reduction in allergen exposure may be needed (12).

Redirecting the immune response toward a modulating T-regulatory cell that would dampen a T-helper type 2 response, which is at the basis of asthmatic /allergic inflammation, could be a strategy for primary prevention. In fact, early-life exposure to cat and dog allergen may protect against the development of allergy through development of immune tolerance (13). There is also a protective effect of endotoxin exposure in early life to the development of asthma. Important gene-environment interactions are at play in the development of asthma (6).

B. Secondary Prevention of Asthma Symptoms and Episodes

The known causes of asthma triggers include allergens to which the asthmatic is allergic to, upper respiratory tract infections usually viral, components of pollutants, and certain medications. Under a special category are patients with aspirin-sensitive asthma who need to avoid salicylates and nonsteroidal anti-inflammatory drugs. Avoidance of allergens includes avoidance of common indoor allergens and outdoor allergens, together with potential allergens encountered at the work place. Irritants such as second-hand smoke or dusty environments (e.g., from building sites) must be avoided. While it is difficult to completely avoid common respiratory viruses and environmental pollution, asthmatic patients need to be made aware that these can be triggers for their asthma (14,15).

Cigarette smoking is an important factor that adversely affects asthma control. Current smokers are nearly three times more likely than nonsmokers to be hospitalized for their asthma over a one-year period (16). In addition, there is a report of increased prevalence of asthma in active adolescent tobacco smokers (17). However, the main reason for poorer control in active smokers is the fact that smoking reduces the effectiveness of corticosteroids as an anti-inflammatory agent. Several studies now indicate that ICSs are not as effective in treating patients with asthma who smoke (18,19).

IV. Comorbidity of Asthma

The presence of concomitant rhinitis with asthma is associated with higher drug use and costs compared with patients without rhinitis. In addition patients with rhinitis have a greater likelihood of being hospitalized with asthma, and more likely to visit their primary care physician (16). Adults and children with asthma and documented concomitant allergic rhinitis experience more asthma-related hospitalizations and physician visits, and incur higher asthma drug costs than adults with asthma alone (20,21). These patients also experience more frequent absence from work and decreased productivity. Thus, it is important to treat concomitant rhinitis, with the concept of one single airway disease extending from the nose to the lungs (22).

Gastroesophageal reflux disease (GERD) and asthma have long been associated together, and GERD may worsen asthma through a direct effect of acid on the airways and through stimulation of vagal nerve endings in the esophagus to cause bronchoconstriction. The prevalence of symptoms of GERD in asthma is higher than in controls, and the prevalence of reflux in asthma is ~60% (23). Whether GERD actually can cause asthma is not clear, but it could be an aggravating comorbidity for asthma (24). There has been no consistent effect of esophageal acid perfusion on asthma symptoms, and specific treatment of GERD in asthma leads to mixed results, with a reduction in asthma medication reported (25). GERD in asthma patients should be treated.

V. Obesity

There is a complex relationship between obesity and asthma and both may emerge during childhood. Epidemiological evidence indicates that obesity may underlie the increase in prevalence and incidence of asthma, and also reduces asthma control (26–28).

VI. The Diagnosis of Asthma

Although recurrent episodes of cough and wheeze are almost always because of asthma in children and adults, one must be aware that there are rarer causes of airways obstruction that can mimic the symptoms and signs of asthma (Table 2). One needs a high degree of suspicion when taking a history and examination to detect any particular unusual features, and be ready to investigate. One of the potentially confusing symptoms in terms of diagnosis of asthma is cough. A cough that occurs at night may or may not be accompanied by wheeze, and this has been classified as "cough variant" asthma, particularly in children who may present with features associated with asthma, such as bronchial hyperresponsiveness, increased diurnal variation in peak flow measurements, and evidence of allergies; the cough usually responds well to ICS therapy. However, if the cough does not have these features, other diagnoses that may be associated with the cough should be sought such as postnasal drip, gastroesophageal reflux, or chronic bronchitis or COPD (29). A condition of eosinophilic bronchitis presenting with a chronic productive cough characterized by sputum eosinophilia but without bronchial hyperresponsiveness, and responding well to corticosteroids has been described (30).

The presence of a wheeze does not always indicate asthma, particularly if the wheeze is not intermittent and auscultation reveals a localized wheeze, in which case one needs to be suspicious of a localized large airway obstruction. Intermittent inspiratory and expiratory wheeze or noises that arise from the larynx are often the indications of the condition of vocal cord dysfunction. Usually, there is marked variability and

Table 2 Diagnoses Masquerading as Asthma

Children
    Obliterative bronchiolitis
    Vocal cord dysfunction
    Tracheobronchomalacia
    Inhaled foreign bodies
    Cystic fibrosis
    Recurrent aspiration
    Developmental abnormality of upper airway
    Immunoglobulin deficiencies
    Primary ciliary dyskinesia
Adults
    Cystic fibrosis
    Bronchiectasis
    Inhaled foreign body
    Tracheobronchomalacia
    Recurrent aspiration
    Chronic obstructive pulmonary disease
    Congestive cardiac failure
    Tumors in or impinging on central airways
    Pulmonary hypertension
    Obstructive bronchiolitis
    Vocal cord dysfunction
    Bronchial amyloidosis
As part of asthmatic diathesis
    Allergic bronchopulmonary aspergillosis
    Pulmonary eosinophilic syndromes (e.g., Churg–Strauss)

lability of symptoms and signs but with normal lung function, without lower airways obstruction, and no response to asthma treatments. Generally, vocal cord dysfunction is associated with psychological or psychiatric disturbances, and management can be difficult and may involve psychological or psychiatric help, voice, and breathing exercises. It is also important to know that there may be some degree of vocal cord dysfunction during genuine episodes of an asthma attack.

    Differentiating asthma from COPD can be difficult, and there is also a general agreement that both conditions may coexist. The differentiation arises when a smoking patient with chronic airflow obstruction presents. A previous history of reversible airflow obstruction may often give support to as diagnosis of asthma. Other pointers toward asthma may include diurnal variation in peak flow measurements and the presence of blood or sputum eosinophilia, which usually indicates a good response of airflow obstruction to a course of oral corticosteroids (31). The presence of emphysema diagnosed on thin-section computed tomographic scans provides some support for a diagnosis of COPD. A study indicated that patients with asthma have significantly lower residual volume, higher carbon monoxide diffusing capacity, higher exhaled nitric oxide, lower high-resolution computed tomography scan emphysema score, and greater reversibility to bronchodilator and corticosteroids than patients with COPD (32).

Table 3 Different Types of Asthma: Asthma Phenotypes

Atopic or nonatopic asthma
Early onset (childhood) or late onset (adult) asthma
Nocturnal asthma
Exercise-induced asthma
Aspirin-induced asthma
Occupational asthma
Seasonal asthma
Cough-variant asthma
Menstrual asthma
Episodic asthma or persistent asthma
Acute severe asthma (exacerbations)
Chronic severe asthma
Asthma and near-asthma deaths
Fixed irreversible asthma
Brittle asthma
Corticosteroid-resistant or -dependent asthma
Eosinophil-predominant or neutrophil-predominant asthma
Churg–Strauss syndrome
Allergic bronchopulmonary aspergillosis

VII. Asthma Phenotypes

Asthma is a disease that presents in varied ways and clinicians often wonder whether these different patterns of presentation represent subclasses of asthma, such that asthma may be best described as a syndrome. This concept is supported further by different patterns of airflow obstruction, varying responses to corticosteroid therapy, and different types of airway inflammation. Table 3 shows different "types" of asthma that are described, although these do not really indicate phenotypes. There is no agreement at present as to how to define a particular phenotype of asthma, and it is likely that certain statistical approaches will be needed together such as cluster analysis (33) with some degree of follow-up of groups. The recognition of phenotypes means that asthma is not one disease but may represent a collection of diseases that end up with a similar presentation of intermittent wheeze with bronchial hyperresponsiveness. Definition of phenotypes will also be helped by a study of the molecular and proteomic profile of the inflammatory process (34).

A potential phenotypic group is the asthmatic patient with chronic (fixed) airflow obstruction that appears to have certain defined characteristics probably related to increased airway wall remodeling and fibrosis, and inflammation (35,36). An increased understanding of the inflammatory mechanisms suggests potential heterogeneity of mechanisms (e.g., the predominantly eosinophilic or neutrophilic inflammation), although there is yet any link established between these and specific phenotypes. Nevertheless, eosinophilic inflammation is usually indicative of a good therapeutic response and neutrophilic of a poorer response to corticosteroid therapy (37). This may become important to define, because this makes it possible that certain specific therapies may only be useful in certain phenotypes. The genomic and proteomic characterization of asthma may bring further light to the separation of asthma into distinct phenotypes.

VIII.   Assessing Asthma: Severity vs. Control

The concepts of asthma severity and control are essential to understand in the context of asthma management and their definitions have been approached in a recent statement (38). The basis for asthma severity definition relates to the characteristics of asthma prior to initiating any treatment, and severity assessed in terms of symptoms, reliever use, night waking, and lung function is categorized as either intermittent, mild persistent, moderate persistent, and severe persistent, as indicated by GINA 1995 guidelines (Fig. 1A). The concept of asthma control, on the other hand, was based on the medication required to maintain control at a certain level, with levels of total control, partly controlled and not controlled being described (Fig. 1B) (39). Levels of control may vary with time such as during an episode of worsening, control may move from well control to not well controlled. These two concepts measure different things, such that there could be patients with severe persistent asthma that have well-controlled asthma if enough medication (e.g., corticosteroids) is given to the patient, or there could be patients with mild intermittent asthma with not well-controlled asthma (e.g., during an exacerbation or if the patient is not compliant with preventive treatments). The definition recommended by the ATS/ERS Task Force is that "severity should be used to refer to the intensity of treatment required to control the patient's asthma," which is a definition that circumvents the necessity to assess severity of treatments. "Asthma control should be used to refer to the extent to which the manifestations of asthma have been reduced or removed by treatment" (38). These definitions are in fact implicit within the definitions of severe or therapy-resistant asthma that have been published (40,41).

Factors that may contribute to increased risk of future life-threatening episodes of asthma include previous intubation for asthma, intensive care unit care for asthma, hospitalization for asthma, excessive use of asthma medications, psychiatric disease, and reduced lung function. A recent episode of severe exacerbation or recent use of a corticosteroid burst is a very strong indicator of future severe exacerbations. These are indicators of severity of asthma.

In practical terms, asthma control is an important component to patients since it assesses current clinical control with symptoms, reliever use, and lung function, and also future risk of exacerbations and loss of lung function. These can be measured simply by asking questions about symptoms and measuring lung function and through regular follow-up. Various tools have now been developed to measure asthma control although there is not enough data yet to widen their use. Validated instruments are the Asthma Control Test (42,43), the Asthma Control Questionnaire (43), the Asthma Therapy assessment questionnaire (44), and the Asthma Control Scoring System (45). The Asthma Control Test scores appear to correlate with the specialist assessment of asthma control (42). Some of these instruments could be used by patients and could improve the assessment of asthma control, and provide an important tool for communication between patient and carer; it has also been suggested as useful as an indicator for stepping up treatments in self-management plans. However, there is still little experience in this usage.

IX.   Pharmacological Treatment

Asthma is treated with two main classes of drugs: controllers and relievers. With good control of asthma achieved by daily use of controllers, there is little need to use reliever therapies.

(A)

	Symptoms	Nighttime Symptoms	PEF
Severe persistent (Step 4)	Continuous Limited physical activity	Frequent	<60% predicted Variability >30%
Moderate persistent (Step 3)	Daily Use B2-agonist daily Attacks affect activity	>1 time a week	>60%–< 80% Variability >30%
Mild persistent (Step 2)	≥1 time a week but <1 time a day	>2 times a month	>80% predicted Variability 20–30%
Intermittent (Step 1)	<1 time a week Asymptomatic & normal PEF between attacks	≤2 times a month	≥80% predicted Variability <20%

(B)

Characteristic	Controlled (All of the following)	Partly Controlled (Any measure present in any week)	Uncontrolled
Daytime symptoms	None (twice or less/week)	More than twice/week	**Three or more features of partly controlled asthma present**
Limitations of activities	None	Any	
Nocturnal symptoms/ awakening	None	Any	
Need for reliever/rescue treatment	None (twice or less/week)	More than twice/week	
Lung function (PEF or FEV1)[a]	Normal	< 80% predicted or personal best (if known)	
Exacerbations	None	One or more/year[b]	One in any week[c]

[a] Lung function is not a reliable test for children 5 years and younger.
[b] Any exacerbation should prompt review of maintenance treatment to ensure that it is adequate.
[c] By definition, an exacerbation in any week makes that an uncontrolled asthma week.

Figure 1 (**A**) Classification of asthma severity according to GINA 1995. (**B**) Levels of asthma control according to GINA 2008.

A. Controllers
Controllers are asthma treatments that are taken daily to keep asthma under constant clinical control. While these treatments best work though anti-inflammatory effects, this may not be the only class of agents in this category. These agents include inhaled glucocorticosteroids (GCS), leukotriene modifiers, long-acting β_2-agonists, slow-release theophylline, anti-immunoglobulin (anti-IgE) monoclonal antibody (Omalizumab), and systemic corticosteroids.

B. Relievers
These medications are taken as needed and are usually quick-acting in relieving bronchoconstriction and symptoms of asthma, and include quick-acting β_2-agonists and anticholinergics.

X. Step Approach to Asthma Treatment
There are five upgrading treatment steps usually advocated for the achievement of control of asthma. This upgrading system is seen with the GINA guidelines as well as with the British Thoracic Society guidelines (46), but the account provided here will be the one published by GINA (39). The step-up guidelines consist of addition of controller medication at each step, emphasizing the concept of additive therapies to control more problematic asthma to the basic controller medication of ICS therapy (Fig. 2). Throughout the steps, the use of an as-needed reliever treatment most often in the form of a short-acting β_2-agonist aerosol is advocated together with controller use.

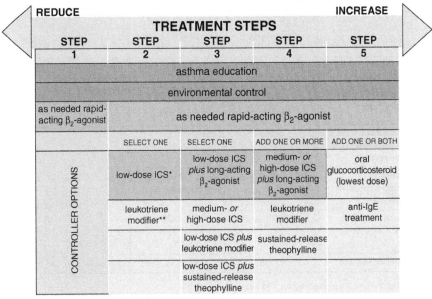

*inhaled glucocorticosteroids
**receptor antagonist or synthesis inhibitors

Figure 2 Treatment steps for asthma according to GINA 2008.

A. Step 1: As-Needed Reliever Medication

Untreated asthma patients with a minimum of symptoms such as occasional daytime symptoms of cough, wheeze, or shortness of breath at the rate of twice or less per week, or less frequently if nocturnal can be treated with an as-needed reliever treatment. In between episodes, there are no symptoms and the patient has normal lung function.

Under this category of treatment, are patients who only experience asthma episodes after exercise, prophylactic use of short-acting β_2-agonists is recommended prior to exercise. Leukotriene receptor antagonists are an alternative. With more troublesome or frequent episodes of exercise-induced asthma, there may be a reason for moving to step 2.

Other options include the early introduction of a low-dose inhaled steroid therapy but the benefits of such therapy are unclear and adherence would be difficult to maintain in this largely asymptomatic group.

B. Step 2: Reliever Medication Plus a Single Controller

At this step, should be considered are patients with asthma whose symptoms are more frequent than twice per week and/or who worsen periodically, or patients needing as-needed bronchodilator therapy more than twice weekly. This group is often categorized as mild persistent asthma, and constitute up to 70% of asthmatics.

The initial controller at step 2 is a low-dose inhaled GCS for asthma patients at all ages, such as beclomethasone dipropionate, budesonide, fluticasone propionate, flunisolide, triamcinolone, mometasone, and ciclesonide (see chap. 6).

The beneficial effects of low-dose ICSs has been shown in several studies, consisting of lesser days with asthma symptoms, reduction in time to exacerbations, small but significant improvement in spirometric measurements, and improved bronchial hyperresponsiveness (47–49). The addition of a long-acting β-agonist at this level of asthma does not provide further benefit on top of low-dose ICSs alone (47).

Other Options

An alternative proposition, but less efficacious, is the use of leukotriene inhibitors (50,51) that may be recommended for those who develop side effects such as hoarseness from ICSs or who do not wish to take ICS therapy.

Other options that have been examined recently are as follows: (*i*) Intermittent short-course corticosteroid treatment of exacerbations alone with reliever therapy, although the control of asthma was not as good as that achieved with regular use of low-dose ICSs (52); (*ii*) intermittent use of a combination inhaler of ICS, beclomethasone, and a short-acting β-agonist, salbutamol, for treatment of exacerbations, which was found to be as useful as regular use of inhaled beclomethasone alone (53); and (*iii*) continuous use of once-daily combined ICS and long-acting β-agonist once asthma has been controlled with twice-daily ICS therapy (54). While these options need to be looked at more carefully, there is no doubt that continuous low-dose inhaled steroid therapy provides the best asthma outcomes so far in this group; the importance of looking at potential alternatives is that patients are often reluctant or unable to take regular treatment with ICS therapy and may prefer to use intermittent treatment when they feel the need for these treatments.

C. Step 3: Reliever Medication Plus One or Two Controllers

At this step, should be considered patients with symptoms at a greater severity than untreated patients at step 2, with worsening of asthma episodes needing treatment with oral corticosteroids or in a hospital setting. Lung function of these patients may show some deterioration. These patients would fall in the moderate persistent asthma category. Some patients may present as such without having used controller medication, or may have had treatment at step 2 level that does not control asthma at all or only partially.

The recommended option at this step for adolescents and adults is to combine low-dose ICS with an inhaled long-acting β_2-agonist such as formoterol or salmeterol, used either from separate inhalers or within a combined inhaler. Combinations within one inhaler currently available are Seretide®, a combination of flixotide and salmeterol; Symbicort®, combination of budesonide and formoterol; and Foster®, combination of beclomethasone and formoterol. One combination at this step 3, Symbicort, can also be used as a reliever during worsening of asthma.

In relation to Symbicort, this is licensed also as use as controller, as well as reliever therapy, in adults aged over 18 years, with a regime of two inhalations per day, with one additional inhalation as needed in response to increased symptoms. Studies have been performed to assess the impact of this approach compared with using combination therapy as a controller alone (55–58). Patients entering these trials had suboptimal control and a recent history of severe exacerbations. This approach was associated with a reduction in the risk of further exacerbations. For every 4 to 14 patients treated using the SMART regimen instead of conventional maintenance and reliever treatment for 12 months, one may expect to prevent one patient having severe exacerbation. This approach was generally associated with a lower average intake of ICS, but there was no generally associated clinically significant improvement in symptom control compared with standard treatment. It may not be an appropriate regime for patients who overuse inhalers, and patients who have difficulty in recognizing worsening of symptoms.

In children aged less than five years old, the place of combination therapy is less certain since the few studies that have been done in this age group do not show any benefit of addition of long-acting β-agonist compared with a higher dose of ICSs.

Other Options

Standard controller medication as advocated at step 3 with combination therapy of ICSs and long-acting β-agonists using low to moderate to high doses of ICSs leads to improved control of asthma, improved quality-of-life measures, and a reduction in exacerbation rates, which is better than that shown by ICSs alone (59,60). Development of once-daily combination ICSs and long-acting β-agonists may improve adherence to treatment.

D. Step 4: Reliever Medication Plus Two or More Controllers

Patients who fall in this category are usually those that fail to be controlled on treatment at step 3, i.e., with combination therapy. It is important at this stage that the patient be referred to a health professional with experience in managing such patients for review of the diagnosis of asthma, any contributory aggravating factors, or concomitant illnesses and for review of treatments used and for adherence to treatment.

At this step, the preferred option may be to increase the dose of ICSs in the combination from low-to-medium or high dose. In general, the dose response to ICSs is shallow and only occasionally will further benefit be observed with increasing the dose from medium-to-high doses, but this should be done on a trial basis of two to four months before reassessing the effects of such an increase in dose of corticosteroids. Addition of other controllers such as leukotriene inhibitors or slow-release theophylline is recommended, probably after increasing from low dose to medium dose of corticosteroids. Other recommendation at this step may be to increase the frequency of ICSs to four times daily from twice daily if budesonide is being used.

E. Step 5: Reliever Medication Plus Additional Controller Options

When addition of controller medication at step 4 does not provide control of asthma, usually associated with recurrent exacerbations needing frequent burst of oral corticosteroids, addition of a regular oral dose of corticosteroids may be indicated. The idea is that a regular dose may be more effective in preventing these exacerbations, although this has yet to be proven. This treatment is associated with important side effects and should be considered as a last resort when all else has failed.

Other Options

This includes a trial of anti-IgE monoclonal antibody treatment for patients with raised circulating total IgE and with evidence of atopy as assessed by positive skin prick tests to one or more aeroallergens (61). In the United Kingdom, because of cost constraints these are reserved for patients who have experienced in the past year at least one admission to hospital and at least one visit to emergency room for treatment of asthma.

For those established on an oral corticosteroid dose, the use of methotrexate or cyclosporine as a steroid-sparing agent is worth trying over a period of four months (62,63).

F. Severe or Difficult-to-Treat Asthma or Therapy-Resistant Asthma

The majority of patients particularly at the lower steps of the GINA guidelines will obtain control of their asthma, often complete control, using pharmacological therapies of ICSs combined with long-acting β-agonists. Addition of other therapies such as leukotriene receptor antagonists or slow-release preparation of theophylline may provide further control, as described at step 4. However, there is now increasing recognition of a group of patients with asthma who still do not experience adequate control of their asthma despite taking maximal anti-asthma treatments, and these patients are now categorized at step 5 because of the maximal therapies they are on. These patients probably form 5% to 10% of asthma patients and are often labeled as having difficult or severe or refractory asthma. There have been several definitions of severe asthma, which emphasize the fact that such patients with asthma have uncontrolled asthma despite treatment with high-dose ICSs or sometimes with oral corticosteroids (40,41). The lack of control of asthma may be characterized by recurrent exacerbations needing treatment with burst of prednisolone or frequent need for acute medical treatment, or by chronic symptoms needing frequent reliever medication perhaps underlined by persistent airflow obstruction (64).

In the management of such patients, it is important that the diagnosis of asthma be reviewed, aggravating factors for asthma identified and dealt with, treatment regimes be maximized, and any issues of treatment adherence be addressed before accepting that the asthma is severe (40,65). In addition, psychiatric factors and conditions that masquerade as severe asthma such as laryngeal stridor or spasm need to be excluded, which is sometimes not easy, as these may be present with a component of asthma. This means that such patients should be systematically reviewed ideally under specific protocols (66). Table 4 summarizes some of the factors that may contribute to loss of control of asthma, which may lead to severe asthma, and Table 5 indicates the range of investigations that can be used in the severe asthma patient. It requires a period of three to six months to entirely investigate and understand the severe asthma patient and his/her disease, time that will allow for a determination of the clinical phenotype of the asthmatic diathesis. There is now a feeling that there may be different types of clinical presentations of severe asthma (phenotypes), such as those which present with recurrent exacerbations or those which have a pattern of chronic airflow obstruction (35,67,68). There may also be different patterns of airway inflammation in these patients, such as an eosinophilic-predominant or a neutrophilic-predominant pattern (69,70), although the effect of therapies particularly corticosteroids may influence the recruitment of these cells to the airways.

The persistence of asthma despite regular medication with ICSs and often with oral corticosteroids indicates some degree of refractoriness to corticosteroids in patients with severe asthma. Such patients do not demonstrate complete corticosteroid resistance since treatment with high-dose corticosteroids often provides improved control of asthma (71,72). This corticosteroid insensitivity has been demonstrated in circulating blood monocytes or in alveolar macrophages obtained from patients with severe asthma (73,74). These patients may require higher doses of inhaled or oral corticosteroids to control their asthma (often only incompletely), which continue to remain their main stay of therapy. Such patients are often described as "corticosteroid-dependent" asthmatics. However, it is important that patients with severe asthma do not escalate their dosage of oral corticosteroids in a futile way but remain at the lowest maintenance dose that keeps their asthma best controlled, accepting a compromise level of control that minimizes exacerbations and need for emergency treatment. Use of bursts of high-dose corticosteroids remains a necessity for patients with severe asthma,

Table 4 Factors That May Contribute to Loss of Control of Asthma

Poor compliance/adherence to therapy
Poor inhaler technique
Psychosocial and emotional factors
Inadequate medical facilities
Poor access to medical facilities
Inadequate treatment
Exposure to allergens
Viral respiratory tract infections
Indoor/outdoor pollution
Gastroesophageal reflux
Rhinosinusitis

Table 5 Investigations of Severe Asthma

1. Assessment of control and severity
   Asthma symptom score chart and use of reliever therapy
   Asthma control score
   Quality-of-life assessment
   Spirometry, lung volumes, and carbon monoxide transfer factor
   Bronchial responsiveness to methacholine or histamine
   Diurnal variation of peak expiratory flow
2. Pharmacological responsiveness
   Compliance/Adherence to therapy
   Bronchodilator response to β_2-adrenergic agonists
   Response to prednisolone
3. Radiology
   Chest radiograph
   Computed tomography of sinuses
   High-resolution computed tomography of thorax
4. Blood tests
   Full blood count, including eosinophil count
   Serum immunoglobulins G, A, and M
   Serum immunoglobulin E
   Specific IgE to common aeroallergens
   Thyroid function tests
5. Biomarkers of inflammation
   Exhaled nitric oxide
   Eosinophils and neutrophils in induced sputum
   Bronchial biopsy examination for inflammatory cells
6. Other tests
   Psychological assessment
   Examination of nasopharynx and vocal cord function
   Sweat test and genetic assessment of cystic fibrosis
   24-hour esophageal pH monitoring
   Tests of ciliary function
   Skin prick tests to common aeroallergens

but throughout the period of observation, patients must reduce maintenance dose of oral corticosteroids as soon as the situation permits. Side effects of corticosteroid therapy particularly with oral corticosteroids need to be attended to, particularly the development of osteoporosis by regular assessment of bone densitometry scans and by the use of bisphosphonates.

Clinical trials have demonstrated the value of low-dose methotrexate, cyclosporine A, and gold salts as steroid-sparing agents in corticosteroid-dependent asthma (62,63). On average, these agents may reduce the maintenance dose of prednisolone by 50% without deterioration in asthma control. While these agents are worth trying in corticosteroid-dependent asthma patients for four to six months, the rate of success observed in the clinical context is rather small, with the risk of side-effects (75,76).

The monoclonal humanized anti-IgE antibody, omalizumab, has been introduced particularly for the treatment of severe allergic asthma, where its addition to currently used drugs led to a significant reduction in exacerbations of asthma, associated with an improvement in quality-of-life scores (77). A therapeutic trial over four months of this treatment given either two- or four-weekly intervals is warranted in suitable patients.

No other treatments are currently available for those with severe asthma, although there have been several candidates that may appear promising such as blocking TNF-α or IL-13 (see chap. 10). Other approaches include reversal of corticosteroid insensitivity (78). A great unmet need for severe asthma is the lack of effective new treatments for severe asthma.

XI. Choice of Inhaler Devices

Because the delivery of drugs by inhalation is an integral component of asthma management, it is important that patients are completely conversant with their proper use and are adherent to the use of their inhalers. There are two main types of inhalers in use: the pressurized metered-dose inhaler (pMDI), which is the most frequently prescribed, and the dry powder inhaler (DPIs). The pMDI is the most difficult to use as it depends on coordination between activation of canister with the inspiratory maneuver to be perfect to provide satisfactory deposition and penetration of the aerosol in the lungs. However, there are pMDIs that can be activated on inhalation and the use of a holding device (spacer) may circumvent the need for this coordination. DPIs are easier to use and are essentially dependent on achieving an adequate inspiratory flow through the device to obtain adequate lung deposition; however, this can be a limitation in many patients with airflow obstruction who cannot generate an adequate inspiratory flow. Inadequate inhaler instruction and poor inhaler technique are important causes of unsatisfactory asthma control. The difficulty in proper use of pMDIs has been emphasized in many studies, even after a period of adequate training (79). The choice of inhaler for delivery of asthma medication particularly controller medication is important, and it is advisable that patients have a say in the choice of device that he/she wishes to use, although this can be constrained by the medication that is chosen. This also allows patients to have a say in their management, which is likely to lead to improved adherence to therapy.

A. Patient's Fears and Hopes
Self-Management

It is clear that with a chronic disease such as asthma for which there is no known cure that the management approach should be considered very much as a partnership between the person suffering from asthma and his health care professional(s). Because asthma is a life-long illness, the aim of this partnership is to allow patients to understand his disease by gaining knowledge that will ultimately allow the patient himself take a major role in the management of his own asthma. In this life-long contract, there will be ample time for (*i*) discussing about the goals of treatment, (*ii*) learning about his/her own asthma and ways of monitoring it, (*iii*) developing a personalized self-management plan, and (*iv*) for periodic review of patient's control and the level of asthma control.

Self-management plans usually in the form of a written action plan may lead to improvement in asthma control and a reduction in morbidity as shown by a reduction in hospitalization for asthma, and requirement for emergency room visits (80–82). There is also support for a reduction in asthma mortality (83). However, a later meta-analysis indicated little benefit derived from written self-management plans (82). Self-management plans can be conducted with varying levels of independence depending on the patient's comfort and willingness to take action when needed. A most common doctor-directed self-management plan will be in the form of a written action plan that may be focused on levels of peak expiratory flow rate measured at the time at which treatments or controller medications are stepped up.

Asthma Education

Education regarding asthma is an essential component of the interactions between the patient and health care professionals. This requires good communication skills on part of the health care professional, and this component often results in better patient satisfaction and reduced use of health care facilities. Information about the diagnosis and the cause of asthma and about the types of treatment available and the way these treatments work, about the avoidance of trigger factors, and about the long-term outcomes of asthma should be provided supplemented by written or pictorial information. Discussion will certainly arise during the course of treatment about the expectations and fears of the patients regarding the long-term outcomes of asthma, and what to expect of regular treatment of asthma.

XII. Adherence to Therapy

Adherence to daily regular medication for asthma particularly controller therapies has been reported to be as low as 50% at least for part of the time (84); in addition there may be regional variations (85). Nonadherence may be defined as the failure of treatment to be taken as agreed upon by the patient and his health care professional. Factors associated with poor adherence include gender with females more nonadherent, ethnicity with African-Americans at higher risk, lower socioeconomic status, patients with depressive illness or anxiety problems, those with less severe disease, and those who have particular fears of side effects particularly with corticosteroid therapy (86). Issues that encourage nonadherence include complex treatment regimens, difficulty with self-monitoring, the route of delivery, in particular the inhaled route that is used for most asthma medications, lack of patient education on asthma and the goals of asthma treatment, and difficulty in mastering the skill for inhalation therapy. Improving adherence can be achieved through regular follow-ups, education, use of self-management plans, good trustworthy carer-patient relationship and dialogue, audiovisual reminders, and simple treatment schedules. While patient adherence is difficult to measure because of lack of reliable methods, the main method remains that of directly questioning the patient and using available techniques such as drug levels (e.g., theophylline or oral corticosteroid), electronic device monitors, or pharmacy records for prescriptions.

Facilitation of optimal adherence is helped by identifying adherence behavior, identification of the perceptual and practical barriers, and tailoring the intervention and support according to the identified barriers and patient preferences. Nonadherence is of course important when asthma symptoms are or remain poorly controlled. Several tools such as The Beliefs about Medicines questionnaire and The Medication Adherence Report Scale have been proposed to measure beliefs and concerns, and to assess adherence, respectively.

XIII. Use of Biomarkers to Monitor Disease and Direct Management

Over the last few years, there have been special efforts directed toward the use of noninvasive biomarkers to help monitor disease severity and control, as a way of determining therapy requirements. These new methodologies may be considered complementary to the clinically based instruments or to assessment of symptoms; however, they would be disadvantageous in necessitating the use of special instruments or procedures that would have to be as straightforward and less cumbersome as possible for patient acceptance. At the moment, the two mostly investigated biomarkers are those of level of nitric oxide gas in exhaled breath, which can be measured instantaneously by exhaling into a nitric oxide sensor and measuring machine, and of the percentage of eosinophil in samples of sputum induced by inhalation of hypertonic saline, determined by examination of sputum supernatants by trained technical staff.

Previous investigators have examined the use of bronchial responsiveness measures using PC_{20} in assessing treatment requirements in asthma, and in comparison to usual clinical target outcomes, the use of PC_{20} in assessing requirements for therapy led to a better outcome in terms of lung function and in terms of reduction in exacerbations of disease, and also in terms of a reduction in subbasement membrane thickness; however, this group of patients needed at least twice as much ICSs to achieve the targeted improvement in PC_{20} (87).

Sputum eosinophilia of >3% has been used as a predictor of clinical improvement with corticosteroid treatment in asthma (88). Reducing prednisolone or ICS therapy, the appearance of sputum eosinophilia usually preceded increased symptoms, airflow limitation, or blood eosinophilia. Sputum eosinophilia has also been used to guide treatment with ICS, and when compared with the use of symptoms and spirometry, it provided more benefit to the patient by reducing the number of exacerbations and reduced the level of maintenance ICS therapy (89,90). One of the advantages of studying induced sputum is the concomitant assessment of neutrophilic inflammation. Sputum neutrophilia may be an indication of asthma severity (69), but their presence could also indicate the involvement of viral or nonviral infective bronchitis. There is also some indication that sputum neutrophilia may be an indication of poor response to ICS therapy (40).

Levels of nitric oxide in exhaled breath (eNO) are raised in a large proportion of symptomatic patients with asthma, although it is not specific for asthma; these levels are reduced by treatment to ICS treatment (91–93). In children with asthma, studies have shown the predictive values for patients requiring or not long-term maintenance with ICS for either high eNO (>50 ppb) or low (<25 ppb) eNO levels to be highly significant (94,95). A raised eNO level may indicate a therapeutic response to ICSs (96), just as induced sputum eosinophilia does. The value of eNO in guiding the dose of ICSs in the treatment of asthma was demonstrated to be safe and practical, allowing for a reduction in steroid dosage of 45% without a concomitant increase in asthma exacerbation (97). However, in another study, no effect was shown on steroid dosage, with a lower but nonsignificant rate of exacerbations (98).

XIV. Summary and Conclusions

The aims of asthma management are to control disease and to prevent episodes of worsening, i.e., exacerbations, and also long-term consequences of asthma. The principles of asthma management are well enunciated in consensus-derived and evidence-based guidelines at both international and national levels, and these have helped to improve the outcomes of asthma in most countries in the world. The pharmacological control of asthma is dependent on the use of controller medication such as ICSs and of reliever medication such as short- and quick-acting β-adrenergic agonists, and a stepwise approach is recommended, with the use of combination of ICSs and long-acting β-agonists in patients with moderate-to-severe asthma. The chronic asthmatic should be initiated to the principles and application of self-management, particularly in aborting deteriorating asthma. This implies a certain amount of asthma education to be imparted to the patient. Although there have been some improvements in asthma outcomes such as a reduction in asthma deaths, probably attributable to the greater use of ICS therapy, asthma continues to be a problem of control in a sizable proportion of asthmatics. These patients need to be assessed as to adequacy of and adherence to treatment, and a proportion will be genuine patients with severe asthma.

Asthma continues to be a chronic disease with considerable morbidity that may come as a surprise given the fact that current treatments are considered to be most effective and capable of controlling disease of most patients. However, it is possible that such impression may be misguided from the controlled trial studies performed using these medications and a restricted population of asthmatics; the effects of these medications in the real-life situation may be different given that patients are no longer under close supervision and may have other concomitant diseases or comorbidities (e.g., smoking or alcohol consumption) that may influence response to therapies. In addition, responses to medications are likely to have responders and not-so-well responding patients, and there is only limited success in predicting the response of a particular patient. This means that we cannot be complacent and there is a lot of work to do to improve asthma management for every asthmatic, and for many asthmatics, improved treatments are also needed.

References

1. Masoli M, Fabian D, Holt S, et al. The global burden of asthma: executive summary of the GINA Dissemination Committee report. Allergy 2004; 59:469–478.
2. Rabe KF, Vermeire PA, Soriano JB, et al. Clinical management of asthma in 1999: the Asthma Insights and Reality in Europe (AIRE) study. Eur Respir J 2000; 16(5):802–807.
3. Rabe KF, Adachi M, Lai CK, et al. Worldwide severity and control of asthma in children and adults: the global asthma insights and reality surveys. J Allergy Clin Immunol 2004; 114:40–47.
4. Haahtela T, Klaukka T, Koskela K, et al. Asthma programme in Finland: a community problem needs community solutions. Thorax 2001; 56:806–814.
5. Eder W, Ege MJ, von Mutius E. The asthma epidemic. N Engl J Med 2006; 355:2226–2235.
6. von Mutius E. Gene-environment interactions in asthma. J Allergy Clin Immunol 2009; 123:3–11.
7. Celedon JC, Milton DK, Ramsey CD, et al. Exposure to dust mite allergen and endotoxin in early life and asthma and atopy in childhood. J Allergy Clin Immunol 2007; 120:144–149.
8. Gotzsche PC, Johansen HK. House dust mite control measures for asthma. Cochrane Database Syst Rev 2008; CD001187.
9. Cloosterman SG, Schermer TR, Bijl-Hofland ID, et al. Effects of house dust mite avoidance measures on Der p 1 concentrations and clinical condition of mild adult house dust mite-allergic asthmatic patients, using no inhaled steroids. Clin Exp Allergy 1999; 29:1336–1346.
10. Schonberger HJ, Dompeling E, Knottnerus JA, et al. The PREVASC study: the clinical effect of a multifaceted educational intervention to prevent childhood asthma. Eur Respir J 2005; 25:660–670.

11. Morgan WJ, Crain EF, Gruchalla RS, et al. Results of a home-based environmental intervention among urban children with asthma. N Engl J Med 2004; 351:1068–1080.
12. van Schayck OC, Maas T, Kaper J, et al. Is there any role for allergen avoidance in the primary prevention of childhood asthma? J Allergy Clin Immunol 2007; 119:1323–1328.
13. Platts-Mills T, Vaughan J, Squillace S, et al. Sensitisation, asthma, and a modified Th2 response in children exposed to cat allergen: a population-based cross-sectional study. Lancet 2001; 357:752–756.
14. McCreanor J, Cullinan P, Nieuwenhuijsen MJ, et al. Respiratory effects of exposure to diesel traffic in persons with asthma. N Engl J Med 2007; 357:2348–2358.
15. Sears MR. Epidemiology of asthma exacerbations. J Allergy Clin Immunol 2008; 122:662–668.
16. Price D, Zhang Q, Kocevar VS, et al. Effect of a concomitant diagnosis of allergic rhinitis on asthma-related health care use by adults. Clin Exp Allergy 2005; 35:282–287.
17. Annesi-Maesano I, Oryszczyn MP, Raherison C, et al. Increased prevalence of asthma and allied diseases among active adolescent tobacco smokers after controlling for passive smoking exposure. A cause for concern? Clin Exp Allergy 2004; 34:1017–1023.
18. Chalmers GW, MacLeod KJ, Little SA, et al. Influence of cigarette smoking on inhaled corticosteroid treatment in mild asthma. Thorax 2002; 57:226–230.
19. Pedersen B, Dahl R, Karlstrom R, et al. Eosinophil and neutrophil activity in asthma in a one-year trial with inhaled budesonide. The impact of smoking. Am J Respir Crit Care Med 1996; 153:1519–1529.
20. Bousquet J, Gaugris S, Kocevar VS, et al. Increased risk of asthma attacks and emergency visits among asthma patients with allergic rhinitis: a subgroup analysis of the investigation of montelukast as a partner agent for complementary therapy [corrected]. Clin Exp Allergy 2005; 35:723–727.
21. Kanani AS, Broder I, Greene JM, et al. Correlation between nasal symptoms and asthma severity in patients with atopic and nonatopic asthma. Ann Allergy Asthma Immunol 2005; 94:341–347.
22. Bousquet J, Khaltaev N, Cruz AA, et al. Allergic Rhinitis and its Impact on Asthma (ARIA) 2008 update (in collaboration with the World Health Organization, GA(2)LEN and AllerGen). Allergy 2008; 63(suppl 86):8–160.
23. Havemann BD, Henderson CA, El Serag HB The association between gastro-oesophageal reflux disease and asthma: a systematic review. Gut 2007; 56:1654–1664.
24. Vakil N, van Zanten SV, Kahrilas P, et al. The Montreal definition and classification of gastroesophageal reflux disease: a global evidence-based consensus. Am J Gastroenterol 2006; 101:1900–1920.
25. Field SK. Gastroesophageal reflux and asthma: are they related? J Asthma 1999; 36:631–644.
26. Saint-Pierre P, Bourdin A, Chanez P, et al. Are overweight asthmatics more difficult to control? Allergy 2006; 61:79–84.
27. Lavoie KL, Bacon SL, Labrecque M, et al. Higher BMI is associated with worse asthma control and quality of life but not asthma severity. Respir Med 2006; 100:648–657.
28. Taylor B, Mannino D, Brown C, et al. Body mass index and asthma severity in the National Asthma Survey. Thorax 2008; 63:14–20.
29. Chung KF, Pavord ID. Prevalence, pathogenesis, and causes of chronic cough. Lancet 2008; 371:1364–1374.
30. Gibson PG, Dolovich J, Denburgh J, et al. Chronic cough: eosinophilic bronchitis without asthma. Lancet 1989; 1:1246–1247.
31. Chanez P, Vignola AM, O'Shaugnessy T, et al. Corticosteroid reversibility in COPD is related to features of asthma. Am J Respir Crit Care Med 1997; 155:1529–1534.
32. Fabbri LM, Romagnoli M, Corbetta L, et al. Differences in airway inflammation in patients with fixed airflow obstruction due to asthma or chronic obstructive pulmonary disease. Am J Respir Crit Care Med 2003; 167:418–424.

33. Haldar P, Pavord ID, Shaw DE, et al. Cluster analysis and clinical asthma phenotypes. Am J Respir Crit Care Med 2008; 178(3):218–224.
34. Woodruff PG, Modrek B, Chay DF, et al. T-helper type 2-driven inflammation defines major subphenotypes of asthma. Am J Respir Crit Care Med 2009; 180:388–395.
35. Bumbacea D, Campbell D, Nguyen L, et al. Parameters associated with persistent airflow obstruction in chronic severe asthma. Eur Respir J 2004; 24:122–128.
36. ten Brinke A, Zwinderman AH, Sterk PJ, et al. Factors associated with persistent airflow limitation in severe asthma. Am J Respir Crit Care Med 2001; 164:744–748.
37. Haldar P, Pavord ID. Noneosinophilic asthma: a distinct clinical and pathologic phenotype. J Allergy Clin Immunol 2007; 119:1043–1052.
38. Taylor DR, Bateman ED, Boulet LP, et al. A new perspective on concepts of asthma severity and control. Eur Respir J 2008; 32:545–554.
39. Bateman ED, Hurd SS, Barnes PJ, et al. Global strategy for asthma management and prevention: GINA executive summary. Eur Respir J 2008; 31:143–178.
40. Chung KF, Godard P, Adelroth E, et al. Difficult/therapy-resistant asthma: the need for an integrated approach to define clinical phenotypes, evaluate risk factors, understand pathophysiology and find novel therapies. ERS Task Force on Difficult/Therapy-Resistant Asthma. European Respiratory Society. Eur Respir J 1999; 13:1198–1208.
41. Proceedings of the ATS workshop on refractory asthma: current understanding, recommendations, and unanswered questions. Am J Respir Crit Care Med 2000; 162:2341–2351.
42. Nathan RA, Sorkness CA, Kosinski M, et al. Development of the asthma control test: a survey for assessing asthma control. J Allergy Clin Immunol 2004; 113:59–65.
43. Juniper EF, O'Byrne PM, Guyatt GH, et al. Development and validation of a questionnaire to measure asthma control. Eur Respir J 1999; 14:902–907.
44. Vollmer WM, Markson LE, O'Connor E, et al. Association of asthma control with health care utilization and quality of life. Am J Respir Crit Care Med 1999; 160:1647–1652.
45. Boulet LP, Boulet V, Milot J. How should we quantify asthma control? A proposal. Chest 2002; 122:2217–2223.
46. British Thoracic SocietyBritish Guideline on the management of asthma. Thorax 2003; 58: i1–i94.
47. O'Byrne PM, Barnes PJ, Rodriguez-Roisin R, et al. Low dose inhaled budesonide and formoterol in mild persistent asthma: the OPTIMA randomized trial. Am J Respir Crit Care Med 2001; 164:1392–1397.
48. Pauwels RA, Pedersen S, Busse WW, et al. Early intervention with budesonide in mild persistent asthma: a randomised, double-blind trial. Lancet 2003; 361:1071–1076.
49. Long-term effects of budesonide or nedocromil in children with asthma. The Childhood Asthma Management Program Research Group. N Engl J Med 2000; 343:1054–1063.
50. Israel E, Rubin P, Kemp JP, et al. The effect of inhibition of 5-lipoxygenase by zileuton in mild- to-moderate asthma. Ann Intern Med 1993; 119:1059–1066.
51. Margolskee D, Bodman S, Dockhorn R, et al. The therapeutic effects of MK-571, a potent and selective leukotriene (LT) D4 receptor antagonist in patients with chronic asthma. J Allergy Clin Immunol 1991; 87:309 (abstr).
52. Boushey HA, Sorkness CA, King TS, et al. Daily versus as-needed corticosteroids for mild persistent asthma. N Engl J Med 2005; 352:1519–1528.
53. Papi A, Canonica GW, Maestrelli P, et al. Rescue use of beclomethasone and albuterol in a single inhaler for mild asthma. N Engl J Med 2007; 356:2040–2052.
54. Peters SP, Anthonisen N, Castro M, et al. Randomized comparison of strategies for reducing treatment in mild persistent asthma. N Engl J Med 2007; 356:2027–2039.
55. Rabe KF, Atienza T, Magyar P, et al. Effect of budesonide in combination with formoterol for reliever therapy in asthma exacerbations: a randomised controlled, double-blind study. Lancet 2006; 368:744–753.

56. O'Byrne PM, Bisgaard H, Godard PP, et al. Budesonide/formoterol combination therapy as both maintenance and reliever medication in asthma. Am J Respir Crit Care Med 2005; 171:129–136.
57. Vogelmeier C, D'Urzo A, Pauwels R, et al. Budesonide/formoterol maintenance and reliever therapy: an effective asthma treatment option? Eur Respir J 2005; 26:819–828.
58. Bousquet J, Boulet LP, Peters MJ, et al. Budesonide/formoterol for maintenance and relief in uncontrolled asthma vs. high-dose salmeterol/fluticasone. Respir Med 2007; 101:2437–2446.
59. Pauwels RA, Lofdahl C, Postma D, et al. Effect of inhaled formoterol and budesonide on exacerbations of asthma. N Engl J Med 1997; 337:1405–1411.
60. Bateman ED, Boushey HA, Bousquet J, et al. Can guideline-defined asthma control be achieved? The Gaining Optimal Asthma ControL study. Am J Respir Crit Care Med 2004; 170:836–844.
61. Chung KF. Anti-IgE monoclonal antibody, omalizumab: a new treatment for allergic asthma. Expert Opin Pharmacother 2004; 5:439–446.
62. Shiner RJ, Nunn AJ, Chung KF, et al. Randomized, double-blind, placebo-controlled trial of methotrexate in steroid-dependent asthma. Lancet 1990; 336:137–140.
63. Alexander AG, Barnes NC, Kay AB. Cyclosporin A in corticosteroid-dependent chronic severe asthma. Lancet 1992; 339:324–327.
64. Moore WC, Bleecker ER, Curran-Everett D, et al. Characterization of the severe asthma phenotype by the National Heart, Lung, and Blood Institute's Severe Asthma Research Program. J Allergy Clin Immunol 2007; 119:405–413.
65. Stirling RG, Chung KF. Severe asthma: definition and mechanisms. Allergy 2001; 56:825–840.
66. Robinson DS, Campbell DA, Durham SR, et al. Systematic assessment of difficult-to-treat asthma. Eur Respir J 2003; 22:478–483.
67. Wenzel SE. Asthma: defining of the persistent adult phenotypes. Lancet 2006; 368:804–813.
68. ten Brinke A, Sterk PJ, Masclee AA, et al. Risk factors of frequent exacerbations in difficult-to-treat asthma. Eur Respir J 2005; 26:812–818.
69. Jatakanon A, Uasuf C, Maziak W, et al. Neutrophilic inflammation in severe persistent asthma. Am J Respir Crit Care Med 1999; 160:1532–1539.
70. Wenzel SE, Schwartz LB, Langmack EL, et al. Evidence that severe asthma can be divided pathologically into two inflammatory subtypes with distinct physiologic and clinical characteristics. Am J Respir Crit Care Med 1999; 160:1001–1008.
71. ten Brinke A, Zwinderman AH, Sterk PJ, et al. "Refractory" eosinophilic airway inflammation in severe asthma: effect of parenteral corticosteroids. Am J Respir Crit Care Med 2004; 170:601–605.
72. Ogirala RG, Aldrich TK, Prezant DJ, et al. High-dose intramuscular triamcinolone in severe, chronic, life- threatening asthma [see comments]. N Engl J Med 324:585–589. Erratum in: N Engl J Med 1991; 324(19):1380.
73. Bhavsar P, Hew M, Khorasani N, et al. Relative corticosteroid insensitivity of alveolar macrophages in severe asthma compared with non-severe asthma. Thorax 2008; 63:784–790.
74. Hew M, Bhavsar P, Torrego A, et al. Relative corticosteroid insensitivity of peripheral blood mononuclear cells in severe asthma. Am J Respir Crit Care Med 2006; 174:134–141.
75. Davies H, Olsan L, Gibson P. Methotrexate as a steroid-sparing agent for asthma in adults. Cochrane Database Syst Rev 2000; (2):CD000391.
76. Evans DJ, Cullinan P, Greddes DM. Cyclosporin as an oral corticosteroid sparing agent in stable asthma. Cochrane Database Syst Rev 2001; (2):CD002993.
77. Humbert M, Beasley R, Ayres J, et al. Benefits of omalizumab as add-on therapy in patients with severe persistent asthma who are inadequately controlled despite best available therapy (GINA 2002 step 4 treatment): INNOVATE. Allergy 2005; 60:309–316.
78. Adcock IM, Caramori G, Chung KF. New targets for drug development in asthma. Lancet 2008; 372:1073–1087.

79. Virchow JC, Crompton GK, Dal Negro R, et al. Importance of inhaler devices in the management of airway disease. Respir Med 2008; 102:10–19.
80. Gibson PG, Coughlan J, Wilson AJ, et al. Self-management education and regular practitioner review for adults with asthma. Cochrane Database Syst Rev 2000:CD001117.
81. Gibson PG, Powell H, Coughlan J, et al. Self-management education and regular practitioner review for adults with asthma. Cochrane Database Syst Rev 2003:CD001117.
82. Toelle BG, Ram FS. Written individualised management plans for asthma in children and adults. Cochrane Database Syst Rev 2004:CD002171.
83. Abramson MJ, Bailey MJ, Couper FJ, et al. Are asthma medications and management related to deaths from asthma? Am J Respir Crit Care Med 2001; 163:12–18.
84. Joshi AV, Madhavan SS, Ambegaonkar A, et al. Association of medication adherence with workplace productivity and health-related quality of life in patients with asthma. J Asthma 2006; 43:521–526.
85. Cerveri I, Locatelli F, Zoia MC, et al. International variations in asthma treatment compliance: the results of the European Community Respiratory Health Survey (ECRHS). Eur Respir J 1999; 14:288–294.
86. Howell G. Nonadherence to medical therapy in asthma: risk factors, barriers, and strategies for improving. J Asthma 2008; 45:723–729.
87. Sont JK, Willems LN, Bel EH, et al. Clinical control and histopathologic outcome of asthma when using airway hyperresponsiveness as an additional guide to long-term treatment. The AMPUL Study Group. Am J Respir Crit Care Med 1999; 159:1043–1051.
88. Brightling CE. Clinical applications of induced sputum. Chest 2006; 129:1344–1348.
89. Green RH, Brightling CE, McKenna S, et al. Asthma exacerbations and sputum eosinophil counts: a randomised controlled trial. Lancet 2002; 360:1715–1721.
90. Jayaram L, Pizzichini MM, Cook RJ, et al. Determining asthma treatment by monitoring sputum cell counts: effect on exacerbations. Eur Respir J 2006; 27:483–494.
91. Kharitonov SA, Yates D, Robbins RA, et al. Increased nitric oxide in exhaled air of asthmatic patients. Lancet 1994; 343:133–135.
92. Jatakanon A, Kharitonov S, Lim S, et al. Effect of differing doses of inhaled budesonide on markers of airway inflammation in patients with mild asthma. Thorax 1999; 54:108–114.
93. Massaro AF, Gaston B, Kita D, et al. Expired nitric oxide levels during treatment of acute asthma. Am J Respir Crit Care Med 1995; 152:800–803.
94. Zacharasiewicz A, Wilson N, Lex C, et al. Clinical use of noninvasive measurements of airway inflammation in steroid reduction in children. Am J Respir Crit Care Med 2005; 171:1077–1082.
95. Pijnenburg MW, Hofhuis W, Hop WC, et al. Exhaled nitric oxide predicts asthma relapse in children with clinical asthma remission. Thorax 2005; 60:215–218.
96. Smith AD, Cowan JO, Brassett KP, et al. Exhaled nitric oxide: a predictor of steroid response. Am J Respir Crit Care Med 2005; 172:453–459.
97. Smith AD, Cowan JO, Brassett KP, et al. Use of exhaled nitric oxide measurements to guide treatment in chronic asthma. N Engl J Med 2005; 352:2163–2173.
98. Shaw DE, Berry MA, Thomas M, et al. The use of exhaled nitric oxide to guide asthma management: a randomized controlled trial. Am J Respir Crit Care Med 2007; 176:231–237.

15

Exacerbations of Asthma in Adults

NEIL BARNES
The London Chest Hospital, Barts and The London NHS Trust and School of Medicine and Dentistry, London, U.K.

SOPHE G. FUIKA
Hospital de Santiago, Vitoria-Gasteiz, Basque Country, Spain

I. Epidemiology

Exacerbations of asthma still remain a relatively common cause of unscheduled medical care. Defining the exact incidence of exacerbations of asthma is difficult as there is no universally accepted definition of an asthma exacerbation. However, if an operational definition of requirement for emergency treatment is used then questionnaire surveys performed in many different countries show a rate of asthma exacerbations varying between 7% and over 40% (1)

There is no universally accepted definition of an asthma exacerbation. Patients almost never use the term asthma exacerbations; they talk about an asthma attack, which for some individuals would mean some wheeze that causes them to take a bronchodilator and for others would mean a severe attack that might lead to attendance at an accident and emergency department or a hospital admission. In clinical trials there has been equally confusing use of the terms asthma attack and asthma exacerbation. In some trials, the term asthma exacerbation has been used to describe an increase in symptoms, up to 20% decrease in peak expiratory flow (PEF), and an increase in rescue β_2-agonist use with the term asthma attack being reserved for requirement for treatment with oral steroids or a larger 30% or more decrease in PEF (2). The FACET study was one of the first trials that had prevention of exacerbations as one of its main outcome measures (3). There were two definitions of exacerbation: severe exacerbation was requirement for a course of oral corticosteroids or a 30% fall in PEF from baseline and a mild exacerbation was an increase in bronchodilator use or an increase in symptoms on two consecutive days. There were about 20 times the number of mild exacerbations compared with severe exacerbations and it is now considered this definition of mild exacerbation is really just an increase in symptoms. Each patient's experience of an asthma exacerbation is different. An individual with well-controlled asthma and good lung function may seek advice and emergency treatment more readily than an individual who has generally poorly controlled asthma, which is used to dealing with a worsening of their asthma without recourse to medical care.

The place where acute exacerbations of asthma are treated depends not only on the severity of the exacerbation but also on a number of other nonmedical factors such as the availability of primary care versus accident and emergency facilities, the type of cost reimbursement system in place, and, in a number of studies, the distance between the patient's home and the nearest hospital. In the United Kingdom, acute severe asthma is responsible for 71,000 accident and emergency attendances and hospital admissions (4). These hospital admissions cost £46 million per year.

II. Causes of Exacerbations

The commonest cause of exacerbations in all age groups is viral upper respiratory tract infections. Viral infections cause an increase in inflammation in the lower airways and an increase in bronchial hyperresponsiveness (5). The common upper respiratory tract viruses causing exacerbations are rhinovirus, adenovirus, respiratory syncytial virus, and influenza viruses (6). The percentage of exacerbation where a virus can be isolated depends on the sensitivity of the method used but where sensitive methods of detecting viruses have been used viral exacerbations account for approximately 70% of exacerbations (6,7).

Allergen exposure is probably the next most frequent cause of asthma exacerbations. Common allergens causing exacerbations vary from country to country but in most developed countries house-dust mite, grass pollen, tree pollen, and cat and dog allergens are common precipitants (8). Mould and fungal spores and cockroach allergy have also been reported as causes of asthma exacerbations (9,10). A particularly striking type of asthma exacerbation has been seen after thunder storms where three- to fourfold increases in the rate in asthma exacerbations have been recorded (11,12). This is thought to be due to massive increase in grass pollen and fungal spores caused by the atmospheric conditions. These exacerbations often occur in individuals with relatively mild asthma or with predominantly allergic rhinitis. They are thought to be due to a very severe early asthmatic response to the inhaled allergen occurring in sensitized individuals.

Epidemiological studies have shown that an increase in the levels of a number of airborne pollutants is associated with an increase in emergency visits and hospital admissions with asthma. A number of different pollutants have been implicated including ozone, nitrogen dioxide (NO_2), sulfur dioxide (SO_2), and particulate pollution (13–16). These airborne pollutants are often present together and it is difficult to be certain whether it is an individual pollutant or a cocktail of the pollutants, which are responsible for the increase in number of exacerbations. It has been estimated in some studies that up to 12% of asthma exacerbations may be related to air pollution (14). There is also evidence that air pollution may interact with exposure to allergens to increase the likelihood of an asthma exacerbation (16).

Another common cause of exacerbations of asthma is poor compliance with medication or stopping treatment, particularly with inhaled corticosteroids (ICSs) (17). Studies of patients with well-controlled asthma whose inhaled steroid dose is titrated down or suddenly stopped show that a proportion of these patients will have an exacerbation associated with an increase in eosinophilic inflammation (18,19). Treatment withdrawal is likely to interact with other precipitants of asthma making an exacerbation more likely on exposure to a virus or allergen.

Exercise, particularly in cold, dry air, causes a decrease in lung function and may lead to presentation with an acute wheezy episode but exercise-induced asthma does not lead to long-term worsening of asthma in contrast to other precipitants such as viruses and allergen (20).

Bacterial infections are not a common cause of asthma exacerbations. Frequently patients will say that they have a "chest infection" and practitioners may erroneously treat them with antibiotics. These chest infections may represent worsening of airflow obstruction often associated with an increase in sputum production because of an increase in eosinophilic or neutrophilic airways inflammation (21).

Stress and anxiety are often mentioned by patients as a cause of asthma exacerbations. It is not clear whether this is due to a genuine worsening of asthma caused by stress and anxiety or whether stress and anxiety lead to an increased awareness of falls in pulmonary function (22).

III. Pathology

The ability to obtain material by bronchoscopy and biopsy during a severe asthma attack is obviously constrained such that much of the information on the pathology of acute severe asthma has been obtained from postmortem studies of deaths from asthma and from studies of induced sputum obtained from milder exacerbations. The commonest finding from these studies is of an eosinophilic airway inflammation with increased mucus production. The mucus is viscid because of the presence of eosinophils, cellular debris, and exuded plasma proteins, and causes blockage of smaller airways and the production of Curschmann's spirals (23). An increase in eosinophilic inflammation can be seen after viral infections, allergen exposure, and reduction in maintenance treatment with corticosteroids. An increase in neurophilic inflammation has been found in some studies, the significance of which remains uncertain (24).

A more unusual pathological finding is of so-called "asthma deaths with clean airways," which is thought to result from intense bronchospasm without a marked increase in inflammation (25).

The airflow obstruction of an acute severe asthma attack is due to a combination of factors including an increase in airway wall inflammation, mucus and eosinophils in the airway, and bronchial smooth muscle spasm. This then leads on to a number of pathophysiological responses. There is an increase in respiratory rate accompanied by tachycardia and in severe asthma attacks by hypotension. The increase in ventilation-perfusion mismatch causes hypoxia. The increase in respiratory rate initially leads to hypocapnia but as airflow obstruction worsens hypercapnia occurs (26). The hyperventilation together with difficulty in eating and drinking because of shortness of breath leads to dehydration. If an asthma attack goes on for long enough it can lead to respiratory muscle fatigue, which is a dangerous development that may lead to respiratory failure.

There is considerable variability in the profile of asthma exacerbations. The commonest pattern is for a gradual increase in symptoms and decrease in lung function over several days before final presentation with an acute severe asthma attack. However, a minority of asthma exacerbations occur suddenly on a background of otherwise well-controlled asthma. The extreme form of this is so-called brittle asthma where patients develop sudden worsening of their lung function over the course of a few minutes (27). A particular problem is of so-called "poor perceivers," who are unable to sense the presence of a marked decrease in lung function.

An examination of the pattern of peak flow, symptom changes, and changes in bronchodilator use was undertaken using data from the FACET study (28). This showed firstly that the mean time between the onset of a worsening of symptoms and a decline in peak flow and the asthma exacerbation was approximately five days. Furthermore, the pattern of both deterioration and recovery was uninfluenced with either treatment with inhaled steroids or with the combination of inhaled steroids and long-acting β_2-agonists. Although these treatments reduced the likelihood of an exacerbation of asthma once the exacerbation asthma occurred, its pathophysiological features seemed unaltered by these treatments (3,28). A further finding from this analysis of exacerbations was of interest. Exacerbations in the FACET study were defined either by a fall in peak flow of 30% or more from baseline on two consecutive days or by requirement for a course of oral corticosteroids. Approximately 70% of the exacerbations were defined by requirement for a course of oral corticosteroids. In those where an exacerbation was defined by requirement for a course of oral corticosteroids, the peak flow decrease was only approximately 20% but there was a more marked increase in symptoms compared with those defined by a fall in peak flow (28). This data suggests that other factors apart from just the fall in lung function are responsible for a patient seeking treatment for an exacerbation of asthma and these may include their sensitivity to bronchoconstriction and possibly the etiology of the exacerbation.

A less common but potentially more dangerous type of acute attack is the so-called "brittle asthma." These are individuals who, on a background of well-controlled asthma with normal or relatively normal lung function, experience sudden severe exacerbations (27). It has been suggested that these are due to sudden episodes of bronchospasm rather than an increase in inflammation as is seen with most asthma exacerbations. This type of asthma exacerbation can be very challenging to prevent.

Another subgroup who are a particular challenge are the poor perceivers (29,30). These are individuals who can have a marked deterioration in pulmonary function before they notice any symptoms of dyspnea or chest tightness. They therefore delay taking rescue bronchodilators and seeking medical help. There is some evidence that it is those patients with the most marked bronchial hyperresponsiveness who are most likely to have poor perception of asthma severity (31). Because of their inability to detect bronchoconstriction peak flow monitoring in this group of individuals may be particularly valuable for early detection of an asthma exacerbation.

IV. Assessment of Acute Severe Asthma

There have been a number of studies investigating the risk of fatal or near-fatal asthma and the assessment of severity in an asthma attack (32–35). These studies come to two important major conclusions. The first is that in assessing the severity of an acute severe asthma attack, objective measurements of severity need to be made, so that the need for urgent treatment can be determined. Of these, the most important are pulse rate, a measure of airway function usually PEF, and a measure of oxygenation such as oxygen saturation or arterial blood gases. The second is that a detailed assessment of the history of previous asthma attacks and psychosocial factors needs to be performed (32–35).

V. Objective Assessment of Asthma Severity

In assessing the severity of an asthma attack the overall state of the patient needs to be taken into account (Figs. 1–3). If they are becoming tired this is a poor sign and any diminished level of consciousness is an ominous sign. The degree of tachycardia is an

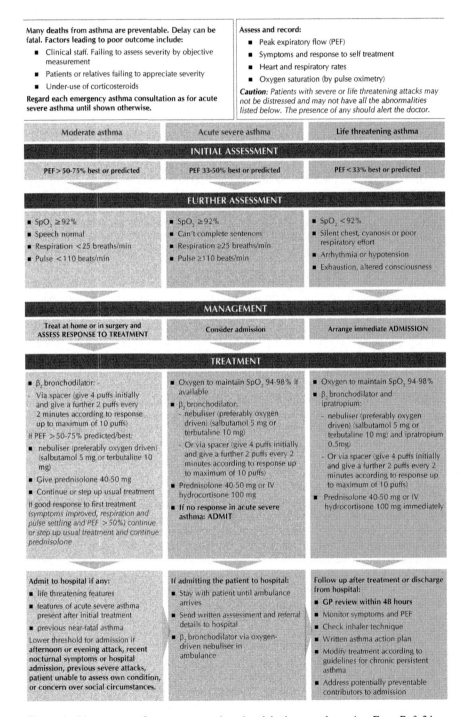

Many deaths from asthma are preventable. Delay can be fatal. Factors leading to poor outcome include:
- Clinical staff. Failing to assess severity by objective measurement
- Patients or relatives failing to appreciate severity
- Under-use of corticosteroids

Regard each emergency asthma consultation as for acute severe asthma until shown otherwise.

Assess and record:
- Peak expiratory flow (PEF)
- Symptoms and response to self treatment
- Heart and respiratory rates
- Oxygen saturation (by pulse oximetry)

Caution: Patients with severe or life threatening attacks may not be distressed and may not have all the abnormalities listed below. The presence of any should alert the doctor.

Moderate asthma	Acute severe asthma	Life threatening asthma

INITIAL ASSESSMENT

PEF > 50-75% best or predicted	PEF 33-50% best or predicted	PEF < 33% best or predicted

FURTHER ASSESSMENT

■ SpO₂ ≥92%	■ SpO₂ ≥92%	■ SpO₂ <92%
■ Speech normal	■ Can't complete sentences	■ Silent chest, cyanosis or poor respiratory effort
■ Respiration < 25 breaths/min	■ Respiration ≥25 breaths/min	■ Arrhythmia or hypotension
■ Pulse < 110 beats/min	■ Pulse ≥110 beats/min	■ Exhaustion, altered consciousness

MANAGEMENT

Treat at home or in surgery and ASSESS RESPONSE TO TREATMENT	Consider admission	Arrange immediate ADMISSION

TREATMENT

■ β₂ bronchodilator: - - Via spacer (give 4 puffs initially and give a further 2 puffs every 2 minutes according to response up to maximum of 10 puffs) If PEF >50-75% predicted/best: ■ nebuliser (preferably oxygen driven) (salbutamol 5 mg or terbutaline 10 mg) ■ Give prednisolone 40-50 mg ■ Continue or step up usual treatment If good response to first treatment *(symptoms improved, respiration and pulse settling and PEF >50%)* continue or step up usual treatment and continue prednisolone	■ Oxygen to maintain SpO₂ 94-98% if available ■ β₂ bronchodilator: - nebuliser (preferably oxygen driven) (salbutamol 5 mg or terbutaline 10 mg) - Or via spacer (give 4 puffs initially and give a further 2 puffs every 2 minutes according to response up to maximum of 10 puffs) ■ Prednisolone 40-50 mg or IV hydrocortisone 100 mg ■ If no response in acute severe asthma: ADMIT	■ Oxygen to maintain SpO₂ 94-98% ■ β₂ bronchodilator and ipratropium: - nebuliser (preferably oxygen driven) (salbutamol 5 mg or terbutaline 10 mg) and ipratropium 0.5mg) - Or via spacer (give 4 puffs initially and give a further 2 puffs every 2 minutes according to response up to maximum of 10 puffs) ■ Prednisolone 40-50 mg or IV hydrocortisone 100 mg immediately

Admit to hospital if any: ■ life threatening features ■ features of acute severe asthma present after initial treatment ■ previous near-fatal asthma Lower threshold for admission if afternoon or evening attack, recent nocturnal symptoms or hospital admission, previous severe attacks, patient unable to assess own condition, or concern over social circumstances.	**If admitting the patient to hospital:** ■ Stay with patient until ambulance arrives ■ Send written assessment and referral details to hospital ■ β₂ bronchodilator via oxygen-driven nebuliser in ambulance	**Follow up after treatment or discharge from hospital:** ■ GP review within 48 hours ■ Monitor symptoms and PEF ■ Check inhaler technique ■ Written asthma action plan ■ Modify treatment according to guidelines for chronic persistent asthma ■ Address potentially preventable contributors to admission

Figure 1 Management of acute severe asthma in adults in general practice. From Ref. 34.

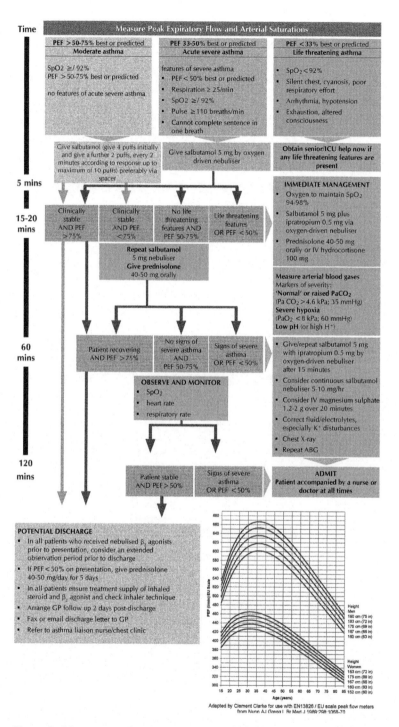

Figure 2 Management of severe acute asthma in adults in emergency department. From Ref. 34.

Features of acute severe asthma

- Peak expiratory flow (PEF) 33-50% of best (use % predicted if recent best unknown)
- Can't complete sentences in one breath
- Respirations ≥ 25 breaths/min
- Pulse ≥ 110 beats/min

Life threatening features

- PEF <33% of best or predicted
- SpO2 <92%
- Silent chest, cyanosis, or feeble respiratory effort
- Arrhythmia or hypotension
- Exhaustion, altered consciousness

If a patient has any life threatening feature, measure arterial blood gases. No other investigations are needed for immediate management.

Blood gas markers of a life threatening attack:

- 'Normal' (4.6-6 kPa, 35-45 mmHg) PaCO2
- Severe hypoxia: PaO2 <8 kPa (60mmHg) irrespective of treatment with oxygen
- A low pH (or high H⁺)

Caution: Patients with severe or life threatening attacks may not be distressed and may not have all these abnormalities. The presence of any should alert the doctor.

Near fatal asthma
- Raised PaCO2
- Requiring mechanical ventilation with raised inflation pressures

IMMEDIATE TREATMENT

- Oxygen to maintain SpO2 94-98%
- Salbutamol 5 mg or terbutaline 10 mg via an oxygen-driven nebuliser
- Ipratropium bromide 0.5 mg via an oxygen-driven nebuliser
- Prednisolone tablets 40-50 mg or IV hydrocortisone 100 mg
- No sedatives of any kind
- Chest X ray if pneumothorax or consolidation are suspected or patient requires mechanical ventilation

IF LIFE THREATENING FEATURES ARE PRESENT:
- Discuss with senior clinician and ICU team
- Consider IV magnesium sulphate 1.2-2 g infusion over 20 minutes (unless already given)
- Give nebulised β₂ agonist more frequently e.g. salbutamol 5 mg up to every 15-30 minutes or 10 mg per hour via continuous nebulisation (requires special nebuliser)

SUBSEQUENT MANAGEMENT

IF PATIENT IS IMPROVING continue:
- Oxygen to maintain SpO2 94-98%.
- Prednisolone 40-50mg daily or IV hydrocortisone 100 mg 6 hourly
- Nebulised β₂ agonist and ipratropium 4-6 hourly

IF PATIENT NOT IMPROVING AFTER 15-30 MINUTES:
- Continue oxygen and steroids
- Use continuous nebulisation of salbutamol at 5-10 mg/hour if an appropriate nebuliser is available. Otherwise give nebulised salbutamol 5 mg every 15-30 minutes
- Continue ipratropium 0.5 mg 4-6 hourly until patient is improving

IF PATIENT IS STILL NOT IMPROVING:
- Discuss patient with senior clinician and ICU team
- Consider IV magnesium sulphate 1.2-2 g over 20 minutes (unless already given)
- Senior clinician may consider use of IV β₂ agonist or IV aminophylline or progression to mechanical ventilation

MONITORING

- Repeat measurement of PEF 15-30 minutes after starting treatment
- Oximetry: maintain SpO2 >94-98%
- Repeat blood gas measurements within 1 hour of starting treatment if:
  - initial PaO2 <8 kPa (60 mmHg) unless subsequent SpO2 >92%
  - PaCO2 normal or raised
  - patient deteriorates
- Chart PEF before and after giving β₂ agonists and at least 4 times daily throughout hospital stay

Transfer to ICU accompanied by a doctor prepared to intubate if:
- Deteriorating PEF, worsening or persisting hypoxia, or hypercapnea
- Exhaustion, altered consciousness
- Poor respiratory effort or respiratory arrest

DISCHARGE

When discharged from hospital, patients should have:
- Been on discharge medication for 12-24 hours and have had inhaler technique checked and recorded
- PEF >75% of best or predicted and PEF diurnal variability <25% unless discharge is agreed with respiratory physician
- Treatment with oral and inhaled steroids in addition to bronchodilators
- Own PEF meter and written asthma action plan
- GP follow up arranged within 2 working days
- Follow up appointment in respiratory clinic within 4 weeks

Patients with severe asthma (indicated by need for admission) **and adverse behavioural or psychosocial features** are at risk of further severe or fatal attacks
- Determine reason(s) for exacerbation and admission
- Send details of admission, discharge and potential best PEF to GP

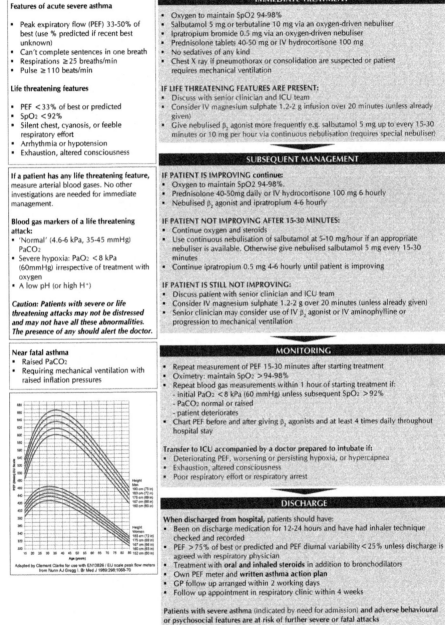

Figure 3   Management of acute severe asthma in adults in hospital. From Ref. 34.

important prognostic sign. A tachycardia of over 100/min indicates a severe attack and over 110/min, a very severe attack (34,35). In the absence of a tachyarrhythmia, a tachycardia should never be attributed to the drugs that have been given, as in most studies that have investigated this, treatment with β_2-agonists or theophyllines only adds approximately 5 to 10 beats/min to the pulse rate. A bradycardia in an asthmatic patient who is obviously having a severe attack is an ominous sign implying impending circulatory collapse.

Pulsus paradoxus used to be recommended as a method of assessing severe asthma attack; however, studies have shown that this is poorly documented and recorded and it is no longer recommended (34,36). Hypotension is also an ominous sign suggesting impending circulatory collapse. Respiratory rate is an important assessment for asthma, particularly in children where objective measures of lung function are difficult.

Examination of the respiratory system is important. The usual finding is of widespread inspiratory and expiratory wheeze. The degree of wheeze is of no value in assessing severity except that if there is a silent chest in somebody with an obvious severe asthma attack this is a poor prognostic sign (34). Examination of the chest may also detect other pathologies such as signs of a pneumothorax or consolidation.

The most important investigation to perform is to measure lung function. This is usually done with a peak flow meter but can also be done with spirometry. Oxygen saturation should be measured while breathing air. If it is below 92, then arterial blood gases should be performed to look for carbon dioxide retention (37). The initial response to a severe asthma attack is hypocapnea due to the increase in respiratory rate. As the attack becomes more severe, CO_2 retention occurs. Therefore, a normal CO_2 in the presence of an obviously severe asthma attack indicates relative CO_2 retention (34,35,37).

Full blood count and differential white cell count are of value. A high neutrophil count may indicate a bacterial infection. The normal finding in a severe asthma attack is an increase in eosinophils but a marked increase in eosinophils may indicate one of the rarer complications of asthma such as pulmonary eosinophilia or Churg–Strauss syndrome. Plasma urea and electrolyte levels should be measured. The effect of the dehydration that may occur during a severe asthma attack plus the effect of drugs, particularly β_2-agonists and steroids, can lead to a fall in plasma potassium levels.

A chest radiograph is very frequently performed in patients with an acute severe asthma attack who attend an accident and emergency department. However, the evidence is that unless there are localizing physical signs the pick-up rate of abnormalities from chest radiographs is low and current guidelines no longer recommend routine chest radiographs in acute severe asthma (34,38).

The important aspects that need to be assessed in an individual with acute severe asthma are psychosocial aspects and the severity of underlying asthma and a previous history of asthma attacks (21,39–44). These features are well set out in the U.K. asthma guidelines (Table 1).

A history of previous ventilation or CO_2 retention during an acute severe asthma attack is a poor prognostic sign, as is a history of previous hospital admissions, particularly if in the last one to two years. The amount of routine treatment should be assessed; the more routine treatment a patient is taking the more concern there should be. When an individual is assessed, he or she may have already been treated in an

Table 1 Patients at Risk of Developing Near-Fatal or Fatal Asthma

A combination of severe asthma recognized by one or more of the following:
   Previous near-fatal asthma, for example, previous ventilation or respiratory acidosis
   Previous admission for asthma especially if in the last year
   Requiring three or more classes of asthma medication
   Heavy use of β_2-agonist
   Repeated attendances at A&E for asthma care especially if in the last year
   Brittle asthma

An adverse behavioral or psychosocial features recognized by one or more of the following:
   Noncompliance with treatment or monitoring
   Failure to attend appointments
   Self-discharge from hospital
   Psychosis, depression, other psychiatric illness, or deliberate self-harm
   Current or recent major tranquillizer use
   Denial
   Alcohol or drug abuse
   Obesity
   Learning difficulties
   Employment problems
   income problems
   Social isolation
   Childhood abuse
   Severe domestic, marital, or legal stress

Abbreviation: A&E, accident and emergency.*Source:* From Ref. 34.

ambulance, by primary care physician, or at his or her first attendance in accident and emergency department with high-dose bronchodilators. Therefore, an assessment of how they were before this is important. Two useful ways of assessing this include the ability to maintain conversation using sentences and the number of puffs of their β_2-agonist inhaler that they have used. Epidemiological studies have shown that an excessive use of short-acting β_2-agonists is associated with an increased risk of asthma death (45–47). Case control studies from New Zealand suggested that this might be a particular problem with fenoterol (33,48). In these epidemiological and case control studies it is always difficult to determine whether a treatment is the cause of an increase in mortality or merely a marker of poorly controlled asthma. It is now generally felt that the excessive use of short-acting β_2-agonists is a marker of poorly controlled asthma, often associated with overreliance on bronchodilators rather than taking regular controller therapy. Guidelines therefore recommend that patients who frequently have to use their short-acting β_2-agonists have their asthma treatment reviewed to try and improve control (34,49).

    Psychosocial features are very important in the assessment of an individual with an acute asthma attack. Individuals with alcohol or drug misuse, poor social circumstances, or psychological problems, particularly depression, are at an increased risk (21). Therefore, in the assessment of whether a patient with a severe asthma attack can be safely managed at home or needs admission to hospital, two components need to be considered: objective evidence of severity and psychosocial factors (34,49).

VI. Drug Treatment of Acute Severe Asthma

Rapidly acting β_2-agonists by the nebulized route are the most important bronchodilators used in the treatment of acute severe asthma (34,49). The principle mode of action of β_2-agonists is to relax airway smooth muscle; they also help to coordinate ciliary function and increase the water content of mucus thus making it less viscid (50). The importance of these nonsmooth muscle relaxant effects of β_2-agonists in the treatment of acute severe asthma is unclear. Because β_2-agonists also have effect on pulmonary vasculature, they may cause a small (and probably clinically insignificant) fall in arterial oxygen tension (PaO_2). The improvement gained from relaxation of airway smooth muscle and therefore bronchodilatation far outweighs the small risk of an increase in hypoxia but if at all possible β_2-agonists should be given concurrently with supplementary oxygen.

β_2-Agonists need to be given in higher doses during an acute severe asthma attack as an effect of worsening asthma is a potential downregulation of β_2-receptor function.

Short-acting and fast-acting β_2-agonists (e.g., salbutamol or terbutaline) are often given by nebulization at a dose of 2.5 or 5 mg. However, particularly in children, 10 to 20 puffs given from a metered-dose inhaler via a large volume spacer set have been shown to be as effective as a nebulizer. The dose of β_2-agonist can be repeated and a technique of continuous nebulization with a low-output nebulizer has been shown to be effective in children.

The long-acting β_2-agonist formoterol has a rapid onset of action, very similar to that of salbutamol and terbutaline. It has been shown to be safe and effective to use as a rescue medication in asthma but is rarely used as a treatment for acute severe asthma in accident and emergency departments.

A. Inhaled Anticholinergics

The short-acting anticholinergic ipratropium bromide causes bronchodilatation by decreasing vagal tone on the airways. It is an effective bronchodilator in acute severe asthma but has the disadvantage of having slower onset of action than inhaled β_2-agonists. When used in combination with inhaled β_2-agonists, there is a small but clinically and statistically significant greater bronchodilatation than compared with that of β_2-agonist administered alone (51,52). Therefore, it is often recommended that ipratropium bromide should be given in addition to a β_2-agonist if there is severe or life-threatening asthma or if the initial response to nebulized β_2-agonist is not sufficient (34,49). Potential disadvantage of ipratropium bromide is that it tends to dry secretions, but in practice this does not appear to be a problem.

B. Methylxanthines

Intravenous (IV) aminophylline is an effective bronchodilator in acute severe asthma; however, its use has fallen in recent years.

The main reason for declining the use of IV aminophylline is the lack of proof that in acute severe asthma treated with adequate doses of β_2-agonists, ipratropium bromide, and systemic steroids, there is the additional effect of IV aminophylline. Meta-analysis of various studies has failed to show any effect overall or any potential advantage in any subgroup such as those with very severe asthma who may benefit (53). The risks of IV aminophylline are well described, and there are case reports and case series of individuals having cardiac arrhythmias and epileptic fits because of overdose with aminophylline (54). Aminophylline is therefore no longer recommended as a routine therapy for acute severe asthma but is reserved for those with life-threatening asthma who may require ventilation.

C. IV Magnesium

There are case reports going back to the 1990s of the efficacy of IV magnesium but a recent Cochrane review has suggested that IV magnesium has beneficial effects in those with very severe acute asthma attacks (55). IV magnesium has a number of pharmacological effects that may give benefit in asthma. Magnesium is a weak bronchodilator and also acts to stabilize a number of inflammatory cells. The data on which the Cochrane review is based have been mainly obtained from studies performed in North America where discharge from the emergency room was the primary outcome measure. Overall the results of the meta-analysis were negative showing no difference between IV magnesium and a placebo. However, a subgroup of patients with more severe asthma attacks was identified and these patients appeared to benefit from a more rapid improvement in PEF. The problem with this meta-analysis is that it is not clear whether the subgroups were identified prospectively and the definition of severe subgroup varies from study to study. The advantage of IV magnesium is that it appears very safe. The dose used is between 1.2 and 2 grams given in 50 mL of normal saline over 15 to 30 minutes. There is no evidence on whether repeated dosing is of value.

D. Leukotriene Receptor Antagonists

There is evidence for increased leukotriene production during acute severe asthma attacks (56). A study of the acute administration of a high oral dose of zafirlukast (160 mg) in patients presenting to an emergency department with acute severe asthma showed a reduction in the number of patients requiring extended care (57). A trial of IV montelukast in patients with acute severe asthma treated with inhaled β_2-agonists and systemic steroids showed a more rapid improvement in PEF (58). At present no leukotriene receptor antagonist is licensed for the treatment of acute severe asthma. As leukotriene receptor antagonists when given to patients with acute severe asthma appear to be safe and well tolerated and have some beneficial effect, they maybe considered in patients with acute severe asthma with an inadequate response to other treatments.

E. Systemic Steroids

Oral or IV corticosteroids are the most important anti-inflammatory drugs for treating acute severe asthma and should be given to all patients with acute severe asthma (34,49,59–61). The mechanism of the beneficial effect of steroids is not fully understood but they cause a decrease in inflammation particularly inflammation involving eosinophils and CD4 positive T cells. There is downregulation of β_2-receptor function in acute severe asthma, and steroids upregulate β_2-receptor function by increasing the synthesis of β_2-receptors. The earliest time that an effect of systemic steroids can be measured is four to six hours but the maximum effect does not come on for several days. Although often given intravenously the limited number of studies that have been performed show no difference in speed of onset of action between IV and oral steroids (62). Therefore, IV steroids should be reserved for patients who are vomiting, who are unconscious, or for some other reason cannot take oral steroids. Evidence for the most appropriate dose of oral steroids to use is poor but there is little evidence for improvement when using doses above approximately 0.5 mg/kg/day of prednisolone. For most acute severe asthma attacks seven days of prednisolone is sufficient, although a small minority of patients may need treatment for a longer duration (63). Gradual weaning of steroids after an acute severe asthma attack is often used but the limited evidence available suggests that this is not routinely necessary. Patients in whom weaning off oral steroids should be considered are patients who are on long-term oral steroids, who have had frequent courses of oral steroids, or those who are on high-dose inhaled steroids.

F. Antibiotics

The commonest causes of exacerbations of asthma are viral infections, allergen exposure, and noncompliance with regular inhaled steroids. Bacterial infections are an infrequent cause of exacerbations. Blinded placebo-controlled trials of antibiotics in acute severe asthma have failed to show any benefit and so antibiotics are not recommended for use in acute severe asthma (34,59,64).

A study of a ketolide antibiotic, telithromycin, has been performed in patients with acute exacerbations of asthma (65). Subjects received telithromycin or placebo for 10 days in addition to their normal asthma treatment. There was a greater improvement in symptoms in the telithromycin-treated group though the difference compared with placebo was only 0.3 on a seven-point scale, which is of doubtful clinical significance. There was no significant effect on morning peak flow but there was a slightly greater FEV_1 (forced expiratory volume in one second) improvement on days 11 to 14 of the study. There was no relationship between the response to treatment and evidence of infection either with *Chlamydia pneumoniae* or *Mycoplasma pneumoniae* suggesting that any benefits from the drug were due to an anti-inflammatory rather than an antibacterial effect. Telithromycin is not available for routine clinical use and this trial does not support the routine use for antibiotics in the management of acute severe asthma.

G. Oxygen

High flow oxygen should be given to all hypoxic asthmatics and it is preferable to use oxygen when giving nebulized β_2-agonists. Chronic carbon dioxide retention is extremely rare in asthma and so controlled oxygen therapy is unnecessary in acute exacerbations of asthma (34,37,49).

H. Helium-Oxygen Mixtures

Helium-oxygen mixtures or heliox has been the subject of a number of small studies. Because heliox has a lower density than air, it can flow more easily through obstructed airways. It is claimed that heliox administration can relieve breathlessness but the evidence for this is weak and heliox cannot at present be recommended for routine treatment in acute severe asthma (66,67).

I. Inhaled Corticosteroids

There are a number of intriguing studies that show that inhaled or nebulized steroids can have an acute bronchodilator effect in exacerbations of asthma (68). The acute bronchodilatation that occurs is far too rapid to be explained by an anti-inflammatory effect. It is well-recognized in the skin that topically applied steroids cause vasoconstriction.

Similarly, inhaled steroids may cause constriction of bronchial wall vasculature and it has been suggested that this acute effect of steroids in acute severe asthma may be due to vasoconstriction decreasing engorgement of the bronchial walls and possibly edema formation (69).

A recent meta-analysis of the use of inhaled steroids in addition to routine treatment for acute severe asthma showed a reduced likelihood of patients being admitted to hospital, which was significant for the subgroup who did not receive oral or IV corticosteroids. For the group receiving concomitant systemic steroids, there was a trend to reduction in hospital admissions, but this was not significant. Patients receiving inhaled steroids showed a small but statistically significant improvement in peak flow and FEV_1 (70).

At present the evidence is not strong enough to recommend the use of ICSs in addition to systemic steroids as a routine treatment for acute severe asthma. However, in patients who have not responded adequately to conventional treatment, as this seems to be safe and well tolerated, the addition of an ICS could be considered.

VII.   Overview of Drug Treatment of Acute Severe Asthma

The principles of treating acute severe asthma are to give bronchodilators to ease dyspnea and keep the patient alive while giving time for the steroids to reduce inflammation. All patients should be given high-dose nebulized β_2-agonists. If these are inadequate or the attack is particularly severe then ipratropium bromide should be added. Steroids should be given either orally or intravenously. If response is inadequate then IV magnesium can be given. If response is still inadequate then increased monitoring in a high dependency unit or intensive care unit should be considered.

A.   Monitoring and Discharge

Monitoring of acute severe asthma should include objective measurements of pulmonary function, usually PEF and pulse rate, and, if hypoxia is present, measurement of oxygen saturation. Patients should continue with oral corticosteroids until discharge. Once a patient has improved ipratropium bromide can be stopped. Before discharge patients should be switched from nebulized to inhaled short-acting bronchodilators. If IV aminophylline has been used this should be stopped once the patient is no longer having a life-threatening attack. Guidelines recommend that discharge can occur when the patient's peak flow is back to 80% of predicted or their best with no marked morning dipping (34,49).

Prior to discharge, the routine management of asthma should be reviewed (34,49,71). Particular attention needs to be paid to any cause of the exacerbation and preventable causes such as allergen exposure need to be addressed. The level of control of their asthma prior to the acute exacerbation should be reviewed. If, as is often the case, the exacerbation has occurred on a background of poor asthma control then routine treatment needs to be increased. Poor compliance with treatment, particularly with ICSs, is a common precipitant of acute severe asthma, and questioning about compliance with treatment and stressing the importance of taking regular treatment are important.

The evidence is strong from individual trial and systematic reviews that any patient admitted to hospital with acute severe asthma should be discharged on ICSs, which reduce the chances of readmission with asthma (34,49,70). The dose of ICSs used will depend on the maintenance dose that was used prior to the attack. In patients who were not on inhaled steroids prior to their acute severe asthma attack, a low-dose inhaled steroid of 400 μg beclomethasone equivalence would be appropriate. In those who were taking higher doses of ICSs prior to admission, an increase in the dose of ICSs or the addition of a long-acting β$_2$-agonist if it is not being used would be appropriate. There is little evidence that the addition of oral aminophylline reduces asthma exacerbations and that the addition of leukotriene receptor antagonists in addition to inhaled steroids and long-acting β$_2$-agonists reduces the chance of exacerbations.

Prior to discharge from hospital, patients inhaler technique should be checked (34,49,72). If their inhaler technique is not optimal then they should be educated in the correct use of inhalers and if this still does not achieve an adequate inhaler technique they should be changed to another device that they can use appropriately.

There is little evidence that in the majority of patients with an acute asthma attack prolongation of use of oral steroids beyond 7 to 10 days is of benefit. The exception to this is patients who have more severe and difficult asthma such as those at step 4 with poorly controlled asthma where slower weaning down of oral steroids may be appropriate.

There is good evidence that asthma education incorporating a written asthma action plan allowing effective self-management should be given to all patients prior to discharge. The Cochrane review of self-management plans showed that they decreased hospital admissions with a trend toward a decrease in asthma deaths (73).

After discharge from hospital, review in either primary or secondary care within two to three weeks is recommended to assess the level of asthma control and reinforce the importance of compliance, plus make any necessary adjustments to treatment (34,71).

VIII. Conclusion

Despite better treatment of asthma, exacerbations of asthma remain a fairly common medical emergency. Patients with an exacerbation of asthma require an assessment of the objective severity of their exacerbation plus recognition of any potential adverse psychological or social factors. The principles of treatment of asthma exacerbations are to relieve symptoms with bronchodilators and oxygen while treating the underlying airway inflammation with systemic corticosteroids. It is important that objective measurements of airway function, usually done with PEF rates, are made to monitor the severity of the attack and the response to treatment. Once the exacerbation has been successfully treated, attention must be paid to minimizing the chance of further exacerbations by examining potential trigger factors and optimizing routine treatment. Of the routine treatment of asthma, the most important remains regular ICSs. Indeed, examination of trends for asthma admission strongly suggests that the increased use of ICSs is associated with a reduction in hospital admissions and a reduction in the number of individuals needing ventilation.

References

1. Rabe KF, Vermeire PA, Soriano JB, et al. Clinical management of asthma in 1999: the Asthma Insights and Reality in Europe (AIRE) study. Eur Respir J 2000; 16:802–807.
2. Reiss TF, Chervinsky P, Dockhorn RJ, et al. Montelukast, a once daily leukotriene receptor antagonist, in the treatment of chronic asthma: a multicenter, randomised, double-blindtrial. Arch Inter Med 1998; 158:1213–1220.

3. Pauwels RA, Löfdahl CG, Postma DS, et al. Effect of inhaled formoterol and budesonide on exacerbations of asthma. N Engl J Med 1997; 337:1405–1411.
4. Asthma UK. Available at: http://www.asthma.org.uk.
5. Gern JE, Busse WW. Relationship of viral infections to wheezing illnesses and asthma. Nat Rev Immunol 2002; 2:132–138.
6. Johnston SL. Viruses and asthma. Allergy 1998; 53:922–932.
7. Johnston SL. The role of viral and atypical bacterial pathogens in asthma pathogenesis. Pediatr Pulmonol 1999(suppl 18):141–143.
8. Atkinson RW, Strachan DP. Role of outdoor aeroallergens in asthma exacerbations: epidemiological evidence. Thorax 2004; 59:277–278.
9. Rosenstreich DL, Eggleston P, Kattan M, et al. The role of cockroach allergy and exposure to cockroach allergen in causing morbidity among inner-city children with asthma. N Engl J Med 1997; 336:1356–1363.
10. Denning DW, O'Briscoll BR, Hogaboam CM, et al. The link btween fungi and severe asthma: a summary of the evidence. Eur Respir J 2006; 27:615–626.
11. Thames Regions Accident and Emergency Trainers Association, Davidson AC, Embrlin J, Cook AD, et al. A major outbreak of asthma associated with a thunderstorm: experience of accident and emergency departments and patients characteristics. BMJ 1996; 312:601–604.
12. Anderson W, Prescott GJ, Packham S, et al. Asthma admission and thunderstorms: a study of pollen, fungal spores, rainfall, and ozone. QJM 2001; 94:429–433.
13. Barnes P. Air pollution and asthma. Postgrad Med 1994; 70:319–324.
14. Swartz J, Slater D, Larson TV, et al. Particulate air pollution and hospital emergency room visits for asthma in Seattle. Am Rev Respir Dis 1993; 147:826–831.
15. Roemer W, Hoek G, Brunekreef B. Effect of ambient winter air pollution on respiratory health of children with chronic respiratory symptoms. Am Rev Respir Dis 1993; 147:118–124.
16. Chen LL, Tager IB, Peden DB, et al. Effect of ozone exposure on airway responses to inhaled allergen in asthmatic subjects. Chest 2004; 125:2328–2335.
17. Ernst P, Spitzer WO, Suissa S, et al. Risk of fatal and near-fatal asthma in relation to inhaled corticosteroid use. JAMA 1992; 268:3462–3464.
18. Belda J, Parameswaran K, Lemiere C, et al. Predictors of loss of asthma control induced by corticosteroid withdrawal. Can Respir J 2006; 13:129–133.
19. Gibson PG, Wong BJ, Hepperle MJ, et al. A research method to induce and examine a mild exacerbation of asthma by withdrawal of inhaled corticosteroid. Clin Exp Allergy 1992; 22:525–532.
20. Randolph C. Exercise-induced asthma: update on pathophysiology, clinical diagnosis, and treatment. Curr Probl Pediatr 1997; 27:53–77.
21. Vanderweil SG, Tsai CL, Pelletier AJ, et al. Inappropriate use of antibiotics for acute asthma in the United States Emergency departments. Acad Emerg Med 2008; 15:736–743.
22. Innes NJ, Reid A, Halstead J, et al. Psychosocial risk factors in near-fatal asthma and in asthma deaths. J R Coll Physicians Lond 1998; 32:430–434.
23. Kay AB, Phipps S, Robinson DS. A role for eosinophils in airway remodelling in asthma. Trends Immunol 2004; 25:477–482.
24. Wenzel S. Mechanisms of severe asthma. Clin Exp Allergy 2003; 33:1622–1628.
25. Tough SC, Green FH, Paul JE, et al. Sudden death from asthma in 108 children and young adults. J Asthma 1996; 33:179–188.
26. Wagner PD, Hechenstierna G, Rodriguez—Roisin R. Gas exchange, expiratory airflow obstruction and the clinical spectrum in asthma. Eur Respir J 1996; 9:1278–1282.
27. Wassertaller JB, Schaller MD, Perret CH. Life threatening asthma with dramatic resolution. Chest 1993; 104:616.
28. Tattersfield AE, Postma DS, Barnes PJ, et al. Exacerbations of asthma: a descriptive study of 425 severe exacerbations. Am J Respir Crit Care Med 1999; 160:594–599.

29. Rubinfield AR, Pain MCF. Perception of asthma. Lancet 1975; 2:822–824.
30. McFadden ER, Kiser R, De Groot WJ. Acute bronchial asthma. Relations between clinical and physiological manifestations. N Engl J Med 1973; 288:221–225.
31. Burdon JGW, Juniper EF, Killian KJ, et al. The perception of breathlessness in asthma. Am Rev Respir Dis 1982; 126:825–828.
32. Turner MO, Noertjojo K, Vedal S, et al. Risk factors for near-fatal asthma. A case-control study in hospitalized patients with asthma. Am J Respir Crit Care Med 1998; 157:1804–1809.
33. Richards GN, Kolbe J, Fenwick J, et al. Demographic characteristics of patients with severe life threatening asthma: comparison with asthma deaths. Thorax 1993; 48:1105–1109.
34. British Guidelines on Asthma Management. Management of acute asthma. Thorax 2008; 63 (suppl 4):51–66.
35. International consensus report on the diagnosis and treatment of asthma. National Heart, Lung, and Blood Institute, National Institutes of Health. Bethesda, Maryland, Publication no. 92-3091, March 1992.
36. Pearson MG, Spence DP, Ryland I, et al. Value of pulsus paradoxus in assessing acute severe asthma. British Thoracic Society Standards of Care Committee. BMJ 1993; 307:659.
37. British Thoracic Society. Guidelines for emergency oxygen use. Thorax 2008; 63(suppl 6): vi 1–vi 68.
38. Findley LJ, Sahn SA. The value of chest roentgenograms in acute asthma in adults. Chest 1981; 80:535–536.
39. Bucknall CE, Slack R, Godley CC, et al. Scottish confidential inquiry into asthma deaths (SCIAD), 1994-96. Thorax 1999; 54:978–984.
40. Burr ML, Davies BH, Hoare A, et al. A confidential inquiry into asthma deaths in Wales. Thorax 1999; 54:985–989.
41. Mohan G, Harrison BD, Badminton RM, et al. A confidential enquiry into deaths caused by asthma in an English health region: implications for general practice. Br J Gen Pract 1996; 46:529–532.
42. Wareham NJ, Harrison BD, Jenkins PF, et al. A district confidential enquiry into deaths due to asthma. Thorax 1993; 48:117–120.
43. Harrison BDW, Slack R, Berrill WT, et al. Results of a national confidential enquiry into asthma. Asthma J 2000; 5:180–186.
44. Jalaludin BB, Smith MA, Chey T, et al. Risk factors for asthma deaths: a population-based, case-control study. Aust N Z J Public Health 1999; 23:595–600.
45. Suissa S, Ernst P, Boivin J-F, et al. A cohort analysis of excess mortality in asthma and the use of inhaled β-antagonists. Am J Respir Crit Care Med 1994; 149:604–610.
46. Spitzer WO, Suissa S, Ernst P, et al. The use of beta-antagonists and the risk of death and near death from asthma. N Engl J Med 1992; 326:501–506.
47. Suissa S, Blais L, Ernst P. Patterns of increasing beta-antagonist use and the risk of fatal or near-fatal asthma. Eur Respir J 1994; 7:1602–1609.
48. Rea HH, Scragg R, Jackson R, et al. A case-control study of deaths from asthma. Thorax 1986; 41(11):833–839.
49. Global Initiative for Asthma. Available at http://www.ginasthma.com. 2008.
50. Lotvall J. Bronchodilators. In: O'Bryne P, Thompson NC, eds. Manual of Asthma Management. 2nd ed. London: W B Saunders, 2001.
51. Rodrigo G, Rodrigo C, Burschtin O. A meta-analysis of the effects of ipratropium bromide in adults. Am J Med 1999; 107:363–370.
52. Rodrigo GJ, Rodrigo C. First-line therapy for adult patients with acute asthma receiving a multiple-dose protocol of ipratropium. Am J Respir Crit Care Med 2000; 161:1862–1868.
53. Parameswaran K, Belda J, Rowe BH. Addition of intravenous aminophylline to beta2-agonists in adults with acute asthma. Cochrane Database Syst Rev 2000; 4:CD002742.

54. Shannon M. Life-threatening events after theophylline overdose: a 10 year prospective analysis. Arch Inter Med 1999; 159:989–994.

55. Rowe BH, Bretzlaff JA, Bourdon C, et al. Magnesium sulfate for treating exacerbations of acute asthma in the emergency department. Cochrane Database Syst Rev 2000; (2):CD001490.

56. Drazen JM, O'Brien J, Sparrow D, et al. Recovery of leukotriene E4 from the urine of patients with airway obstruction. Am Rev Respir Dis 1992; 146:104–108.

57. Silverman RA, Nowak RM, Korenblat PE, et al. Zarirlukast treatment for acute asthma. Chest 2004; 126:1480–1489.

58. Camargo Carlos A Jr., Smithline Howard A, Malice Marie-Pierre, et al. Randomized controlled trial of intravenous montelukast in acute asthma. Am J Respir Crit Care Med 2003; 167:528–533.

59. Rowe BH, FM, Bretzlaff JA, Bota GW. Early emergency department treatment of acute asthma with systemic corticosteroids (Cochrane Review). In: The Cochrane Library. Issue 3. London: John Wiley & Sons Ltd, 2001.

60. Rowe BH, Spooner CH, Ducharme FM, et al. Corticosteroids for preventing relapse following acute exacerbations of asthma (Cochrane Review). In: The Cochrane Library. Issue 3. London: John Wiley & Sons Ltd, 2001.

61. Manser R, Reid D, Abramson M. Corticosteroids, for acute severe asthma in hospitalised patients. Cochrane Database Syst Rev 2000; 2:CD001740.

62. Harrison BD, Stokes TC, Hart GJ, et al. Need for intravenous hydrocortisone in addition to oral prednisolone in patients admitted to hospital with severe asthma without ventilatory. Lancet 1986; 1(8474):181–184.

63. Hasegawa T, Ishihara K, Takakura S, et al. Duration of systemic corticosteroids in the treatment of asthma exacerbation; a randomized study. Intern Med 2000; 39:794–797.

64. Graham VA, Milton AF, Knowles GK, et al. Routine antibiotics in hospital management of acute asthma. Lancet 1982; 1:418–420.

65. Johnston SL, Blasi F, Black PN, et al.; and TELICATS Investigators. The effect of telithromycin in acute exacerbations of asthma. N Engl J Med 2006; 354:1589–1600.

66. Kass JE, Terregino CA. The effect of heliox in acute severe asthma: a randomised controlled trial. Chest 1999; 116:296–300.

67. Henderson SO, Acharya P, Kilaghbian T, et al. Use of heliox-driven nebuliser therapy in the treatment of acute asthma. Ann Emerg Med 1999; 33:141–146.

68. Rodrigo GJ. Comparison of inhaled fluticasone with intravenous hydrocortisone in the treatment of adult acute asthma. Am J Respir Crit Care Med 2005; 171:1231–1236.

69. Hovarth G, Wanner A. Inhaled corticosteroids: effects on the airway vasculature in bronchial asthma. Eur Respir J 2006; 27:172–187.

70. Edmonds M, Camargo CA, Pollack CV, et al. Early use of inhaled corticosteroids in the emergency department treatment of acute asthma. Cochrane Database Syst Rev 2003, (3):CD002308.

71. Grunfeld A, Fitzgerald JM. Discharge considerations in acute asthma. Can Respir J 1996; 3: 322–324.

72. Emerman CL, Woodruff PG, Cydulka RK, et al. Prospective multicenter study of relapse following treatment for acute asthma among adults presenting to the emergency department. MARC investigators. Multicenter Asthma Research Collaboration. Chest 1999; 115:919–927.

73. Gibson PG, Powell H. Written action plans for asthma: an evidence-based review of the key components. Thorax 2004; 59:94–99.

16
Pharmacology and Therapeutics of Cough

ALYN H. MORICE
University of Hull and Castle Hill Hospital, Cottingham, East Yorkshire, U.K.

I. Introduction

The pharmacology of cough may be considered in two separate paradigms: either as a specific treatment of the cause or as a general modulation of cough reflex hypersensitivity. If the origin of the cough can be determined, for example, an inhaled foreign body, specific treatment (by removal of the foreign body) may be curative. Alternatively, ameliorating the consequences of the specific cause, such as reducing the eosinophilic inflammation of cough-variant asthma with corticosteroids, may be the next preferred option. Indeed, current guidelines on the management of chronic cough recommend therapeutic trials of individual agents based on the most likely suspected cause (1–3) (Fig. 1). The second strategy is based on suppression of the cough reflex. The rationale for such a strategy is that in many disease states the cough reflex is hyperresponsive (4); in addition, treatment of the primary associated cause of the cough may not be entirely successful. Cough suppression is the major option used in the treatment of acute cough (1). However, the efficacy of agents used in much of the multimillion pound over-the-counter market in acute cough has a poor scientific base. In intractable chronic cough, which is either treatment resistant or undiagnosed (or "idiopathic"), cough suppression remains the only valuable option. The main thrust of drug development is in the area of cough suppression, with the holy grail of cough therapeutics being the normalization of the cough reflex, suppressing the abnormal cough while retaining this vital reflex, whose main function is to protect the airways against aspiration.

II. The Etiology of Cough

Currently the most successful strategy available for the treatment of cough is a correct diagnosis followed by specific treatment. Unfortunately, in the commonest new presentation with cough, acute bronchitis, even though the cause is known to be the multiple viral pathogens of respiratory tract, there is, as yet, no specific treatment. In contrast, there is now a burgeoning literature describing the diagnosis and successful treatment of chronic cough from specialist cough clinics around the world (5–12), so a search for the specific etiology is usually recommended. This search can be hampered by a number of factors. Firstly disease causing cough often presents in an atypical fashion. Thus, recognizing eosinophilic bronchitis and cough-variant asthma may be difficult for the nonspecialist since the classic asthmatic symptoms of wheeze and airflow obstruction may be entirely absent (13,14). The second barrier to the correct diagnosis and therefore specific treatment is the ignorance of the clinician to the range of possible

Therapeutic algorithm

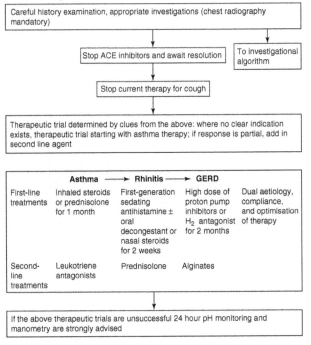

Figure 1 Treatment algorithm for chronic cough.

diagnoses. This is no where better illustrated than in cough associated with gastro-esophageal reflux. Because of the focus on reflux causing heartburn, there has been a lack of appreciation of the effects of extra-esophageal reflux and particularly nonacidic reflux (15). A lack of response to conventional antacid treatment for gastroesophageal reflux disease (GERD) is taken as evidence that the cough cannot be of reflux origin, when in fact the problem is a failure to appreciate that the symptom complex is due to reflux of different composition and timing to that causing dyspepsia (16).

The conventional dogma holds that there are three main causes of chronic cough, namely, GERD, asthma, and postnasal drip (5). In this chapter, the generic term reflux has been used for retrograde flow of gut contents. The forms of chronic cough characterized by eosinophilic infiltration have been given the generic term asthmatic cough and while recognizing that there are important clinical differences between eosinophilic bronchitis, atopic cough, cough-variant asthma, and classic asthma, they will be regarded as separate facets of a single whole, since the pharmacology of specific treatment is based around the suppression of eosinophilic inflammation. Finally, there is no doubt that some patients with chronic cough have predominantly nasal symptoms. The etiological link between these nasal symptoms and the cough is however tenuous (17). Some authors have elevated this to a separate syndrome, the postnasal drip syndrome, which has recently been renamed upper airways cough syndrome (UACS) in the American College of Chest Physicians Guidelines (18). The presence of this separate syndrome has been led by the belief that treatment with "specific" agents was indicative of a separate etiology. As will be discussed later, UACS may be regarded as another extra-esophageal manifestation of reflux disease.

Finally, there has been a number of patients with chronic cough in whom the cough is not associated with asthma or any other recognized cause that have been classified as having an "idiopathic cough" (19). Such patients would usually have had empirical trials of therapy directed at GERD, asthma, and upper airways disease according to the European Respiratory Society (ERS) recommendations without success. Up to 7% to 46% of chronic cough have been identified as idiopathic cough (20). The cause(s) of idiopathic cough remains unclear but could represent continuing enhancement of the cough reflex with disappearance of the initial insult.

III. Cough Receptor Pharmacology

The term receptor has had a dual meaning in cough research. The original term was coined by physiologists who were able to determine that specific nerve fibers responded to specific stimuli associated with cough and cough-like reflex responses (21). Such fibers were usually of the Aδ-subtype of myelinated nerve within the vagus. This use of the word receptor in the description of single nerve fiber recordings and similar techniques therefore describes the hard wiring of the cough reflex rather than what is understood by a receptor in pharmacological terms. While this terminology has been useful in our understanding, it has been superseded by the use of the word receptor as a protein, which usually acts as an ion channel causing neuronal depolarization. A better term to replace receptor is "sensor" since these nerve endings are sensors or sentinels of the respiratory tract. A number of candidates have been proposed as putative cough receptors and drug development is strongly focused around targeting these ion channels.

A. Provoking Cough

Coughing most frequently results from an irritation of the upper airway. Such irritation arises from two main mechanisms. First is physical in the form of aspiration. This is probably the chief role of the cough reflex, particularly in man, since the development of speech has caused us to develop a compromised mechanical defense of the upper airways with the descent of the laryngeal apparatus away from the soft palate (22). The second important stimulus is physicochemical. It is not surprising that in protecting the airway, a family of irritant receptors that is polymodal in sensitivity is utilized. In other areas, these receptors are responsible for the sensation of pain, itch, and temperature. The non-taste, non-smell sensing of chemical stimuli is known as chemesthesis and plays an important role in defining cough receptor pharmacology.

Inhalation of tussigenic stimuli in cough challenge studies broadly defines protussive chemical stimuli into three main categories. The earliest studies by Bickerman et al. (23) demonstrated that inhalation of citric acid is a prominent tussive stimulus. In fact, all complex acids will provoke coughing and the observation that within individuals different acids have the same rank order of potency as tussive agents infers that they act as proton donors rather than through any other mechanism (24). Clearly, within the receptor pharmacology of the cough reflex, acid-sensitive mechanisms must be delineated.

The second inhalational challenge is distilled water. Fog challenge has a markedly different profile in terms of tachyphylaxis and the other chemical challenges. Distilled water cough wears off rapidly during continuous inhalation with most normal subjects no longer coughing after 30 seconds of inhalation (25). Studies using sodium salts have demonstrated that rather than distilled water itself it is the lack of chloride or more correctly a permeant anion that is the crucial stimulus in distilled water cough (26). How this translates into receptor stimulation has not been fully worked out, although osmoreceptors may play a role.

The third receptor type thought to be important in chemosynthesis-induced cough is the nociceptor of the transient receptor potential (TRP) family. The capsaicin receptor, TRP vanniloid-1 (TRPV1), is the archetypal TRP nociceptor. Capsaicin was first used as an agent to produce cough in the 1980s (27). It has become a standardized challenge in the determination of cough reflex sensitivity (28). Other vanilloids such as resin-iferatoxin stimulate cough, and this group of agents represents the most potent tussive agents known (29). Other TRP receptors have now been demonstrated to be important in cough reflex sensitivity and interestingly they have been identified through the per-ception of temperature (30).

IV.   The Molecular Pharmacology of the Cough Reflex
A.   The TRP Family

Twenty-eight mammalian TRP channels have been discovered (31). These channels fall into seven subfamilies but share common structural features, such as tendency to form tetramers, with each subunit containing six transmembrane domains. All channels have the N and C termini on the intracellular side of the membrane and as with voltage-gated channels, to which they are closely related, the TRP are voltage sensitive.

One of the major functions of the TRP channels appears to be temperature sen-sation. Nine channels from three subfamilies have been shown to cover the spectrum of thermal sensation (TRPV1-4, TRPM8, and TRPA1) (Table 1). Bearing in mind the airway membranes exposure to ambient atmospheric conditions, it is perhaps not sur-prising that three members of the thermally active TRP family have been demonstrated to have an important role in the cough reflex sensitivity.

B.   TRPV1

TRPV1 is the most likely candidate of the putative cough receptors. It is polymodal responding not only to the vanilloids but also to low pH and a variety of proinflammatory chemokine such as bradykinin (32). It is regulated (Fig. 2) by activation of phospholipase A2 through lipoxygenase metabolites such as 12-hydroperoxyeicosatetraenoic acid (12-HPETE) (33). As with other respiratory chemesthesis receptors, it is sensitive to temperatures in the moderate noxious range of 42°C to 43°C. The 462 amino acid protein is highly expressed in vagal neurone and ganglia in fibers of the C- and Aδ-subtype. Electrophysiological studies have previously demonstrated these neurones to be typical polymodal nociceptors (34). Activation of TRPV1 causes depolarization of sensory neurones through calcium influx. This generates not only the action potential propagation but also local release of neuropeptides, particularly calcitonin gene-related peptides and the tachykinins substance P and neurokinin A (35). The phenomenon of neurogenic inflammation through these proinflammatory pep-tides may therefore be triggered by activation of TRPV1. The thermal sensitivities of TRPV1

Table 1 Thermosensitive TRP Channels Sense Temperature Over a Range of Values

| | Cold ←→ Pain | | Warm | | | | | Hot → Pain | |
	TRPA1	TRPM8	TRPV3	TRPV4	TRPM2	TRPM4	TRPM5	TRPV1	TRPV2
Activation temperature	<17°C	<25°C	>33°C	>25°C to 34°C	>35°C	Activity increased by heat, threshold undetermined		>42°C	>52°C
Agonist	Cinnamaldehyde acrolein, AITC, THC, gingerol, icillin, allicin, farnesyl-thiosalicylic acid, 4-HNE, menthol, calcium	Menthol, icillin, eucalyptol, geraniol, linalool, isopulegol, l-carvone	2-APB, camphor, menthol, eugenol, thymol, carvacrol	Bisandro-grapholide, 4αPDD	Hydrogen peroxide, ADP-ribose, βNAD	Cytosolic calcium		Capsaicin, resiniferatoxin, piperine, protons (pH below 5.9), ethanol, some lipoxygenase products (e.g. 12-(S)-HPETE), NADA, anandamide, phorbols, camphor, 2-APB, gingerol, eugenol	2-APB, THC

TRPA1, TRPV1, and TRPM8 have been shown to have a role in cough.
Abbreviations: TRP, transient receptor potential; 12-HPETE, 12-hydroperoxyeicosatetraenoic acid.

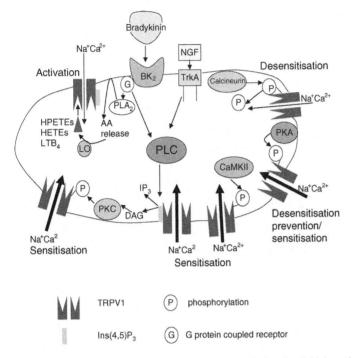

Figure 2   The proposed mechanisms of TRPV1 regulation. Bradykinin and NGF activate specific receptors, BK$_2$ a G protein–coupled receptor (G) and TrkA, respectively, resulting in PLC stimulation and AA release. TRPV1 (*blue crown*) can be sensitized (*thick arrow*) by PLC hydrolysis of Ins(4,5)P$_2$ (PIP$_2$) or phosphorylation (P) by PKC or activated by LO products (*red triangle*). Phosphorylation by PKA and CaMKII sensitizes the channel whereas dephosphorylation by calcineurin desensitizes TRPV1. *Abbreviations*: TRPV1, transient receptor potential vanniloid-1; AA, arachidonic acid; TrkA, tyrosine kinase; LO, lipoxygenase.

may underlie the exquisite sensitivity of patients with chronic cough because of change in atmospheric conditions. It may however provide a negative feature in therapeutics. While TRPV1 antagonists may prove to be therapeutically useful as antitussives, inhibiting temperature sensitivity may lead to a potentially dangerous decrease in thermal sensitivity.

There is marked plasticity in the expression and function of TRPV1. The quantity and density of TRPV1 expressing neurones are thought to be under the regulation of nerve growth factor (35). An increase in density of TRPV1 containing nerves has been demonstrated in patients with chronic cough (36). TRPV1 expression is not only increased in neurones but also in chronic inflammation of chronic cough, expression takes place in nonneuronal tissues, such as bronchial smooth muscle. Expression is not limited to the cell membrane but can be demonstrated by immunohistochemistry in a perinuclear fraction, which is confirmed to be thapsigargin sensitive (37).

At a cellular level TRPV1 is regulated by a wide range of mediators, including products of phospholipase A and C as well as protein kinase A and C. The channel opening probability is altered through a protein kinase C mechanism, decreasing the threshold temperature for thermal activation. Bradykinin through the B2 receptor sensitizes TRPV1 through activation of phospholipase production of lipoxygenase products (10). The production of cough by prostaglandins has been suggested to be through alteration of TRPV1 sensitivity (38). ACE inhibitors may alter cough sensitivity by a bradykinin-induced increase in TPRV1 sensitivity (39). An increase in substance P however is an alternative mechanism (40). Protease-activated receptors (PAR2) when stimulated through cleavage of its extracellular tail by protease (in particular tryptase) provides a mechanism whereby mast cells can directly stimulate the cough reflex through a protein kinase C dependent mechanism (41). The role of TRPV1 in acid sensitization has been much debated. Whether acid-sensitive ion channels provide a main route of acid sensitization causing cough or whether TRPV1 is the major mediator has been indicated by the effect of the antagonist capsazepine and iodoresiniferatoxin on citric acid-mediated cough in animals (42). In contrast, electrophysiological studies suggest acid-sensitive ion channel (ASIC) as being more important (43).

C. TRPA1

TRPA1 was originally identified as the noxious cold receptor, activation being observed at temperatures below 17°C (44). Whether thermal activation does occur at these temperatures has been debated. It appears that its activation is crucially dependent on intracellular calcium levels. This TRP receptor is in the A subclass because of ankyrin repeat sequences within the intracellular domain, which may allow for complex binding with other receptors and mediators. It is particularly promiscuous in the number of ligands, which stimulate the receptor, including a number of natural pungent compounds, such as mustard oil (allyl-isothiocyanate) and cinnamon (cinnamaldehyde), as well as environmental irritants, such as wood smoke (acrolein) (44). It is thought that the common mechanism for TRPA1 activation by these common environmental tussigenic compounds is that they act as electrophiles, which covalently bind to cysteine residues. In the case of isothiocyanates this probably includes lysine residues. These reactive compounds bind nonspecifically to several of the cysteine residues within TRPA1 (45). Thus, TRPA1 appears to be the prime candidate for the major chemesthesis receptor in the airway, and in patients with chronic cough the characteristic precipitation of paroxysms by a range nonspecific of irritants may be via TRPA1. We have recently demonstrated the TRPA1 agonist cinnamaldehyde to be a potent tussive stimulus in man (46).

D. TRPM8

The cold/menthol receptor TRPM8 is activated in the temperature range <23°C to 28°C and by compounds with apparent cooling properties such as icillin, eucalyptol, and menthol (47). The mechanism of activation appears fundamentally similar to that of TRPV1 (48). However, TRPM8 activation inhibits citric acid–induced cough in animals (49) and in man (50). Thus, TRPM8 stimulation probably underlies the inclusion of menthol in many over-the-counter cough remedies. Menthol has several other activities on airway ion channels including activation of calcium channels leading to smooth muscle relaxation (51,52).

E. Acid-Sensitive Ion Channels

In cough, the sensing of acid stimuli is probably the most important role of chemesthesis because the detection of gastric acid by the upper airway may prevent aspiration of this highly toxic mixture. As described earlier, TRPV1 has acid sensitivity but it is unlikely in vivo that it represents the totality of acid sensing mechanisms within the airways. Acid-activated currents that are blocked by amiloride have been reported for many years in sensory neurones (53). ASICs are voltage-insensitive cationic channels, which are activated by extracellular protons. They belong to the ENaC/DEG (epithelial amiloride-sensitive Na+ channels and degenerin) family of ion channels (54). The generic structure of the family is of two hydrophobic transmembrane regions flanking large extracellular domain, which comprises many conserved cysteines. Again, function ASICs probably assemble as tetramers. In addition to their presence on vagal sensory afferents, ASICs are also present in lung epithelial cells (ASIC3).

ASICs are only activated by extracellular protons (55). There are four subtypes of ASICs with differing kinetics and sensitivity to proton stimulation. ASIC3 appears to be the most likely candidate for the acid sensory receptor within the airways, being located on epithelial cells as well as neurones. In addition to the perception of acid it is thought to play a role in mechanoreception. Blockers of ASIC3 include amiloride (which also blocks other ASIC receptors) and nonsteroidal anti-inflammatories (56). Of particular interest is the fact that ASIC3 displays, in addition to a transient current, a sustained component that does not inactivate provided the milieu remains acidic. Thus ASICs are good candidates for the persistent suprasternal irritation described by many patients with chronic cough (57). In addition, ASIC3 current is potentiated by known protussive agents such as bradykinin and arachidonic acid (58). The role of ASIC in human cough reflex has yet to be clearly defined. There may be considerable redundancy in acid sensation since TRPV1 knock out studies have revealed that the proportion of acid response in mice is approximately 50% (59).

F. Mechanoreceptors

Cough evoked by electrical or mechanical stimulation of the trachea and larynx in guinea pigs produces activation of polymodal Aδ fibers, which in addition to mechanical stimulation also respond to acid, but are entirely unresponsive to capsaicin, bradykinin, and distension of the airways (60). These Aδ fibers arise from the vagal nodose ganglia and are a distinct population of neurones supplying the rostral trachea and larynx via the recurrent laryngeal nerves. Further evidence is needed to support this potentially important mechanism in cough.

V. The Clinical Pharmacology of Cough

The key to successful management of chronic cough is to establish a diagnosis and to treat the cause of cough. Various guidelines have been published that distil the lessons mainly from the experience of case-series reports and provide a framework for a logical care pathway for patients with this highly disabling symptom (2,3). The approach is to investigate the cause of cough and then treat any underlying cause, with the knowledge that the most common causes are asthma, gastroesophageal reflux, and postnasal drip or rhinosinusitis. The proposed plan suggested by an ERS Task Force is shown in Figure 3. In patients without asthma and postnasal drip, an empirical two-week treatment trial of

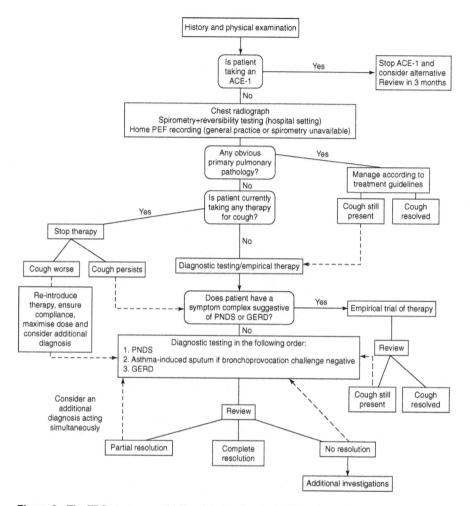

Figure 3 The ERS treatment guideline for chronic cough. Therapeutic trials based on the most likely diagnostic category are recommended. Further treatment options are given in the text. *Abbreviations*: ERS, European Respiratory Society; ACE-I, angiotensin converting enzyme inhibitor 1; PEF, peak expiratory flow; PNDS, postnasal drip syndrome; GERD, gastroesophageal reflux disease. *Source*: From Ref. 2.

high-dose proton pump inhibitor may be more reliable than investigations such as manometry and pH testing in diagnosing patients with reflux-associated cough, with a three- to fivefold cost saving with this empirical approach (61). Combining both laboratory investigation and empirical therapy may offer the best management strategy. The ERS guidelines suggest two pathways, one using an empirical approach and one of recommended investigations, and these strategies should be considered in parallel (2).

VI. Treatment of Asthmatic Cough

Because the eosinophil is the defining cell in cough-associated with TH2 inflammation, it is unsurprising that as in classic asthma the asthmatic cough syndromes are sensitive to inhaled corticosteroids (10). Just as in classic asthma, the usual constraints in terms of inhaler technique and compliance apply. There is no good clinical data defining speed of onset and dose response. The clinical impression is that cough responds more slowly than wheezing (62). One reason may be due to the reported differences in mast cell distribution between classic asthma and eosinophilic bronchitis (63). In classic asthma, mast cells are located within bronchial smooth muscle influencing tone directly, whereas in eosinophilic bronchitis cells are clustered around sensory nerve fibers thus altering cough reflex sensitivity, which as in the case of bronchial hyperresponsiveness may take longer to improve.

If inhaled steroids alone prove inadequate to control symptoms in those forms of asthmatic cough that are characterized by little or no bronchoconstriction, the addition of long acting β-agonists, as is recommended in classic asthma, has a limited place. One exception could be when aspiration is the primary cause of airway response and significant upper airway bronchoconstriction can be present. The leukotriene antagonists have been shown to have little effect on cough challenge in classic asthma (64) but have a substantial effect on cough sensitivity in cough-variant asthma (65). The mechanism for leukotriene antagonist activity in asthmatic cough may be through modulation of TRPV1. The first suggested endogenous mediator of TRPV1 was claimed to be the lipoxygenase product 5HTEPE (66), although these studies were performed in rat cells.

VII. Treatment of Reflux Cough

Reflux causing cough has many characteristics, which differ from reflux causing heartburn (67). Cough may be caused by nonacidic reflux. The reflux episodes can be brief and the extra-esophageal manifestations of reflux produce different symptom complex (68). Guidelines for the treatment of reflux cough recommend therapeutic trials since individual patients seem to respond to a particular modality of treatment and not others.

A. Acid Suppression

Despite the lower reliance on acid as the causative irritant for cough the usual first strategy when reflux cough is suspected is trial of acid suppression (2). The evidence base supporting this is poor with only five controlled trials in this area, which show poor evidence of efficacy (69). Trial design could be criticized with inappropriate use of crossover methodology and inadequate dosing regimen.

It is suggested that when reflux cough is acid dependent then small amounts of acid can precipitate coughing and therefore suppression of acid must be more vigorous. Proton pump inhibitors (PPI) have a relatively short plasma half-life, and while irreversible binding to the proton pump ensures 24-hour suppression of acid, breakthrough acid by the creation of new proton pumps ensures that even with twice-daily PPI dosing gastric acid is below pH 4 in approximately 50% of patients on waking. The recommended regime is therefore twice-daily PPI with nocturnal ranitidine (70). Anecdotal reports have led to the recommendation of prolonged acid suppression as being the norm (71). However, it is difficult to determine whether this is in fact spontaneous remission rather than a therapeutic response.

B. Promotility Agents

The dopamine agonists metoclopramide and domperidone may improve gastro-esophageal motility and increase gastric emptying, thus diminishing the volume of gastric contents liable to reflux (72,73).

C. Baclofen

The gamma aminobutyric acid (GABA) agonist, baclofen, mimics vagal inhibitory tone on the lower esophageal sphincter and reduces episodes of transient opening of the lower esophageal sphincter (74). While this is the most likely mechanism of action of baclofen in reflux cough baclofen has been shown to alter cough reflex sensitivity to inhaled capsaicin so additional central activity is also likely (75,76).

VIII. Cough Suppression

Cough suppression is an important strategy in the management of chronic persistent cough. It is also useful in cough associated with palliative care and is the theoretical strategy behind the treatment of acute cough. In reality however there are few if any convincing studies demonstrating efficacy above placebo in this important therapeutic area. However, effective normalization of a hypersensitive cough reflex has a potential role in all modalities of cough.

A. Opiates

Opiates have long been recommended for the treatment of chronic intractable cough but there is little evidence of efficacy in studies using modern standards. In older studies very high doses of opiates were used (77,78). In the modern era some studies show no effect of codeine in cough associated with COPD (79) and high doses of morphine were required to suppress the cough reflex in normal volunteers (80). Recently, we undertook a study in subjects with chronic treatment unresponsive cough, where morphine sulfate at the dose of 5-mg twice daily was administered in a double-blind randomized placebo-controlled crossover study (81). Morphine led to a reduction by a third in daily diary record card cough counts with an associated rise in the quality-of-life instrument, the Leicester Cough Questionnaire but with no significant difference in cough challenge. Cough responses appear to be dichotomized into responders and nonresponders with approximately one-third of patients achieving a remission. In an open label extension a further third of patients improved with an increase in dose to 10-mg twice daily. Thus, in intractable chronic cough clinically useful cough suppression can be obtained with low-dose opiate therapy, with constipation being the only significant side effect.

A wide range of other opiates have been advocated for the treatment of cough, including codeine, pholcodine, and diamorphine, with codeine, despite the poor evidence base in man being the archetypal opiate standard in many animal and human studies. Oral codeine undergoes first pass metabolism to morphine by cytochrome P450 2D6. Because of the polymorphic nature of this enzyme reliable plasma levels are difficult to obtain within the population (82). Since it probably acts as a prodrug for morphine its continued use seems somewhat of an anachronism.

B. Dextromethorphan

Dextromethorphan, a codeine analog devoid of opiate side effects, is the most widely used over-the-counter cough suppressant. Alteration of the cough reflex sensitivity by dextromethorphan has been demonstrated in healthy subjects using citric acid challenge (83,84). However, when tested on clinical parameters results are less impressive. In the evaluation of antitussive efficacy in acute cough the placebo response may be highly significant (85). A review of eight clinical trials examining the effects of antitussive medicines on cough associated with acute upper respiratory tract infection showed that 85% of the reduction in cough was related to treatment with placebo (86). In a study of children with upper respiratory tract infection, subjective measures were made and neither dextromethorphan nor codeine was significantly more effective than placebo (87). A meta-analysis of three placebo-controlled studies of dextromethorphan in acute cough was required to demonstrate a modest reduction of cough (88). There is surprisingly little evidence to support efficacy of dextromethorphan compared with placebo in the treatment of cough associated with upper respiratory tract infection.

IX. Antihistamines as Antitussives

The American College of Chest Physicians Guidelines on cough recommend antihistamines, and in particular the alkylamine brompheniramine and its dextroisomer, dexbrompheniramine for the treatment of upper airways cough syndrome (UACS) (89). Indeed, response to dexbrompheniramine is taken as an important diagnostic indicator. In contrast, experience in Europe with antihistamines to treat cough has been poor. However, dexbrompheniramine never received a product license in the majority of European countries.

Data from a number of mainly open label studies confirms the efficacy of dexbrompheniramine in acute cough (90,91). Our experience demonstrated a response rate of approximately two thirds in patients with previously intractable cough of a wide range of different etiologies. This response was felt unlikely to be due to antihistamine activity and dexbrompheniramine was may be an antagonist of TRPV1 (92).

X. Other Antitussives

A number of other compounds a have been suggested or promoted for the treatment of cough. There are few if any convincing clinical studies supporting their use. This is partially a problem with the difficulty in performing studies with a symptom which until recently defied objective measurement and where the placebo effect can be responsible for a major therapeutic response. Many drugs however entered clinical practice before there was any need to rigorously demonstrate efficacy. Indeed some prescribing is based on Galenic principles. The expectorants are derived from emetics used to balancing the humors.

A. Guaifenesin

Guaifenesin is the only expectorant thought to be "safe and effective" by the U.S. Food and Drug Administration (93) and as a consequence is found in many over the counter remedies. Studies have purported to demonstrate changes in the characteristics of sputum (94,95) More recently an effect on cough reflex sensitivity has been reported (96).

B. Baclofen

An agonist of the inhibitory neurotransmitter GABA, baclofen, has a number of potential sites of action on the cough reflex. Animal studies have demonstrated a central mode of action (97). In healthy human volunteers baclofen was shown to inhibit capsaicin induced cough (76,98). Baclofen also has a profound effect on the lower esophageal sphincter causing inhibition of transient opening (99) and this activity has been suggested as underlying its role on chronic cough (100).

C. Levodropropizine

A nonopioid agent that has a putative peripheral cough suppressant activity. Studies using subjective endpoints a variety of disease states have claimed significant effects (101,102). This author has conducted three unpublished studies using cough challenge in healthy volunteers using levodropropizine and was unable to demonstrate any beneficial effect over placebo.

D. Moguisteine

Claimed to have a peripheral site of action (103), moguisteine has been shown to be superior to placebo in a subjective study (104) and comparable to placebo in a parallel group comparison (105).

E. Inhaled Anesthetics

Inhalation of local anesthetics has a long history in the treatment of chronic cough (106). More recent isolated reports have confirmed that these agents may be helpful (107–109); however, no randomized studies are available. Anaesthetizing the upper airway comes with the risk of aspiration and many would view this strategy as unsatisfactory in a chronic lifelong condition.

F. Benzonatate

A long-chain polyglycol related to procaine, benzonatate, is a widely used oral antitussive in the Americas. It is suggested to act on "stretch receptors" (110). Clinical studies of a current standard are lacking.

G. Amitriptyline

A recent small clinical study suggests that amitriptyline may have a significant beneficial effect on patients with chronic cough (111). The attractive hypothesis that agents known to effect hyperalgesia may inhibit the hypersensitivity seen in chronic cough, deserves further study.

XI. Conclusion

Current therapeutic options in the treatment of cough are limited. In acute cough there is little evidence of efficacy over and above the effect of placebo. In chronic cough management of the underlying disease offers the best hope of response, particularly in patients with eosinophilic airway inflammation. In reflux cough pharmacological intervention is limited because of the partial role of acid in its etiology and a lack of effective agents to combat esophageal dysmotility. Recent developments in characterization of putative cough receptors have lead to fresh hope of regulating cough reflex sensitivity.

References

1. Morice AH, McGarvey L, Pavord I. Recommendations for the management of cough in adults. Thorax 2006; 61(suppl 1):i1–i24.
2. Morice AH, Fontana GA, Sovijarvi ARA, et al. The diagnosis and management of chronic cough. Eur Respir J 2004; 24(3):481–492.
3. Irwin RS, Baumann MH, Bolser DC, et al. Diagnosis and management of cough executive summary: ACCP evidence-based clinical practice guidelines. Chest 2006; 129(1 suppl):1S–23S.
4. O'Connell F, Thomas VE, Pride NB, et al. Capsaicin cough sensitivity decreases with successful treatment of chronic cough. Am J Respir Crit Care Med 1994; 150:374–380.
5. Irwin RS, Curley FJ, French CL. Chronic cough. The spectrum and frequency of causes, key components of the diagnostic evaluation, and outcome of specific therapy. Am Rev Respir Dis 1990; 141(3):640–647.
6. Irwin RS, Corrao WM, Pratter MR. Chronic persistent cough in the adult: the spectrum and frequency of causes and successful outcome of specific therapy. Am Rev Respir Dis 1981; 123(4 pt 1):413–417.
7. Poe RH, Harder RV, Israel RH, et al. Chronic persistent cough. Experience in diagnosis and outcome using an anatomic diagnostic protocol. Chest 1989; 95(4):723–728.
8. Smyrnios NA, Irwin RS, Curley FJ. Chronic cough with a history of excessive sputum production. The spectrum and frequency of causes, key components of the diagnostic evaluation, and outcome of specific therapy. Chest 1995; 108(4):991–997.
9. McGarvey LP, Heaney LG, Lawson JT, et al. Evaluation and outcome of patients with chronic non-productive cough using a comprehensive diagnostic protocol. Thorax 1998; 53(9): 738–743.
10. Brightling CE, Ward R, Goh KL, et al. Eosinophilic bronchitis is an important cause of chronic cough. Am J Respir Crit Care Med 1999; 160(2):406–410.
11. Kastelik JA, Aziz I, Ojoo JC, et al. Investigation and management of chronic cough using a probability-based algorithm. Eur Respir J 2005; 25(2):235–243.
12. Fujimura M, Abo M, Ogawa H, et al. Importance of atopic cough, cough variant asthma and sinobronchial syndrome as causes of chronic cough in the Hokuriku area of Japan. Respirology 2005; 10(2):201–207.
13. Corrao WM, Braman SS, Irwin RS. Chronic cough as the sole presenting manifestation of bronchial asthma. N Engl J Med 1979; 300(12):633–637.
14. Brightling CE, Woltmann G, Wardlaw AJ, et al. Development of irreversible airflow obstruction in a patient with eosinophilic bronchitis without asthma. Eur Respir J 1999; 14(5): 1228–1230.
15. Irwin RS, Zawacki JK, Curley FJ, et al. Chronic cough as the sole presenting manifestation of gastroesophageal reflux. Am Rev Respir Dis 1989; 140(5):1294–1300.
16. Koufman JA. Laryngopharyngeal reflux is different from classical gastroesophageal reflux disease. Ear Nose Throat J 2002; 81(9 suppl 2):7–9.
17. Morice AH. Post-nasal drip syndrome—a symptom to be sniffed at? Pulm Pharmacol Ther 2004; 17(6):343–345.
18. Pratter MR. Chronic upper airway cough syndrome secondary to rhinosinus diseases (previously referred to as postnasal drip syndrome): ACCP evidence-based clinical practice guidelines. Chest 2006; 129(1 suppl):63S–71S.
19. McGarvey LP. Idiopathic chronic cough: a real disease or a failure of diagnosis? Cough 2005; 1:9.
20. Chung KF, Pavord ID. Prevalence, pathogenesis, and causes of chronic cough. Lancet 2008; 371(9621):1364–1374.
21. Widdicombe JG. Afferent receptors in the airways and cough (review). Respir Physiol 1998; 114(1):5–15.
22. Laitman JT, Reidenberg JS. The human aerodigestive tract and gastroesophageal reflux: an evolutionary perspective. Am J Med 1997; 103(5A):2S–8S.

23. Bickerman HA, Barach AL, Itkin S, et al. Experimental production of cough in human subjects induced by citric acid aerosols. Preliminary studies on the evaluation of antitussive agents. Am J Med Sci 1954; 228:156–163.
24. Wong CH, Matai R, Morice AH. Cough induced by low pH. Respir Med 1999; 93(1):58–61.
25. Morice AH, Higgins KS, Yeo WW. Adaptation of cough reflex with different types of stimulation. Eur Respir J 1992; 5:841–847.
26. Lowry RH, Wood AM, Higenbottam TW. Effects of pH and osmolarity on aerosol-induced cough in normal volunteers. Clin Sci 1988; 74(4):373–376.
27. Collier JG, Fuller RW. Capsaicin inhalation in man and the effects of sodium cromoglycate. Br J Pharmacol 1984; 81(1):113–117.
28. Morice AH, Fontana GA, Belvisi MG, et al. ERS guidelines on the assessment of cough. Eur Respir J 2007; 29(6):1256–1276.
29. Laude EA, Higgins KS, Morice AH. A comparative study of the effects of citric acid, capsaicin and resiniferatoxin on the cough challenge in guinea-pig and man. Pulm Pharmacol 1993; 6:171–175.
30. Clapham DE. TRP channels as cellular sensors. Nature 2003; 426(6966):517–524.
31. Clapham DE, Julius D, Montell C, et al. International union of pharmacology. XLIX. Nomenclature and structure-function relationships of transient receptor potential channels. Pharmacol Rev 2005; 57(4):427–450.
32. Carr MJ, Kollarik M, Meeker SN, et al. A role for TRPV1 in bradykinin-induced excitation of vagal airway afferent nerve terminals. J Pharmacol Exp Ther 2003; 304(3):1275–1279.
33. Chuang HH, Prescott ED, Kong H, et al. Bradykinin and nerve growth factor release the capsaicin receptor from PtdIns(4,5)P2-mediated inhibition. Nature 2001; 411(6840): 957–962.
34. Mazzone SB, Mori N, Canning BJ. Synergistic interactions between airway afferent nerve subtypes regulating the cough reflex in guinea-pigs. J Physiol 2005; 569(pt 2):559–573.
35. Dinh QT, Groneberg DA, Peiser C, et al. Nerve growth factor-induced substance P in capsaicin-insensitive vagal neurons innervating the lower mouse airway. Clin Exp Allergy 2004; 34(9):1474–1479.
36. Groneberg DA, Niimi A, Dinh QT, et al. Increased expression of transient receptor potential vanilloid-1 in airway nerves of chronic cough. Am J Respir Crit Care Med 2004; 170(12): 1276–1280.
37. Mitchell JE, Campbell AP, New NE, et al. Expression and characterization of the intra-cellular vanilloid receptor (TRPV1) in bronchi from patients with chronic cough. Exp Lung Res 2005; 31(3):295–306.
38. Geppetti P, Materazzi S, Nicoletti P. The transient receptor potential vanilloid 1: role in airway inflammation and disease. Eur J Pharmacol 2006; 533(1–3):207–214.
39. Fox AJ, Lalloo UG, Belvisi MG, et al. Bradykinin-evoked sensitization of airway sensory nerves: a mechanism for ACE-inhibitor cough. Nat Med 1996; 2:814–817.
40. Morice AH, Lowry R, Brown MJ, et al. Angiotensin converting enzyme and the cough reflex. Lancet 1987; 2(8568):1116–1118.
41. Gatti R, Andre E, Amadesi S, et al. Protease-activated receptor-2 activation exaggerates TRPV1-mediated cough in guinea pigs. J Appl Physiol 2006; 101(2):506–511.
42. Trevisani M, Milan A, Gatti R, et al. Antitussive activity of iodo-resiniferatoxin in guinea pigs. Thorax 2004; 59(9):769–772.
43. Kollarik M, Undem BJ. Mechanisms of acid-induced activation of airway afferent nerve fibres in guinea-pig. J Physiol 2002; 543(2):591–600.
44. Bandell M, Story GM, Hwang SW, et al. Noxious cold ion channel TRPA1 is activated by pungent compounds and bradykinin. Neuron 2004; 41(6):849–857.
45. MacPherson LJ, Dubin AE, Evans MJ, et al. Noxious compounds activate TRPA1 ion channels through covalent modification of cysteines. Nature 2007; 445(7127):541–545.

46. Faruqi S, Morice AH. Cinnamaldehyde: a novel tussive agent in man. Thorax 2008; 63(suppl VII):A4–A73, A22.
47. McKemy DD, Neuhausser WM, Julius D. Identification of a cold receptor reveals a general role for TRP channels in thermosensation. Nature 2002; 416(6876):52–58.
48. Brauchi S, Orio P, Latorre R. Clues to understanding cold sensation: thermodynamics and electrophysiological analysis of the cold receptor TRPM8. Proc Natl Acad Sci U S A 2004; 101(43):15494–15499.
49. Laude EA, Morice AH, Grattan TJ. The antitussive effects of menthol, camphor and cineole in conscious guinea-pigs. Pulm Pharmacol 1994; 7:179–184.
50. Morice AH, Marshall AE, Higgins KS, et al. Effect of inhaled menthol on citric acid induced cough in normal subjects. Thorax 1994; 49:1024–1026.
51. Wright CE, Laude EA, Grattan TJ, et al. Capsaicin and neurokinin A-induced broncho-constriction in the anaesthetised guinea-pig: evidence for a direct action of menthol on isolated bronchial smooth muscle. Br J Pharmacol 1997; 121(8):1645–1650.
52. Takeuchi S, Tamaoki J, Kondo M, et al. Effect of menthol on cytosolic Ca^{2+} levels in canine airway epithelium in culture. Biochem Biophys Res Commun 1994; 201:1333–1338.
53. Krishtal O. The ASICs: signaling molecules? Modulators? Trends Neurosci 2003; 26(9): 477–483.
54. Kellenberger S, Schild L. Epithelial sodium channel/degenerin family of ion channels: a variety of functions for a shared structure. Physiol Rev 2002; 82(3):735–767.
55. Lingueglia E. Acid-sensing ion channels in sensory perception. J Biol Chem 2007; 282(24): 17325–17329.
56. Voilley N. Acid-sensing ion channels (ASICs): new targets for the analgesic effects of non-steroid anti-inflammatory drugs (NSAIDs). Curr Drug Targets Inflamm Allergy 2004; 3(1): 71–79.
57. Yagi J, Wenk HN, Naves LA, et al. Sustained currents through ASIC3 ion channels at the modest pH changes that occur during myocardial ischemia. Circ Res 2006; 99(5):501–509.
58. Chen CC, Zimmer A, Sun WH, et al. A role for ASIC3 in the modulation of high-intensity pain stimuli. Proc Natl Acad Sci U S A 2002; 99(13):8992–8997.
59. Kollarik M, Undem BJ. Activation of bronchopulmonary vagal afferent nerves with bra-dykinin, acid and vanilloid receptor agonists in wild-type and TRPV1-/- mice. J Physiol 2004; 555(pt 1):115–123.
60. Canning BJ, Mazzone SB, Meeker SN, et al. Identification of the tracheal and laryngeal afferent neurones mediating cough in anaesthetized guinea-pigs. J Physiol 2004; 557(pt 2): 543–558.
61. Ours TM, Kavuru MS, Schilz RJ, et al. A prospective evaluation of esophageal testing and a double-blind, randomized study of omeprazole in a diagnostic and therapeutic algorithm for chronic cough. Am J Gastroenterol 1999; 94(11):3131–3138.
62. Brightling CE, Ward R, Wardlaw AJ, et al. Airway inflammation, airway responsiveness and cough before and after inhaled budesonide in patients with eosinophilic bronchitis. Eur Respir J 2000; 15(4):682–686.
63. Brightling CE, Bradding P, Symon FA, et al. Mast cell infiltration of airway smooth muscle in asthma. N Engl J Med 2002; 346:1699–1705.
64. Dicpinigaitis PV, Dobkin JB. Effect of zafirlukast on cough reflex sensitivity in asthmatics. J Asthma 1999; 36(3):265–270.
65. Dicpinigaitis PV, Dobkin JB, Reichel J. Antitussive effect of the leukotriene receptor antagonist zafirlukast in subjects with cough-variant asthma. J Asthma 2002; 39:291–297.
66. Hwang SW, Cho H, Kwak J, et al. Direct activation of capsaicin receptors by products of lipoxygenases: endogenous capsaicin-like substances. Proc Natl Acad Sci U S A 2000; 97(11):6155–6160.

67. Morice AH. Gastro-oesophageal reflux and tachykinins in asthma and chronic cough. Thorax 2007; 62(6):468–469.
68. Everett CF, Morice AH. Clinical history in gastroesophageal cough. Respir Med 2007; 101(2): 345–348.
69. Chang AB, Lasserson TJ, Kiljander TO, et al. Systematic review and meta-analysis of randomised controlled trials of gastro-oesophageal reflux interventions for chronic cough associated with gastro-oesophageal reflux. Br Med J 2006; 332(7532):11–17.
70. Xue S, Katz PO, Banerjee P, et al. Bedtime H2 blockers improve nocturnal gastric acid control in GERD patients on proton pump inhibitors. Aliment Pharmacol Ther 2001; 15 (9):1351–1356.
71. Irwin RS, Zawacki JK, Wilson MM, et al. Chronic cough due to gastroesophageal reflux disease: failure to resolve despite total/near-total elimination of esophageal acid. Chest 2002; 121(4):1132–1140.
72. Poe RH, Kallay MC. Chronic cough and gastroesophageal reflux disease: experience with specific therapy for diagnosis and treatment. Chest 2003; 123(3):679–684.
73. Jiang SP, Liang RY, Zeng ZY, et al. Effects of antireflux treatment on bronchial hyper-responsiveness and lung function in asthmatic patients with gastroesophageal reflux disease. World J Gastroenterol 2003; 9(5):1123–1125.
74. Lidums I, Lehmann A, Checklin H, et al. Control of transient lower esophageal sphincter relaxations and reflux by the GABA(B) agonist baclofen in normal subjects. Gastroenterology 2000; 118(1):7–13.
75. Dicpinigaitis PV, Rauf K. Treatment of chronic, refractory cough with baclofen. Respiration 1998; 65(1):86–88.
76. Dicpinigaitis PV, Dobkin JB, Rauf K, et al. Inhibition of capsaicin-induced cough by the gamma-aminobutyric acid agonist baclofen. J Clin Pharmacol 1998; 38(4):364–367.
77. Woolf CR, Rosenberg A. Objective assessment of cough suppressents under clinical conditions using a tape recorder system. Thorax 1964; 19:125–130.
78. Woolf CR, Rosenberg A. The cough suppressant effect of heroin and codeine: a controlled clinical study. Can Med Assoc J 1962; 86:810–812.
79. Smith J, Owen E, Earis J, et al. Effect of codeine on objective measurement of cough in chronic obstructive pulmonary disease. J Allergy Clin Immunol 2006; 117(4):831–835.
80. Fuller RW, Karlson JA, Choudry NB, et al. Effect of inhaled and systemic opiates on responses to inhaled capsaicin in Humans. J Appl Physiol 1988; 65(3):1125–1130.
81. Morice AH, Menon MS, Mulrennan SA, et al. Opiate therapy in chronic cough. Am J Respir Crit Care Med 2007; 175(4):312–315.
82. Vree TB, Verwey-van Wissen CP. Pharmacokinetics and metabolism of codeine in humans. Biopharm Drug Dispos 1992; 13(6):445–460.
83. Grattan TJ, Marshall AE, Higgins KS, et al. The effect of inhaled and oral dextromethorphan on citric acid induced cough in man. Br J Clin Pharmacol 1995; 39:261–263.
84. AbdulManap R, Wright CE, RostamiHodjegan A, et al. Cytochrome P450 2D6 (CYP2D6) activity in relation to the antitussive effect of dextromethorphan. Br J Clin Pharmacol 1999; 47(5):586–587.
85. Rostami-Hodjegan A, Abdul-Manap R, Wright CE, et al. The placebo response to citric acid-induced cough: pharmacodynamics and gender differences. Pulm Pharmacol Ther 2001; 14(4):315–319.
86. Eccles R. The powerful placebo in cough studies? Pulm Pharmacol Ther 2002; 15(3):303–308.
87. Taylor JA, Novack AH, Almquist JR, et al. Efficacy of cough suppressants in children. J Pediatr 1993; 122(5 pt 1):799–802.
88. Parvez L, Vaidya M, Sakhardande A, et al. Evaluation of antitussive agents in man. Pulm Pharmacol 1996; 9(5–6):299–308.

89. Irwin RS, Baumann MH, Bolser DC, et al. Diagnosis and management of cough executive summary: ACCP evidence-based clinical practice guidelines. Chest 2006; 129(1 suppl):1S–23S.
90. Curley FJ, Irwin RS, Pratter MR, et al. Cough and the common cold. Am Rev Respir Dis 1988; 138(2):305–311.
91. Arroll B. Non-antibiotic treatments for upper-respiratory tract infections (common cold). Respir Med 2005; 99(12):1477–1484.
92. Sadofsky LR, Campi B, Trevisani M, et al. Transient receptor potential vanilloid-1-mediated calcium responses are inhibited by the alkylamine antihistamines dexbrompheniramine and chlorpheniramine. Exp Lung Res 2008; 34(10):681–693.
93. Expectorant Drug Products for Over-the-Counter Human Use: Final Monograph. Federal Register 54. Washington, D.C.: US Department of Health and Human Services, 1989: 8494–8509.
94. Hirsch SR, Viernes PF, Kory RC. The expectorant effect of glyceryl guaiacolate in patients with chronic bronchitis. A controlled in vitro and in vivo study. Chest 1973; 63(1):9–14.
95. Houtmeyers E, Gosselink R, Gayan-Ramirez G, et al. Effects of drugs on mucus clearance. Eur Respir J 1999; 14(2):452–467.
96. Dicpinigaitis PV, Gayle YE. Effect of guaifenesin on cough reflex sensitivity. Chest 2003; 124(6):2178–2181.
97. Bolser DC, DeGennaro FC, O'Reilly S, et al. Peripheral and central sites of action of GABA-B agonists to inhibit the cough reflex in the cat and guinea pig. Br J Pharmacol 1994; 113(4):1344–1348.
98. Dicpinigaitis PV, Dobkin JB. Antitussive effect of the GABA-agonist baclofen. Chest 1997; 111(4):996–999.
99. Zhang Q, Lehmann A, Rigda R, et al. Control of transient lower oesophageal sphincter relaxations and reflux by the GABA(B) agonist baclofen in patients with gastro-oesophageal reflux disease. Gut 2002; 50(1):19–24.
100. Menon MS, Mulrennan SA, Everett CF, et al. Experience with baclofen in cough secondary to gastro-oesophageal reflux disease. Proc Am Thorac Soc 2005; 2:A323 (abstr).
101. Bariffi F, Tranfa C, Vatrella A, et al. Protective effect of levodropropizine against cough induced by inhalation of nebulized distilled water in patients with obstructive lung disease. Drugs Exp Clin Res 1992; 18(3):113–118.
102. Allegra L, Bossi R. Clinical trials with the new antitussive levodropropizine in adult bronchitic patients. Arzneimittelforschung 1988; 38(8):1163–1166.
103. Gallico L, Borghi A, Dalla RC, et al. Moguisteine: a novel peripheral non-narcotic antitussive drug. Br J Pharmacol 1994; 112(3):795–800.
104. Aversa C, Cazzola M, Clini V, et al. Clinical trial of the efficacy and safety of moguisteine in patients with cough associated with chronic respiratory diseases. Drugs Exp Clin Res 1993; 19(6):273–279.
105. Barnabe R, Berni F, Clini V, et al. The efficacy and safety of moguisteine in comparison with codeine phosphate in patients with chronic cough. Monaldi Arch Chest Dis 1995; 50:93–97.
106. Howard P, Cayton RM, Brennan SR, et al. Lignocaine aerosol and persistent cough. Br J Dis Chest 1977; 71(1):19–24.
107. Trochtenberg S. Nebulized lidocaine in the treatment of refractory cough. Chest 1994; 105:1592–1593.
108. Udezue E. Lidocaine inhalation for cough suppression. Am J Emerg Med 2001; 19(3):206–207.
109. Peleg R, Binyamin L. Practice tips. Treating persistent cough. Try a nebulized mixture of lidocaine and bupivacaine. Can Fam Physician 2002; 48:275.
110. Banner AS. Pharmacologic Treatment of Cough. New York: McGraw-Hill, 1996:673–679.
111. Jeyakumar A, Brickman TM, Haben M. Effectiveness of amitriptyline versus cough suppressants in the treatment of chronic cough resulting from postviral vagal neuropathy. Laryngoscope 2006; 116(12):2108–2112.

Index